Office Gynecology

Office Gynecology

A Case-Based Approach

Edited by

David Chelmow, MD
Virginia Commonwealth University
Richmond, VA

Nicole W. Karjane, MD
Virginia Commonwealth University
Richmond, VA

Hope A. Ricciotti, MD
Harvard Medical School
Boston, MA

Amy E. Young, MD
The University of Texas at Austin, Dell Medical School
Austin, TX

CAMBRIDGE
UNIVERSITY PRESS

CAMBRIDGE
UNIVERSITY PRESS

University Printing House, Cambridge CB2 8BS, United Kingdom

One Liberty Plaza, 20th Floor, New York, NY 10006, USA

477 Williamstown Road, Port Melbourne, VIC 3207, Australia

314–321, 3rd Floor, Plot 3, Splendor Forum, Jasola District Centre, New Delhi – 110025, India

79 Anson Road, #06–04/06, Singapore 079906

Cambridge University Press is part of the University of Cambridge.

It furthers the University's mission by disseminating knowledge in the pursuit of education, learning, and research at the highest international levels of excellence.

www.cambridge.org
Information on this title: www.cambridge.org/9781108400220
DOI: 10.1017/9781108227469

© Cambridge University Press 2019

First published 2019
Reprinted 2019

Printed in the United Kingdom by TJ International Ltd. Padstow Cornwal

A catalogue record for this publication is available from the British Library.

Library of Congress Cataloging-in-Publication Data
Names: Chelmow, David, editor. | Karjane, Nicole, editor. | Ricciotti, Hope, editor. | Young, Amy. editor.
Title: Office gynecology : a case-based approach / edited by David Chelmow, Nicole Karjane, Hope Ricciotti, Amy Young.
Other titles: Office gynecology (Chelmow)
Description: Cambridge, United Kingdom ; New York, NY : University Press House, 2019. | Includes bibliographical references and index.
Identifiers: LCCN 2018031737 | ISBN 9781108400220 (paperback)
Subjects: | MESH: Genital Diseases, Female | Ambulatory Care | Pelvic Pain | Preconception Care | Pregnancy | Mastodynia | Case Reports
Classification: LCC RG101 | NLM WP 140 | DDC 618.1–dc23
LC record available at https://lccn.loc.gov/2018031737

ISBN 978-1-108-40022-0 Paperback

....

Contents

List of Contributors   ix

Preface   xiii

Section 1 Pelvic Pain

1   **A 27-Year-Old Woman with Recurrent Visits for Severe Pelvic Pain**   1
Lee A. Learman

2   **A 25-Year-Old Woman with Deep Dyspareunia**   4
Kate A. McCracken

3   **A 16-Year-Old Adolescent with Ongoing Dysmenorrhea Despite Oral Contraceptive Pill Use**   7
Geri D. Hewitt

4   **A 37-Year-Old Woman with Pain at the Lateral Aspect of Her Pfannenstiel Incision**   10
Christopher M. Morosky

5   **A 26-Year-Old Woman with Chronic Pelvic Pain and Negative Work-Up**   13
Misa Perron-Burdick

6   **A 30-Year-Old Woman with Endometriosis with Worsening Pelvic Pain Despite Continuous Oral Contraceptives**   16
William D. Po

7   **A 47-Year-Old Woman with Severe Menstrual Cramps and Painful Intercourse**   19
Abimbola Famuyide

Section 2 Vaginal Discharge and Sexually Transmitted Infections

8   **A 28-Year-Old Woman with Metronidazole Allergy and Trichomonas Infection**   23
Anita Tamirisa

9   **A 24-Year-Old Woman with Mucopurulent Cervicitis**   26
Jaime J. Alleyn

10   **A 27-Year-Old Woman with Trichomonas Requesting a Prescription for Her Partner**   29
Rita Tsai

11   **A 33-Year-Old Woman with Multiple Visits for Vaginal Discharge and Itching**   32
Shelly Holmstrom

12   **A 24-Year-Old Woman with Trichomonas in the First Trimester of Pregnancy**   36
Mark Turrentine

13   **A 16-Year-Old Adolescent Requesting Confidential Treatment for Chlamydia Exposure (Understanding State Laws Regarding Minors and Resources)**   39
Kavita Shah Arora

14   **A 75-Year-Old Woman Complaining of Greenish Discharge**   42
Amy R. Stagg

Section 3 Amenorrhea and Abnormal Vaginal Bleeding

15   **A 32-Year-Old Woman with Friable Cervix**   45
Julianna Schantz-Dunn

16   **A 28-Year-Old Woman with Secondary Amenorrhea and Family History of Mental Retardation (Fragile X Premutation)**   47
Frederick Friedman, Jr.

17   **A 27-Year-Old Female Runner with Secondary Amenorrhea**   51
Janeen L. Arbuckle

18   **A 38-Year-Old Woman with Secondary Amenorrhea Six Months after Gastric Bypass**   54
Kyle Andrew Biggs

19   **A 25-Year-Old Woman with a Levonorgestrel Intrauterine Device (LNG-IUD), New Onset Spotting, and a Positive Pregnancy Test**   57
Jeffrey Rothenberg

20   **A 30-Year-Old Woman with Irregular Periods (Hypothyroidism)**   59
Scott Graziano

21 **A 25-Year-Old Woman with Midcycle Spotting** 61
Ann Lee Chang and Tod C. Aeby

Section 4 Contraception and Abortion

22 **A 25-Year-Old Woman with No IUD String Visible One Year after Placement (IUD in Uterus)** 65
Adrianne Dade

23 **A 29-Year-Old HIV-Positive Woman Requesting Oral Contraceptive Pills** 68
Patricia Huguelet

24 **A 42-Year-Old Woman with IUD and *Actinomyces* on Cervical Cytology** 71
Regan N. Theiler

25 **A 25-Year-Old Woman with a History of Pulmonary Embolism on OCPs Who Desires Contraception** 73
Hedwige Saint Louis

26 **A Pregnant 22-Year-Old Woman Who Desires Long-Acting Postpartum Birth Control** 76
Stacey L. Holman

27 **A 33-Year-Old G4P4 Unable to Palpate Implant Desiring Removal** 79
Michael K. Chinn

28 **A 24-Year-Old Woman with a Contraceptive Implant Placed Three Weeks Ago Presents with Positive Pregnancy Test** 82
Roxanne Jamshidi

29 **A 32-Year-Old HIV-Positive Woman Requesting IUD** 85
Christy M. Boraas

30 **A 23-Year-Old Woman Presents Two Hours after Sexual Assault** 88
Shandhini Raidoo

31 **A Woman with a BMI of 40 kg/m² Requests Oral Contraceptive Pills (Efficacy of Contraceptive Methods with Obesity)** 91
Sara Whetstone

Section 5 Breast Problems

32 **A 41-Year-Old Woman with Bilateral Clear Nipple Discharge (Physiologic Discharge)** 95
Christine Robillard Isaacs

33 **A 38-Year-Old Woman with New-Onset, Unilateral Bloody Nipple Discharge** 98
Esther Fuchs

34 **A 34-Year-Old Newly Pregnant Woman with a Breast Mass** 101
Asha Bhagsingh Bhalwal and Pamela D. Berens

35 **A 29-Year-Old Woman with Lactational Mastitis and Persistent Fevers and Erythema** 104
Pamela D. Berens

36 **A 45-Year-Old Woman with Unilateral Green Nipple Discharge (Duct Ectasia)** 107
Tricia Camille Yusaf and Katherine Chua

37 **A 35-Year-Old Woman Who Complains of Cyclic Breast Pain (Idiopathic Mastodynia)** 111
Dorota Kowalska

Section 6 Cancer Screening and Prevention

38 **A 22-Year-Old Woman with LSIL on Initial Cervical Cytology** 115
Mark K. Hiraoka

39 **A 25-Year-Old Woman Who Has Received a Letter from an Aunt Recommending Lynch Testing (Cascade Testing)** 118
Jessica M. Kingston

40 **A 30-Year-Old Woman with Positive Margins on LEEP for HSIL** 122
Jordan B. Hylton

41 **A 32-Year-Old Woman Whose Paternal Aunt and Grandmother Had Ovarian Cancer** 125
Roopina Sangha

42 **A 23-Year-Old Woman with HSIL on Cervical Cytology** 129
Florencia Greer Polite

43 **A 35-Year-Old Woman with a Strong Family History of Breast Cancer Not Linked to BRCA Mutation** 132
Natalie A. Bowersox

44 **A 25-Year-Old Woman with LSIL Desiring HPV Vaccination** 136
Christine Conageski

Section 7 Vulvar Disease

45 **A 55-Year-Old Woman with a White, Itchy Lesion on the Vulva (Lichen Sclerosus)** 139
Nancy D. Gaba

46 **A 55-Year-Old Woman with a New Wart (Vulvar High-Grade Squamous Intraepithelial Lesions)** 142
Diana Curran

47 **A 25-Year-Old Woman with Perineal Pain and Inability to Have Intercourse (Vestibulodynia)** 145
Vanessa M. Barnabei

48 **A 30-Year-Old Woman with New Vulvar Lesions (Condyloma Accuminata)** 149
Christopher Maguire

49 **A 50-Year-Old Woman with Lichen Sclerosus, Fused Labia, and UTIs** 152
Dawn Palaszewski

50 **A 25-Year-Old Woman with Recurrent *Candida* Vaginitis** 155
Kimberly Carter

51 **A 35-Year-Old Woman Complaining of a "Knot" in the Vulva (Bartholin's Cyst)** 158
D. Scott Wiersma

Section 8 Infertility

52 **A Couple with Medicaid and No Conception after Two Years (Cost Conscious Infertility Evaluation)** 161
Merielle Stephens

53 **A 33-Year-Old Woman with Infertility (Bilateral Hydrosalpinx)** 164
Elizabeth E. Puscheck

54 **A 26-Year-Old Woman with Irregular Menses and Infertility** 167
Helen Dunnington

55 **A 32-Year-Old Woman with a 3 cm Endometrioma and Infertility** 170
Michael T. Breen

56 **A 32-Year-Old Woman with Recurrent Pregnancy Loss** 173
Debra A. Taubel

Section 9 Preconception Planning

57 **A Couple Planning Pregnancy Who Have Just Returned from Brazil (Zika Virus)** 177
Michael Nix

58 **A 26-Year-Old Woman with a History of Depression Planning Pregnancy** 181
Jonathan Schaffir

59 **A 25-Year-Old Woman with a History of DVT Presents for Preconception Counseling** 184
Erica Oberman

60 **A 25-Year-Old Ashkenazi Jewish Woman Who Desires Pregnancy** 187
Jessica C. Arluck

61 **A 40-Year-Old Woman with Chronic Hypertension on Atenolol Planning Pregnancy** 190
L. David Moore

62 **A 30-Year-Old Woman with a History of Diabetes Controlled on Oral Agents Planning Pregnancy** 194
Saul D. Rivas

Section 10 Pediatric and Adolescent Problems

63 **A 14-Year-Old Adolescent with a Large Labia** 197
Roshanak Zinn

64 **A 16-Year-Old Adolescent with Acne, Hirsutism, and Irregular Menses** 200
Eduardo Lara-Torre

65 **An Eight-Year-Old Girl with Persistent Vulvar Itching** 203
Laura A. Parks

66 **A Four-Year-Old Girl with Recurrent Vulvar Discharge and Itching** 206
Sarah H. Milton

67 **A 15-Year-Old with Painful Vulvar Ulcers** 209
Sarah A. Shaffer

68 **A 15-Year-Old Adolescent Who Is Unable to Use a Tampon** 213
Celeste Ojeda Hemingway

69 **A Six-Year-Old Girl with Breast Development (Precocious Puberty)** 216
Shelly Holmstrom

70 **A 13-Year-Old Adolescent with Primary Amenorrhea and Cyclic Abdominal Pain (Imperforate Hymen)** 221
James Casey

71 **A 17-Year-Old Adolescent with Secondary Amenorrhea** 224
Courtney Rhoades

Section 11 Pelvic Masses and Cysts

72 **A 53-Year-Old Woman with a 3 cm Dermoid Cyst Noted as an Incidental Finding on CT** 227
Jacob Lauer

73 **A 60-Year-Old Woman with a 4 cm Simple Ovarian Cyst** 230
Tara Harris

74 **A 25-Year-Old Woman with a 2 cm Simple Asymptomatic Cyst Noted Incidentally on Ultrasound** 233
Sarah A. Wagner

Contents

75 **A 25-Year-Old Woman with Endometriosis and a 4 cm Endometrioma** 236
Mostafa A. Borahay

76 **A 25-Year-Old Woman with Abrupt Onset of Pelvic Pain, Nausea and Vomiting, and Adnexal Mass (Torsion)** 239
Todd R. Jenkins

77 **A 30-Year-Old Woman with Fever, Abdominal Pain, Vaginal Discharge, and Adnexal Mass (Tubo-Ovarian Abscess)** 242
Joseph E. Peterson

78 **A 45-Year-Old Woman with Pelvic Pain One Year after TLH/BSO for Endometriosis (Ovarian Remnant)** 246
Todd R. Griffin

79 **A 21-Year-Old Woman at Five Weeks EGA with Left Lower Quadrant Pain** 249
Lisa M. Keder

Section 12 Incontinence and Prolapse

80 **A 30-Year-Old Woman with Postpartum Flatal and Fecal Incontinence** 253
K. Lauren Barnes and Lori R. Berkowitz

81 **A 46-Year-Old Woman with Leakage of Urine** 256
Cynthie K. Wautlet

82 **A 48-Year-Old Woman with Microscopic Hematuria and Negative Urine Culture** 260
Kimberly S. Gecsi

83 **A 55-Year-Old Woman with Urinary Urgency and Negative Urinalysis and Culture** 263
Julie Zemaitis DeCesare

84 **A 30-Year-Old Woman with Frequency, Urgency, Nocturia, and Pressure Relieved by Urination** 266
Jaclyn van Nes

85 **A 25-Year-Old Woman with Recurrent Urinary Tract Infections** 269
Jonathan Emery

86 **An 80-Year-Old Woman with Total Procidentia with Vaginal Irritation** 272
Madhurima Krishna Keerthy

87 **A 60-Year-Old Woman Presenting with Difficulty with Defecation (Posterior Wall Defect)** 276
Erica Nelson

Section 13 Behavioral, Sexual, and Social Health

88 **A 25-Year-Old Woman with Recurrent STDs (Human Trafficking)** 279
Fay Chelmow and David Chelmow

89 **A 41-Year-Old Woman with Loss of Interest in Having Sex** 285
Tracy E. Irwin

90 **A 28-Year-Old Transgender Woman Requesting Well-Woman Visit** 288
Ghazaleh Moayedi

91 **A 35-Year-Old Female-to-Male Transgender Patient with Vaginal Spotting on Testosterone** 291
Beth Cronin

92 **A 23-Year-Old Woman Who Reports Inability to Consummate Her Marriage Due to Vaginal Pain (Vaginismus Due to Sexual Abuse)** 294
Cristina Wallace Huff

93 **A Tearful 32-Year-Old Woman Requesting a Sleeping Aid Two Weeks after Delivery (Postpartum Depression)** 297
Enid Yvette Rivera-Chiauzzi

Section 14 Menopause and Aging

94 **A 50-Year-Old Breast Cancer Survivor with Severe Hot Flashes** 301
Myrlene Jeudy

95 **A 56-Year-Old Woman with Dyspareunia** 304
Nan G. O'Connell

96 **A 60-Year-Old Woman with FRAX® Score Indicating a 10 Percent Probability of Osteoporotic Fracture** 307
Kathryn I. Marko

97 **A 45-Year-Old Woman with Menses Every 60–90 Days and Hot Flashes** 311
Makeba Williams

98 **A 70-Year-Old Victim of Elder Abuse** 315
Nguyet A. Nguyen

Index 318

Contributors

Tod C. Aeby, MD, MEd
University of Hawai'i John A. Burns School of Medicine
Honolulu, HI

Jaime J. Alleyn, MD
Louisiana State University Health Sciences Center
New Orleans, LA

Janeen L. Arbuckle, MD, PhD
University of Alabama at Birmingham
Birmingham, AL

Jessica C. Arluck, MD
Emory University
Atlanta, GA

Kavita Shah Arora, MD, MBE
Case Western Reserve University
Cleveland, OH

Vanessa M. Barnabei, MD, PhD
Jacobs School of Medicine and Biomedical Sciences, University at Buffalo
Buffalo, NY

K. Lauren Barnes, MD
Brigham and Women's Hospital and Massachusetts General Hospital
Boston, MA

Pamela D. Berens, MD
McGovern Medical School, The University of Texas Health Science at Houston
Houston, TX

Lori R. Berkowitz, MD
Harvard Medical School and Massachusetts General Hospital
Boston, MA

Asha Bhagsingh Bhalwal, MD, MRCOG
McGovern Medical School, The University of Texas Health Science at Houston
Houston, TX

Kyle Andrew Biggs, DO
University of Texas
Edinburg, TX

Christy M. Boraas, MD, MPH
University of Minnesota Medical School
Minneapolis, MN

Mostafa A. Borahay, MD, PhD
Johns Hopkins School of Medicine
Baltimore, MD

Natalie A. Bowersox, MD
Cleveland Clinic
Cleveland, OH

Michael T. Breen, MD
University of Texas at Austin, Dell Medical School
Austin, TX

Kimberly Carter, MD, MPP
University of Texas at Austin, Dell Medical School
Austin, TX

James Casey, MD
Vanderbilt University Medical Center
Nashville, TN

Ann Lee Chang, MD, MPH
University of Hawai'i John A. Burns School of Medicine
Honolulu, HI

David Chelmow, MD
Virginia Commonwealth University School of Medicine
Richmond, VA

Fay Chelmow, BSN
ImPACT Virginia: People Against Child Sex Trafficking
Richmond, VA

Michael K. Chinn, MD
Madigan Army Medical Center
Tacoma, WA

Katherine Chua, MD
School of Medicine, St George's University
Grenada, West Indies

Christine Conageski, MD
University of Colorado
Aurora, CO

Beth Cronin, MD
The Warren Alpert Medical School of Brown University
Providence, RI

Diana Curran, MD
Michigan Medicine, University of Michigan
Ann Arbor, MI

Adrianne Dade, MD
University of Chicago
Chicago, IL

Julie Zemaitis DeCesare, MD
University of Florida College of Medicine
Pensacola, FL

Helen Dunnington, MD
Baylor College of Medicine
Houston, TX

Jonathan Emery, MD
Cleveland Clinic
Cleveland, OH

Abimbola Famuyide, MBBS
Mayo Clinic College of Medicine and Science
Rochester, MN

Frederick Friedman Jr., MD
Icahn School of Medicine at Mount Sinai
New York, NY

Esther Fuchs, MD
University of Washington
Seattle, WA

Nancy D. Gaba, MD
The George Washington University School of Medicine and
Health Sciences
Washington, DC

Kimberly S. Gecsi, MD
University Hospitals Cleveland Medical Center
Case Western Reserve University School of Medicine
Cleveland, OH

Scott Graziano, MD, MS
Stritch School of Medicine at Loyola University Chicago
Maywood, IL

Todd R. Griffin, MD
Stony Brook University Hospital
Stony Brook, NY

Tara Harris, MD
Baylor College of Medicine and Texas Children's Hospital
Pavilion for Women
Houston, TX

Celeste Ojeda Hemingway, MD, MHPE
Vanderbilt University Medical Center
Nashville, TN

Geri D. Hewitt, MD
The Ohio State University College of Medicine
Columbus, OH

Mark K. Hiraoka, MD, MSCR
John A. Burns School of Medicine at University of Hawaii
Honolulu, HI

Stacey L. Holman, MD
Louisiana State University Health Sciences Center
New Orleans, LA

Shelly Holmstrom, MD
University of South Florida
Tampa, FL

Cristina Wallace Huff, MD
McGovern Medical School, University of Texas Health Science
Center at Houston
Houston, TX

Patricia Huguelet, MD
University of Colorado and Children's Hospital Colorado
Aurora, CO

Jordan B. Hylton, DO
Virginia Commonwealth University School of Medicine
Richmond, VA

Tracy E. Irwin, MD, MPH
University of Washington
Seattle, WA

Christine Robillard Isaacs, MD
Virginia Commonwealth University School of Medicine
Richmond, VA

Roxanne Jamshidi, MD, MPH
The George Washington University School of Medicine and
Health Sciences
Washington, DC

Todd R. Jenkins, MD, MSHA
University of Alabama at Birmingham School of Medicine
Birmingham, AL

Myrlene Jeudy, MD
Virginia Commonwealth University School of Medicine
Richmond, VA

Lisa M. Keder, MD, MPH
Ohio State University
Columbus, OH

Madhurima Krishna Keerthy, MD
Henry Ford Health System, Wayne State University Medical
School
Detroit, MI

Jessica M. Kingston, MD
University of California San Diego Health
San Diego, CA

Dorota Kowalska, MD
Stony Brook University Hospital
Stony Brook, NY

Eduardo Lara-Torre, MD
Virginia Tech-Carilion School of Medicine
Roanoke, VA

Jacob Lauer, MD, MPH
School of Medicine and Public Health, University of Wisconsin
Madison, WI

Lee A. Learman, MD, PhD
Florida Atlantic University
Boca Raton, FL

Christopher Maguire, DO
Texas Tech University Health Sciences Center-Permian Basin
Lubbock, TX

Kathryn I. Marko, MD
The George Washington School of Medicine and Health Sciences
Washington, DC

Kate A. McCracken, MD
The Ohio State University College of Medicine
Columbus, OH

Sarah H. Milton, MD
Virginia Commonwealth University School of Medicine
Richmond, VA

Ghazaleh Moayedi, DO
University of Hawai'i John A. Burns School of Medicine
Honolulu, HI

L. David Moore, MD
Texas Tech Health Sciences Center at the Permian Basin
Odessa, TX

Christopher M. Morosky, MD, MS
University of Connecticut School of Medicine
Farmington, CT

Erica Nelson, MD
Southern Illinois University, SIU School of Medicine
Springfield, IL

Nguyet A. Nguyen, MD
Denver Health Medical Center
Denver, CO

Michael Nix, MD
The University of Texas at Austin, Dell Medical School
Austin, TX

Erica Oberman, MD
David Geffen School of Medicine at the University of
California Los Angeles
Santa Monica, CA

Nan G. O'Connell, MD
Virginia Commonwealth University School of Medicine
Richmond, VA

Dawn Palaszewski, MD
Morsani College of Medicine, University of South Florida
Tampa, FL

Laura A. Parks, MD
University of Kansas School of Medicine
Kansas City, KS

Misa Perron-Burdick, MD, MAS
University of California San Francisco
San Francisco, CA

Joseph E. Peterson, MD
University of Florida
Pensacola, FL

William D. Po, MD
Oklahoma State University Center for Health Sciences
Tulsa, OK

Florencia Greer Polite, MD
Perelman School of Medicine University of Pennsylvania
Philadelphia, PA

Elizabeth E. Puscheck, MD, MS, MBA
Wayne State University School of Medicine
Detroit, MI

Shandhini Raidoo, MD, MPH
University of Hawai'i John A. Burns School of Medicine
Honolulu, HI

Courtney Rhoades, DO, MBA
University of Florida
Jacksonville, FL

Saul D. Rivas, MD, MSPH
The University of Texas Rio Grande Valley School of
Medicine
Edinburg, TX

Enid Yvette Rivera-Chiauzzi, MD
Mayo Clinic College of Medicine
Rochester, MN

Jeffrey Rothenberg, MD, MS
Marian University College of Medicine
Indianapolis, IN

Hedwige Saint Louis, MD, MPH
Morehouse School of Medicine
Atlanta, GA

Roopina Sangha, MD, MPH
Henry Ford Hospital, Wayne State University School of Medicine
Detroit, MI

Jonathan Schaffir, MD
The Ohio State University
Columbus, OH

Julianna Schantz-Dunn, MD, MPH
Harvard Medical School
Boston, MA

Sarah A. Shaffer, DO
University of Iowa Carver College of Medicine
Iowa City, IA

Amy R. Stagg, MD
Harvard Medical School
Boston, MA

Merielle Stephens, MD
Tufts Medical Center
Boston, MA

Anita Tamirisa, DO
Emory University
Atlanta, GA

Debra A. Taubel, MD
Western Michigan University Homer Stryker M.D. School of Medicine
Kalamazoo, MI

Regan N. Theiler, MD, PhD
Dartmouth-Hitchcock Medical Center
Lebanon, NH

Rita Tsai, MD
University of Texas at Austin, Dell Medical School
Austin, TX

Mark Turrentine, MD
Baylor College of Medicine
Houston, TX

Jaclyn van Nes, MD, MBA
University of Tennessee Medical Center Knoxville
Knoxville, TN

Sarah A. Wagner, MD
Stritch School of Medicine at Loyola University Chicago
Maywood, IL

Cynthie K. Wautlet, MD, MPH
University of Wisconsin School of Medicine and Public Health
Madison, WI

Sara Whetstone, MD, MHS
University of California San Francisco
San Francisco, CA

D. Scott Wiersma, MD
Walter Reed National Military Medical Center
Bethesda, MD

Makeba Williams, MD, NCMP
School of Medicine and Public Health, University of Wisconsin
Madison, WI

Tricia Camille Yusaf, MD
Mount Sinai Medical Center
New York City, NY

Roshanak Zinn, MD
University of Texas at Austin, Dell Medical School
Austin, TX

Preface

As OB/GYN specialists, we spend the bulk of our time in office practice. In the office, we see a broad array of primary, preventive, prenatal, and problem visits. Evaluation and management vary from areas with widely accepted guidelines to ones based on expert opinion. Many of these areas are old and continue to slowly evolve. Others, like Zika virus and awareness of human trafficking, are new. Some areas are acutely transforming, such as chronic pain and the opioid epidemic.

The intent of this book is to help practitioners of women's health care, including OB/GYNs, family practitioners, and internal medicine women's health specialists, with these many changes. The book is intended for physicians, trainees, nurse midwives, nurse practitioners, and physician's assistants. We chose nearly 100 important ambulatory gynecology problems and present them in a case-based format. They are intended to be easy to read and suitable as a quick office reference for providers seeing similar patients. The book is meant to supplement the many other journals, electronic references, and textbooks available, but in a real-life format suitable for adult learners.

The book was a project of the Society for Academic Specialists in General Obstetrics and Gynecology (SASGOG). SASGOG was formed in 2012 as a professional society for academic faculty specializing in OB/GYN ("academic generalists"). The organization has several missions, which include both faculty development and enhancing care in the areas not within the scope of the many subspecialty societies. Well-woman care, the subject of our first book, and office practice, the subject of this one, fall squarely into SASGOG's domain.

SASGOG members were invited to write cases. As academic faculty, they had the skills to review and assess the available recommendations and evidence. As physicians who take care of patients in the office on a regular basis, they had the clinical experience to allow them to synthesize this information to make it applicable for practice. Each chapter presents a sample case with description of appropriate evaluation and management. The case is followed by a discussion explaining the basis for management. When major society evidence-based recommendations are available, they are incorporated, with discussion of their nuances and application. These recommendations come from widely accepted organizations including the American College of Obstetricians and Gynecologists (ACOG), ASCCP, Centers for Disease Control and Prevention (CDC), and the United States Preventive Services Task Force (USPSTF). When consensus recommendations are not available, the basis for expert opinion is described, with current references and systematic reviews whenever available. Distributing the topics among so many medical school faculty allowed careful fact checking, literature review, and synthesis.

We hope to expand this book into a series of case-based books written by SASGOG authors and editors. *Acute and Emergency Care Gynecology: A Case-Based Approach* was the first in this format. It was also written largely by SASGOG authors and the organization is credited, but it was not an "official" SASGOG book as it was started just before SASGOG was incorporated. In the future, we hope to add books on operative gynecology and obstetrics.

As editors, we are deeply grateful to the original officers and board of SASGOG, who recognized book projects as a way to combine its missions of developing faculty through providing writing opportunities and enhancing care of women through development of high-quality educational material for practitioners. We are equally grateful to Nicholas Dunton and Cambridge University Press for seeing the potential in our new organization and being willing to partner with us on *Well Woman Visit* and *Office Practice: A Case-Based Approach*. We especially want to thank our spouses, Fay, Damian, Charles, Vincent, and our families for their support and indulgence while we disappeared for several months of editing.

As we were nearly done with the book, Hope developed a major medical problem. She was an essential team member. We deeply missed her knowledge, energy, organizational skills, and enthusiasm as the book finally came together. We are thinking of her, and hoping for continued recovery.

A 27-Year-Old Woman with Recurrent Visits for Severe Pelvic Pain

Lee A. Learman

History of Present Illness

A 27-year-old woman returns to your office with severe pelvic pain that has persisted since her initial visit three months ago. Assessment at that time identified dysmenorrhea and pelvic floor myalgia as the leading pain generators. Screening for depression was negative. Pelvic ultrasound did not show uterine or adnexal abnormalities. The treatment plan included 84-day extended-cycle birth control pills, a referral for pelvic physiotherapy, and a high-dose regimen of a nonsteroidal anti-inflammatory drug (NSAID). The patient returned three months later with fewer bleeding days and improvement in pain, from 10 out of 10 to 8 out of 10. She had not made an appointment for physiotherapy. The patient was encouraged to continue her current regimen and urged to begin physical therapy, with follow-up planned in two to three more months.

The patient called the practice two weeks later asking for an urgent appointment and was scheduled the following day. At this visit she reported no improvement in pain since her visit one month ago. She has not had any further vaginal bleeding. She found physical therapy intolerably painful and could not get through the first session. It hurt so much that she took a 10 mg oxycodone pill left over from her partner's postoperative prescription. The oxycodone was very effective in reducing her pain, but has worn off. She says she is "miserable" and requests a prescription for oxycodone.

Review of systems is positive for occasional bloating and constipation. The patient has smoked one pack of cigarettes per day since age 15 and drinks alcohol with friends over the weekend. She denies use of other drugs. She has no other medical problems or prior surgeries.

Physical Examination

Vital Signs

Temperature	98.6°F (37.0°C)
Pulse	72 beats/min
Blood pressure	122/70 mmHg
Respirations	18 breaths/min
Body mass index (BMI)	24.8 kg/m^2
General	Well-developed, well-nourished woman in no acute distress.
Abdomen	Soft, no masses, mild lower quadrant tenderness without rebound or guarding. Normal bowel sounds.
External genitalia	Unremarkable.
Vagina	No lesions. Scant discharge. Tight, tender bands of pelvic floor muscles bilaterally, which when palpated reproduce the patient's pain.
Cervix	Nulliparous. No bleeding or discharge.
Bimanual exam	Limited by tenderness.

How Would You Manage This Patient?

The patient has been seen three times in the past three months for severe pelvic pain likely from dysmenorrhea and pelvic floor myalgia. Her dysmenorrhea has been adequately managed with extended-cycle birth control pills. Her pelvic floor myalgia has not been treated due to a delay, and then intolerance of physical therapy.

Rather than focusing exclusively on the patient's request for oxycodone, the visit focused on supporting adherence to the recommended course of treatment and establishing realistic expectations for symptom improvement. The patient was counseled that severe pelvic floor myalgia may require 12 or more weeks of skilled pelvic physical therapy once or twice a week. There are no more rapid alternatives for restoring normal muscle tone and flexibility, and for correcting any contributing biomechanical issues. She was counseled that opioid medications are effective for acute pain and have potential harms when used for chronic pain, particularly constipation, nausea, somnolence, tolerance requiring higher doses over time to achieve the same analgesia, chemical dependence, and opioid addiction [1]. In light of the patient's use of her partner's oxycodone, she was counseled that it is not safe to use medications prescribed for other individuals.

Short-term use of opioid medication may be necessary to manage this patient's reactive muscle pain after physical therapy visits. Screening for addiction risk is indicated in all patients, and may be particularly useful in light of this patient's chronic tobacco use and potential nicotine addiction. The patient's history of prior opioid use should be obtained, and her current use should be verified by performing a baseline urine drug screen (UDS) and searching available prescription monitoring registries.

If the patient is at low risk for opioid addiction, and additional analgesia is needed to make the physical therapy more tolerable, a short-term regimen can be prescribed according to evidence-based guidelines. The high-dose NSAIDs should be continued to provide baseline analgesia, and a short-acting opioid in doses up to 40 morphine milligram equivalents (MME) prescribed for pain exacerbations. The recommended starting dose of oxycodone is 5–15 mg (7.5–22.5 MME) every 4–6 hours [2]. Patients receiving opioid medications should not use other central nervous system depressants, such as benzodiazepines or alcohol, and cytochrome P450 3A4 inhibitors that impede opioid metabolism, such as amiodarone, cimetidine, fluoxetine, grapefruit juice, protease inhibitors, azoles, and macrolide antibiotics other than azithromycin. The patient should be advised that the opioid prescription is just one part of a comprehensive treatment plan. Adherence to the NSAID regimen, menstrual suppression, and physical therapy will be required for the patient's pain to improve and should be made a condition for prescribing the opioid medication.

After three months of physical therapy the patient's pelvic floor myalgia is greatly improved. She reports fewer flares, and only needs to take oxycodone once a week after a physically active day. A search of available prescription registries shows she has filled no other prescriptions for controlled substances. The oxycodone is refilled, adjusting the number of pills downward to accommodate her current use. She agrees with the plan to discontinue the oxycodone at her next follow-up visit and understands that a repeat urine drug screening will become necessary if opioid use becomes chronic (six months or longer) or if there is a suspicion of nonprescription drug use.

Initial Screening and Monitoring

The epidemic of prescription drug abuse in the United States has many negative effects on women's health [3]. When a patient comes to the office asking for an opioid prescription, it can be difficult to determine the root cause of the request. Frustration and urgency to find relief are normal reactions to severe pain, but these behaviors can raise clinicians' concerns about drug-seeking behavior. A few simple approaches can be used to rule out current use of illicit substances and misuse of prescription medication, and to stratify a patient's risk of future addiction.

First, a patient's current prescriptions for opioid and other controlled medications can be confirmed using searchable web-based prescription monitoring systems. Once an opioid medication is prescribed, the same monitoring systems can be checked periodically to confirm there are no other controlled substance prescriptions.

Second, a UDS can establish the absence of common drugs of abuse before an opioid is prescribed. A UDS is not commonly required before prescribing opioids for acute pain, as in the case of major surgical procedures or traumatic injuries. In contradistinction, UDS is an evidence-based recommendation before prescribing opioids for pain in the ambulatory setting and is generally repeated annually or semiannually, or when the patient's behavior raises concern about medication misuse or substance abuse [1].

Third, risk stratification is important for preventing opioid abuse and misuse. Many screening instruments exist for opioid risk assessment [4]; however, evidence of limited reliability and validity does not support their routine use [1]. Stratification can be done instead using clinical characteristics. High-risk features include pain involving more than three regions of the body without objective signs; severe pain exacerbations and limited coping strategies; major psychological disorders; younger age (<45 years old); resistance to participation in multimodal therapy; and severe limitations in usual activities. Patients with a history of drug abuse, misuse, addiction, diversion, dependency, alcoholism, tolerance with hyperalgesia, or HIV-related pain are also at high risk [1].

Pain Medication Agreements and Best Practices

In this case, the patient was able to participate in multimodal therapy, which effectively reduced her pain and her need for opioid medication. When patients require continuation of opioid medication for chronic pelvic pain, periodic prescription monitoring and UDS testing are safeguards for detecting and preventing opioid abuse and misuse. In addition, many practices routinely use long-term opioid agreements to align treatment expectations. Examples are publicly available and include a common set of statements signed by the patient, her physician, and a witness (Box 1.1). Failure to adhere to the agreement results in discontinuation of opioid therapy [5]. One study in a primary care clinic followed patients with a variety of chronic pain syndromes who were placed on opioid contracts and reported 63 percent adherence with median follow-up of 22.5 months. Seventeen percent of the contracts were canceled for noncompliance or substance abuse, and the other 20 percent of patients discontinued the use of opioid medication [5].

Box 1.1 Example of elements included in opioid agreements (contracts)

To not use illegal substances, street drugs, abuse alcohol, or take opioids prescribed for others.

To not be involved in the sale, illegal possession, diversion, or transport of controlled substances.

To take drug screening tests when requested by the physician.

To obtain all opioid prescriptions from a single physician and take other medications prescribed.

To use only one pharmacy for filling opioid prescriptions (specify name and phone number).

To follow up as scheduled regarding pain control and keep all scheduled appointments related to pain treatment (e.g., physical therapy, psychotherapy).

To allow the primary physician to communicate with other physicians and pharmacists regarding pain management as needed.

To use an effective method of contraception during the course of opioid treatment.

To contact the practice within 24 hours if an emergency occurs requiring a prescription for opioids.

Accepting that no allowances will be made for lost prescriptions, drugs, or any problems related to transportation or dates of medication pickup.

Accepting the possible adverse effects and dependencies associated with opioids as outlined by the physician.

To provide at least seven days of lead time for all refills and to schedule an appointment for pickup.

Accepting that opioid medication will be stopped if any of the following occurs:

Box 1.1 (cont.)

- giving away, selling, or misusing the drugs or using other people's drugs or substances
- not complying with any of the terms of the agreement
- disrespecting or harassing clinic personnel
- not following up regularly or as requested
- not participating in other aspects of the treatment plan
- if pain and function do not improve

The Centers for Disease Control (CDC) published guidelines for opioid prescribing for chronic pelvic pain in 2016 [6], and the CDC website provides open access to a dozen clinical tools supporting evidence-based practice (www.cdc.gov/drugoverdose/prescribing/clinical-tools.html, accessed 5/3/2017). Best practices for chronic opioid prescribing expand beyond the clinician's role to a full-scale reengineering of the ambulatory care setting, similar to models of care for other complex chronic conditions. The Robert Wood Johnson Foundation funded a program called "Primary Care Teams: Learning from Exemplar Ambulatory Practices" (LEAP). A study of team-based approaches to improve chronic opioid therapy management in 30 LEAP clinics across the United States identified six building blocks for optimizing care. Of these components opioid contracts, registry tracking and planned visits with patients may be the most feasible to implement in Ob/Gyn practice [7].

Key Teaching Points

- Opioids are not first-line medications for pain in the ambulatory setting, but can be used short term if around-the-clock non-opioid analgesics do not provide adequate relief during pain exacerbations.
- Safe opioid prescribing requires baseline screening for drug abuse or misuse and appraisal of addiction risk.
- Risk stratification relies on clinical characteristics, including a history of prior drug dependence or addiction.
- Urinary drug screens and prescription registry searches should be done before prescribing opioid medications and periodically thereafter if opioid use exceeds six months.
- Pain medication agreements establish a shared understanding of expectations with patients requiring long-term opioid prescribing.

References

1. Manchikanti L, Kaye AM, Knezevic NN et al. Responsible, safe, and effective prescription of opioids for chronic non-cancer pain: American Society of Interventional Pain Physicians (ASIPP) Guidelines. *Pain Physician: Opioid Special Issue* 2017;20: S3–S92.

2. CDC Guideline for Prescribing Opioids for Chronic Pain – United States, 2016. Morphine milligram equivalent (MME) doses for commonly prescribed opioids. Adapted from Von Korff M, Saunders K, Ray GT et al. *Clin J Pain* 2008;24:521–527 and Washington State Interagency Guideline on Prescribing Opioids for Pain (www.agencymeddirectors.wa.gov/Files/2015AMDGOpioidGuideline.pdf).

3. American College of Obstetricians and Gynecologists. Nonmedical use of prescription drugs. Committee Opinion No. 538. *Obstet Gynecol* 2012;120:977–982.

4. Sehgal N, Manchikanti L, Smith HS. Prescription opioid abuse in chronic pain: a review of opioid abuse predictors and strategies to curb opioid abuse. *Pain Physician* 2012;15:ES67–ES92.

5. Hariharan J, Lamb GC, Neuner JM. Long-term opioid contract use for chronic pain management in primary care practice. A five year experience. *JGIM* 2007;22:485–490.

6. Dowell D, Haegerich TM, Chou R. CDC guideline for prescribing opioids for chronic pain – United States, 2016. *MMWR Recomm Rep* 2016;65(No. RR-1):1–49.

7. Parchman ML, Von Korff M, Baldwin L et al. Primary care clinic re-design for prescription opioid management. *J Am Board Fam Med* 2017;30:44–51.

A 25-Year-Old Woman with Deep Dyspareunia

Kate A. McCracken

History of Present Illness

A 25-year-old woman, gravida 0, presents with the complaint of painful intercourse. She is sexually active with one male partner with whom she has vaginal-penile intercourse. She complains of pain with insertion of the penis and with deep thrust. She reports trying "different positions" during intercourse, but continues to experience pain. She also notes intermittent pain that she localizes to the anorectal region. She reports a history of sexual assault. She denies any domestic violence and feels safe with her current male partner. She denies a history of pelvic trauma. She denies any other bowel or bladder symptoms.

Her only medication is a combined oral contraceptive pill, which she uses for contraception. She has regular menses, occurring during placebo pills, with five days of flow, and no dysmenorrhea. She has no significant past medical or surgical history. She has no known drug allergies. She reports consistent latex condom use. She has completed college and is working full time. She lives with her male partner. She drinks two alcoholic beverages per week. She denies tobacco and illicit drug use. Her family history is noncontributory.

Physical Examination

General appearance	Well-developed, well-appearing female in no acute distress

Vital Signs

Pulse	75 beats/min
Blood pressure	118/64 mmHg
Height	65 inches
Weight	140 pounds
BMI	23.3 kg/m^2
Abdomen	Soft, non-distended, non-tender, no masses

Pelvic Exam

External genitalia	Normal appearing. Pubic hair Tanner V. Normal urethral meatus.
Vagina	Normal mucosa. No atrophy, no lesions, no masses, scant clear vaginal discharge (no odor).
Cervix	Normal appearing nulliparous cervix without masses or discharge.
Bimanual exam	No urethral or bladder base tenderness. Bilateral levator ani tenderness. Uterus small, anteverted, mobile, non-tender. Cervix palpably normal and without cervical motion tenderness. No adnexal masses or tenderness bilaterally.
Rectal exam	Normal tone, no masses. Tenderness of the puborectalis musculature is present.

Gonorrhea/chlamydia/ trichomonas DNA amplification probes	Negative
Urine pregnancy test	Negative

How Would You Manage This Patient?

This patient has dysmenorrhea and chronic pelvic pain, which impacts her quality of life. A complete history identified no associated gastroenterologic, urologic, or psychiatric symptoms. A urine pregnancy test was negative and sexually transmitted infection screening was negative. A pelvic exam was notable for bilateral levator ani tenderness. The absence of other causes and presence of levator ani tenderness strongly suggest levator spasm as the source of her deep dyspareunia. She was referred for pelvic physical therapy. Three months after starting pelvic floor physical therapy, she reported significant improvement in her symptoms and was able to engage in vaginal-penile intercourse without difficulty.

Levator Ani Spasm Causing Dyspareunia

Definition, Pathogenesis, and Prevalence

Levator ani spasm syndrome is a particular type of myofascial pelvic pain, in which spasm of the levator ani muscle group leads to chronic or recurrent vaginal, rectal, or pelvic pain. Myofascial pain is characterized by hyperirritable areas within a muscle leading to persistently contracted fibers that cause pain. The primary reactive area within the muscle is termed a "trigger point." These areas typically manifest as a palpable, contracted, taut band or nodule. The pelvic floor musculature may develop trigger points and pain because the pelvic girdle is involved in a multitude of activities, including sexual function, bowel and bladder control, and musculoskeletal support of the upper and lower body, placing these muscles at risk for overuse injury. Pelvic floor myofascial pain may be a primary condition, or secondary to underlying conditions such as endometriosis or interstitial cystitis/painful bladder syndrome. Women with chronic pelvic pain may have reduced thresholds to pain in the pelvic floor musculature [1]. In some cases of levator ani muscle spasm, the pain may manifest as dyspareunia, which is defined as recurrent or persistent genital pain associated with sexual intercourse that is not caused exclusively by lack of lubrication or by vaginismus and causes marked distress or interpersonal difficulties [2, 3]. Dyspareunia is common, and although classified as a sexual pain disorder, it can be characterized as pain disorder that interferes with sexuality, rather than a sexual disorder characterized by pain [2]. The differential diagnosis of chronic pelvic pain and dyspareunia includes gynecologic (endometriosis, adenomyosis, uterine fibroids, pelvic inflammatory disease [PID], malignancy), urologic (interstitial cystitis, cystitis, nephrolithiasis, malignancy), gastroenterologic (irritable bowel syndrome [IBS], inflammatory bowel disease [IBD], constipation, celiac disease, hernias, malignancy), musculoskeletal (abdominal wall myofascial pain/trigger points, fibromyalgia), neurologic (nerve entrapment), and vascular (varicosities, pelvic congestion syndrome) causes. A population-based survey based on symptoms noted the prevalence of levator ani syndrome in women to be 7.4 percent [4, 5].

Presentation and Diagnostic Criteria

Patients typically describe pain from levator ani spasm syndrome as aggravated by a specific activity, often sexual activity. Common precipitating factors include sexual intercourse, sitting for long periods of time, stress, defecation, childbirth, prior trauma, and prior surgical procedures. In general, trigger points within the pelvis may refer pain to the vagina, vulva, perineum, bladder, rectum, buttocks, lower abdomen, or even the upper thighs. Patients may describe a pressure sensation, ache, or burning sensation. The symptoms may be intermittent or continuous and acute or chronic. In addition, patients may experience concomitant bladder symptoms or constipation. Specific diagnostic criteria for levator ani syndrome, set forth primarily by gastroenterologists, are known as the Rome III criteria. The criteria are:

- symptoms are present for more than three months;
- episodes of pain should last at least 20 minutes; and
- symptoms are associated with puborectalis muscle tenderness when palpated [6, 7].

Evaluation/Examination

Evaluation begins with a comprehensive patient history. Particular attention should be paid to gynecologic, sexual, gastrointestinal, and urinary symptoms. The pain should be characterized in terms of onset, location, radiation, severity, and timing. Provoking or relieving factors should be elicited. Providers should inquire about the impact of certain positions on the pain, as myofascial pain is often aggravated by specific positions and relieved by others. Menstrual history and impact of menses on the pain should be reviewed. A history of trauma such as prior pelvic surgeries, back or hip injuries, and childbirth may also be relevant. A psychosocial history is also important as patients may have other contributing conditions such as depression or post-traumatic stress disorder from history of sexual assault or interpersonal violence. Any prior treatments and their impact on symptoms should be noted.

The physical exam should include assessment of the patient's abdomen and trunk; pelvic exam including external genitalia, internal genitalia, and pelvic floor musculature; and anorectal exam. The exam has the potential to trigger the patient's pain and be very uncomfortable. The patient should be allowed to be in control of the exam by communicating that she may ask the examiner to stop at any time. An external genital exam should be performed. The examiner should ask the patient to contract her pelvic floor or bear down. Women with myofascial pelvic pain disorders may have weak musculature, which will be detectable by an asymmetric contraction

when bearing down. An anal wink should be elicited to evaluate for other neurologic conditions. A speculum exam should be performed to assess the vaginal mucosa and cervix. Tests for gonorrhea, chlamydia, trichomonas, and yeast can be obtained if appropriate, based on risk factors or physical findings. This is particularly important in sexually active women to rule out an infectious etiology like gonorrhea, chlamydia, trichomonas, or pelvic inflammatory disease. Bimanual exam should include palpation of the urethra, bladder base, cervix, uterus, and adnexa to help rule out other etiologies of pain.

The pelvic floor muscles should be systematically palpated to identify trigger points or contracted muscle bands. Examiners should first insert one finger into the introitus and palpate the bulbocavernosus muscle, located just lateral to the introitus. Next, the superficial transverse perineal muscles should be palpated by moving the finger inferiorly. Last, the levator ani muscle complex should be examined. The levators are the "pelvic floor" surrounding the rectum. Moving medial to lateral, the complex is composed of the pubococcygeus, puborectalis, and iliococcygeus muscles. The examiner may picture the vagina as a face of a clock with the pubococcygeus muscle from 7 to 11 o'clock and 1 to 5 o'clock. The puborectalis is slightly more lateral within the distal vagina (Figure 2.1) and the iliococcygeus is from 4 to 8 o'clock [7]. Each muscle group should be palpated and note taken of whether palpation elicits pain. Trigger points are tender to palpation, and palpation may cause involuntary spasm. With levator ani spasm, palpation of the levators will elicit pain. Unilateral or bilateral tenderness may be present. The patient should be asked to rate the pain throughout the exam and whether palpation of the trigger points reproduces her presenting symptoms. A rectovaginal exam should be performed, noting any decreased tone, masses, tenderness, rectovaginal septum nodularity, or trigger points involving the pubococcygeus and puborectalis muscles.

Pelvic ultrasound is not usually required for the diagnosis of levator ani spasm, but can be useful when ruling out other underlying structural causes of pain such as ovarian cysts or masses and uterine masses. Diagnostic gastrointestinal procedures such as colonoscopy or upper GI endoscopy may be useful if the patient's history or physical exam suggests a functional or structural gastrointestinal condition.

Treatment

Treatment of levator ani spasm typically involves a combination of therapies. A multidisciplinary approach may be beneficial. Commonly used modalities include pelvic floor physical therapy with trigger point release maneuvers, biofeedback, heat, massage, warm sitz baths, cognitive-behavioral therapy, and pharmacologic agents such as nonsteroidal anti-inflammatory drugs and other analgesics and muscle relaxants [6].

First-line therapy includes pelvic floor physical therapy. Referral to a pelvic floor physical therapist with specific experience treating dyspareunia and pelvic floor disorders is important. The therapist may use a variety of techniques including strengthening exercises, stretching (e.g., sitting with hips

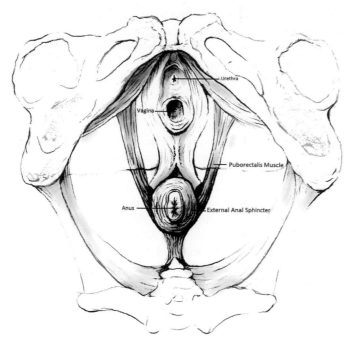

Figure 2.1 Pelvic bones and muscles of pelvic floor. Anatomic structures are indicated (illustration by Joseph Werkmeister).

flexed), transcutaneous nerve stimulation, and biofeedback. Pelvic floor physical therapy should be initiated as soon as the diagnosis is made and continued while other adjuvant therapies are added.

Cognitive-behavioral therapy ("systemic desensitization") may help the patient gain a sense of control over penetration into the vagina. This is a useful tool in many cases of dyspareunia, as it helps reduce automatic vaginal muscle contractions. This therapy can be initiated simultaneously with a pelvic floor physical therapy referral. Vaginal dilators are commonly used during desensitization and pelvic floor physical therapy. Dilator therapy begins by teaching Kegel exercises

and relaxation. The patient is then instructed to start with the smallest dilator and progressively increase the diameter as she becomes more comfortable and notes a reduction in vaginal muscle spasms. It is important to confirm the patient understands that the therapist is not actually physically dilating her vagina, but gradually desensitizing her reaction to vaginal penetration.

Alternative therapies such as massage and relaxation techniques may be appropriate adjunctive interventions for many patients and enhance the effectiveness of traditional therapy. These should be discussed with the patient and integrated into her treatment plan early on. Muscle relaxants such as cyclobenzaprine and baclofen are useful adjuncts, but should be primarily used short term and typically only as second-line therapies if the patient is not coping well with pelvic floor physical therapy. The psychological effect of dyspareunia and pelvic pain on relationships and sexual function should be addressed in the treatment plan. Partners may be involved with therapeutic measures like using vaginal dilators, but only after the patient has gained a sense of control over her symptoms and is ready to welcome partner participation.

Key Teaching Points

- Levator ani spasm is a form of myofascial pelvic pain that may lead to dyspareunia.
- Evaluation involves identification of trigger points, tender or taut muscle foci within the levator ani muscle complex, which are signs of levator ani spasm.
- Treatment is multifactorial.
- First-line therapies include pelvic floor physical therapy, heat, massage, and cognitive-behavioral therapy with vaginal dilator use.
- Second-line therapies include pharmacologic therapies such as nonsteroidal anti-inflammatory drugs and muscle relaxants.

References

1. Tu FF, Fitzgerald CM, Kuiken T et al. Comparative measurement of pelvic floor pain sensitivity in chronic pelvic pain. *Obstet Gynecol* 2007;110:1244–1248.

2. American College of Obstetricians and Gynecologists Committee on Practice Bulletins – Gynecology. ACOG Practice Bulletin No. 119: Female sexual dysfunction. *Obstet Gynecol* 2011 April;117(4):996–1007.

3. American Psychiatric Association. *Diagnostic and Statistical Manual of Mental Disorders* (4th edn Text rev.). Washington, DC: APA, 2000.

4. Bharucha AE, Lee TH. Anorectal and pelvic pain. *Mayo Clin Proc* 2016 October;91(10):1471–1486.

5. Drossman DA, Li Z, Andruzzi E et al. U.S. householder survey of functional gastrointestinal disorders:

prevalence, sociodemography, and health impact. *Dig Dis Sci* 1993;38 (9):1569–1580.

6. Williams JW, Hoffman BL. *Williams Gynecology* (2nd edn). New York, NY: McGraw-Hill Education LLC, 2012.

7. Hull M, Corton MM. Evaluation of the levator ani and pelvic wall muscles in levator ani syndrome. *Urologic Nursing* 2009;29(4):225–232.

A 16-Year-Old Adolescent with Ongoing Dysmenorrhea Despite Oral Contraceptive Pill Use

Geri D. Hewitt

History of Present Illness

A 16-year-old adolescent, gravida 0, presents with ongoing lower abdominal cramping pain that worsens with vaginal bleeding. She underwent menarche at age 14 and within six months began having regular monthly cycles with dysmenorrhea. Her pediatrician prescribed nonsteroidal anti-inflammatory drugs (NSAIDs), which initially provided some improvement in her symptoms. Six months later, the patient reported worsening dysmenorrhea and the patient was started on low-dose combination hormonal oral contraceptive pills. After three months, the patient still reported dysmenorrhea, and her pediatrician switched her to extended cycle combined hormonal contraception pills. The patient reports good compliance over the last three months on the new regimen, but reports still experiencing lower abdominal crampy pelvic pain, which worsens with unscheduled bleeding. At times, her pain is so significant that despite taking NSAIDs she has had to leave school early or miss sports practices. She denies dysuria, constipation, nausea, vomiting, fever, and ever being sexually active.

She has no medical problems and has never had surgery. She has no known drug allergies, and her only medications are her combined hormonal contraceptive pill and NSAIDs. She does well academically in school, lives with both parents and two siblings, and denies alcohol, tobacco, or marijuana use. Her family history is significant for endometriosis in her mother, which required infertility treatment to achieve conception.

Physical Examination

General appearance	Well-developed, well-nourished teen who is engaged, is communicative, and appears to be in no acute distress

Vital Signs

Pulse	78 beats/min
Blood pressure	108/62 mmHg
Height	65 inches
Weight	130 pounds
BMI	21.6 kg/m^2
Abdomen	Soft and non-tender, no masses

How Would You Manage This Patient?

This patient has dysmenorrhea and chronic pelvic pain, which is impacting her quality of life and ability to function despite six months of combined hormonal contraceptives and NSAIDs and therefore needs additional evaluation. A focused history identified no associated gastrointestinal (GI), urologic, musculoskeletal, or psychological symptoms. A urine specimen was collected for pregnancy testing and sexually transmitted infection (STI) screening. Both were negative. After pelvic examination education, consent was obtained from both the patient and her mother, and a pelvic examination was performed. No abnormalities were noted. A pelvic ultrasound identified no anatomic abnormalities.

The patient underwent diagnostic laparoscopy with peritoneal biopsies, coagulation of possible endometriotic implants, and insertion of a levonorgestrel-releasing intrauterine system (LNG-IUS). Pathologic examination of the peritoneal biopsies confirmed endometriosis. Three months after surgery, she reported her symptoms have improved. She is using less NSAIDs and no longer experiencing disruption in school or sports practices.

Adolescent Endometriosis

Dysmenorrhea is the most common gynecologic complaint and the leading cause of school absenteeism among adolescents and young adult women [1]. In epidemiologic studies, 60 to 70 percent of adolescents reported experiencing painful periods and 15 percent reported interruption of their daily activities due to severe menstrual pain [2]. Up to 90 percent of adolescents experiencing dysmenorrhea have primary dysmenorrhea or painful menses without an identifiable etiology [2]. Primary dysmenorrhea may be caused by an overproduction of prostaglandins within the endometrium. Both prostaglandins and leukotrienes are biochemical by-products of ovulation and inflammatory modulators known to cause myometrial contractions and vasoconstriction leading to local tissue ischemia and crampy pain [2]. Secondary dysmenorrhea is painful menses due to an identifiable abnormality, most commonly endometriosis, and the next most common, outflow tract obstructions (Box 3.1) [2]. Types of outflow tract obstructions that present with pain at the time of or shortly after menarche include imperforate hymen, transverse vaginal septum, obstructed hemivagina and ipsilateral renal anomaly syndrome, lower vaginal atresia, cervicovaginal agenesis/dysgenesis, and obstructed uterine horn [3].

The initial evaluation of dysmenorrhea focuses on menstrual history and associated symptoms. A family history of endometriosis should be elicited, particularly in first-degree relatives, and if present should raise clinical suspicion [4]. A pelvic examination is not necessary in patients who have never been sexually active and have a history compatible with primary dysmenorrhea [1]. A trial of empiric therapy is a reasonable first step. NSAIDs are the initial pharmacologic intervention in patients with primary dysmenorrhea not needing contraception. NSAIDs lead to a reduction in prostaglandin production and improvement in symptoms [1]. In patients who need contraception, do not tolerate or cannot take NSAIDs, or need additional symptom relief, hormonal therapies including combined hormonal contraceptives, progestin-only contraceptive

7

Box 3.1 Causes of secondary dysmenorrhea

- Endometriosis, including endometrioma
- Outflow tract obstruction
  - Imperforate hymen
  - Distal vaginal atresia
  - Vaginal/cervical atresia
  - Transverse vaginal septum
  - Cervical stenosis
  - Obstructive mullerian anomaly
- Ovarian cysts
- Uterine polyps
- Uterine leiomyomata
- Adenomyosis
- Pelvic inflammatory disease
- Pelvic adhesions

pills, transdermal patch and vaginal ring, depot medroxyprogesterone intramuscular injection, etonogestrel subdermal implant, and LNG-IUS are all effective in treating primary dysmenorrhea [1]. While safe and effective strategies for treating primary dysmenorrhea are available, many symptomatic teens do not seek treatment and rely on less effective over-the-counter or non-pharmacologic interventions [5].

Patients who do not respond to standard therapy for primary dysmenorrhea, have onset of severe symptoms with onset of menarche or shortly thereafter, or experience atypical symptoms such as heavy or abnormal menstrual bleeding, mid-cycle pain, or dyspareunia require further evaluation (Table 3.1) [5].

Patient history should review symptoms related to GI, urologic, musculoskeletal, and psychosocial etiologies, which may contribute to the pain. Evaluation for other causes of dysmenorrhea should include a pelvic examination, particularly if the patient is sexually active. Many adolescents who are not sexually active are able to tolerate a pelvic examination with education and support. The pelvic examination can identify signs of pelvic inflammatory disease, outflow track obstruction, and adnexal masses, and allow for assessment of tenderness and uterosacral nodularity. Pelvic imaging should be ordered regardless of the findings on pelvic examination. Ultrasound is the preferred initial imaging modality. There is no evidence that MRI is more advantageous as the initial study. Although a normal pelvic ultrasound does not eliminate the possibility of endometriosis, it can identify mullerian abnormalities and ovarian masses including endometriomas.

Patients with dysmenorrhea or chronic pelvic pain with no other identified etiology based on careful history, physical examination, and pelvic ultrasound and who have not improved after at least three months of initial medical therapy with NSAIDs and hormonal medications should undergo laparoscopy. Up to 70 percent of girls and adolescents with dysmenorrhea unresponsive to initial medical treatment will be diagnosed with endometriosis at the time of laparoscopy [6]. Endometriosis remains a surgical and pathologic diagnosis in adolescents, requiring the presence of endometrial glands and stroma in the biopsy specimen. There is no role for empiric use of gonadotropin-releasing hormone (GnRH) agonists in this patient population. Laparoscopy should be performed for diagnostic (both visual inspection and peritoneal biopsies) as well as therapeutic purposes with coagulation, ablation, or resection of visible implants. Endometriotic implants can appear different in adolescents. Moving the laparoscope within millimeters of the peritoneum to identify the clear or red

Table 3.1 Diagnostic and therapeutic considerations in adolescents with dysmenorrhea

Historical or physical findings	Things to consider in differential diagnosis	Interventions to consider
Persistent, significant dysmenorrhea despite good compliance with at least 3–6 months of hormonal agents and NSAIDs	Secondary causes of dysmenorrhea	Pelvic examination Pelvic ultrasound Diagnostic laparoscopy
Concomitant symptoms such as abnormal or heavy vaginal bleeding, pain with intercourse, noncyclic pain, painful defecation	Endometriosis	Pelvic examination Diagnostic laparoscopy
Cyclic abdominal pain with primary amenorrhea or early onset dysmenorrhea shortly after menarche	Obstructed outflow tract	Pelvic examination Pelvic ultrasound
History of endometriosis in first-degree relative	Endometriosis	Diagnostic laparoscopy
Known renal abnormality	Mullerian anomaly	Pelvic ultrasound
Adnexal mass	Ovarian cyst or endometrioma	Pelvic ultrasound
Vaginal discharge, cervical motion tenderness, uterine or adnexal tenderness	Pelvic inflammatory disease	STI testing Pelvic ultrasound Antibiotics

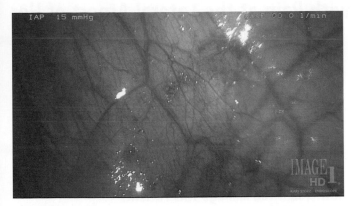

Figure 3.1 Laparoscopic images of adolescent endometriosis. The lesions are clear and vesicular. Peritoneal biopsies of the lesions were performed. Pathological examination confirmed endometriosis.

lesions in the anterior or posterior cul-de-sacs or on the pelvic side walls may increase sensitivity of the diagnostic laparoscopy (Figure 3.1) [7]. Most adolescents have American Society of Reproductive Medicine Stage 1 or 2 disease at the time of diagnosis. Stage of endometriosis does not predict the extent of painful symptoms. The clear or red endometriotic implants more common in adolescents are more likely to be associated with pain than are the black or blue lesions typically seen in adult women [7]. Many pediatric and adolescent gynecologists recommend placing an LNG-IUS at the time of laparoscopy to decrease discomfort with insertion and perforation risk. An LNG-IUS can be beneficial regardless of intraoperative findings, as it has been shown to help decrease pain associated with both dysmenorrhea not responsive to hormonal contraceptives and pain associated with endometriosis [7].

Adolescent endometriosis is considered chronic and progressive. The goals of therapy include symptom relief, suppression of progression of disease, and protection of future fertility. There is no cure, nor is there one single best treatment option. Therapy must be individualized [7]. Adolescent endometriosis is best treated with a combination of conservative surgical therapy for both diagnosis and treatment and ongoing medical therapies, such as hormonal therapies or possibly GnRH agonists. Regardless of symptomatology, adolescents with endometriosis should continue on hormonal therapy to suppress disease progression until attempting conception. Hormonal

therapies include both combined hormonal contraceptives, preferably administered continuously to suppress menses, or continuous progestins in oral (such as progestin-only contraceptive pills or norethindrone acetate 5 mg daily or twice daily), IM, or IUS form. If a patient has continuous pain attributed to endometriosis and is over 16 years old, GnRH agonists can be used with addback therapy to diminish side effects and protect bone health [7]. NSAIDs should be the mainstay of pain relief. Adolescents should not be prescribed narcotics chronically outside of a specialized pain management team. Adolescents with endometriosis often benefit from ongoing education and support as well as integration of other services such as biofeedback, pain management teams, acupuncture, and herbal therapy [7].

Key Teaching Points

- The vast majority of adolescents with dysmenorrhea have primary dysmenorrhea, which responds well to standard medical therapy with NSAIDs and hormonal contraceptives.
- Patients with ongoing symptoms despite treatment with NSAIDs and hormonal contraceptives require further evaluation including pelvic examination and pelvic ultrasound.
- The most common cause of secondary dysmenorrhea in adolescents is endometriosis, followed by outflow tract obstruction.
- Diagnostic laparoscopy should be considered in adolescents with significant dysmenorrhea despite treatment with NSAIDs and hormonal contraceptives. In appropriately selected patients, most will have pathologically proven endometriosis at the time of their laparoscopy. Visible lesions should be biopsied to confirm diagnosis and surgically treated with excision or ablation.
- GnRH agonists should not be prescribed to adolescents unless the diagnosis of endometriosis is confirmed.
- Once the diagnosis of endometriosis is confirmed by laparoscopy, the patient should be maintained on suppressive therapy, which may include hormonal agents or possibly GnRH agonists with addback. The patient may also require supplementary symptomatic therapy with NSAIDs.

References

1. Harel Z. Dysmenorrhea in adolescents and young adults: an update on pharmacological treatments and management strategies. *Expert Opin Pharmacother* 2012;13:2157–2170.

2. Sanfilippo J, Erb T. Evaluation and management of dysmenorrhea in adolescents. *Clin Obstet Gynecol* 2008;51:257–267.

3. Deitrich J, Millar D, Quint E. Obstructive reproductive tract anomalies. *J Pediatr Adolesc Gynecol* 2014;27:396–402.

4. Laufer M, Sanfilippo J, Rose G. Adolescent endometriosis: diagnosis and treatment approaches. *J Pediatr Adolesc Gynecol* 2003;16: S3–S11.

5. Allen L, Lam A. Premenstrual syndrome and dysmenorrhea in adolescents. *Adolesc Med* 2012;23:139–163.

6. Janssen E, Rijkers A, Hoppenbrouwers K, Meuleman C, D'Hooghe T. Prevalence of endometriosis diagnosed by laparoscopy in adolescents with dysmenorrhea or chronic pelvic pain: a systematic review. *Human Reprod Update* 2013;19:1–13.

7. Laufer M. Helping "adult gynecologists" diagnose and treat adolescent endometriosis: reflections on my 20 years of personal experience. *J Pediatr Adolesc Gynecol* 2011;24: S13–S17.

A 37-Year-Old Woman with Pain at the Lateral Aspect of Her Pfannenstiel Incision

Christopher M. Morosky

History of Present Illness

A 37-year-old female, gravida 3, para 3, presents with a nine-month history of right lower quadrant pain in the lateral aspect of her prior Pfannenstiel incision. She describes the pain as 9/10 in severity, piercing and stabbing in quality, with radiation into her right upper medial thigh and vulva. Bending to lift objects and walking make the pain worse. The pain is improved with sitting and leaning forward slightly. She has had no relief with over-the-counter analgesics or with two short courses of different prescription opiates.

Her past medical history is unremarkable. She is currently taking only occasional ibuprofen for her pain. She has undergone three cesarean deliveries all through Pfannenstiel incisions. She has had no other surgeries or hospitalizations. Her last cesarean delivery was two years ago and included a bilateral tubal ligation. She initially had lingering pain for six months after the surgery, which resolved for three months and then returned at the lateral aspect of her incision. Two pelvic ultrasounds, a CT scan of the abdomen and pelvis, and a diagnostic laparoscopy have been unable to identify the source of her pain.

Physical Examination

General appearance	An alert and oriented woman who is in moderate discomfort
Vital Signs	
Temperature	98.7°F (37.1°C)
Pulse	72 beats/min
Blood pressure	124/82 mmHg
Respirations	18 breaths/min
Oxygen saturation	99% on room air
Height	64 inches
Weight	123 lb
BMI	21.1 kg/m^2
Abdomen	Soft and non-distended. Well-healed low-transverse scar. Moderate shooting pain elicited with light palpation of the right lateral aspect of the scar. No hernia present.
External genitalia	Numbness and decreased sensation of the right groin and mons pubis compared to the left using gentle palpation with a cotton swab. No rashes, lesions, or skin changes.
Bimanual exam	Normal-sized anteverted uterus. Non-tender. No pelvic masses.
Speculum exam	No lesions on the vagina or cervix. Physiologic discharge present without blood.
Provoking procedure	The patient is asked to lie supine on her back. She is then asked to raise her head and neck slightly from the exam table, causing mild contraction of her abdominal muscles. This maneuver causes a significant increase in her right lower quadrant pain.

How Would You Manage This Patient?

The patient has entrapment of the right ilioinguinal-iliohypogastric nerves. She is experiencing all three components of the diagnostic triad associated with ilioinguinal-iliohypogastric nerve entrapment or neuroma formation. As a diagnostic and therapeutic office-based procedure, she was consented for a neuronal blockade. Using a 25-gauge needle, a total of 3 cc of 1 percent lidocaine buffered with sodium bicarbonate was injected into the area of the patient's pain at the right lateral aspect of her Pfannenstiel incision. Ten minutes after injection, she reported being pain-free for the first time in nine months.

Ilioinguinal-Iliohypogastric Nerve Entrapment

Injury to the ilioinguinal-iliohypogastric nerves can occur through severing the nerve, causing neuroma formation, stretch, compression with retractors, entrapment with suture, fibrosis, and scarring [1, 2]. Ilioinguinal-iliohypogastric nerve injury can occur after transverse incisions in the lower abdomen, inguinal herniorrhaphy, and laparoscopy. It is estimated that 6–18 percent of patients following cesarean delivery and 5–32 percent of patients following hysterectomy will suffer from chronic postsurgical pain, and approximately 2–4 percent of patients will suffer from chronic lower abdominal pain due to ilioinguinal-iliohypogastric nerve entrapment following a Pfannenstiel incision [1].

The ilioinguinal nerve is a mixed nerve with both motor and sensory functions. It arises from the L1 and L2 spinal nerve roots with variable contribution from T12. The iliohypogastric nerve is also a mixed nerve arising from the L1 and often the T12 spinal nerve roots [3, 4]. Both nerves emerge from the upper part of the lateral border of the psoas muscle. Although there is variation in location, these nerves pierce the transversus abdominis muscle approximately one centimeter above the anterior superior iliac spine. The nerves travel in an inferior-medial course, and eventually pierce the aponeurosis of the internal and external oblique muscles. The iliohypogastric nerve goes on to provide sensory innervation to the superomedial thigh, mons pubis, and labia majora. The iliohypogastric nerve divides into lateral and anterior cutaneous branches. The lateral cutaneous branch provides sensory innervation to the gluteal region. The anterior cutaneous branch provides sensory innervation to the hypogastric region (Figure 4.1). Transverse incisions in the lower abdomen and laterally placed laparoscopic trochar ports can cause direct injury to these nerves or entrapment of these nerves with suture placement and scarring.

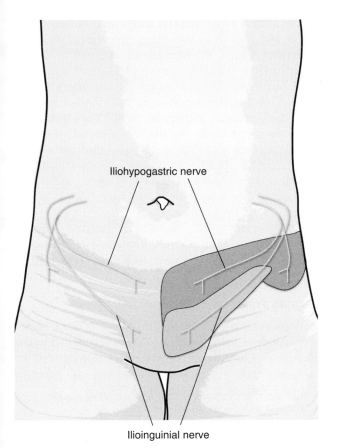

Iliohypogastric nerve

Ilioinguinial nerve

Figure 4.1 Nerve paths and innervation distribution of the ilioinguinal and iliohypogastric nerves.

Patients with entrapment of the ilioinguinal-iliohypogastric nerve have a diagnostic triad consisting of:

(1) lancinating or shooting pain near the original surgical site and radiating to the area innervated by the ilioinguinal-iliohypogastric nerves,

(2) clear evidence of sensory perception impairment in the area supplied by the nerves, and

(3) pain relief with infiltration of a local anesthetic near the painful portion of the surgical site or along the path of the nerves [3, 5].

The diagnostic evaluation of a patient presenting with symptoms of ilioinguinal-iliohypogastric nerve entrapment includes a thorough history and complete examination of the abdomen and pelvis. Special attention should focus on the details of all surgical procedures performed in the lower abdomen, groin, and pelvis. Patients may report their pain immediately following their surgery or months to years later. The neuropathic pain is often sharp, stabbing, burning, or shooting and radiates from the area of injury into the groin, pubic area, and medial thigh. Increased pain with Valsalva or truncal movements such as bending, twisting, or walking is common. Patients may report that sitting up with a slight lean forward at the hips helps to alleviate the pain. Traditional over-the-counter analgesics and prescription opiate medications often do not provide adequate pain relief.

On physical exam, pressure along the lateral edges of the abdominal incision scar may elicit trigger point tenderness. Patients may have allodynia (pain elicited by sensations that are not usually painful) including light touch from a cotton swab. The same cotton swab can be used to assess for numbness (hypoesthesia) or a pins and needles sensation (dysesthesia) in the area of reported pain or along the distribution of the injured nerve. Provoking dysesthesia through the compression of a suspected entrapped nerve is known as Tinel's sign. This is performed by gently tapping repeatedly over the more proximal course of the nerves, such as at the anterior superior iliac spine. Worsening of pain with contraction of the abdominal muscles is known as a positive Carnett's sign, and localizes the pain to the anterior abdominal wall [6].

While quantitative sensory testing using electrical, thermal, or ultrasonic stimulation is available to evoke specific nerve, electromyographic, and cortical potentials, it is rarely used. This costly and time-consuming testing is not superior to physical examination and bedside testing.

Patients benefit diagnostically and therapeutically from neuronal blockade using a local anesthetic with or without steroids. One option is to inject 2–3 milliliters of 1 percent lidocaine subcutaneously at the trigger point of tenderness or 5–10 milliliters of lidocaine deeper within the fascia planes more proximal along the path of the suspected injured nerve [6]. Another option is to use a linear high-frequency ultrasound probe (6–13 MHz) to guide the tip of the needle within the transversus abdominis and internal oblique muscles. At the area three centimeters medial to the anterior superior iliac spine, 5–10 milliliters of lidocaine placed in the space between these two muscles can anesthetize both of the ilioinguinal-iliohypogastric nerves [2, 7]. Improvement of the pain lasting 2–4 hours is clinically assumed to be associated with ilioinguinal-iliohypogastric nerve entrapment. If initially successful, the pain can be managed with injections repeated weekly to monthly. Some patients may experience long-term relief from their pain with local injections alone.

Neurectomy can be considered as a long-term treatment option. In the setting of a prior Pfannenstiel incision, patients are brought to the operating room where the lateral margin of their original skin incision is opened. The incision is further lateralized and dissected down to the underlying external oblique aponeurosis. The fascia and muscle are incised and dissected up to the anterior superior iliac spine to identify the ilioinguinal-iliohypogastric nerves. The nerves are excised up to the level of the anterior superior iliac spine, and the remaining ends are buried in the underlying muscle to prevent neuroma formation. In a number of small case series, 70–90 percent of patients experienced long-lasting pain relief [1, 3, 8, 9]. Similar procedural interventions with less published data available include smaller neurectomy procedures, surgical neurolysis, and cryoneurolysis. Unfortunately, some patients experience long-lasting pain, numbness, or hypersensitivity despite undergoing invasive procedures.

Surgical interventions are not appropriate or suitable for all patients and treatment algorithms have been suggested (Figure 4.2). Several medical treatment options are

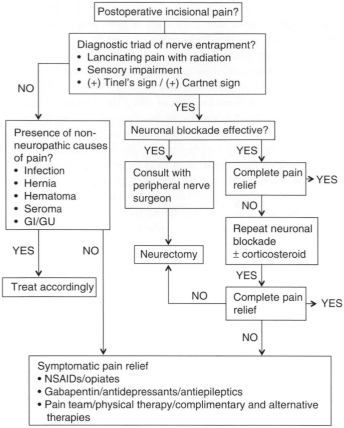

Figure 4.2 Treatment algorithm for patients with suspected ilioinguinal-iliohypogastric nerve entrapment.

therapy, connective tissue release, and transcutaneous electrical nerve stimulation is also being investigated as treatment options for ilioinguinal-iliohypogastric nerve entrapment [6].

Several techniques should reduce risk of injury to the ilioinguinal-iliohypogastric nerves at the time of surgery involving the anterior abdominal wall. For transverse abdominal incisions such as the Pfannenstiel incision, care should be taken to avoid lateral dissection out farther than the lateral border of the anterior rectus muscles. Surgeons should also avoid placement of their fascial closure stitches farther lateral than the lateral apex of the facial incision [4]. Blunt dissection of the anterior rectus fascia as performed in the Joel-Cohen incision may be associated with less injury to the ilioinguinal-iliohypogastric nerves compared to the sharp dissection performed in the Pfannenstiel incision [10].

Key Teaching Points

- The diagnostic triad for ilioinguinal-iliohypogastric nerve injury includes lancinating pain in the area supplied by the ilioinguinal-iliohypogastric nerves, clear evidence of sensory impairment of the nerves, and relief with injection of a local anesthetic in the area of maximal pain.
- Confirmatory findings on physical exam include hyperesthesia (increased sensation to pain), allodynia (increased pain with light touch), hypoesthesia (numbness), and dysesthesia (pins and needles) in the regions supplied by the ilioinguinal and iliohypogastric nerves.
- Neuronal blockade with an injection of local anesthetic with or without steroids can be both diagnostic and therapeutic for many patients.
- Neurectomy has good success for treating the pain associated with ilioinguinal-iliohypogastric nerve entrapment, with several medical treatments and multimodal therapies available to patients with persistent symptoms or who cannot or do not want to undergo a repeat surgical procedure.

available for patients who cannot undergo a repeat surgical procedure, those who decline surgical intervention, and those who continue with ilioinguinal-iliohypogastric nerve pain following neurectomy. Tricyclic antidepressants, selective serotonin/norepinephrine reuptake inhibitors, and anticonvulsants have been used to treat ilioinguinal-iliohypogastric nerve entrapment pain. Topical treatment with capsaicin or lidocaine patches is an additional nonsurgical therapeutic option. Multimodal treatment with physical

References

1. Loos MJ, Scheltinga MR, Mulders LG et al. The Pfannenstiel incision as a source of chronic pain. *Obstet Gynecol* 2008;111:839–846.

2. Recker D, Perry PM. Postsurgical pain syndromes: chronic pain after hysterectomy and cesarean section. *Tech Reg Anesth Pain Manag* 2011;15:133–139.

3. Kim D, Murovic JA, Tiel RL et al. Surgical management of 33 ilioinguinal and iliohypogastric neuralgias at Louisiana State University Health Sciences Center. *Neurosurgery* 2005;56(5):1013–1020.

4. Rahn DD, Phelan JN, Roshanravan SM et al. Anterior abdominal wall nerve and vessel anatomy: clinical implications for gynecologic surgery. *Am J Obstet Gynecol* 2010;202:234.e1–e5.

5. Melville K, Schultz EQ, Dougherty JM. Ilioinguinal-Iliohypogastric nerve entrapment. *Ann Emerg Med* 1990;19 (8):925–929.

6. Tu FF, Hellman KM, Backonja MM. Gynecologic management of neuropathic pain. *Am J Obstet Gynecol* 2011;205(5):435–443.

7. Wieczorek PM. Regional analgesic techniques for postoperative cesarean section pain. *Int Anesthesiol Clin* 2014;52 (2):111–128.

8. Ducic I, Moxley M, Al-Attar A. Algorithm for treatment of postoperative incisional groin pain after cesarean delivery or hysterectomy. *Obstet Gynecol* 2006;108:27–31.

9. Madura JA, Madura JA, Copper CM et al. Inguinal neurectomy for inguinal nerve entrapment: an experience with 100 patients. *Am J Surg* 2005;185: 283–287.

10. Gizzo S, Andrisani A, Noventa M et al. Caesarean section: could different transverse abdominal incision techniques influence postpartum pain and subsequent quality of life? A systematic review. *PloS ONE* 2015;10(2):e0114190.

A 26-Year-Old Woman with Chronic Pelvic Pain and Negative Work-Up

Misa Perron-Burdick

History of Present Illness

A 26-year-old, gravida 1, para 0, woman presents with pelvic pain for several years. The pain is 6/10 on most days of the month. She calls in sick to work three to four days per month. The pain is focused in the right lower abdomen and radiates throughout the pelvis. It is constant and aching, and worsens throughout the day. It is not associated with her period, which she describes as occurring every month with a normal amount of bleeding. She does not have pain with intercourse. She has no vaginal discharge, pain with urination, or change in bowel habits. The patient is unable to identify exacerbating factors because the pain is "always there." She has tried acetaminophen and ibuprofen, without relief. She has tried hormonal contraception, but found the side effects intolerable and does not know if it helped her pain.

The patient denies a history of depression, but she feels "down" lately due to pain. She has trouble sleeping and does not exercise regularly because of the pain. She is in a long-term monogamous relationship with a male partner and feels very supported and safe. She denies a history of sexual or physical abuse. The patient had a diagnostic laparoscopy several years ago when the pain first started, which did not identify the cause for her pain. She is very frustrated that no one has been able to tell her what is causing the pain.

Physical Examination

General appearance No acute distress but tearful at times

Vital Signs

Temperature	37.0°C
Pulse	82 beats/min
Blood pressure	122/71 mmHg
Weight	64 kg
Height	160 cm
BMI	25 kg/m^2
Abdomen	Soft, no masses, tender to deep palpation in both lower quadrants, no rebound or guarding, pain does not worsen with contraction of abdominal muscles during palpation (negative Carnett's sign)
External genitalia	Normal vulva, no pain with light touch of the vestibule using a cotton swab
Vagina	Normal vaginal epithelium, no bleeding or vaginal discharge
Cervix	Nulliparous, no cervical motion tenderness
Uterus	Small, anteverted, mildly tender
Adnexa	No masses, adnexa tender mildly bilaterally
Pelvic floor muscles	Non-tender, no vaginismus.

Laboratory Studies

Urine pregnancy test	Negative
Urinalysis	Normal
Gonorrhea and chlamydia nucleic acid amplification tests	Negative

How Would You Manage This Patient?

This patient has chronic pelvic pain with a negative work-up. A patient-centered approach was used to discuss the unclear etiology of her pain and the need for a multidisciplinary approach that including both behavioral and medical therapies. The provider discussed treatment goals, focusing on symptom improvement rather than complete relief. The patient's goals were to be pain-free on some days and rarely needing to call in sick from work because of pain. The patient was started on low-dose amytriptyline. She was given literature on relaxation breathing and stretching exercises, and was referred for cognitive-behavioral therapy to learn pain management techniques. The patient was recommended to manage pain exacerbations with warm or cold compresses, relaxation and stretching, and either acetaminophen or ibuprofen. The patient returned to clinic two months later reporting no significant relief in her pain. However, upon further questioning, she noted that her pain had improved to a 4/10 and she was calling in sick to work less frequently. The patient was reassured by this improvement. The amitriptyline was increased, and the patient was encouraged to continue cognitive-behavioral therapy until completion. The patient returned three months later reporting continued improvement of pain; however, she had not reached her goal of some pain-free days. The patient was recommended to increase her physical activity now that her pain was no longer prohibitive. She was offered a referral for physical therapy or transcutaneous electrical nerve stimulation, but she chose to pursue acupuncture as the next line of therapy. The recurring and remitting nature of chronic pain was discussed and a plan was made for the patient to return to clinic if the acupuncture therapy was ineffective or if she experienced worsening pain.

Chronic Pelvic Pain

Chronic pelvic pain is defined as pain in the lower abdomen and pelvis that lasts longer than six months. It is usually noncyclic in nature. Chronic pelvic pain affects one in seven reproductive-age women and accounts for up to 10 percent of gynecology visits [1, 2]. Chronic pelvic pain has many etiologies. Common gynecologic causes include endometriosis, adenomyosis, and vulvodynia. Common non-gynecologic etiologies include irritable bowel syndrome, painful bladder syndrome, and musculoskeletal pelvic floor disorders. Sixty-one percent of patients with chronic pelvic pain never receive a diagnosis for their pain [3].

Patients with chronic pelvic pain should have an initial evaluation including a detailed health history, psychosocial screening, and full physical exam. Patients should be evaluated for the common gynecologic and non-gynecologic causes of chronic pelvic pain. Imaging is recommended for patients with a history or exam concerning adenomyosis or adnexal or uterine masses, and should also be considered for patients with pain that is worsening, new, or refractory to treatment. However, most patients with chronic pelvic pain will have a negative ultrasound and so imaging is not necessary prior to initiating long-term management. Ultrasound is the recommended imaging modality because of its low cost and invasiveness and high sensitivity for detecting pelvic pathology. Diagnostic laparoscopy has limited value in patients with chronic pelvic pain, even those with no clear etiology. More than a third will have no visible pathology and those who do most commonly have endometriosis or adhesions for which surgical intervention does not have long-term benefits [4, 5]. It is recommended to begin empiric treatment at the first visit even if the diagnosis is unclear, as it may aid in diagnosis and bring the patient immediate relief. First-line treatments include over-the-counter analgesics such as acetaminophen and nonsteroidal anti-inflammatory drugs (NSAIDs), hormonal contraception, and pelvic floor physical therapy.

Negative evaluation is common in chronic pain patients. In patients who have completed an initial evaluation, including imaging if indicated, the provider should focus on a long-term treatment plan using a multidisciplinary approach that includes behavioral, pharmacologic, and physical therapies (Table 5.1). This approach is appropriate for patients with an unknown etiology for their pain as well as those with a known diagnosis who have failed usual treatment. Foremost is the therapeutic relationship with the clinician. Chronic pain patients report symptom improvement when they feel that their condition is taken seriously and that adequate time is taken to explain exam findings and management recommendations [6]. The provider should establish treatment goals that focus on improving quality of life rather than complete resolution of pain, and explain that treatment may take several months and require significant patient participation. Underlying psychosocial disorders such as depression, anxiety, or post-traumatic stress disorder that could worsen or be a result of pain symptoms should be addressed. Even in patients without an underlying psychosocial disorder, working with a mental health therapist experienced in chronic pain is very beneficial. Cognitive-behavioral training is very effective for managing chronic pain conditions because it uses a problem-focused approach that teaches patients to identify pain triggers and modify their responses in a way that ameliorates the pain experience.

Options for pharmacologic treatments depend on the nature of the pain. Patients with unclear etiology often have a combination of visceral and musculoskeletal pain. First-line pharmacologic therapy for all types of pelvic pain includes NSAIDs or acetaminophen. NSAIDs are favored if there is a strong musculoskeletal component. Many chronic pain patients experience sensitization of the peripheral or

Table 5.1 Treatment of chronic pelvic pain with unknown etiology

Treatment class	Treatment
Behavioral therapy	Relaxation breathing Meditation Exercise Cognitive-behavioral therapy
Pharmacologic therapy	Acetaminophen NSAIDs Hormonal contraception Tricyclic antidepressants (amitriptyline or nortriptyline) Serotonin norepinephrine reuptake inhibitors (venlafaxine or duloxetine) Antiepileptic medications (gabapentin)
Physical therapy	Stretching Massage Heat and icing Acupuncture Transcutaneous electrical nerve stimulation Biofeedback Myofascial physical therapy (e.g., trigger point release)

central nervous system and benefit from a low-dose antidepressant or anticonvulsant medication. Tricyclic antidepressants such as amitriptyline (25–150 mg daily) and nortriptyline (10–150 mg daily) are commonly used in the treatment of chronic pain and are especially useful in patients with insomnia, due to their sedating side effects. Selective norepinephrine reuptake inhibitors such as venlafaxine (37.5–225 mg daily) and duloxetine (30–120 mg daily) are also effective. Antidepressants should be started at the lowest dose and slowly titrated up every few weeks until a therapeutic level or maximum dose is reached. Patients who fail to improve or experience intolerable side effects may be changed to a different antidepressant medication. Anticonvulsants such as gabapentin may be slightly more effective and have fewer side effects than low-dose tricyclic antidepressants when used for pelvic pain [7]. Gabapentin is associated with significant side effects, so it is recommended to start at a low dose of 300 mg per day and increase weekly by 300 mg daily increments until a therapeutic level or maximum dose of 2,700 mg is reached. Patients should be made aware of the potential need to taper medications should they wish to discontinue. Hormonal therapy is considered the mainstay treatment for patients with cyclic pain or endometriosis and it may be beneficial in patients with pelvic pain of unclear origin. Hormonal options include combined oral contraceptives with high progestin potency dosed continuously, depo medroxyprogesterone acetate, the etonogestrel implant, and the levonorgestrel intrauterine device.

Opioids are not recommended for the management of chronic pain because of the risk of opioid use disorder and overdose. There is a lack of evidence supporting the effectiveness of long-term opioid use in the treatment of chronic pain with respect to pain or quality of life. Initiation of opioid use should be avoided whenever possible, especially in patients at high risk of opioid use disorder, including those with younger age, major depression, substance use disorder, or psychotropic medication use. Patients who are taking opioids for chronic pain should be encouraged to taper if possible. All patients receiving opioids for chronic pain should be managed by a clinician who is experienced in assessing and mitigating the risk of opioid use disorder and overdose. Initiation of opioid treatment should be done selectively in patients who are simultaneously pursuing non-pharmacologic and non-opioid pharmacologic treatment and should include a discussion of treatment goals, review of the risks of opioid treatment, and a plan for reevaluation and cessation if opioids are ineffective or the risks outweigh the benefits. Immediate-release opioids are preferred over extended-release and should be prescribed at the lowest possible therapeutic dose, ideally reserved for acute exacerbations [8].

Patients with chronic pelvic pain of unknown etiology often experience pelvic floor dysfunction and myofascial pain as muscle spasms and ligament strain develop in response to pain. Physical therapy treats pain with relaxation and breathing exercises, stretching, self-massage, and self-awareness exercises for patient to learn how to identify and relax tense muscles that exacerbate pain. Small studies also suggest that transcutaneous electrical nerve stimulation and acupuncture reduce pain and improve the quality of life for patients with chronic pelvic pain [9, 10]. While hysterectomy can be an effective treatment for chronic pain in patients with a uterine etiology, such as adenomyosis or leiomyoma, there is a lack of evidence that it improves pain in patients with pelvic pain of other etiologies [11].

Key Teaching Points

- Up to 60 percent of patients with chronic pelvic pain will not receive a diagnosis for their pain.
- Diagnostic imaging or laparoscopy is not required prior to initiating long-term treatment; however, it may be indicated in some patients.
- Treatment goals should focus on improving symptoms and quality of life rather than complete relief.
- The mainstays of treatment include over-the-counter analgesics, cognitive-behavioral therapy, low-dose antidepressants, and physical therapy.
- Opioids are not recommended for the long-term management of chronic pelvic pain.

References

1. Latthe P, Latthe M, Say L, Gulmezoglu M, Khan KS. WHO systematic review of prevalence of chronic pelvic pain: a neglected reproductive health morbidity. *BMC Public Health* 2006;6(6):177.

2. Reiter RC. A profile of women with chronic pelvic pain. *Clin Obstet Gynecol* 1990;33(1):130–136.

3. Mathias SD, Kupperman M, Liberman RF, Lipschutz RC, Steege JF. Chronic pelvic pain: prevalence, health-related quality of life, and economic correlates. *Obstet Gynecol* 1996;87(3):321–327.

4. Howard FM. The role of laparoscopy in the chronic pelvic pain patient. *Clin Obstet Gynecol* 2003;46(4):749.

5. Swank DJ, Swank-Bordewijk SC, Hop WC et al. Laparoscopic adhesiolysis in patients with chronic abdominal pain: a blinded randomised controlled multi-centre trial. *Lancet* 2003;361 (9365):1247.

6. Price J, Farmer G, Harris J et al. Attitudes of women with chronic pelvic pain to the gynaecological consultation: a qualitative study. *BJOG* 2006;113(4):446.

7. Carey ET, Till SR, As-Sanie S. Pharmacological management of chronic pelvic pain in women. *Drugs* 2017;77: 285–230.

8. Dowell D, Haegerich TM, Chou R. CDC guidelines for prescribing opioids for chronic pain–United States, 2016. *MMWR Recomm Rep* 2016;65 (RR-1):1–49.

9. Sharma N, Rekha K, Srinivasan JK. Efficacy of transcutaneous electrical nerve stimulation in the treatment of chronic pelvic pain. *J Midlife Health* 2017;8(1):36–39.

10. Arnouk A, De E, Rehfuss A et al. Physical, complementary, and alternative medicine in the treatment of pelvic floor disorders. *Curr Urol Rep* 2017;18:47.

11. Lamvu G. Role of hysterectomy in the treatment of chronic pelvic pain. *Obstet Gynecol* 2011 May;117(5):1175–1178.

A 30-Year-Old Woman with Endometriosis with Worsening Pelvic Pain Despite Continuous Oral Contraceptives

William D. Po

History of Present Illness

A 30-year-old, gravida 0, is a new patient to your office. She has a history of endometriosis diagnosed by laparoscopy several years ago, which was demonstrated on biopsy. At that surgery, all visible lesions were cauterized by electrocautery. Until recently, she had been stable with minimal pain on continuous combined hormonal contraceptive (OC) pills. However, over the last six months, she reports increasing dysmenorrhea and dyspareunia. She is unsure about her plans for having children. She has an otherwise unremarkable medical history. Her only surgery was the diagnostic laparoscopy. She would like to discuss other treatment options for endometriosis.

Physical Examination

General appearance	Well-developed, well-nourished woman in no discomfort, alert and oriented

Vital Signs

Temperature	37.0°C
Pulse	80 beats/min
Blood pressure	120/74 mmHg
Respiratory rate	16 breaths/min
Oxygen saturation	100% on room air
Height	66 inches
Weight	140 lb
Abdomen	Soft, non-tender, non-distended, no guarding, no rebound. Mild tenderness in LLQ and RLQ, left greater than right
External genitalia	Unremarkable
Vagina	Well estrogenated, normal rugae
Cervix	Nulliparous, no lesions or discharge, moderately tender
Uterus	Anteverted, mobile, normal size, moderate tenderness on bimanual examination. Nodularity along uterosacral ligaments
Adnexa	No masses, moderate discomfort bilaterally with palpation

Laboratory Studies

Urine pregnancy test	Negative
WBC	Unremarkable
Gonorrhea and chlamydia nucleic acid amplification tests (NAATs)	Negative

Imaging

Transvaginal ultrasound	Normal uterus, no adnexal masses, no free fluid

How Would You Manage This Patient?

A thorough history was performed to rule out other causes of pelvic pain and dyspareunia, such as sexually transmitted infections, cystitis, and irritable bowel syndrome, which were negative. The ultrasound did not demonstrate endometriomas, adnexal masses, or uterine pathology. NAATs for chlamydia and gonorrhea were negative. The history, coupled with the findings of nodularity along the uterosacral ligaments and tender bimanual examinations, and the normal ultrasound suggested that her pain was likely due to endometriosis.

Continuous OC use was no longer controlling her pain, and future fertility may still be important to the patient. Depot Leuprolide, a gonadotropin-releasing hormone (GnRH) agonist, 3.75 mg injection, given intramuscularly, once a month was recommended, along with norethindrone, 5 mg, orally once a day as add-back therapy to mitigate hypoestrogenic side effects (vaginal dryness and hot flashes). The patient was instructed to try this therapy for three to six months and to monitor her pain levels as well as medication side effects. She was encouraged to continue nonsteroidal anti-inflammatory drugs (NSAIDs) such as ibuprofen and also advised to take calcium supplements. If this therapy does not work or is not tolerated, the next step may involve surgical options depending on the severity of her symptoms. She was instructed to return for a follow-up in four weeks.

Evaluation

With any chronic pain condition, it is important to consider all etiologies despite the established diagnosis of endometriosis. A thorough history and physical examination can help determine if there are any coexisting conditions such as interstitial cystitis, irritable bowel syndrome, or pelvic infection. A detailed discussion with the patient regarding desire for future pregnancies should be made, as that may help determine the course of therapy. Evaluation can be complicated, as endometriosis can have many presentations and be unpredictable in its course. Dysmenorrhea, chronic pelvic pain, dyspareunia, uterosacral ligament nodularity, and an adnexal mass are typical. However, a large number of women can also be asymptomatic [1].

Endometriosis is a common gynecological condition characterized by deposits of endometrial tissue outside the endometrial cavity, including liver, diaphragm, umbilicus, and pleural cavity. The prevalence of endometriosis is as high as 10 percent in the general population and as high as 40 percent in subfertile women. Pain is a common presenting feature and often recurs, even after treatment. There is a familial component, and there seems to be no racial predisposition [2]. The American Society for Reproductive Medicine Practice Committee states that "endometriosis should be viewed as a chronic disease that requires a lifelong management plan with the goal of maximizing the use of medical treatment and avoiding repeated surgical procedures" [3].

The type of pain that is classic for endometriosis can be described as secondary dysmenorrhea. Pain frequently starts before the onset of menses; there may be deep dyspareunia (which is often worse during menses) or sacral backache during menses. Organs affected by endometriosis may result in pain or physiologic dysfunction of those organs, such as perimenstrual tenesmus, diarrhea or constipation, cramping and dyschezia in cases of bowel involvement, or dysuria and hematuria in cases of bladder involvement. The pain from endometriosis may not correlate with the stage of disease, and instead may be due to the depth of infiltration of endometrial lesions. Painful defecation during menses and severe dyspareunia can be an indication of deeply infiltrating endometriosis.

Imaging has limited utility in the diagnosis of endometriosis. Ultrasound may be useful in the diagnosis if a pelvic mass consistent with an endometrioma is identified. Transvaginal ultrasonography can help to detect the presence of deeply infiltrating endometriosis of the rectum, rectovaginal septum, and bladder lesions. MRI is superior to ultrasound in diagnosing rectosigmoid lesions and endometriosis of the bladder, and may help diagnose indeterminate pelvic masses, as well as guide surgical approaches. CT scan is not useful in the diagnosis of endometriosis. Biomarkers such as CA125 lack specificity, and routine testing with them is not recommended [1, 4].

The gold standard for diagnosing endometriosis remains laparoscopic evaluation, preferably with tissue biopsy. While it is reasonable to treat endometriosis based upon a presumptive diagnosis from history and physical examination findings, laparoscopy is indicated for severe symptoms or failed medical management. Histology should confirm endometrial glands and stroma with varying amounts of inflammation and fibrosis. The lesions themselves may have several appearances and not just the classic black powder-burn lesions [5].

Treatment

In women who have pain from endometriosis and desire future fertility, a number of different medications may help. These include combined OCs, progestins, danazol, GnRH agonists, and NSAIDs. Dysmenorrhea on OCs can be avoided with the use of extended-cycle pills. In a two-year prospective study of women with endometriosis-associated dysmenorrhea that was not responsive to cyclic combined OCs, continuous combined OC administration was found to provide significant pain reduction from baseline ($P < .001$) [6].

Two randomized controlled trials (RCTs) have shown that subcutaneous depot medroxyprogesterone acetate (DMPA) was equivalent to GnRH agonists in reducing pain with substantially less bone loss. The bone loss that occurred with DMPA returned to pretreatment levels by 12 months [6]. Intrauterine progestin use with the levonorgestrel intrauterine system also has been shown to be effective in reducing endometriosis-associated pelvic pain. Three-year follow-up data showed a persistent benefit of the levonorgestrel intrauterine system, although approximately 40 percent of patients discontinued use because of unacceptable irregular bleeding or persistent pain. In an RCT comparing a GnRH agonist and the levonorgestrel intrauterine system, there was no significant difference between the two groups in control of pain [6]. Danazol is an androgenic drug that has been used for the treatment of endometriosis-associated pain. Although highly effective, Danazol has a significant side-effect profile, which includes acne, hirsutism, and myalgias, that is more severe than other treatments [6].

Gonadotropin-releasing hormone agonists are highly effective in reducing the pain syndromes associated with endometriosis. However, they are not superior to other methods such as combined OCs as first-line therapy. Gonadotropin-releasing hormone agonists may have significant hypoestrogenic side effects, including hot flashes, vaginal dryness, and osteopenia. Osteopenia has been shown to be reversible with short-term use, but may not be with long-term use or use of multiple cycles. As with other suppressive therapy, recurrence of symptoms is common after the medication is discontinued. The recurrence rate at five-year follow-up, after discontinuing GnRH agonist treatment, ranges from 53 percent to as high as 73 percent in women with advanced disease. There may be an option for prolonged use of the GnRH agonist for up to one year if add-back therapy is used [1, 6].

Add-back therapy reduces or eliminates GnRH agonist-induced bone mineral loss and provides relief from the symptoms of hypoestrogenism without reducing the efficacy of pain relief. Add-back regimens (using either sex-steroid hormones or other specific bone-sparing agents) have been advocated for use in women undergoing long-term therapy (more than six months). Such treatment strategies have included progestins alone, progestins and bisphosphonates, low-dose progestins, and estrogens. The US Food and Drug Administration has approved the daily use of norethindrone, 5 mg, as add-back therapy with add-back treatment does not diminish the efficacy of pain relief observed during three months or six months of GnRH agonist therapy. Therefore, the add-back regimen can be started immediately with the GnRH agonist. There appears to be no disadvantages to the use of an add-back regimen in combination with a GnRH agonist other than the small cost associated with the additional medication. However, a Cochrane review found little or no difference between GnRH agonist and other medical treatments for endometriosis, suggesting again that this regimen is not recommended as a primary treatment approach [6].

Laparoscopic surgery (ablation and excision; ablation and uterine nerve transection) was associated with increased live births and ongoing pregnancies compared with diagnostic laparoscopy. In women with endometriomas receiving surgery for infertility or pain, excision of the endometrioma capsule increased the rate of spontaneous postoperative pregnancy compared with drainage and electrocoagulation of the endometrioma wall. Surgery to endometriomas, however, can also reduce ovarian reserve and fertility due to removal of normal ovarian tissue. A Cochrane review based on four RCTs concluded that surgical treatment to endometriomas before assisted laparoscopic excision of the endometrioma cyst wall was associated with increased clinical pregnancy rates compared with ablation [6].

For patients who do not desire future pregnancies, definitive surgical therapy may be indicated. Prospective observational studies indicate that hysterectomy with bilateral salpingo-ophrectomy is a successful strategy for women who are not pursuing pregnancy, but results in surgical menopause. Retrospective data suggest that hysterectomy alone (with ovarian conservation) reduces pain, since dysmenorrhea no longer occurs. Around a third of women, however, will require further surgery for symptoms at five years, compared with 10 percent of those who undergo hysterectomy with oophorectomy for endometriosis. In younger women (aged 30–39), however, removal of the ovaries did not significantly improve the surgery-free time and is likely to lead to adverse symptomatic and health consequences associated with surgical menopause [6, 7].

Key Teaching Points

- Dysmenorrhea, chronic pelvic pain, dyspareunia, uterosacral ligament nodularity, and an adnexal mass are typical findings in women with endometriosis.
- Endometriosis is a chronic disease that requires a lifelong management plan with the goal of maximizing the use of medical treatment and avoiding repeated surgical procedures.
- It is reasonable to treat endometriosis based upon a presumptive diagnosis from history and physical examination findings. Imaging has limited utility in the diagnosis of endometriosis.
- The gold standard for diagnosing endometriosis remains laparoscopic evaluation, preferably with tissue biopsy.

Laparoscopy is indicated for severe symptoms or failed medical management.

- Treatments that may help endometriosis pain include combined OCs, progestins, danazol, GnRH agonists, NSAIDs, and the levonorgestrel intrauterine device.
- Continuous combined OC administration provides significant pain reduction compared to cyclic use.
- DMPA is equivalent to GnRH agonists in reducing pain with substantially less bone loss.
- GnRH agonists and the levonorgestrel intrauterine system are equivalent in control of pain.
- Gonadotropin-releasing hormone agonists, while highly effective, are not superior to other methods and should not be a first-line treatment option. Add-back therapy reduces or eliminates GnRH agonist–induced bone mineral loss and provides relief from the symptoms of hypoestrogenism without reducing the efficacy of pain relief.
- Surgical management of endometriosis-related infertility does improve pregnancy rates, but the magnitude of improvement is unclear.
- Excision of an endometrioma increases the rate of spontaneous postoperative pregnancy compared to simple drainage and ablation of the cyst wall.
- For patients who do not desire future pregnancies, hysterectomy with bilateral salpingo-ophrectomy is a successful strategy. Hysterectomy alone (with ovarian conservation) reduces pain, but a third of women will require further surgery for symptoms at five years. In younger women, removal of the ovaries does not significantly improve the surgery-free time.

References

1. The American College of Obstetricians and Gynecologists. Management of endometriosis. Practice Bulletin No, 114. *Obstet Gynecol* 2010;116(1): 223–36.

2. Hickey M, Ballard K, Farquhar C. Endometriosis. *BMJ* 2014;348.

3. Practice Committee of the American Society for Reproductive Medicine. Treatment of pelvic pain associated with endometriosis: a committee opinion. *Fertil Steril* 2014 April; 101(4): 927–35. Epub 2014 Mar 13. Brown J, Farquhar C,

An overview of treatment for endometriosis. *JAMA* 2015; 313(3):296–297.

4. Hsu Al, Khachikyan I, Stratton P. Invasive and non-invasive methods for the diagnosis of endometriosis. *Clin Obstet Gynecol* 2010;53: 413–419.

5. Brosens I, Puttemans P, Benagiano G, Endometriosis: a life cycle approach? *Am J Obstet Gynecol* 2013 October;209 (4):307–316.

6. Brown J, Farquhar C, Endometriosis: an overview of Cochrane reviews. *Cochrane Database Syst Rev* 2014 March;10(3): CD009590.

7. Brosens I, Puttemans P, Benagiano G, Endometriosis: a life cycle approach? *Am J Obstet Gynecol* 2013 October;209 (4):307–316.

8. Kodaman PH, Current strategies for endometriosis management. *Obstet Gynecol Clin North Am* 2015 March;42 (1):87–101.

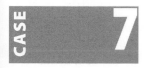

A 47-Year-Old Woman with Severe Menstrual Cramps and Painful Intercourse

Abimbola Famuyide

History of Present Illness

A 47-year-old G4P4 woman presented with a two-year history of worsening heavy menstrual bleeding (HMB) associated with use of double sanitary products during the heavy days of bleeding. A pictorial blood loss assessment chart showed a score of 380, indicating heavy menstrual blood loss. She also reported crampy pelvic pain that began one day before her menstrual flow and lasted two to three days. Intercourse was painful with deep penetration. She had been on combined oral contraceptive pills (OCPs) in the past, which improved her pain and HMB, but she stopped this because of persistent irregular vaginal bleeding. Her past medical history was significant for a seizure disorder, post-concussion syndrome, and depression. Her current medications included low-dose aspirin and an anti-seizure medication, Levetiracetam. She reported allergies to ondansetron and adhesive tape. She is married and her husband had a vasectomy for contraception. She has never smoked cigarettes.

Physical Examination

General appearance: Healthy, not in discomfort

Vital Signs

Pulse	88 beats/min
Blood pressure	125/79 mmHg
Height	150 cm
Weight	49.1 kg
Body mass index	21.82 kg/m^2
Abdomen	Soft, non-tender, no masses
Pelvis	Normal external genitalia, vagina, and cervix. Uterus uniformly bulky, approximately ten weeks' size, anteverted, and tender to palpation. No adnexal masses or tenderness.

Laboratory Studies

Urine pregnancy test	Negative
Hemoglobin	13.4 g/dl
Hematocrit	40.7%

Imaging

Transvaginal ultrasound – small intramural fibroids, largest measuring 1.3 × 1.4 × 1.2 cm. Myometrium diffusely heterogenic with striations arising from the endometrium and extending into posterior junctional zone. Tiny subendometrial cysts with endometrial thickness of 4 mm. Both ovaries visualized and normal (Figure 7.1).

How Would You Manage This Patient?

The patient's most likely diagnosis is adenomyosis, based upon the symptom triad of HMB, dysmenorrhea, and deep

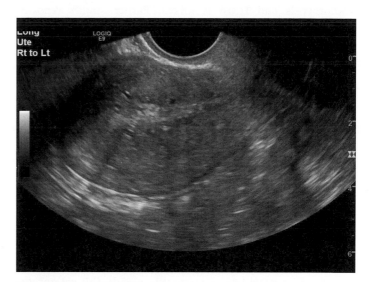

Figure 7.1 Sagittal 2D TVUS of uterus demonstrates heterogeneous myometrium with indistinct endometrial/myometrial border, with small cysts and small hyperechoic nodules in the inner myometrium, features typical of adenomyosis.

dyspareunia. On physical examination, the bulky tender uterus also supports the diagnosis. Finally, the finding of an ill-defined junctional zone and myometrial cysts on transvaginal imaging provides additional diagnostic support for the diagnosis of adenomyosis. The differential diagnosis also includes symptomatic fibroids although this is unlikely given the small size and intramural location of the fibroids. Endometriosis is also a consideration, but this is not typically associated with HMB. Because of her prior response to combined OCPs albeit with irregular bleeding, she was offered the etonogestrel/ethinyl estradiol vaginal ring and levonorgestrel intrauterine device (LNG-IUD). She preferred to try the vaginal ring, and she was counseled regarding her age-related risk of thromboembolic disorders. At the four-month reevaluation visit, she noted bloating and persistent lower quadrant pain with her menses. She was offered definitive surgical therapy for failed medical treatment and had an uneventful total laparoscopic hysterectomy. Pathology showed a uterus weighing 150 g with adenomyosis and small fibroids, the largest measuring 1.6 cm. Peritoneal biopsies did not show endometriosis.

Symptomatic Adenomyosis

Adenomyosis is a common benign condition defined by the presence of endometrial glands and stroma surrounded by hyperplastic and hypertrophied myometrial fibers in the myometrium. The condition typically afflicts multiparous women in the fourth and fifth decades of life. Estimating the prevalence of adenomyosis has been problematic in part because it is a histological diagnosis, but also as a result of its common association and shared symptomatology with leiomyomas.

The classic triad of HMB, dysmenorrhea, and dyspareunia is often diagnostic; however, leiomyoma and endometriosis can also present with similar features. Pain is a prominent symptom of adenomyosis, often presenting as painful menses with or without dyspareunia; however, evidence for the association of adenomyosis and HMB is mixed. Earlier studies reported a positive correlation, but recent studies failed to find any correlation. Most of the older studies were retrospective in design with inherent biases involved in attempts to correlate hysterectomy diagnosis with symptoms patients had before undergoing surgery. A more recent prospective study that involved ultrasound diagnosis of adenomyosis and assessment of menstrual blood loss showed a strong positive relationship between increasing severity of adenomyosis and menstrual blood loss [1]. The exact mechanism for increased menstrual blood loss in adenomyosis is unknown, but it may be related to the increased vascularization of the endometrium or from the increased bleeding surface of a globally bulky uterus. Adenomyosis is recognized in the recently adopted PALM-COEIN classification abnormal uterine bleeding (AUB) as abnormal uterine bleeding-adenomyosis (AUB-A) [2].

As in this case, leiomyoma often coexists with adenomyosis in up to 57 percent of hysterectomy cases. In this patient, the small size of the leiomyomas, their intramural location, and prominence of pain in the presentation made it less likely that these symptoms were due to leiomyoma. Some studies have suggested that women with adenomyosis have more pain and smaller uteri compared to leiomyoma alone [3]. If pain appears in excess of what is expected for a given burden of leiomyoma lesions, consideration should be given to the existence of adenomyosis. The mechanisms for pain may also be different for leiomyoma and adenomyoma. Leiomyoma often presents with painful episodes in the context of episodic degenerative changes, whereas adenomyoma lesions are more associated with chronic pain that may result from the increased prostaglandin production found in the ectopic tissue compared to normal myometrium.

Given its enigmatic nature, it is not surprising that there are a number of purported risk factors associated with adenomyosis. Many of these risk factors should be interpreted with caution because of retrospective study designs and selection bias. For example, increasing age has traditionally been described as a risk factor; however, older women are more likely to be offered hysterectomy, which increases the likelihood of confounding. In fact, some studies show that younger women, including adolescents, may also be at risk for adenomyosis. Similarly, multiparity is a reported risk factor. Like age, the association of multiparity with adenomyosis may be related to their higher likelihood of being offered and accepting hysterectomy. However, it is also possible that pregnancy may be a predisposing factor, possibly related to trophoblastic invasion of the myometrium aiding deposits of endometrium and formation and sustenance of glands and stroma in the myometrium. Prior uterine surgery, for example, dilation and curettage for pregnancy termination, has been proposed as a risk factor. In theory, surgical trauma may disrupt endometrial–myometrial interface, allowing for invasion of the myometrium by endometrial tissues. Others have also reported increased prevalence of adenomyosis in nonpregnant women who had dilatation and curettage and in those with prior cesarean delivery. However, an equal number of studies failed to find any association between adenomyosis and prior surgery; therefore, this association remains controversial. Tamoxifen therapy has also been associated with increased risk of adenomyosis in postmenopausal women with breast cancer. It is hypothesized that the agonist action of Tamoxifen on the endometrium may predispose postmenopausal women to adenomyosis. Other associated factors include smoking, ectopic pregnancy, and use of antidepressants.

The diagnosis of adenomyosis may be aided by imaging studies: two-dimensional transvaginal ultrasound (2D TVUS) or magnetic resonance imaging (MRI) of the pelvis. Ultrasound features of adenomyosis include a globally enlarged uterus with myometrial cysts, heterogenous myometrial echotexture, indistinct endometrial-myometrial border, and presence of diffuse vascularity in the myometrium. When compared with hysterectomy specimens, 2D TVUS showed sensitivity and specificity of 75 percent and 90 percent with an overall accuracy of 83 percent [4]. The most sensitive ultrasound finding of adenomyosis is a heterogenous myometrium; however, the most specific finding is the presence of myometrial cysts. Three-dimensional ultrasound (3D US) allows for visualization of the junctional zone – the uniformly hypoechoic area surrounding the endometrium – where the findings of thickening and disruption strongly correlate with the presence of adenomyosis. When reconstructed in the coronal plane, 3D US may have a better diagnostic accuracy than 2D TVUS. MR diagnostic criteria relate to the features of the junctional zone: increased thickening, increased ratio of the junctional zone compared to the myometrium, and the finding of a difference of >5mm between the maximum and minimum thickness of the junctional zone. Although MRI has a high specificity and accuracy, 2D TVUS has comparable diagnostic performance and is superior in cost, affordability, and access. The American College of Obstetricians and Gynecologists recommends ultrasonography as the initial screening test for AUB and MRI as a second step if initial results are inconclusive or when leiomyomas are suspected [5].

There are a variety of medical options for treating adenomyosis. Nonsteroidal anti-inflammatory agents inhibit prostaglandin production and may be effective in treating dysmenorrhea and HMB; however, gastrointestinal intolerance can be problematic. Combined OCPs suppress ovarian steroidogenesis and cause endometrial decidualization and atrophy in the ectopic endometrial tissue, thus reducing menstrual blood flow and pain. However, OCP use in older patients, especially in smokers, elevates the risk of thromboembolic disorders. Other effective therapies include Danazol or gonadotropin-releasing hormone (GnRH) agonist/analog, which acts by reducing pituitary gonadotropins, causing atrophy of the endometrium and the adenomyotic tissue. Danazol is associated with significant side effects including acne, hirsutism, deepened voice, breast atrophy, and decreased high-density lipoprotein. GnRH use may cause hot flashes, and use greater than six months may result in vaginal atrophy and bone density loss. Aromatase inhibitors have been cited in a few case reports to be effective by inhibiting the upregulated conversion of androgens to estrogen in ectopic endometrial tissues. Further validating studies are needed.

The levonorgestrel intrauterine system (LNG-IUS) is an effective treatment choice for adenomyosis that is associated with high patient satisfaction rates and improvement in quality-of-life indices. The LNG-IUS downregulates estrogen receptors in the ectopic endometrium, leading to a reduction in size of adenoymosis, decidualizes the endometrium, and reduces prostaglandin production in the endometrium. Side effects may include irregular vaginal bleeding, simple ovarian cysts, risks of expulsion (greater with uterine cavity sound >10 cm), and perforation. The LNG-IUS is a particularly attractive treatment option for younger women who wish to retain their fertility.

Hysterectomy remains a tried and tested solution for older women who have failed initial medical alternatives and do not desire for future fertility. Minimally invasive approaches including vaginal and laparoscopic hysterectomy are favored over laparotomy for costs, morbidity, and length of hospital stay. Since adenomyosis is confined to the uterus, ovarian conservation can be employed, as was the case with this patient.

Risks of surgical morbidity aside, newer evidence suggesting hysterectomy with ovarian conservation diminishes ovarian reserve with long-term cardiovascular risks increasingly places emphasis on non-hysterectomy therapeutic options for women with benign gynecological disorders [6, 7].

For older women who wish to retain their uterus but do not desire future childbearing, uterine artery embolization (UAE) is an effective option. A number of case series reported symptom improvement in up to 78 percent in the short and medium term (up to three years) with no major safety concerns. However, nearly a quarter of patients ultimately required hysterectomy, and patients should also be informed of the risks of premature ovarian failure and transient increase in vaginal discharge. Similarly, there are a few reports of early successes with MRI-guided high-intensity-focused ultrasound treatment for adenomyosis. Further validation studies are needed [8].

Non-hysterectomy surgical treatment options include endometrial resection or ablation. However, results are inconsistent. Adenomyosis may, in fact, be a significant risk factor for failure of the global endometrial ablation procedure [9]. More aggressive myometrial or adenomyoma resection procedures aimed at removing diseased myometrial tissue by wedge resections and metroplasty can be performed in the context of infertility. Improved pregnancy rates have been reported following these procedures.

Key Teaching Points

- The classic diagnostic triad for adenomyosis is HMB, dysmenorrhea, and deep dyspareunia.
- 2D TVUS can provide reliably accurate diagnostic support for the diagnosis of adenomyosis.
- Nonsurgical treatment options include NSAIDs, combined oral contraceptives, Danazol, GnRH agonists, and the LNG-IUS.
- Hysterectomy should be offered only as a last resort since there are effective non-hysterectomy treatment options.
- UAE is an effective option for older women who wish to retain their uterus but do not desire future childbearing.

References

1. Naftalin J, Hoo W, Pateman D et al. Is adenomyosis associated with menorrhagia? *Hum Reprod* 2014;29 (3):473–479.

2. Munro MG, Critchley HO, Broder MS, Fraser IS. FIGO classification PALM COEIN for causes of abnormal uterine bleeding in non gravid women of reproductive age group. *Int Gynecol Obstet* 2011;111:3–13.

3. Taran FA, Stewart EA, Brucker S. Adenomyosis: epidemiology, risk factors, clinical phenotype and surgical and interventional alternatives to hysterectomy. *Geburtshilfe Frauenheilkd* 2013;73(9):924–931.

4. Exacoustos C, Manganaro L, Zupi E. Imaging for the evaluation of endometriosis and adenomyosis. *Best Pract Res Clin Obstet Gynaecol* 2014;28:655–681.

5. American College of Obstetricians and Gynecologist Practice Bulletin 128, July 2012 (reaffirmed 2016). Diagnosis of abnormal uterine bleeding in reproductive aged women.

6. Trabuco E, Moorman P, Algeciras-Schimnick A et al. Association of ovary-sparing hysterectomy with ovarian reserve. *Obstet Gynecol* 2016;127 (5);819–827.

7. Laughlin-Tommaso S, Khan Z, Weaver A et al. Cardiovascular risk factors and diseases in women undergoing hysterectomy with ovarian conservation. *Menopause* 2016;23 (2):121–128.

8. Struble J, Reid S, Bedaiwy M. Adenomyosis: a clinical review of a challenging gynecologic condition. *JMIG* 2015;23: 164–185.

9. El-Nashar S, Hopkins MR, Creedon DJ et al. Prediction of treatment outcomes after global endometrial ablation. *Obstet Gynecol* 2009;113 (1):97–106.

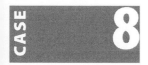

A 28-Year-Old Woman with Metronidazole Allergy and Trichomonas Infection

Anita Tamirisa

History of Present Illness

A 28-year-old, gravida 0, presents due to worsening of dysuria, dyspareunia, and purulent vaginal discharge that started three weeks ago after being sexually active with a new male partner. She initially thought the vaginal irritation and discharge were due to yeast infection. However, after using an over-the-counter medication to treat the yeast infection, the symptoms worsened. She denies other medical conditions. She is currently using oral contraception for birth control, and she did not use condoms when they had intercourse. She denies any past surgical history. Her family history is notable for hypertension on her mother's side. She drinks alcohol occasionally and denies tobacco or illicit drug use. She reports that she developed a diffuse rash and itching immediately after taking oral metronidazole last year.

Physical Examination

General appearance	Well-developed, well-nourished woman, mildly anxious, but otherwise in no acute distress, alert and oriented
Vital Signs	
Temperature	98.6°F (37°C)
Pulse	70 beats/min
Blood pressure	110/80 mmHg
Respirations	18 breaths/min
Abdomen	Thin, soft, non-tender, non-distended, no guarding, no rebound, mild supra-pubic tenderness
External genitalia	Unremarkable
Vagina	Mucosa mildly erythematous, moderate amount of thin green-yellow, frothy discharge
Cervix	Punctate hemorrhages
Uterus	Anteverted, small, mobile, normal size, non-tender on bimanual examination
Adnexa	No masses, non-tender

Laboratory Studies

Urine pregnancy test	Negative
Urinalysis	Negative
Wet mount	Numerous trichomonads, no candida or clue cells
GC/CT	Negative
HIV	Negative

How Would You Manage This Patient?

This patient presents with classic symptoms of trichomonas infection, which include green-yellow frothy discharge, dyspareunia, pruritus, and dysuria. This was most likely transmitted from her new male partner. It is important after diagnosis of a trichomonas infection for patients to be screened for other sexually transmitted infections, since these frequently coexist. Her tests for gonorrhea, chlamydia, and HIV were all negative.

The Centers for Disease Control and Prevention recommendations for treatment of trichomonas infection are for metronidazole 2 g orally or tinidazole 2 g orally in a single dose [1]. Nitromidazoles are the only family of anti-protazoal medications that have been shown to be effective in treating trichomonas. Because of this patient's history of metronidazole allergy, she was referred to a specialist (an allergist/immunologist) for metronidazole desensitization. The patient was counseled on the use of barrier protection, on the need for her partner to be treated, and to abstain from intercourse until both are treated and symptoms resolved. She was instructed to return in three months to be rescreened due to the high rate of reinfection among women treated for trichomoniasis.

Trichmonas Infection with Metronidazole Allergy

Trichomonas vaginalis (*T. vaginalis*), along with bacterial vaginosis and vulvovaginal candidiasis, is one of the three most common causes of vaginitis among reproductively aged women and the most common nonviral sexually transmitted infection in the United States. While not a reportable sexually transmitted infection, the annual incidence is estimated to be 7.4 million cases in the United States, with an overall prevalence of 3.1 percent [1]. There are significant differences in prevalence between non-Hispanic black women (13.5 percent) compared to non-Hispanic white women (1.2 percent) [2, 3].

T. vaginalis is a flagellated protozoan most commonly transmitted from men to women through penile-vaginal intercourse. Women can acquire the infection from other women, and it is only rarely transmitted between men. Trichomonas favors the squamous epithelium of the female lower genitourinary tract, affecting mainly the vagina, urethra, and paraurethral glands. Less common sites include the cervix, bladder, and Bartholin glands. Humans are the only natural host [4, 5].

Women are most commonly asymptomatic (50 percent) and may remain so for as long as three months. The most common symptom is a purulent, malodorous discharge, which may be associated with pruritus, irritation, dysuria, lower abdominal pain, increased frequency of urination, dyspareunia, or postcoital bleeding. Green, frothy, malodorous discharge is seen on examination in approximately 30 percent of symptomatic women. A minority of patients will have punctate hemorrhages on the vagina and cervix, known as "strawberry cervix." Pain with bimanual examination may or may not be present. Complications of the infection are rare, and may include urethritis, cystitis, cervical neoplasia, posthysterectomy cuff cellulitis or abscess, pelvic inflammatory disease, HIV infection, and infertility. Pregnancy-related complications may also occur [1, 2].

Saline microscopy may be used to diagnose infection via direct visualization of motile trichomonads, and is commonly used due to ease and low cost. However, microscopy has a sensitivity of only 55–60 percent [1]. To diagnose the infection with microscopy, a sample of vaginal discharge is mixed with one to two drops of 0.9 percent normal saline solution at room temperature on a glass slide. A cover slip is placed over the mixture and examined under low and high power. Trichomonads may remain motile for 10–20 minutes outside of their natural human host. Vaginal pH is nondiagnostic, but typically elevated >4.5. One may also see an increased number of neutrophils.

Nucleic acid amplification tests (NAATs) have become the gold standard for diagnosing trichomonas infection due to high sensitivity and specificity. NAATs detect RNA by transcription-mediated amplification. Multiple assays are available. The Aptima *T. vaginalis* assay uses vaginal swab or urine specimens and has a sensitivity and specificity as high as 95–100 percent. If available, the "inPouch" *T. vaginalis* culture system has high sensitivity and takes <3 days to report. Rapid antigen and DNA hybridization probes have been found to have high sensitivity and specificity; results are obtained the same day, and have been approved by the Food and Drug Administration (FDA) for women [1, 5, 6]. The OSOM trichomonas rapid test is an antigen-detecting test that gives results in 10 minutes. The Affirm VP III is a DNA hybridization probe test that also evaluates for bacterial vaginitis and *candida albicans*. These methods are particularly useful in areas of high prevalence [5]. Culture was once considered gold standard for the diagnosis of *T. vaginalis*, but turnaround time for results may take up to one week to obtain. *T. vaginalis* cultures still have a role in situations where there are concerns for infection, but trichomonads are not seen on microscopy and NAAT is unavailable [1, 5].

Incidental findings of trichomonads may be reported on cervical cancer screening reports. Liquid-based cytology has a high specificity with a low false positive rate (and a low sensitivity), making it reasonable to offer as treatment to patients. In contrast, conventional Papanicalaou smears have higher false positive rates compared to liquid-based cervical cytology and therefore treatment should be withheld on asymptomatic women until evaluation is completed by wet mount, NAAT, culture, or rapid test [6]. Asymptomatic screening for *T. vaginalis* should be performed in all HIV-positive women annually and at their initial prenatal visits, and may be considered in individuals at high risk for infection (new or multiple partners, history of STI, illicit drug use, sex workers) [1]. Treatment of *T. vaginalis* infections reduces symptoms, transmission, and adverse outcomes in HIV-positive women.

Nitroimidazoles, which include metronidazole and tinidazole, are the only class of medications known to effectively treat *T. vaginalis* infections, are FDA approved for oral and parenteral treatment, and should be utilized in both asymptomatic and symptomatic women. To reduce the incidence of a disulfiram-like reaction, patients should be instructed to avoid alcohol (for 24 hours after completing metronidazole and 72 hours after tinidazole). Typically, a 2 g single oral dose of metronidazole or tinidazole is recommended due to ease of use, better compliance, and shorter period of alcohol avoidance. Alternatively, metronidazole 500 mg orally twice daily for seven days may be prescribed if the higher dose is not tolerated or if compliance is not a concern. Cure rates are comparable; however, tinidazole is associated with decreased gastrointestinal side effects but at higher cost. Metronidazole gel is not recommended because it does not reach therapeutic drug levels in anatomic locations that can act as reservoirs, such as the Bartholin and Skene's glands, urethra, and periurethral glands. Both partners should be instructed to abstain from intercourse until seven days after antibiotic completion. Patients should also be screened for other STIs, including gonorrhea, chlamydia, and HIV. Because of high rates of reinfection, retesting within three months following initial treatment is recommended. Testing with NAAT can be conducted as soon as two weeks after treatment [1, 5].

Metronidazole Allergy

Adverse IgE-mediated allergic reactions to metronidazole are rare, but can include flushing, urticaria, fever, angioedema, and anaphylactic shock [7]. Due to their similar molecular structures, and thus high likelihood of hypersensivity reaction, tinidazole is not a recommended alternative to metronidazole. This overlap has been noted in case reports; however, data are still lacking. Alternative intravaginal treatments, such as betadine douche, paromomycin, clotrimazole, furazolidone, and acetersol, are not effective or are associated with adverse reactions, and so are not recommended. While intravaginal paromomycin was noted to successfully treat 25 percent of women, it was associated with ulceration of the vaginal mucosa [6]. Clotrimazole was found to only be 11 percent successful in eradicating infection, according to a recent multicenter trial [6]. Given this, nitromidazoles are the best options for treatment [7–9].

Patients with an IgE-mediated-type allergy to nitromidazoles should have metronidazole desensitization according to published regimens and in consultation with an allergy specialist [1]. Oral and intravenous dosing protocols have been used with 100 percent effectiveness [7]. Desensitization is the process of reintroducing a medication to which an individual has had an allergic response in order to allow for temporary tolerance. Once the medication is discontinued, the hypersensitivity to the medication returns. An allergist/immunologist should conduct the process, which may occur in either an inpatient or outpatient setting. After confirmation of the allergic reaction with skin testing, the total dose of medication is divided into very small dilutions. The medication is then delivered over a period of time, typically 15 minutes. The dose is doubled with each step until a full therapeutic dose has been delivered. By administering the medication in this manner, the immune system is inhibited.

If a reaction is observed, the medication is held and symptoms are treated, and then the protocol is reinitiated. While no standard protocol has been developed for the class of nitromidazoles, both oral and IV metronidazole desensitization regimens have been used with 100 percent success in the management of trichomonas infections [7]. Desensitization is not a permanent cure for the drug allergy and the nitromidazoles should be avoided after treatment is completed and must be performed again if the drug is required for treatment in the future.

Key Points

- Adverse IgE-mediated allergic reactions to metronidazole are rare, but can include flushing, urticaria, fever, angioedema, and anaphylactic shock.

- Due to their similar molecular structures, and thus high likelihood of hypersensivity reaction, tinidazole is not a recommended alternative to metronidazole.

- There are currently no safe and effective alternatives to metronidazole and tinidazole, and therefore desensitization according to published regimens and in consultation with an allergy specialist is recommended.

- Desensitization is the process of reintroducing a medication to which an individual has had an allergic response in order to allow for temporary tolerance. Once the medication is discontinued, the hypersensitivity to the medication returns.

- Both oral and IV metronidazole desensitization regimens have been used with 100 percent success in the management of trichomonas infections.

References

1. Centers for Disease Control and Prevention. 2015 Sexually Transmitted Diseases Treatment Guidelines. Trichomonas. Available at: www.cdc.gov/std/tg2015/trichomoniasis.htm [accessed 8/10/17].

2. Vaginitis. ACOG Practice Bulletin Number 72. American College of Obstetricians and Gynecologists. *Obstet Gynecol* 2006; 107: 1195–1206.

3. Sutton M, Sternberg M, Koumans EH et al. The prevalence of *Trichomonas vaginalis* infection among reproductive-age women in the United States, 2001–2004. *Clin Infect Dis* 2007;45(10): 1319–26.

4. Kissinger P. Epidemiology and treatment of trichomonas. *Curr Infect Dis Rep* 2015;17:484.

5. Centers for Disease Control and Prevention. Sexually transmitted diseases treatment guidelines, 2015. *MMWR Morb Mortal Wkl Rep* 2015;64:1.

6. Lara-Torre E, Pinkerton JS. Accuracy of detection of *Trichomonas vaginalis* organisms on a liquid-based papanicolaou smear. *Am J Obstet Gynecol* 2003;188:354.

7. Helms DJ, Mosure DJ, Secor E, Workowski KA. Management of *Trichomonas vaginalis* in women with suspected metronidazole hypersensitivity. *Am J Obstet Gynecol* 2008; 370: e1–e7.

8. Nyirjesy P, Sobel JD, Weitz MV, Leamn DJ, Gelone SP. Difficult to treat trichomoniasis: results with paromycin cream. *Clin Infect Dis* 1998;26: 986–8.

9. duBouchet L, Spence MR, Rein MF, Danzig MR, McCormack WM. Multicenter comparison of clotrimazole vaginal tablets containing sulfanilamide, aminacrine hydrochloride, and allantoin in the treatment of symptomatic trichomoniasis. *Sex Transm Dis* 1997;24: 156–60.

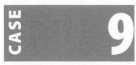

A 24-Year-Old Woman with Mucopurulent Cervicitis

Jaime J. Alleyn

History of Present Illness

A 24-year-old nulliparous female presents to the office complaining of vaginal discharge for the past week. She also reports vaginal spotting after intercourse. Her last menstrual period was one week ago. The patient denies abdominal pain, fever, or chills. Her past medical and surgical history is negative. The patient is heterosexual and is not in a committed relationship. She denies any prior history of sexually transmitted infections. She reports having had three sexual partners within the last year and sporadic condom use. Her most recent intercourse was two weeks ago and was with a new partner. Her family history is noncontributory. The patient has no known drug allergies and does not take any regular medications.

Physical Examination

General appearance   Well-developed, well-nourished woman in no apparent distress. She is alert and oriented.

Vital Signs

Temperature	37.0°C
Pulse	80 beats/min
Blood pressure	110/72 mmHg
Respiratory rate	16 breaths/min
Height	65 inches
Weight	120 lb
Abdomen	Thin, soft, non-tender, non-distended, no guarding, no rebound
External genitalia	Unremarkable
Vagina	No abnormalities
Cervix	Mucopurulent discharge at the external os, cervix bleeds easily when touched with a cotton swab, no cervical motion tenderness
Uterus	Anteverted, mobile, non-tender
Adnexa	No masses or tenderness

Laboratory Studies

Urine pregnancy test	Negative
Wet prep	Many leukocytes, no clue cells or trichomonads

How Would You Manage This Patient?

Based on the patient's clinical presentation with mucopurulent cervical discharge and endocervical bleeding (friability) with gentle touch, this patient has acute cervicitis. There is no foreign body in the vagina, and the non-tender uterus and adnexae exclude pelvic inflammatory disease. To distinguish infectious from noninfectious acute cervicitis, the evaluation includes a swab of the discharge for microscopy (wet prep) and vaginal pH to identify bacterial vaginosis and trichomonas, and nucleic acid amplification test (NAAT) for chlamydia, gonorrhea, and trichomonas (if the wet prep is negative for trichomonas).

The patient was managed empirically with antibiotic therapy at the time of initial evaluation, without waiting for results of laboratory tests. In a 24-year-old, the empiric treatment regimen for cervicitis should include coverage of chlamydia at a minimum, as the prevalence in women ≤25 years old is high. This patient also has other risk factors, including more than one sexual partner and inconsistent use of condoms. Therefore, she was also treated empirically for gonorrhea, with ceftriaxone 250 mg IM in a single dose plus azithromycin 1 g orally in a single dose in the office the day she was evaluated. The patient was also offered testing for HIV and syphilis. In addition, the patient should receive counseling about prevention of STIs, including a description of high-risk behaviors and education about prevention methods. All partners for the past 60 days should be referred for evaluation and treatment. The patient should be given follow-up to ensure that the cervicitis has resolved.

Cervicitis

Acute cervicitis is an inflammation of the columnar epithelial cells of the endocervical glands and can also affect the squamous epithelium of the ectocervix. It may be due to an infectious or noninfectious etiology. Chlamydia and gonorrhea are the most common organisms identified, with chlamydia cervicitis the most common. It is important to note that a large proportion of women with chlamydia and gonorrhea are asymptomatic and do not develop mucopurulent cervicitis [1]. Cervicitis can also be caused by *Trichomonas vaginalis*, bacterial vaginosis, or genital herpes (particularly primary herpes simplex virus-2 infection). Noninfectious cervicitis may be caused by retained foreign bodies (condoms, tampons) or chemical irritation from latex, vaginal douches, or contraceptive creams. Risk factors for cervicitis include women ≤ 25 years of age, history of sexually transmitted infections, new or multiple sexual partners, lack of barrier protection, drug use, and commercial sex work.

Patients often present with vaginal discharge, postcoital spotting, or intermenstrual bleeding. Some patients are asymptomatic. Cervicitis is diagnosed on physical examination by the presence of a mucopurulent discharge visualized at the external os or endocervical bleeding that is present with gentle manipulation of the os. It is important to determine if the patient has associated upper genital tract symptoms such as pelvic pain, cervical motion tenderness, abdominal pain, or fever that would suggest pelvic inflammatory disease. This will guide treatment options.

Testing for infectious causes of cervicitis includes a swab of the discharge for microscopy and vaginal pH to test for bacterial vaginosis and trichomonas, as well as NAAT testing for chlamydia and gonorrhea. Because sensitivity of microscopy to detect trichomonas is only approximately 50 percent, women with cervicitis and negative wet preps should also be tested for trichomonas by NAAT, which has a sensitivity of at least 95 percent and can be performed on the same swab used for chlamydia and gonorrhea testing [2].

Most women with mucopurulent cervicitis should be treated empirically at the time of initial evaluation with antibiotics even before the results of diagnostic tests are available. For some low-risk patients, treatment can be deferred until the results are available. The Centers for Disease Control and Prevention (CDC) guidelines for treating cervicitis recommend antibiotic coverage for chlamydia at a minimum [2]. For women at higher risk, treatment should also add coverage for gonorrhea. There is no strict definition of which patients are defined as high risk, and clinicians should consider risk factors such as age ≤25 years old (the prevalence is highest in this age group), local prevalence of gonorrhea, previous chlamydial or gonorrhea infection in the prior months, new or more than one sexual partner, and inconsistent use of condoms in making this decision. If reliable patient follow-up of test results is a concern, it is also reasonable to treat empirically for both chlamydia and gonorrhea. Empiric therapy for acute cervicitis includes azithromycin 1 g orally in a single dose or doxycycline 100 mg orally twice a day for seven days [2].

Neisseria gonorrhoeae is a gram-negative coccobacillus that invades the columnar cells of the endocervix. There are an estimated 820,000 new infections each year in the United States and it is the second most common reported communicable disease [2]. Gonococcal infections are frequently asymptomatic in women. Annual screening is recommended in women ≤ 25 years old and in older women who are at risk for infection. NAATs have replaced cultures in most laboratories to diagnose gonococcal infections. Samples can be obtained from the vagina, the endocervix, or urine. In 2007, there was an emergence of fluoroquinolone-resistant *N. gonorrhoeae*. This prompted the CDC to change its recommendation of fluoroquinolones for the treatment of gonorrhea. In order to prevent the development of resistance to cephalosporins, the CDC recommends dual therapy first-line treatment of gonorrhea with ceftriaxone (250 mg, single IM dose) and azithromycin (1 g, single oral dose), regardless of the results of chlamydia testing. These treatments should be administered together on the same day. If ceftriaxone is not available, an alternative is cefixime 400 mg orally in a single dose plus azithromycin 1 g orally in a single dose, but this should be second line due to concerns about decreased susceptibility of the organism for orally delivered antibiotics [2].

Chlamydial infection is the most frequently reported infectious disease in the United States, and its prevalence is highest in persons ≤ 24 years [2]. Chlamydia trachomatis is an obligate intracellular parasite that can cause columnar epithelial infection. As with gonorrhea, infection is usually asymptomatic and screening is recommended annually for women ≤ 25 years old and for older women who are at risk for infection (new partner, more than one partner, a partner with concurrent partners, or partner with sexually transmitted infection). Diagnosis is made using NAAT on vaginal, endocervical, or urine specimens.

First-line treatment for chlamydial infection is azithromycin 1 g orally in a single dose or doxycycline 100 mg orally twice a day for seven days. There appears to be comparable efficacy between these regimens. Alternatives for patients with allergies or adverse reactions to these drugs include erythromycin base 500 mg orally four times a day for seven days, levofloxacin 500 mg orally once daily for seven days, and ofloxacin 300 mg orally twice daily for seven days [2]. Posttreatment infections are generally not from therapeutic failure, but are from reinfection caused by partners not receiving treatment or sexual activity with a new infected partner. Therefore, test-of-cure to detect therapeutic failure is not indicated, and retesting less than three weeks after treatment with NAAT may result in false positives because the continued presence of nonviable organisms. Women who have been treated for chlamydia should follow up three months after treatment to be tested for reinfection [2].

Trichomoniasis is one of the most common sexually transmitted infections in the United States, affecting an estimated 3.7 million persons [2]. *Trichomonas vaginalis* is a single-cell, anaerobic, flagellated protozoan. Infection is characterized by a discharge that is often foul-smelling, thin, and yellow or green. Inflammation of the cervix, resulting in subepithelial hemorrhages (strawberry cervix), is commonly noted. Diagnosis is made by microscopic identification of the mobile parasites. Treatment consists of metronidazole in a 2 g, single oral dose, or tinidazole in a 2 g, single oral dose. For patients who cannot tolerate 2 g at once, an alternative is metronidazole 500 mg orally twice daily for seven days. Options are limited for patients with allergy to metronidazole and tinidazole, and referral for desensitization is recommended [2].

Bacterial vaginosis is a clinical syndrome resulting from changes in the vaginal flora, including an overabundance of anaerobic bacteria along with a decrease of the normal lactobacillus species. Risk factors include oral sex, douching, black race, cigarette smoking, sex during menses, intrauterine device, early age of sexual intercourse, new or multiple sexual partners, and sexual activity with other women [3]. The most common symptom is a nonirritating, malodorous discharge. Clinical diagnosis can be made using Amsel's criteria, which requires three of the following signs or symptoms to be present:

(1) homogenous, white discharge
(2) clue cells on microscopic evaluation
(3) vaginal pH >4.5
(4) fishy odor after addition of 10 percent KOH (whiff test) [2]

Alternatively, the diagnosis can be made with a gram stain.

First-line treatment regimens for bacterial vaginosis include metronidazole 500 mg, orally twice a day for seven days, or gel 0.75 percent, 5 g, intravaginally, once a day for five days; or clindamycin intravaginal cream 2 percent, 5 g, intravaginally at bedtime for seven days. Patients taking metronidazole should be instructed to avoid alcohol during treatment and for 24 hours after completion of treatment with metronidazole to avoid a disulfiam-like reaction [2]. The data on the performance of alternative regimens are limited, but options include tinidazole 2 g orally once daily for two days or 1 g orally once daily for five days, or clindamycin 300 mg orally twice daily for seven days or 100 mg ovules intravaginally once at bedtime for three days. Patients should be warned that clindamycin ovules use an oleaginous base that can weaken condoms and diaphragms, so these should not be used within 72 hours following treatment with clindamycin ovules.

Sexual partners of women with chlamydia, gonorrhea, or trichomoniasis should be treated for the infection for which the woman received treatment. Patients and their sex partners should be advised to abstain from sexual intercourse until seven days after a single-dose regimen or after completion of a seven-day regimen. All patients should be offered counseling and testing for HIV and syphilis. Repeat testing three to six months after a diagnosis of either chlamydia or gonorrhea is recommended, due to high rates of recurrent infection [2].

Key Teaching Points

- Cervicitis is defined as presence of a mucopurulent discharge from the endocervical os or the presence of endocervical bleeding/friability.
- The two most common infectious etiologies of mucopurulent cervical discharge are chlamydia and gonorrhea.
- Cervicitis should be treated empirically, before results of chlamydia and gonorrhea are available. At a minimum, antibiotic treatment should be for chlamydia with azithromycin 1 gram × 1. For higher-risk patients, treatment includes azithromycin 1 g PO × 1 dose or doxycycline 100 mg PO BID × seven days.
- Women should follow up in three months to be tested for reinfection.

References

1. Marrazzo JM, Handsfield HH, Whittington WL. Predicting chlamydial and gonococcal cervical infection: implications for management of cervicitis. *Obstet Gynecol* 2002;100 (3):579.

2. Workowski KA, Bolan GA. Centers for Disease Control and Prevention. Sexually Transmitted Diseases Treatment Guidelines, 2015. *MMWR Recomm Rep* 2015;64(RR-03):1–137.

3. Hoffman BL. *Williams Gynecology* (3rd edn). New York, NY: The McGraw-Hill Companies, 2016.

4. Dual Therapy for Gonococcal Infections. Committee Opinion No. 645. American College of Obstetricians and Gynecologists. *Obstet Gynecol* 2015;126: e95–e99.

5. Centers for Disease Control and Prevention. 2015 Sexually Transmitted Treatment Guidelines. Chlamydial Infections in Adolescents and Adults. 2015. Available at https://www.cdc.gov/ std/tg2015/chlamydia.htm.

6. United States Preventative Services Task Force. Final Recommendation Statement – Chlamydia and Gonorrhea: Screening. 2014.

A 27-Year-Old Woman with Trichomonas Requesting a Prescription for Her Partner

Rita Tsai

History of Present Illness

A 27-year-old, gravida 0, woman presents to the office complaining of vaginal discharge. She has been sexually active since age 18, and she has been with her current partner for about three months. She reports she was seen at an urgent care center about one month ago with a similar complaint and diagnosed with trichomonas and treated with a single dose of 2 g oral metronidazole. The patient is uncertain if her partner was ever tested or treated, although she did tell him that she had an infection. She reports that she has had unprotected intercourse with her partner since being treated.

Physical Examination

General appearance	Well-developed, well-nourished, alert and oriented
Vital Signs	
Temperature	37.0°C
Pulse	76 beats/min
Blood pressure	114/70 mmHg
Height	65 inches
Weight	130 lb
BMI	21.6 kg/m2
Abdomen	Thin, soft, non-tender, non-distended, no guarding, no rebound
External genitalia	Unremarkable
Vagina	Erythema of mucosa with green, frothy, malodorous discharge noted in vault
Cervix	Nulliparous, has punctate hemorrhages with a "strawberry cervix" appearance, no cervical motion tenderness
Uterus	Anteverted, mobile, normal size, non-tender
Adnexa	No masses, non-tender bilaterally
Laboratory	Wet mount with motile trichomonads, increase in white blood cells noted on saline microscopy; pH 5

How Would You Manage This Patient?

The patient is diagnosed with trichomonas vaginitis, most likely from reinfection, since her partner was not treated. The patient is counseled regarding her diagnosis and the risk of other sexually transmitted infections (STIs). Safe sex practices for prevention of STIs are reviewed with the patient. She is screened for gonorrhea, chlamydia, HIV, and syphilis at the time of her evaluation. She is treated with single-dose therapy with 2 g oral metronidazole. She is instructed to notify her sexual partners for the past two months to seek evaluation and treatment and to avoid intercourse for one week after both she and her partner have completed therapy.

The patient asks if she can be given a prescription today for her partner to be treated. Given this patient's history of prior treatment, the patient was likely reinfected by an untreated sexual partner. The patient is questioned regarding barriers to her partner obtaining evaluation and treatment. She did not indicate any limitations to this access. In the absence of any barriers, EPT (expedited partner therapy) is not performed, and the patient is given the information for the city STI clinic for her partner.

Expedited Partner Therapy

To ensure adequate treatment, patients with STIs need to avoid reinfection by untreated sexual partners. Ideally, partner treatment should occur through clinical evaluation in a health-care setting. In the United States, partner notification and referral to treatment are most commonly performed by the patient. However, this method has been unsuccessful in ensuring treatment of sexual partners. In order to improve prevention and control the spread of STIs, particularly given the problems untreated STIs can cause young women with future fertility and chronic pain, partner management with EPT has been recommended [1–5]. EPT is the practice of treating the sexual partners of patients diagnosed with STIs without medical evaluation or counseling. Typically, EPT is performed through patient-delivered partner therapy, in which medication is provided by clinicians through direct dosing or prescription to the patient that includes treatment of both the patient and her partner.

Currently, only EPT for treating gonorrhea and chlamydia have data supporting its use [1]. The Centers for Disease Control and Prevention (CDC) sponsored four randomized controlled trials between 2000 and 2004 to compare EPT with standard partner management approaches and also assess behavioral predictors of treatment and reinfection. These trials demonstrated an approximately 20 percent reduction in recurrent infections among patients with chlamydia infections and a 60 percent or better reduction rate among patients with gonorrhea infections. The studies also noted increased notification and treatment of sexual partners and decreased rates of unprotected intercourse with EPT. In conjunction with the findings of two expert consultations convened in 2004 and 2005, the CDC issued a report in February 2006 supporting the use of EPT as an option for the management of heterosexual sex partners with gonorrhea or chlamydia infection.

The 2006 CDC recommendations state that EPT is at least equivalent to, if not better than, standard patient partner management in preventing recurrent or persistent gonorrhea or chlamydial infection. The CDC concluded that EPT can be used to treat the male sex partners of females infected with gonorrhea and chlamydia when other management strategies are not practical or successful. EPT can also be used to treat the female partners of male patients infected with gonorrhea and chlamydia when other management strategies are similarly deemed impractical or unsuccessful, with the understanding that female recipients of EPT are strongly encouraged to seek medical attention – particularly in cases of patients exhibiting symptoms of acute pelvic inflammatory disease, such as abdominal or pelvic pain.

In 2012, due to concern over increasing resistance of gonorrhea to oral cefixime and possible treatment failures, the CDC updated its gonorrhea treatment recommendations [2, 3]. The current CDC-recommended treatment for uncomplicated gonorrhea infections is combination therapy with a single intramuscular dose of ceftriaxone 250 mg plus a single dose of azithromycin 1 g orally. Given that the treatment regimen involves an injection, the potential use of EPT is limited in the treatment of gonorrhea. The current recommendation is for the patient's sexual partners to be evaluated and treated with ceftriaxone and azithromycin; however, the CDC still approves the use of EPT in cases where the provider is concerned for timely evaluation and treatment of the partner. In such cases, oral cefixime and azithromycin can still be considered.

Historically, EPT is believed to have been widely employed in the treatment of the partners of women with trichomonas. Currently, there is not sufficient evidence to support the use of EPT for the treatment of trichomoniasis [1]. EPT is not routinely recommended for treatment of female patients with trichomoniasis due to the high risk of STI comorbidity in sex partners. Undiagnosed gonorrhea and chlamydia infection are common in the partners of women with trichomoniasis. The CDC advises the use of EPT for trichomonal infection with caution only in selective cases where other strategies again are impractical or unsuccessful.

The CDC 2006 statement also notes that EPT is not suggested for use in the treatment of patients with syphilis [1]. Treatment of syphilis frequently requires injection, as penicillin is the current recommended therapy. Concern for penicillin allergy and anaphylaxis limits its use for EPT when compared to cephalosporins and macrolides used to treat gonorrhea or chlamydia. Typically, partner notification services are also available at state and local health departments for syphilis infections through mandatory notification requirements.

Studies evaluating EPT use are largely limited to heterosexual adults, although EPT can be used for other populations. The CDC advises that EPT should not be used in gonorrhea and chlamydial infection in men who have sex with men due to the high risk of comorbidity, particularly undiagnosed HIV, in partners. There is no specific statement regarding the use of EPT in homosexual women. No data exist to demonstrate the efficacy or role of EPT among women who have sex with women. However, the American College of Obstetricians and Gynecologists (ACOG) states that EPT may be an appropriate management option for same-sex partners of female patients [4].

The ACOG has endorsed the use of EPT for a patient's partners who are unable or unwilling to seek medical care as a method of preventing gonorrhea and chlamydial reinfection [4]. EPT has also been supported by other medical professional organizations, including the Society for Adolescent Medicine and the American Academy of Family Physicians [5]. Guidelines have been published for the practice of EPT by the CDC, as well as several state health departments [1–3].

Use of EPT includes education of the patient for her partner. This education should include the indication for the partner treatment, instructions for administration, and warnings regarding adverse reactions. It should also include STI counseling with the recommendation for referral to a local testing center for a full STI evaluation. Furthermore, instructions should include abstinence from intercourse for seven days after treatment.

EPT is recommended for all sexual partners in the last 60 days [1]. Additionally, it is important for providers to assess the risk of intimate partner violence with partner notification. EPT is not recommended in situations of suspected child abuse, sexual assault, or other situations in which the patient's safety may be compromised [4].

EPT has not been studied in pregnant women in isolated trials. Pregnancy may be a key time to implement EPT given the potential adverse effects of infection with gonorrhea and chlamydia on the pregnancy and on neonatal health. Conversely, there may be less need for EPT in pregnancy; traditional partner treatment may be more successful due to increased access to care for pregnant women, as well as a desire of the patient and partner to protect the health of the fetus. EPT may be important in adolescents, but is not well studied. Rates of gonorrhea and chlamydia infection in female adolescents are much higher than in other age groups.

The legal status of EPT has not always been certain, resulting in a large barrier to the use of EPT. While no specific rule of law prohibited the use of EPT, EPT use can be prevented indirectly through licensing, public health, or prescription drug laws that require examination of patients or direct patient–physician relationships as specific requirements for a pharmacist to dispense drugs. To help clarify the legal framework to allow state and local programs to institute EPT in their areas, the CDC developed a website in conjunction with the Center for Law and the Public's Health that contains state information [6]. Included are the key legal provisions in six areas that were found to relate to EPT implementation for each state; a final conclusion indicates whether EPT is supported legally in that jurisdiction. As of December 2016, EPT is permissible in 38 states, potentially allowable in eight states, and prohibited in four states. The website can be accessed at www.cdc.gov/std/ept/legal for further information. Of note, variation exists by state as to which diseases may be treated with EPT. For example, in New York, EPT can only be used to treat chlamydia.

Key Teaching Points

- EPT may be used to treat the male partners of women with gonorrhea and chlamydia infection.
- Because of gonorrhea resistance to oral cefixime and possible treatment failures, partners with gonorrhea should be encouraged to seek evaluation and treatment, as first-line therapy requires an intramuscular injection

of ceftriaxone 250 mg plus a single dose of azithromycin 1 g orally.

- EPT is not recommended for routine use in the management of women with trichomoniasis. Use should be limited to selective cases where other partner management strategies are not felt to be successful or practical options.

- EPT is not well studied in pregnancy and in adolescents.
- EPT is not to be used for the management of patients with syphilis.
- Providers should be aware of the legal status of EPT in the area where they practice.

References

1. Centers for Disease Control and Prevention. Expedited partner therapy in the management of sexually transmitted diseases: review and guidance. Available at www.cdc.gov/std/treatment/eptfinalreport2006.pdf.

2. Centers for Disease Control and Prevention. Guidance on the use of expedited partner therapy in the treatment of gonorrhea. Available at www.cdc.gov/std/ept/gc-guidance.htm.

3. Workowski KA, Bolan GA; Centers for Disease Control and Prevention. Sexually transmitted diseases treatment guidelines, 2015. *MMWR Recomm Rep* 2015; 64(RR-03):1–137.

4. The American College of Obstetricians and Gynecologists. Committee Opinion No. 632. Expedited partner therapy in the management of gonorrhea and chlamydial infection. *Obstet Gynecol* 2015;125:1526–1528.

5. Burstein GR, Eliscu A, Ford K et al. Expedited partner therapy for adolescents diagnosed with chlamydia or gonorrhea: a position paper of the Society for Adolescent Medicine. *J Adolesc Health* 2009;45:303–309.

6. Centers for Disease Control and Prevention. Legal status of expedited partner therapy (EPT). Available at www.cdc.gov/std/EPT/legal.

A 33-Year-Old Woman with Multiple Visits for Vaginal Discharge and Itching

Shelly Holmstrom

History of Present Illness

A 33-year-old woman, gravida 2, para 2, presents to your office with her fourth episode in the last 12 months of complaints of vaginal discharge associated with intense vulvar itching. She reports that vaginal discharge has been present for the last three days and is white, thick, and non-malodorous. The patient denies any pelvic or abdominal pain and any change in bladder or bowel habits.

Her past medical history is significant for uncontrolled diabetes mellitus type 2 and obesity. Her past surgical history includes two previous cesarean deliveries. She has been in a mutually monogamous relationship with her husband for the last four years and uses oral contraceptive pills for contraception. They have vaginal intercourse approximately four times during a typical week. She has no known drug allergies, and her medications include a combined oral contraceptive pill and insulin.

Physical Examination

General appearance	Well-developed, well-nourished obese woman in no acute distress

Vital Signs

Temperature	37°C
Pulse	80 beats/min
Blood pressure	125/84 mm Hg
Respiratory rate	14 breaths/min
Oxygen saturation	100% on room air
Height	65 inches
Weight	250 lb
BMI	41.6 kg/m^2
Abdomen	Obese, soft, non-tender, non-distended, no guarding, no rebound
External genitalia	Erythema and edema of labia majora bilaterally and excoriations located in the folds between the labia minora and majora bilaterally
Vagina	Moderate, thick, white vaginal discharge in the vault and on the vaginal sidewalls
Cervix	No lesions
Uterus	No cervical motion tenderness, the size and contour of her uterus limited by her body habitus
Adnexa	Cannot be palpated/limited by her body habitus

Laboratory Studies

Urine pregnancy test	Negative
Random glucose level	233 mg/dl
Hemoglobin A1C	8.2%
Vaginal pH	4.2

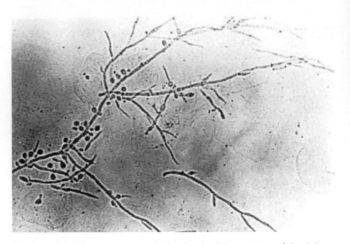

Figure 11.1 Wet mount – pseudo-hyphae budding pattern of *Candida*, no Trichomonas or clue cells.
Source: Gynecologic Disorders, *Current Medical Diagnosis and Treatment 2017* [5]

Wet mount	+pseudo-hyphae, no trichomonas or clue cells (Figure 11.1)
Yeast culture	+*Candida albicans*, sensitive to azoles

How Would You Manage This Patient?

This patient has recurrent vulvovaginal candidiasis (VVC) based on her fourth episode of symptomatic candida infection in the last 12 months. She has several risk factors for VVC, including uncontrolled diabetes, estrogen-containing oral contraceptive pills, and frequent intercourse. She was treated with fluconazole 150 mg every three days for three doses followed by once weekly for six months. She was counseled about alternative contraceptive methods and chose to have a copper-containing intrauterine device inserted. Her primary care physician worked with her to improve her glucose control with a different insulin regimen. She was seen six months later and reported that her symptoms had resolved. This patient was asked to follow up every three months for the next year.

Introduction

VVC is a disease process characterized by symptoms of vulvovaginal inflammation in the presence of *Candida* species and is the second most common cause of vaginitis symptoms (bacterial vaginosis is the most common). The vast majority (80–92 percent) of VVC episodes are caused by *Candida albicans* [1, 2]. The prevalence of this disorder is difficult to determine since the diagnosis is often clinically determined and not based on microscopy or culture. Moreover, unreliable self-diagnosis of VVC and widespread availability of over-the-counter antifungal medications contribute to an overestimation of the prevalence of the disease.

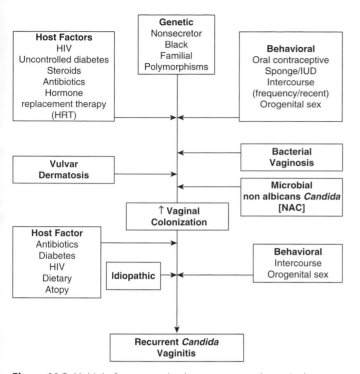

Figure 11.2 Multiple factors can lead to recurrent vulvovaginal candidiasis.
Source: Sobel. Recurrent vulvovaginal candidiasis. *Am J Obstet Gynecol* 2016 [3]

Recurrent VVC occurs when a woman experiences four or more episodes of symptomatic infection within 12 months [1]. Additionally, these women are asymptomatic between episodes of infection.

Risk Factors

A number of factors can predispose a woman to VVC, including diabetes mellitus, antibiotic use, increased estrogen levels, immunosuppression, contraceptive devices, and behavioral factors (Figure 11.2). These risk factors are contributory to a minority of cases of recurrent VVC. The majority of women with recurrent VVC have abnormalities in their local vaginal mucosal immunity and genetic susceptibility. Azole-sensitive *Candida albicans* is the causative organism in approximately 85–95 percent of cases of recurrent VVC, implying that host immunity as opposed to the pathogen plays a role in the pathophysiology of recurrent VVC [3, 4]. Sexual transmission does not play a role in recurrent infections and research does not support the treatment of sexual partners [5].

Clinical Presentation

Symptoms of VVC include vulvar pruritus, burning, irritation, soreness, dyspareunia, and vaginal discharge. Physical examination of the genital tract of a woman with VVC often reveals erythema of the vulva and vaginal mucosa as well as vulvar edema. Patients have vulvar fissures or excoriations in about 25 percent of cases. A vaginal discharge may or may not be present on examination and when present is typically white, thick, curd-like, and non-malodorous. However, the discharge associated with VVC may also be thin, watery,

and/or homogeneous. However, clinical findings are relatively nonspecific and should not be used as the means of diagnosis.

Evaluation and Diagnosis

Initial evaluation of patients with recurrent VVC consists of a thorough history and physical examination. Physical examination findings consistent with VVC should be confirmed with testing, which includes vaginal pH testing and wet mount or yeast culture. Vaginal pH is typically in the normal range of 4–4.5 in the setting of VVC, as opposed to an elevated pH observed with bacterial vaginosis and trichomoniasis. A wet mount is prepared by adding saline and potassium hydroxide to separate samples of vaginal discharge. Microscopy of the saline slide is used to examine for clue cells and trichomonads, which are present in bacterial vaginosis and trichomoniasis, respectively. The addition of 10 percent potassium hydroxide dissolves cellular elements and assists in the identification of budding yeast and pseudohyphae (Figure 11.2). It is important to be aware that microscopy is negative in up to half of culture-positive VVC [4]. A yeast culture should be obtained in the following two situations:

1. Clinical suspicion of VVC is high, vaginal pH is in a normal range, and the wet mount demonstrates no pathogens.
2. Persistent or recurrent symptoms of VVC since these infections may be caused by azole-resistant non-*albicans* species.

Management

Once the diagnosis of recurrent VVC is made, attempts should be made to reduce or eliminate risk factors for infection, such as improving glycemic control or changing to a lower estrogen dose oral contraceptive pill or to an intrauterine system. Women with recurrent VVC triggered by antibiotic use can be prescribed concurrent antifungal prophylaxis for the duration of antibiotic treatment. An example of antifungal prophylaxis is oral fluconazole 150 mg with the commencement of antibiotic use and then every three to four days until the antibiotics are completed [4]. Behavioral changes, including avoidance of panty liners, cranberry juice, and vaginal lubricants, rarely succeed in preventing recurrent episodes of VVC [6, 7].

Optimal therapy for recurrent vulvovaginal candidiasis consists of induction therapy with fluconazole 150 mg every three days for three doses followed by once weekly for six months (see Box 11.1). Some patients are able to achieve long-term remission once this regimen is completed, while others will have a relapse of symptoms. Relapse shortly after completion of the six months of weekly fluconazole necessitates a yeast culture to confirm the diagnosis. Approximately 50 percent of women will experience a culture-positive recurrence of VVC within 3–4 months of discontinuation of the weekly suppressive therapy [4]. Induction with 3 doses of fluconazole 150 mg every 3 days is repeated by weekly fluconazole for another 6–12 months. Fortunately, this low-dose fluconazole regimen is considered safe and does not require

Box 11.1 Treatment of recurrent vulvovaginal candidiasis

1. Regimens for *Candida albicans*, *Candida tropicalis*, and *Candida parapsilosis*

    a. Oral

    Fluconazole induction 150 mg q 72 hours for 3 doses

    Fluconazole maintenance regimen 150 mg q weekly for 6 months

    Itraconazole induction 200 mg bid × 3 days

    Itraconazole maintenance regimen 100–200 mg/day for 6 months

    b. Topical regimens:

    Induction

    Clotrimazole 1% vaginal cream for 7 nights

    Clotrimazole 2% vaginal cream for 3 nights

    Miconazole 2% vaginal cream for 7 nights

    Miconazole 4% vaginal cream for 3 nights

    Tioconazole 6.5% ointment for 1 night

    Terconazole 0.4% vaginal cream for 7 nights

    Terconazole 0.8% vaginal cream for 3 nights

    Terconazole 89 mg vaginal suppository for 3 nights

    Butoconazole 2% vaginal cream single dose

    Maintenance regimen

    Miconazole 1,200 vaginal suppository once weekly for 6 months

2. Regimens for *Candida glabrata*

    a. Boric acid vaginal suppository/capsule 600 mg daily for 14 days

    b. Nystatin induction therapy 100,000 units suppository per vagina for 14 d

    Maintenance regimen in same dose should be considered

3. *C. krusei* – any of the above regimens except fluconazole

4. Azole-resistant *Candida* species (based on MIC studies)

    Boric acid (see above)

    Nystatin (see above)

    Amphotericin B vaginal cream/suppositories 5–10% nightly for 14 days

    Flucytosine cream 17% per vagina, nightly for 14 days

    Combination amphotericin B/flucytosine

bid, twice daily; MIC, minimal inhibitory concentration; q, every

Source: Sobel. Recurrent vulvovaginal candidiasis. *Am J Obstet Gynecol* 2016 [4]

laboratory monitoring of liver function tests. Moreover, drug–drug interaction with other medications (i.e., warfarin or rifampin) is rare when fluconazole is used once weekly and does not require additional monitoring.

Frequent or prolonged use of fluconazole can lead to fluconazole-resistant strains of *Candida albicans* in a minority of women. In these cases, the minimum inhibitory concentration (MIC) for the *Candida albicans* isolate should be used to guide further therapy. Fluconazole MIC values of 2 or 4 µg/mL can be treated using fluconazole 200 mg twice weekly. If the fluconazole MIC is > 8, cross-resistance to itraconazole should be evaluated. If the *Candida albicans* isolate is sensitive to itraconazole, this medication is prescribed at 200 mg twice daily for 3 days followed by 100–200 mg daily for 6 months. Long-term use of itraconazole requires periodic liver function testing to screen for hepatotoxicity. Recurrent VVC caused by pan-resistant azole *Candida albicans* can be successfully treated with 14 days of vaginal boric acid suppositories made at a compounding pharmacy, or over-the-counter nystatin suppositories (see Box 11.1).

Topical gentian violet may be useful in refractory cases of VVC, especially in the setting of azole-resistant forms of *Candida*. Moreover, this medication can be used as a vulvar antipruritic. Gentian violet is applied with care to affected areas of the vulva and vagina for 10 to 14 days. Patients need to be warned that the drug is messy and permanently stains clothing.

Non-*albicans* *Candida* Species

The approach to treatment of *Candida glabrata*, *Candida krusei*, or *Candida Saccharomyces* is quite different from the treatment for *Candida albicans* described earlier. Recurrent vulvovaginal candidiasis from these species is due to lack of susceptibility to topical and oral azole drugs, which often do not eradicate infection. Treatment with vaginal boric acid 600 mg daily for 7–14 days made at a compounding pharmacy may offer relief to women suffering from recurrent VVC. Additionally, over-the-counter intravaginal nystatin or compounded flucytosine 17 percent cream or compounded amphotericin B alone or in combination may be necessary for treatment success of non-*albicans* *Candida* (see Box 11.1 for dosing). Chronic and recurrent VVC secondary to *Candida glabrata* is often seen in the setting of uncontrolled type 2 diabetes. Resolution of infection from *Candida glabrata* is unlikely without appropriate glucose control [1].

Key Teaching Points

- VVC is a disease process characterized by symptoms of vulvovaginal inflammation in the presence of *Candida* species, with the vast majority of cases caused by *Candida albicans*.
- Symptoms of VVC include vulvar pruritus, burning, irritation, soreness, dyspareunia, and vaginal discharge.
- Evaluation includes a physical examination to look for discharge consistent with VVC, vaginal pH testing, and wet mount or yeast culture.
- Recurrent VVC occurs when a woman experiences four or more episodes of symptomatic infection within 12 months.

- Optimal therapy for recurrent vulvovaginal consists of induction therapy with fluconazole 150 mg every 3 days for 3 doses followed by once weekly for 6 months.
- Several alternative therapies exist in cases of fluconazole-resistant strains of *Candida albicans*: oral itraconazole, compounded vaginal boric acid suppositories, over-the-counter nystatin suppositories, or gentian violet.

- Recurrent vaginitis from *Candida glabrata, Candida krusei,* or *Candida Saccharomyces* is different from the treatment for *Candida albicans* and is due to lack of susceptibility to azole medications, and should be treated with compounded vaginal boric acid, over-the-counter nystatin suppositories, compounded amphotericin B cream/suppositories, compounded flucytosine cream, or combined amphotericin B/flucytosine cream.

References

1. Vaginitis. American College of Obstetricians and Gynecologists Practice Bulletin No. 72. *Obstet Gynecol* 2006;107 (5):1195–1206.

2. Workowski KA, Bolan GA, Centers for Disease Control and Prevention. Sexually transmitted diseases treatment guidelines, 2015. *MMWR Recomm Rep* 2015; 64:1.

3. Odds, FC. Candidosis of the genitalia. In: Odds, FC. *Candida and Candidosis: A Review and Bibliography*, 2nd edn, Bailliére Tindall, London 1988, p. 124.

4. Sobel JD. Recurrent vulvovaginal candidiasis. *Am J Obstet Gynecol* 2016;214(1):15–21.

5. Fong IW. The value of treating the sexual partners of women with recurrent vaginal candidiasis with ketoconazole. *Genitourin Med* 1992;68:174.

6. Papadakis MA, McPhee SJ, Rabow MW. *Current Medical Diagnosis and Treatment 2017;* 2016 Available at http://accessmedicine.mhmedical.com/content .aspx?bookid=1843&sectioni d=135712463&jumpsectionI D=135712826 Accessed: April 11, 2017.

7. Patel DA, Gillespie B, Sobel JD et al. Risk factors for recurrent vulvovaginal candidiasis in women receiving maintenance antifungal therapy: results of a prospective cohort study. *Am J Obstet Gynecol* 2004;190:644.

A 24-Year-Old Woman with Trichomonas in the First Trimester of Pregnancy

Mark Turrentine

History of Present Illness

A 24-year-old female, gravida 1, para 0, presents for her initial prenatal care visit at eight weeks gestation. She reports that for the past five days, she has been experiencing vaginal itching with a copious "frothy" vaginal discharge, which is greenish-yellow in color and has a "fishy" odor. She denies any abdominal pain, vaginal bleeding, or fever. She has no medical problems. Her past surgical history is negative. She reports a past history of chlamydia, but no history of other sexually transmitted infections. She has been with the same partner for one year. She has no known drug allergies. Her only medication is a daily prenatal vitamin.

Physical Examination

General appearance	Well-developed, well-nourished woman, who is in no distress. She is alert and oriented.
Vital Signs	
Temperature	37.1°C
Pulse	78 beats/min
Blood pressure	110/70 mmHg
Height	63 inches
Weight	164 lb
Abdomen	Soft, non-tender
External genitalia	Unremarkable
Vagina	A purulent, foul-smelling discharge is present
Cervix	Closed, with some punctate hemorrhagic lesions
Uterus	Anteverted, mobile, eight weeks in size, non-tender
Adnexa	Non-tender

Laboratory Studies

Vaginal pH	6.0
Wet mount microscopy	Motile flagellated protozoan parasites (Figure 12.1)

Gonorrhea, chlamydia, syphilis, and human immunodeficiency virus (HIV) all return negative.

How Would You Manage This Patient?

This patient has symptomatic *Trichomonas vaginalis*. Patients with this infection frequently have a combination of vulvar pruritus; copious, frothy, malodorous vaginal discharge; and petechiae of the cervix ("strawberry cervix"). The motile flagellated protozoan parasites (trichomonads) on wet mount confirm the diagnosis. Tests for other sexually transmitted infections were negative.

The patient was counseled of the potential risks and benefits of treatment. She consented and was prescribed metronidazole 2 g orally in a single dose. She was recommended

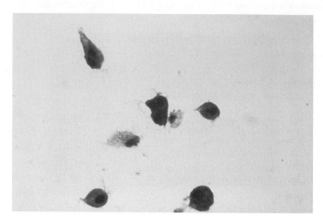

Figure 12.1 Trophozoites of *T. vaginalis* obtained from in vitro culture, stained with Giemsa.
Reprinted from the Centers for Disease Control and Prevention Public Health Image Library (https://phil.cdc.gov/Details.aspx?pid=5237)

that her sexual companion undergo evaluation and receive similar treatment. She indicated he did not have health insurance and would have difficulty seeing a health-care provider. The patient was provided a second prescription for 2 g of metronidazole for expedited partner therapy. She was counseled to abstain from intercourse until both she and her sexual partner had taken their antibiotics and all symptoms have resolved. She returned for a routine four-week follow-up prenatal visit and had reported no further vaginal discharge. Speculum examination demonstrated no vaginal discharge and wet mount was negative for trichomonads. She underwent repeat wet mount microscopy testing in three months, which was negative. She was retested in the third trimester for gonorrhea, chlamydia, syphilis, and HIV, all of which returned negative.

Trichomonas Infection during Pregnancy

T. vaginalis is an anaerobic parasitic flagellated protozoan that adheres to epithelial cells of the urogenital tract. Generally, infection is restricted to the genitourinary region. It is unsure whether the rectum or oral cavity can be a reservoir for *T. vaginalis* parasites, or if the occasional discovery of the organism in these areas is from recent deposition of organism during anal or oral sex.

Trichomoniasis is the most prevalent nonviral sexually transmitted infection in the United States, with an estimated 3.7 million infected individuals annually [1]. Approximately 3.1 percent of US women of reproductive age are infected [2]. Prevalence is increased in women ≥40 years old, in non-Hispanic black women, and in symptomatic women among sexually transmitted infection clinic patients [3].

T. vaginalis infection during pregnancy has been associated with an increased risk of preterm birth. A meta-analysis of nine studies (cohort studies and secondary analyses of randomized controlled trials) with 81,001 women reported a greater risk of preterm birth less than 37 weeks gestation (relative risk [RR] 1.42, 95 percent confidence interval [CI], 1.15–1.75, P = 0.001); however, the heterogeneity between studies was moderate [4]. An increased risk of preterm prelabor rupture of membranes (RR 1.41, 95 percent CI, 1.10–1.82, P = 0.007, two studies, n = 14,843) and small for gestation-age infants (RR 1.51, 95 percent CI, 1.32–1.73, P < 0.001, two studies, n = 72,077) were noted [4].

T. vaginalis is frequently diagnosed through microscopic evaluation of saline preparations of genital secretions because of convenience and low cost. Wet mount visualization of flagellated protozoan parasites (trichomonads) has a sensitivity of 55–70 percent [5]. Immunoassay rapid antigen and nucleic acid amplification tests for *T. vaginalis* combine high sensitivities (82–99 percent) with a rapid turnaround time (10–45 minutes), though at a greater cost [5, 6]. Although *T. vaginalis* may be an incidental finding on a Papanicolaou screening test, neither conventional nor liquid-based Papanicolaou test is considered diagnostic for trichomoniasis. Cytology has a high specificity (99 percent) but a low sensitivity (60 percent) with a false positive rate of 4–8 percent for this organism. If feasible, when trichomonas is identified on a Papanicolaou test, a wet mount microscopy should be performed [7].

Although treatment with metronidazole during pregnancy produces a greater than 90 percent parasitological cure, a Cochrane meta-analysis of two randomized controlled trials (n = 842) showed no evidence that treatment with metronidazole reduced preterm birth or delivery of low-birthweight infants in asymptomatic pregnant women with trichomoniasis [8]. In one of these two trials, a tendency toward an increased risk of preterm birth at less than 37 weeks gestation was noted with metronidazole treatment (RR 1.78, 95 percent CI 1.19–2.66, P = 0.004). While it is not clear why metronidazole should cause adverse pregnancy outcomes when it is effective in clearing the infection, the authors concluded that there is no evidence to support the use of metronidazole in pregnant asymptomatic women with *T. vaginalis* [8].

Standard therapy for *T. vaginalis* in any trimester of pregnancy is metronidazole 2 g orally in a single dose [6]. Parasitological cure following treatment with this regimen during pregnancy is 93 percent [8]. The superiority of this treatment regimen compared to multiple dose regimens has been recently questioned. In a meta-analysis of six trials, which included 937 nonpregnant women, women who received a single 2 g dose of metronidazole were more likely to experience treatment failure compared with those who were prescribed multidose metronidazole treatment (RR 1.87, 95 percent CI 1.23–2.82, P < 0.003) [9]. Metronidazole vaginal gel is only half as efficacious as oral metronidazole and is not recommended [6, 10]. Side effects of oral metronidazole may include nausea, stomach upset, vomiting, headache, dizziness, dry mouth, and an unpleasant metallic taste.

Symptomatic pregnant women diagnosed with *T. vaginalis* infection, regardless of gestational age, should be treated. Treatment of *T. vaginalis* infection can relieve symptoms of vaginal discharge in pregnant women and reduce sexual transmission to partners. However, treatment in symptomatic or asymptomatic women does not prevent adverse pregnancy sequelae. There is no benefit to treating otherwise healthy asymptomatic women during pregnancy, and unless symptomatic, treatment is usually deferred until after delivery. Metronidazole is secreted in breast milk. Because of demonstrated genotoxicity in bacteria and carcinogenicity in animals, concern has been raised about exposure of healthy infants to metronidazole via breast milk. Opinions vary among experts, but some sources recommend discontinuing breastfeeding for 12–24 hours after single 2 g dose treatment while other data suggest that lower doses over a longer period of time (400 mg three times daily for seven days) result in a lower concentration of metronidazole in breast milk and consider it compatible with breastfeeding [6]. *T. vaginalis* infection is a risk factor for vertical transmission of HIV, and treatment of trichomoniasis is associated with a 66 percent reduction (RR 0.34, 95 percent CI 0.12–0.92, P = 0.03) in genital-tract HIV shedding. HIV-infected women should have trichomonas treated regardless of symptoms [6].

Symptomatic pregnant women with trichomoniasis should be counseled regarding the potential risks for (such as side effects of oral metronidazole) and benefits of treatment (e.g., elimination of genital symptoms and spread of infection). The use of metronidazole in pregnancy is considered safe, and studies have shown no increased risk of teratogenic effects [11].

Infected patients should also be counseled about the importance of partner treatment and condom use in the prevention of recurrence. While screening of sexual partners is not recommended, concurrent partner treatment is necessary for symptom relief, parasitological cure, and prevention of spread and reinfection. While patient-delivered (i.e., expedited) partner therapy may have a role in partner management, no specific intervention has been shown to be superior in reducing reinfection rates [6]. Because of the increased rate of reinfection among women treated for trichomoniasis, retesting for *T. vaginalis* is recommended within three months following initial treatment [6]. Women at increased risk for sexually transmitted infections should be rescreened for gonorrhea, chlamydia, syphilis, and HIV in the third trimester of pregnancy [6].

Key Teaching Points

- Trichomoniasis is the most prevalent nonviral sexually transmitted infection in the United States.
- Wet mount visualization of trichomonads has a sensitivity of 55–70 percent whereas immunoassay rapid antigen and nucleic acid amplification tests for *T. vaginalis* combine

high sensitivities (82–99 percent) with a rapid turnaround time (10–45 minutes), though at a greater cost.

- Trichomoniasis during pregnancy is associated with an increased risk of preterm delivery, preterm rupture of membranes, and low birth rate.
- Symptomatic pregnant women diagnosed with *T. vaginalis* infection, regardless of gestational age, should be offered treatment, although treatment does not appear to prevent adverse associated sequelae.

- Asymptomatic pregnant women diagnosed with *T. vaginalis* infection need not be treated until after delivery.
- Standard therapy for *T. vaginalis* in any trimester of pregnancy is metronidazole 2 g orally in a single dose.
- Because of the increased rate of reinfection among women treated for trichomoniasis, retesting for *T. vaginalis* is recommended within three months following initial treatment.

References

1. Satterwhite CL, Torrone E, Meites E et al. Sexually transmitted infections among US women and men: prevalence and incidence estimates, 2008. *Sex Transm Dis* 2013;40:187–193.

2. Sutton M, Sternberg M, Koumans EH et al. The prevalence of *Trichomonas vaginalis* infection among reproductive-age women in the United States, 2001–2004. *Clin Infect Dis* 2007;45:1319–1326.

3. Meites E, Gaydos CA, Hobbs MM et al. A review of evidence-based care of symptomatic trichomoniasis and asymptomatic *Trichomonas vaginalis* infections. *Clin Infect Dis* 2015;61 Suppl 8: S837–S848.

4. Silver BJ, Guy RJ, Kaldor JM, Jamil MS, Rumbold AR. *Trichomonas vaginalis* as a cause of perinatal morbidity:

a systematic review and meta-analysis. *Sex Transm Dis* 2014;41(6):369–376.

5. Nye MB, Schwebke JR, Body BA. Comparison of APTIMA *Trichomonas vaginalis* transcription-mediated amplification to wet mount microscopy, culture, and polymerase chain reaction for diagnosis of trichomoniasis in men and women. *Am J Obstet Gynecol* 2009;200:188.e1–188.e7.

6. Centers for Disease Control and Prevention. Sexually Transmitted Diseases Treatment Guidelines, 2015. *MMWR Recomm Rep* 2015;64(No. RR-3):1–137.

7. Vaginitis. American College of Obstetricians and Gynecologists Practice Bulletin No. 72. *Obstet Gynecol* 2006;107 (5):1195–1206.

8. Gülmezoglu AM, Azhar M. Interventions for trichomoniasis in

pregnancy. *Cochrane Database Syst Rev* 2011, Issue 5. Art. No.: CD000220. DOI:10.1002/14651858.CD000220. pub2.

9. Howe K, Kissinger PJ. Single-dose compared with multidose metronidazole for the treatment of trichomoniasis in women: a meta-analysis. *Sex Transm Dis* 2017;44:30–35.

10. duBouchet L, McGregor JA, Ismail M, McCormack WM. A pilot study of metronidazole vaginal gel versus oral metronidazole for the treatment of *Trichomonas vaginalis* vaginitis. *Sex Transm Dis* 1998;25 (3):176–179.

11. Sheehy O, Santos F, Ferreira E, Berard A. The use of metronidazole during pregnancy: a review of evidence. *Curr Drug Saf* 2015;10(2):170–179.

A 16-Year-Old Adolescent Requesting Confidential Treatment for Chlamydia Exposure (Understanding State Laws Regarding Minors and Resources)

Kavita Shah Arora

History of Present Illness

A 16-year-old, gravida 0, para 0, adolescent with last menstrual period three weeks ago presents to the office requesting treatment for chlamydia exposure. She is a new patient to the office, is unaccompanied by a parent/guardian, and is requesting confidential treatment. She reports having unprotected intercourse with her partner several times over the last few months. The partner was recently evaluated at a public health clinic and the patient notified of a positive chlamydia test. The patient denies any discharge, vulvovaginitis, fever, or pelvic pain.

She has no medical problems. Prior surgeries include a tonsillectomy and adenoidectomy as a child. She denies tobacco, alcohol, or intravenous drug abuse. She does not take any medications.

Physical Examination

General appearance	Well-appearing adolescent in no acute distress

Vital Signs

Temperature	37.0°C
Pulse	80 beats/min
Blood pressure	110/65 mm Hg
Respiratory rate	18 breaths/min
Height	65 inches
Weight	130 lb
BMI	21.6 kg/m^2
Abdomen	Soft, non-tender, non-distended, no rebound, no guarding
Pelvic Exam	Deferred

How Would You Manage This Patient?

The patient was informed that in this state, confidential treatment of sexually transmitted infections for adolescents is permitted. However, the patient's care was covered by her mother's health insurance, and therefore confidentiality could not be guaranteed, since the explanation of benefits or bill from the visit sent to her parents may contain information about her care. Information regarding public health clinics that could offer confidential treatment was given. The patient opted to continue her care with this limitation in mind.

In addition to the medical history, a complete sexual, abuse, intimate partner violence, and mood history was obtained. No pelvic examination was necessary given the lack of symptoms of pelvic inflammatory disease or other pelvic complaints. The patient's urine was tested via nucleic acid amplification testing (NAAT) for chlamydia and gonorrhea, and she was offered testing for trichomonas, HIV, hepatitis C,

and syphilis. Given the patient's risk factors (age, multiple episodes of unprotected intercourse, known infected partner) as well as the risk of progression to pelvic inflammatory disease, treatment was not delayed while the diagnosis was confirmed. The patient was given empiric treatment for *Chlamydia trachomatis* (azithromycin 1 g orally in a single dose) on the day of presentation. The patient was counseled regarding emergency contraception, the importance of condoms to prevent transmission of sexually transmitted infections, and contraception to prevent unintended pregnancy. Expedited partner therapy was offered. The patient was counseled to abstain from intercourse for seven days as well as the possible need for her partner to be retreated if they had unprotected intercourse between the courses of antibiotics. She was instructed to return to the clinic in three months to undergo a repeat NAAT for chlamydia to rule out reinfection.

Clinical Considerations for the Adolescent with Chlamydia

Gonorrhea and chlamydia are the two most commonly reported bacterial infections in the United States. High-risk sexual behaviors are common in adolescents, and gynecologists will frequently encounter the need to test and treat sexually transmitted infections in adolescents in the office [1]. The gynecologist needs to be aware of recommendations for screening, treatment, and counseling, as well as local state legal considerations for confidential treatment of sexually transmitted infections in adolescents.

The Centers for Disease Control and Prevention (CDC) and United States Preventative Services Task Force recommend annual screening for gonorrhea and chlamydia in sexually active adolescents (Grade B recommendation) [2, 3]. An internal pelvic examination is not necessary to screen or test for chlamydia in an adolescent unless a patient is symptomatic, there is concern for pelvic inflammatory disease, or the patient reports other pelvic symptoms. NAAT is most sensitive via urethral or cervical swabs, though urine and patient-collected vaginal swabs are also possible [4]. Screening for other sexually transmitted infections such as trichomoniasis, HIV, syphilis, and hepatitis C in high-risk individuals or locations should also be offered. Routine herpes simplex virus or human papilloma virus screening is not recommended in adolescents.

Treatment for chlamydia should be offered in line with CDC recommendations. Treatment may include single dose (azithromycin 1 g orally once) or multiple dose (doxycycline 100 mg orally twice daily for seven days). To maximize adherence, onsite, directly observed single-dose therapy is preferred. Alternative recommendations are available per the CDC in the case of allergies or microbial resistance. Warning signs of pelvic inflammatory disease should be discussed. Repeat testing in three months should be performed given the high rate of reinfection in the adolescent population.

Ideally, partners should undergo clinical evaluation, sexually transmitted infection STI screening and HIV testing, counseling, and treatment by a health-care provider. However, when this is not practical, expedited partner therapy (giving prescriptions or medications to patients to take to their partners without first examining these partners) should be offered if legal in the office's state [5, 6]. Partners receiving expedited partner therapy should also be encouraged to seek care to discuss screening for other sexually transmitted infections, including HIV. Expedited partner therapy can decrease reinfection rates when compared with standard partner referrals for examination and treatment.

It is important that a full sexual, abuse, intimate partner violence, and mood history be obtained in the adolescent with a sexually transmitted infection. Adolescents should also be counseled regarding emergency contraception (if applicable based upon timing of sexuality and last menstrual period), condom use, and contraception.

Privacy, Confidentiality, and Legal Considerations for the Adolescent with a Sexually Transmitted Infection

Adolescents should be offered privacy for their care that is separate from parents/guardians. Privacy is different from confidentiality. Confidentiality includes protection of information shared during a health-care encounter from parents, and also includes a method of keeping information from the encounter confidential in the medical record (e.g., if medical record requests by parents or guardians are obtained, confidential encounters should be placed as private sections in electronic records, or documented with special ink that cannot be copied in paper records) [7]. Adolescents should be made aware of limitations of confidentiality that may arise if their care is billed to their parents' health insurance, since insurance billing and explanation of benefits sent to parents may contain information about diagnosis or tests ordered.

The American Congress of Obstetricians and Gynecologists recognizes the importance of confidentiality in caring for adolescents [8, 9]. Gynecologists need to be aware of their state's policies surrounding informed consent, emancipation, and sexual health for adolescents. Adolescents who are under the age of 18 are considered minors and require parental consent to receive health-care services. However, in all 50 states and the District of Columbia, minors are permitted to consent to services (diagnosis and treatment) for sexually transmitted infections. Each state has differing policies on an adolescent's ability to consent to the remainder of sexual and reproductive health services apart from sexually transmitted

infections, and gynecologists should be aware of these federal and state laws [10]. In some states, adolescents can consent to health care through emancipated minor rules such as when an adolescent is married or is an active duty member of the military, or by court order. In other states, physicians can deem an adolescent to be a mature minor, or one who has the capacity to provide informed consent. Some states allow minors to consent for contraception or other pregnancy-related care, screening and treatment for sexually transmitted diseases, HIV and AIDS, outpatient mental health care, or substance abuse counseling and treatment. There is a wide variation in the laws by state [8]. Some states have minimum age requirements, and some states allow physicians to notify parents that sexual health services were sought. However, no state mandates that physicians notify parents about screening and treatment for sexually transmitted infections, other than one state that mandates it in the case of a positive HIV test [10]. In contrast, laws addressing minors' access to abortion services are more restrictive.

Privacy and confidentiality due to administrative and billing practices remains a separate concern for adolescent health care. Office bills, insurance explanation of benefits, and a parent's/guardian's ability to visualize a child's electronic health record through patient portals all serve as potential avenues for confidentiality and privacy to be inadvertently violated. Ideally, both the adolescent and the parent/guardian are informed of the importance of confidentiality in the patient-physician relationship and these potential breaches proactively. Title X–funded family planning clinics, however, are required to provide truly confidential care with no associated administrative or billing practices that will breach confidentiality in these settings and, as such, should be offered as a referral to adolescents concerned about administrative confidentiality and privacy.

Key Teaching Points

- Screening and treatment of sexually transmitted infections in the asymptomatic adolescent does not require a pelvic examination, since screening for chlamydia and gonorrhea can be done by urine NAAT.
- Comprehensive sexually transmitted infection screening that includes HIV and syphilis, as well as counseling regarding sexual health, abuse, mood, and contraception, should be provided.
- Providers should be aware of federal and state laws regarding consent, confidentiality, and privacy for adolescent sexual and reproductive health.
- Providers should be aware that confidentiality can be inadvertently breached through administrative and billing practices when adolescents are using parents' health insurance.
- Title X–funded family planning clinics can be offered to adolescents concerned about administrative confidentiality and privacy.

References

1. Mansouri R, Santos XM. Sexually transmitted infections in adolescents. *Contemporary Ob/Gyn.* 2013. Available at http://contemporaryobgyn .modernmedicine.com/contemporary-obgyn/news/user-defined-tags/hiv/sexually-transmitted-infections-adolescents? page=full (Accessed April 9, 2017).

2. Centers for Disease Control and Prevention. 2015 Sexually Transmitted Disease Treatment Guidelines. Screening recommendations and considerations referenced in treatment guidelines and original sources. 2016. Available at www .cdc.gov/std/tg2015/screening-recommendations.htm (Accessed April 9, 2017).

3. United States Preventative Services Task Force. Final Recommendation Statement – Chlamydia and Gonorrhea: Screening. 2014. Available at www .uspreventiveservicestaskforce.org/Page/ Document/RecommendationStatement Final/chlamydia-and-gonorrhea-screening (Accessed April 9, 2017).

4. Centers for Disease Control and Prevention. Chlamydial Infections in Adolescents and Adults. 2015. Available at www.cdc.gov/std/tg2015/chlamydia .htm (Accessed April 9, 2017).

5. American College of Obstetricians and Gynecologists. Committee Opinion No. 632. Expedited partner therapy in the management of gonorrhea and chlamydial infection. *Obstet Gynecol.* 2015;125:1526–1528.

6. Centers for Disease Control and Prevention. Legal Status of Expedited Partner Therapy. www.cdc.gov/std/ept/ legal/default.htm. (Accessed June 13, 2017).

7. Ford C, English A, Sigman G. Confidential health care for adolescents: position paper for the Society for Adolescent Medicine. *J Adolesc Health* 2004;35:160–167.f

8. American College of Obstetricians and Gynecologists. Committee Opinion No. 599. Adolescent confidentiality and electronic health records. *Obstet Gynecol* 2014;**123**: 1148–1150.

9. American College of Obstetricians and Gynecologists. Confidentiality in adolescent health care. In: Guidelines for Adolescent Health Care. 2nd edn. Washington, DC: American College of Obstetricians and Gynecologists; 2011. pp. 9–17.

10. Guttmacher Institute. An overview of minors' consent law. 2017. www .guttmacher.org/state-policy/explore/o verview-minors-consent-law (Accessed April 9, 2017).

A 75-Year-Old Woman Complaining of Greenish Discharge

Amy R. Stagg

History of Present Illness

The patient is a 75-year-old, gravida 2, para 2, who presents with vaginal burning and greenish vaginal discharge. The patient reports that she has had these symptoms for the past two years, and notes that they have been worse for the past six months. She was widowed ten years ago, and for the past two years she has been sexually active in a monogamous relationship with a male partner and has noted increasing pain with intercourse. She uses water-based lubrication with intercourse with some, but not complete, relief of her pain. When her symptoms first started, she noted an occasional flare of vaginal burning and pain, especially with intercourse, but over the past six months she notes vaginal burning and discharge almost daily. On review of systems, she also notes urinary urgency for the past five years, but no urinary, flatal, or fecal incontinence. Her last gynecology examination and pap smear were five years ago and were normal.

Her past medical history is only significant for hypertension with no other medical issues. She had routine pap smear screening until five years ago, all of which were normal. She had two vaginal deliveries with no complications.

Physical Examination

General appearance	Well-developed, well-nourished woman in no current apparent discomfort
Vital Signs	
Temperature	37.0°C
Pulse	80 beats/min
Blood pressure	137/86 mmHg
Height	62 inches
Weight	125 pounds
Abdomen	Soft, non-tender, non-distended, no masses, and normal bowel sounds
External genitalia	Pale labia majora with no lesions, no apparent labia minora, and mild erythema of vaginal introitis. Pale urethral opening with no lesions and normal mobility of the urethra with valsalva.
Vagina	Pale vaginal tissue with flattening of the vaginal rugae and small amount of watery yellow-green vaginal discharge. No prolapse with valsalva.
Cervix	Normal with no lesions
Uterus	Anteverted, small, non-tender
Adnexa	No tenderness or masses

How Would You Manage This Patient?

The patient has atrophic vaginitis, more currently described as "genitourinary syndrome of menopause (GSM)" [1]. The clinical presentation of vaginal burning and discharge with increased symptoms over time is suggestive of symptomatic decreased estrogen levels affecting the vulvar, vaginal, and urologic tissue. Additionally, the urinary urgency as well as the vaginal symptoms with the onset of sexual activity two years ago is consistent with the diagnosis of GSM. On exam, she has noted atrophy of the vulva, vagina, and urethra, which are also consistent with the diagnosis. During her initial visit, she was offered sexually transmitted infection screening due to her history of a new partner since her last gynecologic evaluation. She agreed to the screening, which was negative, and after discussion of her options for therapy (Table 14.1), she chose to be treated with topical vaginal estrogen cream twice weekly. She was instructed to place 1 g vaginally at night just prior to sleep using a vaginal applicator. For this patient, only the topical estradiol cream was covered by her insurance, and was still 50 dollars for one tube. The other formulations of topical estrogen would have cost three hundred dollars. Given these choices, the patient opted for the estradiol cream knowing that no one formulation was more effective. She was counseled that the cream may not take effect until after six weeks of use and that discontinuation might result in return of her symptoms. The patient followed up after three months of topical estrogen therapy with resolution of her symptoms. On examination, she had resolution of introital erythema and only had mild urethral and vulvovaginal atrophy. She was instructed to continue vaginal topical estrogen cream therapy twice weekly with counseling that her symptoms may return with cessation of the treatment. The patient followed up in one year for routine gynecologic care with return of symptoms over the past month as she had discontinued the estrogen therapy. She hoped that after nine months of use she might not need the estrogen and could use lubrication only. Unfortunately, on examination, she had recurrence of the vulvovaginal atrophy and she was counseled to resume the estradiol cream twice weekly.

Table 14.1 Local vaginal estrogen therapy

Medication	Trade name	Dose of medication	Frequency of use
Conjugated equine estrogen cream	Premarin	0.625 mg of conjugated equine estrogen per gram	0.5-1 g 2 × weekly
Estradiol cream	Estrace	0.1 mg of estradiol per gram	1 g 1–3 × weekly
Estradiol tablet	Vagifem	10 µg tablet	1 tablet 2 × weekly
Estradiol ring	Estring	2 mg of estradiol reservoir with 7.5 µg daily	Change every 90 days

Atrophic Vaginitis

Atrophic vaginitis, currently described as GSM, involves vulvovaginal, sexual, and urinary symptoms [1]. This is a chronic progressive syndrome resulting from a hypoestrogenic state typical with menopause or less commonly during lactation, hormonal suppression, or various cancer treatments. GSM is thought to affect 15 percent of premenopausal women and 40–50 percent of postmenopausal women, although this still may be underreported. Studies suggest that only 25–50 percent of patients present to their provider for GSM symptoms, but that it significantly affects a patient's quality of life [1]. Provider and patient education is essential to increase the rate of early diagnosis and treatment.

Due to common embryologic development, hypoestrogenism affects both the urologic and genital systems. Estrogen is a vasoactive hormone that increases blood flow and lubrication to the vagina. Additionally, estrogen promotes proliferation of urethral, bladder, and vaginal epithelium, as well as increases smooth muscle tissue, collagen, elastin, and hyaluronic acid, which are all essential for vaginal strength and distention. In the hypoestrogenic state, the epithelium thins with decreased exfoliation of epithelial cells and decreased glycogen release. Glycogen is converted into glucose in the vagina, which is then converted into hyaluronic acid by local *Lactobacillus*. This maintains a low pH (3.5–4.5) in the vagina that is essential to prevent vaginal and urinary infections. With the hypoestrogenic state, there is less lubrication, less plasticity of the vagina, and pathogenic bacteria can overgrow, increasing vaginal and urinary infections [2].

GSM is a clinical diagnosis that is based upon a patient's history and physical examination. Patients with GSM can present with genital dryness, irritation, pain, as well as urinary urgency and frequency, and stress urinary incontinence (SUI). They can also have dyspareunia, and decreased libido and orgasm [3]. Screening all menopausal patients who present for a well-woman visit or with any of these symptoms for GSM is essential, given the significant prevalence in this population. Symptoms of GSM are often progressive over time and early treatment can halt the progression. Patients with GSM may get frequent urinary tract infections and may be given antibiotics unnecessarily, as estrogen therapy can prevent recurrence of infection [3].

Patients with GSM often do not present for care or report their symptoms as they are embarrassed or unaware that there is effective treatment. Providers should screen for GSM as a routine part of the evaluation of a menopausal or otherwise hormonally suppressed patient. Additionally, providers should be aware that when patients do present, they may complain about issues such as decreased libido or vaginal discharge, leading one to think of an alternative diagnosis other than GSM.

A thorough urogenital examination is essential for diagnosis. Typically, the vulva is pale with a decrease in size of the labia majora, and shrinking or disappearance of the labia minora. The urethra is often pale and the vagina may have decreased or loss of rugae and areas of erythema where irritation has occurred. The cervix may be flush with the vagina and there can be vaginal shortening and a decrease in diameter.

Given the associated urinary symptoms of SUI and urgency with GSM, a thorough evaluation for urethral hypermobility and pelvic organ prolapse is important to evaluate for urogynecologic issues other than GSM [4]. Patients can also present with postmenopausal bleeding and in this case, in addition to an examination, a work-up for endometrial hyperplasia and cancer, including endometrial biopsy and pelvic ultrasound, must be done. Other diagnoses that should be considered in the differential are bacterial vaginosis, contact dermatitis, candidiasis, trichomoniasis, and vulvar or vaginal neoplasia [5].

There are several laboratory tests that can be helpful to support the diagnosis of GSM. On cytology, the vaginal epithelium has an increase in parabasal cells and a decrease in superficial cells in women with GSM (Figure 14.1). A vaginal maturation index, which assesses the relative proportion of parabasal, intermediate, and superficial vaginal epithelial cells, is the standard test used to determine vaginal atrophy, but is often not used or necessary in clinical practice. A vaginal pH of 5–7 (in the absence of bacterial vaginosis) is also typical for patients with GSM. On wet mount, there is a paucity of *Lactobacillus* in the presence of leukocytes. On pelvic ultrasound, an endometrial echo of <5 mm supports the diagnosis of an atrophic hypoestrogenic state [1].

For patients with mild symptoms or who are concerned about topical estrogen therapy, over-the-counter vaginal moisturizers can be effective treatments. These are water based and come as gels or ovules that can be inserted vaginally every few days. Vaginal lubricants can also be used, but are short-acting and are best for patients whose main concern is

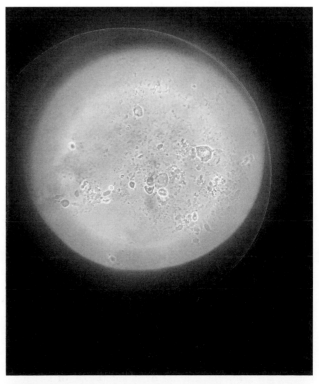

Figure 14.1 Slide from patient with atrophic vaginitis with increased parabasal cells (high nuclear to cytoplasmic ratio).

dypareunia. Increased intercourse frequency and mechanical vaginal dilation have also been shown to decrease symptoms of GSM, as they promote vaginal elasticity and lubrication [1].

The primary treatment for GSM, especially with moderate to severe symptoms, is local estrogen therapies to the vagina (Table 14.1). Studies of these various formulations suggest that no treatment is superior to another, and patient preference, ease of use, and cost should dictate choice [6]. The available estrogen formulations are creams – conjugated equine estrogen or estradiol – tablets, or a vaginal ring. These have been shown to be far better than vaginal moisturizers for symptom relief, with about 90 percent of patients noting relief of symptoms within six weeks of starting these medications. Patients need to continue these treatments indefinitely, as discontinuation results in recurrence of symptoms in most patients. Additionally, patients with vaginal prolapse, especially those using a pessary, are at higher risk of GSM and often need ongoing topical estrogen therapy to maintain the integrity of the vaginal tissue [3].

Contraindications to local estrogen therapy include abnormal vaginal or uterine bleeding of unknown origin and untreated uterine or vaginal cancer. For patients with estrogen-dependent cancers such as breast cancer, topical estrogen therapy remains controversial [3]. An ACOG Committee Opinion suggests that nonhormonal-based therapies should be first-line therapy for these patients, but topical estrogens can be used if nonhormonal therapies are not sufficient. Due to the variable absorption of creams, ACOG recommends the use of the vaginal estradiol tablet or ring if hormonal therapy is needed [7]. Alternative non-estrogen therapies for GSM include SERMs such as Ospemifene, laser therapy, Tibolone, oxytocin gel, and intra-vaginal dehydroepiandrosterone.

Key Teaching Points

- Genitourinary syndrome of menopause (GSM), previously known as atrophic vaginitis, affects 50 percent of menopausal women, but only 25–50 percent of these patients present to a provider for this issue.
- Screening for GSM should be an essential part of a complete gynecologic evaluation in a postmenopausal patient and one should consider this diagnosis when patients present with any sexual or urologic issues.
- Early treatment of GSM can halt and reverse the progression of symptoms in the majority of patients.
- Topical vaginal estrogen therapy is the mainstay of treatment and no one formulation is superior in efficacy, and choice of therapy should be steered by availability, insurance coverage, as well as patient preference.

References

1. Gandhi J, Chen A, Dagur G et al. Genitourinary syndrome of menopause: an overview of clinical manifestations, pathophysiology, etiology, evaluation, and management. *Am Journal of Obstet Gynecol* 2016;215(6): 704–711.

2. Macbride MB, Rhodes DJ, Shuster LT. Vulvovaginal atrophy. *Mayo Clinc Proc* 2010; 85(1):87–94.

3. Hyun-Kung K, So-Yeon K, Youn-Jee C et al. The recent review of the genitourinary syndrome of menopause. *J Menopausal Med* 2015;21:65–71.

4. Goldstein I, Dicks B, Kim NN et al. Multidisciplinary overview of vaginal atrophy and associated genitourinary syndrome of menopausal women. *Sex Med* 2013; 1:44–53.

5. American College of Obstetricians and Gynecologists. Vaginitis. Practice Bulletin No. 72. *Obstet Gynecol* 2006;107:1195–1206.

6. Rahn DD, Carberry C, Sanses TV et al. Vaginal estrogen for genitourinary syndrome of menopause. *Obstet Gynecol* 2014;124:1147–1156.

7. American College of Obstetricians and Gynecologists. The use of vaginal estrogen in women with a history of estrogen-dependent breast cancer. Committee Opinion No. 659. *Obstet Gynecol* 2016;127(3):618–619.

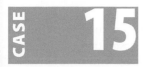

A 32-Year-Old Woman with Friable Cervix

Julianna Schantz-Dunn

History of Present Illness

A 32-year-old G0 presents with complaints of postcoital bleeding for the past three years. She reports a two-year history of levonorgestrel intrauterine device (LNG IUD) use and is currently amenorrheic with the exception of the postcoital bleeding. Prior to using the NG IUD, she used combination oral contraceptive pills. She states the bleeding occurs immediately after intercourse and is now occurring more regularly. The bleeding will fill several pads and takes a day or two to resolve. A year ago, she had her cervix chemically treated with Monsel's solution, which she said reduced the bleeding for approximately eight weeks before it returned. She has a history of an abnormal Pap test in her early 20s, but reports that her most recent cytology was normal and co-testing was negative for high-risk human papilloma virus (HPV). She is unsure of the date of her most recent evaluation. She is sexually active with one male partner, denies a history of sexually transmitted infections, and uses the IUD for contraception.

Her medical history is otherwise unremarkable. She denies any other history of easy bleeding or coagulopathy. She drinks alcohol occasionally and has never used tobacco. She denies any history of sexual or physical abuse. She works as a school teacher. Her family history is negative for any gynecologic, breast, or colon cancers.

Physical Examination

General appearance   Comfortable, well appearing

Vital Signs

Temperature	98.6°F
Pulse	72 beats/min
Weight	135 lbs
Height	65 inches
Respirations	16 breaths/min
BMI	23 kg/m^2
Abdomen	Soft, non-tender, non-distended. No rebound or guarding.
Vulva/Vagina	Normal external genitalia and urethra, no vulvar lesions, pink, well-ruggated vagina. Small amount of blood in the vault.
Cervix	IUD strings are visualized at external cervical os, small area on posterior cervix with increased vasculature versus transformation zone. Area bleeds easily when touched with a Q-tip. Spatula and cytobrush are used to collect Pap smear, HPV, gonorrhea, chlamydia, and trichomonas probe. After Pap sample is collected, a moderate amount of blood is noted from the posterior cervix. Silver nitrate is applied with excellent hemostasis.
Uterus	Small anteverted, normal cervical contour
Adnexa	No masses or tenderness.

Laboratory Studies

Urine hCG	Negative
Wet prep	pH 4.5, negative for yeast, clue cells, or trichomonads
Pap smear	Satisfactory for evaluation, negative for intraepithelial lesion or malignancy. High-risk HPV negative

Gonorrhea, chlamydia, trichomonas negative

Imaging

Pelvic ultrasound demonstrates a normal size uterus with endometrial thickness of 5 mm and an IUD in correct location. Normal ovaries bilaterally.

How Would You Manage This Patient?

This patient has postcoital spotting from an area of increased vascularity on her cervix. Initial work-up did not reveal an underlying medical, infectious, or pathologic cause of the cervical friability. The patient returned for colposcopy, with a targeted biopsy of the area, which returned as squamous metaplasia with reactive epithelial changes. She was prescribed 1 g of azithromycin for empiric treatment of nongonococcal, non-chlamydial cervicitis in a final attempt at conservative management. When this failed and she continued to be bothered by the ongoing postcoital bleeding, she presented for a loop electrosurgical excision procedure (LEEP). A shallow LEEP of the posterior cervix was successfully performed in the office, with roller ball cautery of the LEEP bed to achieve hemostasis, followed by application of Monsel's solution. She maintained pelvic rest for six weeks following the procedure and her symptoms resolved. Pathology on the LEEP specimen showed squamous metaplasia with severe chronic inflammation.

Friable Cervix with Negative Evaluation

A "friable cervix" refers to a cervix that bleeds easily, and often presents as postcoital or post-traumatic bleeding. Postcoital bleeding is not an uncommon complaint of reproductive-aged women presenting for gynecologic care. Surveys of reproductive-aged women have reported the annual incidence of postcoital bleeding to be between 3.4 and 12.6 percent, with a higher incidence in younger women and lower incidence in postmenopausal women [1, 2]. While it is important to rule out underlying pathology, such as cervical cancer, the cause of cervical friability and postcoital bleeding is more commonly a benign etiology. In fact, over 60 percent of women who report postcoital bleeding will have resolution of their symptoms with expectant management alone [3].

Bleeding originating from the cervix should be distinguished from abnormal uterine bleeding or structural causes such as polyps, as the evaluation and management differ. If abnormal uterine bleeding is suspected, the work-up may include a pelvic ultrasound or endometrial biopsy, especially if no lesion is identified on the cervix. Structural causes, such as cervical or endometrial polyps, can be removed. Cervical polyps can typically be removed easily with forceps in the office and the base cauterized as necessary.

A common cause of postcoital bleeding or cervical friability is cervical ectropion, which can be secondary to the physiologic process of endocervical columnar epithelium replacing squamous epithelium on the external cervical os. The columnar epithelium is more fragile than the squamous epithelium and therefore more prone to bleeding with contact [4]. Cervical ectropion is often associated with estrogen high states, such as pregnancy or estrogen-containing oral contraceptive pills. Therefore, in evaluating patients with ectropion, thorough history taking including medication history and exposure to hormonal changes is an important initial step. Of note, there is no indication for evaluation or treatment of asymptomatic women with cervical ectropion outside of routine screening, as ectropion alone is not necessarily pathologic or symptomatic [5].

The patient should also be evaluated for vaginal or cervical infections. Though postcoital bleeding has been reported as a predictor for chlamydia cervicitis [6], screening should also rule out infection with gonorrhea, trichomoniasis, and bacterial vaginosis. Herpes simplex virus should also be ruled out if there is evidence of cervical ulcerations. If a specific infectious cause cannot be identified, azithromycin or doxycycline can be used as empiric treatment for cervicitis [7].

A Pap test with HPV co-testing should be collected on women with postcoital bleeding, or cervical friability, though there are no consensus guidelines on whether or not colposcopy needs to be performed in the setting of normal cytology and negative HPV [4]. Visible lesions should be biopsied. The incidence of cervical intraepithelial neoplasia and invasive cancer associated with postcoital bleeding is dependent on the baseline risk of cervical pathology in the specific population being screened; in countries with adequate cervical cancer screening programs, the risk of CIN 2 or greater is extremely low [1].

Once the above etiologies have been ruled out and an area of cervical friability is identified, resolution or induction of squamous metaplasia can be achieved with topical hemostatic agents such as silver nitrate, Monsel's solution, or Amino-cerv. Monsel's (ferric subsulfate) solution penetrates denuded mucosa and causes a coagulation necrosis via thrombosis in the small vessels supplying the traumatized area. It has no effect on the normal surrounding epithelium; complete re-epithelialization and healing takes four weeks [8]. Amino-cerv is an alternative topical agent, which is reported to promote cervical healing. It is a combination of amino acid, antifungal, and urea, which work to promote cell growth. In one study, it was reported to improve cervical healing by four weeks in 83 percent of the women who received the treatment [9]. In settings where available, cryotherapy (the application of carbon dioxide or nitrous oxide via a probe at −89°C) has also been reported to be efficacious in over 72 percent of women with postcoital bleeding as a result of ectropion [10]. Cryotherapy may be more readily available in resource-limited settings. However, if these modalities are unavailable or result in inadequate treatment, a shallow LEEP procedure may be performed. Patients are counseled on the importance of pelvic rest after the procedure. The depth of the excised specimen should be minimized as the procedure is done for therapeutic and not diagnostic purposes, optimizing cervical integrity and future fertility outcomes.

Key Teaching Points

1. Malignancy, infection, pregnancy, and structural abnormalities should be ruled out prior to empiric treatment of postcoital bleeding
2. Conservative treatment includes altering hormonal medications, prescribing a course of antibiotics, application of Amino-cerv, or topical cauterization with silver nitrate or Monsel's solution
3. A small loop electrosurgical excision procedure (LEEP), roller ball ablation, or cryotherapy may be necessary for ultimate resolution of the symptoms

References

1. Shapley M, Jordan K, Croft PR, A systematic review of postcoital bleeding and risk of cervical cancer. *Br J Gen Pract* 2006;**56**:453–460.

2. Shapley M, Jordan K, Croft PR, An epidemiological survey of symptoms of menstrual loss in the community. *Br J Gen Pract* 2004;**54**(502):359–363.

3. Shapley M, Blagojevic-Bucknall M, Jordan K, Croft P. The epidemiology of self-reported intermenstrual and postcoital bleeding in the perimenopausal years. *BJOG* 2013;**120**:1348–1355.

4. Tarney CM, Han J. Postcoital bleeding: a review on etiology, diagnosis and management. *Obstet Gynecol Int* 2014;**2014**:1–8.

5. Yang K, Li J, Liu Y et al. Microwave therapy for cervical ectropion. *Cochrane Database Syst Rev* 2007;4.

6. Gotz HM et al. A prediction rule for selective screening of Chlamydia trachomatis infection. *Sex Transm Infect* 2005;**81**(1):24–30.

7. Center for Disease Control and Prevention. Sexually transmitted diseases treatment guidelines, 2015. *MMWR* 2015;**64**(3).

8. Davis JR et al. Effects of Monsel's solution in the uterine cervix. *Am J Clin Patho* 1984; **82**(3):332–335.

9. Gimpelson RJ, Graham B. Using amino-cerv after cervical LEEP. *J Reprod Med* 1999;**44**(3):275–278.

10. Kong et al. Cryotherapy as the treatment modality of postcoital bleeding: a randomized clinical trial of efficacy and safety. *Aust N Z J Obstet Gynaecol* 2009; **49**:517–524.

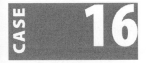

A 28-Year-Old Woman with Secondary Amenorrhea and Family History of Mental Retardation (Fragile X Premutation)

Frederick Friedman Jr.

History of Present Illness

A 28-year-old nulliparous patient presents with a complaint of absent menses for the past six months. She states she has occasional hot flashes and some vaginal dryness with associated dyspareunia. She performed a home pregnancy test that was negative. She notes no headache, visual changes, or galactorrhea. She exercises regularly, but has not noted any weight changes, or hot or cold intolerance. Her hair and skin are unchanged. She is engaged to be married next spring, and has been mutually monogamous with her fiancé for the past two years. She currently works as a social worker and enjoys her job. She does not smoke or use illicit drugs, and she only rarely drinks alcohol. She reports having a younger sister, who is well, but a brother and a male cousin with mental retardation.

Physical Examination

General appearance	Well-appearing young woman, alert and oriented, in no apparent distress

Vital Signs

Temperature	37.0°C
Pulse	68 beats/min
Blood pressure	110/70 mmHg
Respiratory rate	14 breaths/min
Height	66 inches
Weight	130 lb
BMI	21.0 kg/m²
HEENT	Normocephalic, anicteric sclerae, no oral cavity lesions, good dentition
Neck	Supple, full range of motion, no thyromegaly, bruits, or adenopathy
Cardiovascular	Normal S1 and S2, no murmurs, regular rate and rhythm
Lungs	Clear to auscultation bilaterally
Abdomen	soft, non-tender, no masses, no inguinal adenopathy

Pelvic

External genitalia and escutcheon	Normal
Vagina	Decreased rugae with mild atrophic changes; physiologic leukorrhea
Cervix	Nulliparous, closed/long/posterior, no cervical motion tenderness
Uterus	Normal size, anteverted, mobile, non-tender
Adnexae	No palpable masses or tenderness
Extremities	No cyanosis, clubbing, or edema; normal reflexes

Lab Values

Urine pregnancy test	Negative
FSH	42 mIU/ml
Estradiol	45 pg/ml
TSH	1.25 mIU/ml
Prolactin	13 ng/ml
Electrolytes	Sodium 140 mEq/ml, Potassium 4.2 mEq/ml
Hematocrit	39%
Pelvic sonogram	7 cm uterus with no fibroids, endometrium normal with 3.5 mm thickness; ovaries normal size bilaterally measuring 1.3 × 1.7 × 1.6 cm; a few subcentimeter follicles are seen; no free fluid in the cul-de-sac.

How Would You Manage This Patient?

This patient has secondary amenorrhea with a history, physical examination, and initial laboratory testing that are concerning for primary ovarian insufficiency (POI). Her FSH and estradiol were repeated in one month and resulted as 56 mIU/mL and 30 pg/mL, respectively, confirming a diagnosis of POI. At this point, a karyotype was ordered and confirmed 46 XX, Fragile X mutation testing (FMR1) was positive for 70–85 CGG repeats, and adrenal antibodies were negative. The patient was extensively counseled about the diagnosis of being a Fragile X premutation carrier and referred for genetic counseling.

The patient and her partner opted to pursue conception and were referred to the Reproductive Endocrinology team. Following controlled ovarian hyperstimulation with FSH, several eggs were harvested and fertilized, and five showed sufficient maturation and development. Pre-implantation genetic diagnosis (PGD) yielded three females and two males, and the patient underwent single embryo transfer of one of the female embryos. She subsequently conceived, and a second-trimester amniocentesis confirmed a 46 XX fetus, with no expansion of the CGG repeats. The patient was followed up for an uneventful pregnancy, and she delivered a baby girl at 39 weeks gestation. Following cessation of lactation, she started combination oral contraceptives with 30 mcg ethinyl estradiol and 1 mg of norethindrone acetate, and continues to be well three years later.

Secondary Amenorrhea

Secondary amenorrhea is defined as the absence of menses for three months after the establishment of regular cycles, or after six months in patients with irregular menses. After pregnancy, menopause is the second most common reason for cessation of menstruation. Other causes that must be considered include endocrine (thyroid disease, hyperprolactinemia, hypothalamic or pituitary dysfunction, primary ovarian failure, androgen excess), traumatic or iatrogenic (postsurgical, such as uterine synechiae), hypothalamic (anorexia, bulimia, stress), environmental (toxins), pharmacologic (exogenous hormones or certain psychotropic medications), infectious (e.g., tuberculous endometritis), immunologic, or genetic. This case will focus on secondary amenorrhea caused by POI resulting from Fragile X premutation.

Primary Ovarian Insufficiency Due to Fragile X Premutation

POI is the term used to describe accelerated ovarian senescence before the age of 40 years. Prior names for this clinical condition include "premature ovarian failure" and "premature menopause." Both of these terms are somewhat misleading and have fallen out of favor because many such patients express some residual folliculogenesis, and hence may not be entirely infertile [1]. Other authors have advocated the term "Premature Ovarian Dysfunction"[2, 3, 4].

The exact prevalence of POI is not known; however, as many as 1–2 percent of women will experience a significant decline in ovarian activity prior to age 40 [3]. While most causes are idiopathic or presumably autoimmune, one must exclude abnormalities of the X chromosome or other genetic causes that may indicate systemic disease. In the absence of historic environmental or infectious exposures, a karyotype and microarray analysis will help define the etiology. See Box 16.1 for a complete list of potential causes of POI.

The association of Fragile X premutations and POI was first reported by Conway and colleagues [5]. Numerous subsequent reports confirmed those observations and expanded upon them. Although the prevalence of Fragile X premutation as the etiology of sporadic POI is approximately 1–8 percent, the incidence is much higher in those patients with a related family history [1, 3].

The gene for Fragile X syndrome (FMR-1) is located on the long arm of the X chromosome. It codes for production of the fragile X mental retardation protein that has been found to suppress translation of messenger RNA in the brain [6, 7]. As a result, untranslated mRNA may accumulate in the dendrites, thus disrupting function. The disorder results from an increase in the number of cytosine–guanine–guanine (CGG) repeats in the noncoding region of the gene. In the normal case, there are fewer than 55 such repeats; when the number of repeats exceeds 200, the Fragile X syndrome results. The "intermediate number," between 55 and 200 repeats, is referred to as the premutation state (see Table 16.1). Males are affected far more than females because they have only one X chromosome; if they have more than 200 CGG repeats, they will suffer from Fragile X syndrome. As a result of having a second X chromosome, with inactivation or underexpression of the abnormal X chromosome, women rarely have the full disorder. They may, however, have a variety of other conditions, including ataxia or mild cognitive disorders.

Although women who have the premutation are typically asymptomatic, they are at risk for developing premature

Box 16.1 Causes of primary ovarian insufficiency

- Chromosomal
  - X chromosomal abnormalities (absence or mutations)
    - Turner's Syndrome (45, XO)
    - Fragile X premutations (FMR-1)
    - Other mutations of the X chromosome
  - XY gonadal dysgenesis
  - Autosomal abnormalities
    - Galactosemia
    - 17α-hydroxylase deficiency
    - Mutations of receptor coding
    - Autoimmune polyendocrine syndrome, type 1
    - Certain inherited leukodystrophies
    - Hereditary disorders of glycosylation
    - Bloom's syndrome
    - Fanconi's anemia
    - Werner's syndrome
- Environmental causes
  - Ionizing radiation
  - Other systemic toxin exposure
- Traumatic/Iatrogenic
  - Chemotherapy
  - Radiation therapy
  - Surgical
- Infectious
  - Tuberculosis
  - Viral (e.g., mumps)
- Immunologic
  - Autoimmune disorders
- Idiopathic

ovarian insufficiency, as in the patient described above. There is debate as to whether the underlying pathophysiology of ovarian dysfunction associated with FMR-1 premutation is caused by an accelerated rate of follicle atresia or a diminished initial number of follicles [8]. In addition, women with the Fragile X premutation may pass off an expanded number of CGG repeats to their offspring. This generational increase in number of CGG repeats appears to occur during oogenesis and post-zygotic mitosis and means that a woman who carries a premutation is likely to pass along the full mutation and thus have an affected child. When a male has the premutation, he typically will develop tremor and ataxia; however, males who carry the premutation are less likely to pass on an amplified number of CGG repeats to their progeny.

In addition to discussion with the patient, family members should be informed and counseled about the possibility of carrying the premutation and offered testing accordingly. It is important for women with the Fragile X premutation to understand that unlike in true menopause, when follicles have

Table 16.1 Classification of FMR-1 gene repeats

# CGG repeats	Nomenclature
5–44	Unaffected
45–54	Intermediate
55–200	Premutation
>200	Full mutation

been exhausted, there may still be active follicles, even in the face of an early decline in ovarian function. As a result, women with POI due to the Fragile X premutation may continue to be fertile for several years, but the exact likelihood of fertility preservation is hard to predict.

Counseling of couples is extremely important. It is advised that women be counseled prior to pregnancy about reproductive options and the potential risk to their offspring. Women with the Fragile X premutation may opt to undergo genetic testing of the fetus via chorionic villus sampling (CVS) or amniocentesis. It should be noted that the placenta may not always reflect the exact number of CGG repeats, so amniocentesis is more reliable than CVS in this situation. Alternatively, with the development of PGD, couples may choose to undergo in vitro fertilization (IVF) with PGD and implant only unaffected embryos [6]. Couples may also choose to undergo IVF with donor eggs, particularly if POI has already been diagnosed.

In addition to reproductive concerns in Fragile X premutation carriers, there are emotional changes that may accompany any woman faced with declining estrogen, which may be even more important when it occurs significantly earlier than anticipated or than in her cohorts and friends. The principal medical issues that should be addressed include bone loss, cardiovascular disease, and an increased risk of endocrine and/or autoimmune dysfunction (hypothyroidism and diabetes) [1, 3, 9, 10]. Since endocrine disorders are more commonly found in women who suffer from idiopathic or immune-mediated POI, screening for hypothyroidism and diabetes mellitus with an annual TSH and Hemoglobin A1 C is appropriate.

Estrogen deprivation in young women causes vasomotor symptoms and urogenital atrophy in addition to increasing the risk of bone loss and excess cardiovascular morbidity and mortality; therefore, women with POI require estrogen replacement. These patients may benefit from doses found in combination estrogen–progestin oral contraceptives (OCPs), especially in those wishing to avoid pregnancy. It is also reasonable to use the lower doses in postmenopausal hormone replacement regimens, but these options are less reliable at preventing ovulation in patients who desire contraception. Transdermal estradiol 0.025–0.05 mg per day or oral regimens including estradiol 1 mg daily or combined equine estrogens 0.625 mg daily will provide sufficient bone support and may reduce cardiovascular risk in young patients. In patients with an intact uterus, progestogens in the form of a progestin-containing IUD or oral progesterone (100 mg daily or cyclic for at least 12 days per month) must be added to avoid endometrial hyperplasia or adenocarcinoma. The combination of transdermal estrogen with concomitant use of a progesterone-containing IUD is a good alternative to oral progestin administration and is gaining popularity, as it may be a safer approach by avoiding "first pass" metabolism. Patients should be counseled about reported risks of combination HRT [11]; however, it does not appear that younger patients have the same degree of risks as do older women. Vitamin D and calcium supplementation might also provide additional bone support when used in concert with a regular, weight-bearing exercise regimen.

Key Teaching Points

- As many as 1–2 percent of women will experience POI defined as ovarian dysfunction prior to age 40 years.
- Testing for premutation of the FMR-1 gene is indicated in young women with hypergonadotropic amenorrhea and is more likely to be positive when there is a family history of mental retardation.
- Counseling is indicated to provide emotional stability and reproductive likelihood; many such patients are not truly "menopausal" and hence they are not infertile.
- Referral to genetic counselors and reproductive endocrinologists should be offered to assist patients and their partners in understanding options for future fertility and risks of expansion to full mutation in offspring.
- To avoid complications of estrogen deprivation, supplementation with either OCPs or HRT is indicated.

References

1. Persani L, Rosetti Raffaella, Cacciatore C et al. Primary ovarian insufficiency: x chromosome defects and autoimmunity. *J Autoimmun* 2009;33:35–41.

2. Nelson LM. Primary ovarian insufficiency. *N Engl J Med* 2009;360:606–614.

3. Rebar RW. Premature ovarian failure. *Obstet Gynecol* 2009;113:1355–1363.

4. Panay N, Kalu. Management of premature ovarian failure. *Best Pract Res Clin Obstet Gynaecol* 2009;23:129–140.

5. Conway GS, Hettiarachchi S, Murray, A et al. Fragile X premutation in familial

premature ovarian failure. *Lancet* 1995;346:309–310.

6. Conway GS. Premature ovarian failure and FMR1 gene mutations: an update. *Ann Endocrin* 2010;71:215–217.

7. Cornish K, Turk J, Hagerman R. The fragile X continuum: new advances and perspectives. *J Intellect Disabil Res* 2008;52:469–482.

8. Ryan JR, Arici A. Fragile X and reproduction. *Curr Opin Obstet Gynecol* 2008 June;20(3):216–220.

9. Hoyos LR, Thakur M. Fragile X premutation in women: recognizing the health challenges beyond primary ovarian insufficiency. *J Assist Reprod Genet* 2017;34:315–323.

10. American College of Obstetricians and Gynecologists. Primary ovarian insufficiency in adolescents and young women. Committee Opinion No. 605. *Obstet Gynecol* 2014;123:193–197.

11. Rossouw JE, Anderson GL, Prentice RL et al. Risks and benefits of estrogen plus progestin in healthy postmenopausal women: principal results from the Women's Health Initiative randomized controlled trial. *JAMA* 2002;288:321–333.

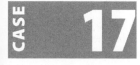

A 27-Year-Old Female Runner with Secondary Amenorrhea

Janeen L. Arbuckle

History of Present Illness

A 27-year-old female, gravida 0, presents as a new patient for her annual gynecology exam. She reports her last menstrual period as very light and occurred approximately four months prior to this visit. She reports menarche at age 12. She describes fairly regular, monthly periods while in high school. Her periods, however, became increasingly erratic while in college. She notes that at first she would skip her period for a month or so at a time but then would go several months without having a cycle. Her longest period without a cycle was eight months. She reports having been seen at her college's clinic for evaluation of her periods but cannot recall what labs were drawn. She was started on a birth control pill at that time with resumption of periods every 28 days. She continued the pill until approximately one year ago and has only had three spontaneous periods since.

She reports the provider she saw at the college clinic attributed her irregular cycles to her cross-country runs. Though she has always been athletic, she became increasingly so while in college, running at least five miles daily. She was especially mindful of her diet during training and admits to having restricted calories to maintain a slimmer figure in the past.

Her past medical history is notable for a prior stress fracture in her right foot, sustained while training for a marathon. She has had no prior surgeries. She does not smoke but does drink one or two glasses of wine per week. She is currently in law school and applying for a federal clerkship. She continues to be an active runner, running approximately 30 miles per week. When asked about her self-image, she reports feeling as though she is at her ideal body weight and is fearful of weight gain. She is sexually active in a committed relationship and anticipates getting engaged within the year. She and her boyfriend inconsistently use condoms for contraception.

Physical Examination

Vital Signs

Temperature	37.0°C
Pulse	58 beats/min
Blood pressure	107/55 mmHg
Respiratory rate	18 breaths/min
Height	69 inches
Weight	127 lb
BMI	18.8 kg/m^2
General appearance	Well-developed, lean female in no acute distress
Integumentary	No rash, hirsutism, or acanthosis nigricans
Cardiovascular	Bradycardic, regular rhythm
Pulmonary	Clear lung fields bilaterally
Breast	Symmetric, without mass, focal tenderness, or nipple discharge
Abdomen	Normoactive bowel sounds, soft, non-tender, non-distended, no rebound or guarding
External genitalia	Normal external female genitalia
Vagina	Estrogenized, without lesion
Cervix	Nulliparous
Uterus	Retroverted, mobile, non-tender
Adnexa	No masses or tenderness to palpation

Laboratory Studies

Urine pregnancy test	Negative
Hb	14.7 g/dL
FSH	5.7 mIU/mL
LH	5 IU/L
Estradiol	<30 pg/mL
Prolactin	14 ng/dL
TSH	1.4 0 mU/L
Free T4	6.2 mcg/dL
	CBC, CMP, and liver function tests all within normal limits

Imaging

Dual-energy radiograph absorptiometry (DXA)	Z-score −1.3 at the hip and −1.7 at the spine

How Would You Manage This Patient?

The patient has functional hypothalamic amenorrhea due to an imbalance of energy requirements and energy expenditure. Hypothalamic amenorrhea should be considered in the evaluation of women with a history of intense exercise and low body weight. Hypothalamic amenorrhea is a diagnosis of exclusion and can only be made when other anatomic and organic causes of amenorrhea have been excluded. The patient's presentation is suggestive of the female athlete triad. She describes a history of secondary amenorrhea and disordered eating, and her DXA scan is consistent with low bone mineral density. Importantly, her laboratory evaluation excludes the possibility of other endocrinopathies associated with amenorrhea.

The goals for this patient include a correction of her energy imbalance, either with a decrease in her energy expenditure or an increase in her daily caloric intake. These changes may be difficult for her to make given her concerns regarding her body image and fear of weight gain. In addition to being followed up by her physician, she will benefit from the guidance of a nutritionist and psychological counseling. Given the risk of bone loss in the setting of amenorrhea, she will benefit from estrogen support. There is controversy regarding the best means of estrogen supplementation, and the patient's need for contraception must be balanced with her goals for bone health. A traditional oral contraceptive pill may be used in this setting [1]. Though 100 µg transdermal estrogen coupled with cyclic medroxyprogesterone may result in superior bone health relative to an oral contraceptive, this regimen is not an effective form of contraception. Transdermal estrogen combined with a long-acting reversible form of contraception containing a progesterone such as a levonorgestrel intrauterine device would optimize both bone health and contraceptive efficacy. Though she is likely anovulatory, restoration of her energy balance will eventually restore ovulation.

Hypothalamic Amenorrhea

Maintenance of the female reproductive system relies on the hypothalamic-pituitary-ovarian axis. In well-nourished females, the pulsatile secretion of gonadotropin-releasing hormone and pituitary gonadotropins, coupled with ovarian feedback, establishes cycle regularity. Normal cycle length varies from 21 to 45 days in adolescents and from 21 to 35 days in adult women [2, 3]. Hypothalamic hypogonadism occurs when this axis is disrupted, which may be a result of weight loss, vigorous exercise, stress, or as a combination of two or more of these factors [4]. Hypothalamic hypogonadism may manifest by lengthening of the menstrual cycle, resulting in cycles lasting >45 days, or amenorrhea [3]. Hypothalamic amenorrhea may present as either primary or secondary amenorrhea. Primary amenorrhea is defined as the absence of menarche by age 15. Concerns for menstrual dysfunction should also be raised in those patients without signs of secondary sexual characteristics by age 14 [5]. Secondary amenorrhea is defined as three or more months without a menstrual cycle in a postmenarchal female [5]. The prevalence of hypothalamic amenorrhea has not been well established, but has been estimated to affect 2–5 percent of collegiate athletes and may be more prevalent in those sports which favor a lean body build [3, 4].

The diagnosis of hypothalamic amenorrhea is one of exclusion. The presence of pregnancy, thyroid disorders, prolactinemia, and premature ovarian insufficiency should be evaluated. Important diagnostic tests include a urine pregnancy test and tests for thyroid-stimulating hormone (TSH), free thyroxine (T4), prolactin, luteinizing hormone (LH), follicle-stimulating hormone (FSH), and estradiol. A complete blood count, complete metabolic profile, liver profile, and C-reactive peptide level are also recommended. In those women with hirsute features, assessment of total and free testosterone, dehydroepiandrosterone sulfate, and 17-hydroxyprogesterone should be a part of the diagnostic evaluation to rule out polycystic ovarian syndrome and late-onset congenital adrenal hyperplasia. Typical laboratory findings in the patient with hypothalamic amenorrhea are a low or low-normal FSH and a low estradiol level with otherwise normal labs. In women with a history of prior uterine instrumentation such as a prior dilation and curettage, an ultrasound to rule out occult accumulation of menstrual fluid due to synechiae can be performed [4].

Patients with hypothalamic amenorrhea often meet criteria for the female athlete triad (Figure 17.1). This triad, first described in 1997, includes amenorrhea, osteoporosis, and disordered eating [5]. The triad has since been revised to include variable presentations along a spectrum of disorders of the menstrual cycle, bone mineral density, and energy availability

[5, 6]. Patients may present anywhere along a continuum of optimal health to disease in any one or more of the three components. The prevalence of any one component of the triad has been estimated to be 16–54 percent among high school athletes while the presence of two or more components is less common with a prevalence of 4–18 percent [5]. When a patient presents with any one of the three elements, evaluation for the presence of the other elements of the triad is indicated. The Female Athlete Triad Coalition has developed a screening tool for the identification of women at risk for the triad (Box 17.1) [6].

The general health sequelae of hypothalamic amenorrhea are predominantly manifested in decreased bone mineral density and compromised cardiovascular health. Amenorrhea is associated with lower total bone density, unfavorable bone microarchitecture, and lower trabecular number [5]. Women with hypothalamic amenorrhea who have been amenorrheic for greater than six months, have a history of energy deficit, or have a history of prior fragility fracture should undergo evaluation of their bone mineral density by DXA [4]. Because athletes typically have a higher bone mineral density than the general population, a Z-score between −1 and −2 is considered low bone mineral density in athletes [5]. Women with

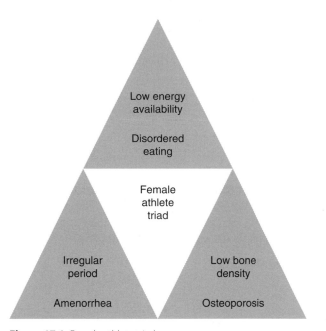

Figure 17.1 Female athlete triad.

Box 17.1 2014 Female athlete triad coalition consensus panel screening questions

Have you ever had a menstrual period?

How old were you when you had your first menstrual period?

When was your most recent menstrual period?

How many periods have you had in the last 12 months?

Are you presently taking any female hormones (estrogen, progesterone, and birth control pills)?

Box 17.1 (cont.)

Do you worry about your weight?

Are you trying to or has anyone recommended that you gain or lose weight?

Are you on a special diet or do you avoid certain types of foods or food groups?

Have you ever had an eating disorder?

Have you ever had a stress fracture?

Have you ever been told you have low bone density (osteopenia or osteoporosis)?

Joy E, De Souza MJ, Nattive A et al. 2014 Female Athlete Triad Coalition Consensus Statement on Treatment and Return to Play of the Female Athlete Triad. Current Sports Medicine Reports: 2014 July/August 13(4):219–232

hypothalamic amenorrhea may also be at increased risk for cardiovascular disease. Specifically, endothelial dysfunction has been shown to be more prevalent in amenorrheic athletes when compared to those with normal cycle intervals [3, 5]. In addition, amenorrheic athletes demonstrated higher total cholesterol and low-density lipoprotein levels [5]. The long-term impact of these changes on the development of cardiovascular disease has yet to be determined.

The primary treatment of hypothalamic amenorrhea is a correction of the energy imbalance. This can be achieved by a decrease in energy expenditure or an increase in caloric intake. A multidisciplinary approach involving the patient, physician, nutritionist, and a clinical psychologist is often required to implement the changes necessary to restore a normal energy balance [4, 5]. Improvement in energy balance may ultimately require weight gain though the exact amount of weight gain required for a return of menses has not been well established. It has been suggested that a weight gain of 2 kg higher than the weight at which menses were lost is required for a restoration of the menstrual cycle [4]. In addition, it may take up to 12 months of normalized energy balance for menses to resume [4, 5].

Bone density may be compromised after 6–12 months of amenorrhea. Maintaining adequate calcium and vitamin D stores is especially important for a patient's bone health [3–6]. In addition, treatment of the hypoestrogenic state is beneficial in those women who have not had a return to menses after behavioral modification. Transdermal preparations of estrogen, administered with a cyclic progesterone, appear to have a more beneficial effect on bone mineral density than oral preparations. Though oral contraceptive pills may be used in these patients, they may have a deleterious effect on bone mineral density. As such, oral contraceptive pills should not be used for the sole indication of restoration of menses or for improved bone mineral density [4, 6]. It should be noted, however, that as the energy balance is restored in women undergoing treatment, ovulation will resume, and sexually active women may be at risk for unintended pregnancy. An oral contraceptive pill may therefore be considered in these patients [1].

Key Teaching Points

- Hypothalamic amenorrhea is commonly associated with disordered eating and changes in bone mineral density. Once a diagnosis of hypothalamic amenorrhea has been made, evaluation for these concurrent disorders is indicated.
- In patients who have been amenorrheic for six or more months, a DXA scan should be done for assessment of bone health.
- Prevention of bone loss is best achieved with transdermal estrogen therapy, coupled with a cyclic progesterone, and calcium and vitamin D supplementation.
- Reversal of hypothalamic amenorrhea requires improvement in energy balance and may take up to a year following a return to a positive energy balance.
- Successful therapy for the patient with hypothalamic amenorrhea involves a team approach including the patient, physician, nutritionist, and psychologist and/or psychiatrist.

References

1. American College of Obstetricians and Gynecologists. Committee Opinion No. 702. Female athlete triad. *Obstet Gynecol* 2017; (6): e160–e1676.

2. American College of Obstetricians and Gynecologists. Committee Opinion No. 651. Menstruation in girls and adolescents: using the menstrual cycle as a vital sign. *Obstet Gynecol* 2015; 126(6): e143–e146.

3. Mountjoy M, Sundgot-Borgen J, Burke L et al. The IOC Consensus Statement: beyond the female athlete triad – Relative Energy Deficiency in Sport (RED-S). *Br J Sports Med* 2014;48:491–497.

4. Gordon CM, Ackerman KE, Berga SL et al. Functional hypothalamic amenorrhea: an Endocrine Society Clinical Practice Guideline. *J Clin Endocrinol Metab* May 2017;102(5):1–27.

5. Weiss Kelly AK, Hecht S; Council on Sports Medicine and Fitness. The female athlete triad. *Pediatrics* 2016;137(6): e20160922.

6. Joy E, De Souza MJ, Nattive A et al. 2014 Female athlete triad coalition consensus statement on treatment and return to play of the female athlete triad. *CurrSports Med Report* 2014 July/August 13 (4):219–232.

A 38-Year-Old Woman with Secondary Amenorrhea Six Months after Gastric Bypass

Kyle Andrew Biggs

History of Present Illness

A 38-year-old gravida 1, para 0010 woman presents to the office with eight weeks of amenorrhea.

She underwent a Roux-en-Y gastric bypass six months earlier and has lost 16 pounds since her surgery. The patient does desire pregnancy, but is not planning to conceive until after additional weight loss occurs. She is currently taking combined oral contraceptive pills for contraception. Prior to her bariatric surgery, she weighed 234 pounds, with a body mass index (BMI) of 44.2 kg/m^2. In addition to amenorrhea, review of systems is positive for nausea, breast tenderness, and fatigue.

Her past medical history is unremarkable. In addition to her bariatric surgery, her past surgical history is notable for one dilation and curettage for a miscarriage at eight weeks gestation. Menarche occurred at 11 years of age. Her menstrual cycles are typically irregular, but had normalized in the last three months. She is sexually active with her spouse and they do not use barrier contraception. She does not smoke or drink, and she takes no medications other than OCPs.

Physical Examination

Height	61 inches
Weight	218 pounds
BMI	41.2 kg/m^2
General	Well appearing

Vital Signs

Temperature	98.8°F
Heart rate	87 beats/min
Blood pressure	138/85 mmHg
Respiratory rate	16 breaths/min
Cardiovascular	Regular rhythm, no rubs or gallops
Pulmonary	Clear to auscultation bilaterally
Abdomen	Soft, obese, non-tender, healed laparoscopic scars
Extremities	No calf tenderness bilaterally

Laboratory Studies

Urine pregnancy test	Positive
Hemoglobin	10.5 g/dL (11 g/dL)*
Hematocrit	31% (33%)
Ferritin	5 µg/dL (>10 µg/dL)
Iron	35 µg/dL (40–175 µg/dL)
Vitamin B12	400 pg/mL (200–500 pg/mL)
Folate	6 ng/mL (2–20 ng/mL)
Thiamine	3 µg/mL (2.5–7.5 µg/mL)
Calcium	8.5 mg/dL (8.5–10.2)
Vitamin D	45 ng/mL (12–50 ng/mL)

* Values in parentheses represent normal ranges.

Imaging

Transvaginal ultrasound shows an eccentrically located gestational sac, yolk sac, and fetal pole with positive fetal cardiac activity. Crown-rump length measures 10 mm consistent with seven weeks gestation.

How Would You Counsel This Patient?

This patient became pregnant in the first year following bariatric surgery. Rapid return to fertility is not uncommon after such procedures, and fertility rates have been shown to double in certain populations [1]. Special attention is required for such cases, and prenatal care should be coordinated among an obstetrician-gynecologist (Ob/Gyn), a bariatric surgeon, and a nutritionist. Evaluation and correction of identified nutrient deficiencies with supplementation should be employed to optimize perinatal outcomes.

Historically, perinatal outcomes have not been found to be worsened in patients with a history of bariatric surgery [2]. However, more recent evidence suggests that infants of mothers with prior bariatric surgery have increased risk of prematurity, small-for-gestational-age status, neonatal intensive care unit admission, and congenital malformations [3]; thus, the obstetrician should have increased awareness for these conditions and screen where appropriate.

Vigilance for bariatric procedural complications is warranted in pregnancy, as diagnosis may be delayed. Computed tomography and surgical consultation are warranted with gastrointestinal complaints.

Pregnancy and Bariatric Surgery

Obesity, defined as a BMI of $\geq$30 kg/m^2, affects more than 1 out of every 3 people in the United States and approximately 500 million adults worldwide. Frequently overlooked as a serious medical condition by health-care providers, obesity is now the most common health problem in women of reproductive age. While diet, exercise, behavioral therapy, and pharmacotherapy serve as first-line treatment options for overweight and obese individuals, bariatric surgery, including restrictive and malabsorptive procedures, remains the most effective therapy for morbid obesity (BMI $\geq$40). Candidates for bariatric surgery include patients with a BMI of $\geq$40 or a BMI of $\geq$35 and comorbid conditions [4]. Successful weight loss following bariatric surgery can lead to resolution of obesity-associated comorbidities, including hypertension and type 2 diabetes mellitus. Given these well-demonstrated benefits, bariatric procedures have increased significantly over the past two decades; more than 80 percent of these patients are female [5]. Ideally, patients should wait between 12 and 24 months before attempting pregnancy after a bariatric procedure to minimize fetal risk during the rapid weight loss that occurs. Moreover, patients can safely achieve their weight loss goals prior to conception.

Bariatric procedures are divided into two main types: restrictive and malabsorptive.

Restrictive procedures (e.g., gastric banding, sleeve gastrectomy) limit the amount of food one can eat by narrowing the lumen of the stomach. Malabsorptive procedures (e.g., biliopancreatic diversion) reduce absorption by diverting caloric intake past large portions of the small intestine. The Roux-en-Y gastric bypass has both restrictive and malabsorptive components.

Prenatal care of the patient with prior bariatric surgery presents unique considerations for the health-care provider. For example, approximately 50 percent of gastric bypass surgery patients experience dumping syndrome. Attributed to the rapid transit of incompletely digested food from the stomach into the small intestine, dumping syndrome can lead to nausea, vomiting, bloating, cramping, and diarrhea in the period immediately following consumption of a glucose load. Delayed symptoms, thought to be due to a hyperinsulinemic state and a reactive hypoglycemia, include diaphoresis, weakness, and palpitations. As a result, many patients with a prior bariatric procedure are unable to tolerate the 50-gram glucose beverage used to screen for gestational diabetes and require an alternative screening method. One commonly employed alternative requires home glucose monitoring of fasting and postprandial blood glucose levels for 1 week between 24 and 28 weeks of gestation [6]. If the results are consistently elevated, a diagnosis of gestational diabetes can be made and appropriate treatment can be initiated.

Significant nutritional abnormalities can occur in patients with prior bariatric surgery and can be exacerbated by the demands of pregnancy. Common nutrient deficiencies include protein, iron, vitamin B12, folate, vitamin D, and calcium. Additional micronutrient deficiencies in patients with malabsorptive-type procedures include thiamine, vitamin K, zinc, and biotin. A broad evaluation of these potential derangements should be performed at the first prenatal visit, and deficiencies should be corrected and then monitored in every trimester. Oral supplementation is typically adequate, but parenteral replacement may be required if laboratory values do not improve during monitoring. It has been suggested that supplementation with both a prenatal vitamin and a multivitamin be considered in patients who become pregnant after bariatric surgery; however, special attention should be paid to limiting the maximum daily dose of vitamin A to 5,000 international units to avoid teratogenicity. Vitamin B12 can be given as a daily oral dose or weekly through intramuscular or intranasal routes; oral absorption is dependent on the presence of intrinsic factor and may be reduced in patients with partial gastrectomy [7].

Additional issues that result from malabsorption in patients with a prior Roux-en-Y gastric bypass surgery can impact the use of various medications. A reduction in functional intestinal length reduces the time for absorption of extended release medications, for example nifedipine, which should therefore be avoided and replaced with oral solutions or immediate release formulations that can be more appropriately absorbed. Oral medications that require specific serum levels (e.g., certain antibiotics and anticoagulants) should be monitored to ensure that the levels are therapeutic. Restrictive procedures result in a small gastric pouch and increase the

Table 18.1 Institute of Medicine weight gain recommendations for pregnancy

Prepregnancy weight category	Body mass index (kg/m²)	Recommended range of total weight (lb)	Recommended rates of weight gain in the second and third trimesters (lb) (mean range [lb/wk])
Underweight	Less than 18.5	28–40	1 (1–1.3)
Normal weight	18.5–24.9	25–35	1 (0.8–1)
Overweight	25–29.9	15–25	0.6 (0.5–0.7)
Obese (all classes)	30 and greater	11–20	0.5 (0.4–0.6)

Institute of Medicine (US). Weight gain during pregnancy: reexamining the guidelines.
Washington DC National Academies Press. 2009. National Academy of Sciences (used with permission).

risk of gastric ulceration from nonsteroidal anti-inflammatory agents, and their use should be limited in the postpartum period.

Recommended maternal gestational weight gain in patients with prior bariatric surgery follows the Institute of Medicine's weight gain recommendations for pregnancy (Table 18.1). Even for patients who do not achieve their weight loss goal after bariatric surgery, caloric restriction is not recommended during pregnancy as it has been shown not to reduce perinatal comorbidities. Limited evidence supports an association between caloric restriction and impaired fetal growth. If minimal weight gain goals during pregnancy are not being met in the second and third trimesters, ultrasound evaluation for fetal growth and dietary consultation should be considered. Risk for excess or inadequate weight gain is increased in this population, and evidence supports the involvement of a nutritional counselor and a bariatric surgery care team throughout the prenatal period to optimize weight gain for these patients.

Irregular menstrual patterns are often associated with obesity, specifically due to oligo- and anovulation, which in turn may contribute to infertility. Obese patients also have decreased responses to fertility treatments such as clomiphene citrate for ovulation induction. Thus, weight loss, whether achieved surgically or by nonsurgical means, has shown to improve fertility rates in obese infertile females. A rapid return to fertility following weight loss from a bariatric procedure is not uncommon, and fertility rates have shown to double in certain populations. Moreover, patients can safely achieve their weight loss goals prior to conception. Oral contraceptive pills, used for contraception in patients with malabsorptive procedures, have demonstrated increased failure rates and should be avoided. Nevertheless, bariatric surgery is currently not indicated as a primary treatment for infertility in obese women.

Patients who undergo bariatric surgery and go on to achieve pregnancy demonstrate lower rates of several adverse pregnancy outcomes as compared to their obese counterparts, including miscarriage, preeclampsia, gestational diabetes, cesarean delivery, and still birth. However, these patients are at increased risk for complications related to their bariatric surgery [8]. Procedure-related operative complications include anastomotic leak, bowel obstruction, ventral and internal hernia, internal bleeding, band erosion, and band migration. Complications are most commonly described within the first two years of surgery. Pregnancy may delay the diagnosis of one of these complications, and there are case reports of maternal and fetal death [9]. As such, a pregnant patient with a history of bariatric surgery and any gastrointestinal complaint, particularly severe abdominal pain, should undergo a thorough and complete evaluation, with a high index of suspicion and a low threshold for computed tomography.

Bariatric surgery is not an indication for cesarean delivery, and standard obstetrical indications are reserved for this population. Yet retrospective data have identified a history of bariatric surgery as an independent risk factor for cesarean section. Patients who have undergone a bariatric procedure often still suffer from obesity in pregnancy and experience its ensuant risks and complications, including a need for induction and prolonged labor. If a patient's bariatric surgery was complicated or atypical, consultation with a bariatric surgeon or general surgeon with knowledge of bariatric procedures may be prudent to optimize perioperative outcome if cesarean delivery is indicated.

Key Teaching Points

- Successful weight loss after bariatric surgery can eliminate chronic morbidities and improve fertility rates.
- Pregnancy should be delayed for at least 12 months after bariatric surgery and non-oral hormonal contraceptives used primarily.
- Special attention should be paid to nutrient deficiencies and consultation with a nutritionist.
- Maternal pregnancy risk is not increased after bariatric surgery, though certain surgery-specific complications warrant urgent evaluation and consultation.
- Perinatal risk may be elevated in patients who conceive after bariatric surgery and should be reviewed during preconception counseling.

References

1. The American College of Obstetricians and Gynecologists. Bariatric surgery in Pregnancy. Practice bulletin No. 105. *Obstet Gynecol* 2009;113(**6**):1405–1413.

2. Sheiner E. Pregnancy after bariatric surgery is not associated with adverse perinatal outcome. *Amer Jour of Obstet Gynecol* 2004;190(**5**):1335–1340.

3. Brodie P et al. Bariatric surgery in women of child bearing age, timing between an operation and birth, and associated perinatal complications. *JAMA Surg.* 2017 (February);152(**2**):1–8.

4. National Institutes of Health. The practical guide to the identification, evaluation, and treatment of overweight and obesity in adults. The North American Association for the Study of Obesity, National Heart, Lung, and Blood Institute, National Institutes of Health Publication no. 00–4084; 2000. www.nhlbi.nih.gov/guidelines/obesity/prctgd_c.pdf. Accessed June 23, 2017.

5. The American College of Obstetricians and Gynecologists. Obesity in Pregnancy. Practice bulletin No. 156. *Obstet Gynecol* 2013;121 (**1**):213–217.

6. Kominiarek MA. Preparing for and managing a pregnancy after bariatric surgery. *Semin Perinatol* 2011;35(**6**): 365–361.

7. Ziegler O et al. Medical follow up after bariatric surgery: nutritional and drug issues. General recommendations for the prevention and treatment of nutritional deficiencies. *Diabetes Metab* 2009;35 (**6–2**):544–557.

8. Stuart A, Kallen K. Risk of abdominal surgery in pregnancy among women who have undergone bariatric surgery. *Obstet Gynecol* 2017;129(**5**):887–895.

9. Maggard MA et al. Pregnancy and fertility following bariatric surgery: a systematic review. *JAMA* 2008;300 (**19**):2286–2296.

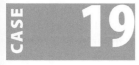

A 25-Year-Old Woman with a Levonorgestrel Intrauterine Device (LNG-IUD), New Onset Spotting, and a Positive Pregnancy Test

Jeffrey Rothenberg

History of Present Illness

A 25-year-old gravida 2, para 1, had an LNG-IUD placed eight months prior to this visit. She presents with symptoms of nausea and vaginal spotting that began this week. She took a home pregnancy test, which was positive. She was amenorrheic prior to the recent bleeding episode. She has had one normal full-term vaginal delivery without complications. She informs you that although unexpected and unplanned, she would like to continue the pregnancy.

Physical Examination

General appearance	Well-developed, well-nourished woman in no discomfort who is alert and oriented

Vital Signs

Temperature	36.9°C
Pulse	82 beats/min
Blood pressure	106/72 mmHg
Respiratory rate	14 breaths/min
Oxygen saturation	100 percent on room air
Height	63 inches
Weight	122 lb
BMI	21.6 kg/m^2
Abdomen	Soft and non-tender. No peritoneal signs, normal bowel sounds
External genitalia	Normal
Vagina	Rugose with a small amount of dark blood in the posterior fornix
Cervix	Parous, closed with scant amount of dark blood at the os, IUD strings clearly visible
Uterus	Anteverted, mobile and slightly enlarged, non-tender
Adnexa	No masses or fullness appreciated, small right adnexa, unable to palpate the left

Laboratory Studies

Urine pregnancy test	Positive
Blood group and Rh	O+
Hemoglobin	12.9 g/dL
Hematocrit	39.3%

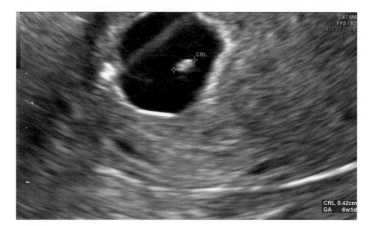

Figure 19.1 US image: 6 1/7 week IUP with IUD visible within endometrium.

Imaging	Transvaginal ultrasound reveals an intrauterine pregnancy of 6 weeks, 1 day with positive cardiac activity located in the uterine fundus with an intrauterine device located in the lower segment (Figure 19.1)

How Would You Manage This Patient?

The patient has a viable intrauterine gestation in the fundus and an LNG-IUD in the lower segment. A woman using an intrauterine device for contraception who becomes pregnant is at risk for complications in pregnancy, including miscarriage and preterm labor [1, 2]. Overall, it is important to remember that pregnancy is a rare event in IUD users. The reported failure rate for the LNG-IUD is 0.2 [1, 2]. Pregnancy associated with an IUD user has higher risks associated with it in both women who elect to have their IUD removed and those who leave it in place during the pregnancy [3]. This patient chose to have the IUD removed, which was easily performed in the office. The pregnancy progressed without any complications and she had a successful second vaginal delivery of a healthy 3,660-gram female infant.

Pregnancy Resulting from IUD Failure

Clinically, providers need to be able to articulate to patients that if pregnancy should occur with an IUD in place, removal or manipulation may result in pregnancy loss; however, leaving it in place increases the risk of spontaneous abortion and preterm labor. It is of paramount importance to evaluate these women for the possibility of having an ectopic pregnancy due to the increased incidence in this population [4]. The practical management of the IUD when a Cu-IUD or LNG-IUD user is found to be pregnant is to first exclude ectopic pregnancy, which has an incidence of approximately 0.1 percent per year.

Once an ectopic pregnancy is excluded, the patient must then be counseled that she is at an increased risk of miscarriage. This is more commonly seen in the first or second trimester and can be associated with a septic abortion. Later in the third trimester, preterm delivery risks increase if the IUD is left in place. While removing the IUD decreases these risks, unfortunately, patients do need to understand that the removal of the IUD also causes a small risk of miscarriage. Whether the IUD is removed or retained, patients must seek care urgently if they should have heavy bleeding, cramping, pain, abnormal vaginal discharge, or fever. In patients that desire to continue the pregnancy and the IUD strings are visible or the IUD can be retrieved safely from the cervical canal, it is best to remove the IUD by pulling on the strings gently. In those cases that the IUD strings are not visible, ultrasound is useful in determining the location of the IUD. In those instances when the IUD is not visualized on ultrasound, expulsion or perforation of the IUD may have occurred. It appears that many of the pregnancies in women with an IUD in situ may result from a malpositioned or missing device when evaluated by ultrasound [5, 6].

If a woman chooses to leave an LNG-IUD in situ for the remainder of the pregnancy, in addition to the risk of preterm delivery, there is a theoretical concern for an increased risk of fetal abnormalities secondary to fetal exposure to the progesterone in the LNG. This should also be discussed with patients. The exact risk however is unknown [7, 8]. Observational data support a small increased risk of masculinization of the external genitalia of the female fetus following exposure to progestins at doses greater than those currently used for oral contraception; however, whether these data apply to the LNG-IUD is unknown.

The published literature's evidence about pregnancy outcomes of levonorgestral IUD users is limited to case series [3], and no study has directly compared pregnancy outcomes with those of women whose IUDs were removed. In addition, there are insufficient data on timing of removal.

Most physicians offer removal as soon as the diagnosis is made after proper counseling since adverse pregnancy outcomes are increased by leaving the IUD in situ and early IUD removal appears to improve outcomes, but does not entirely eliminate risks.

Key Teaching Points

- In a patient using an IUD for contraception who becomes pregnant, an ectopic pregnancy must first be excluded.
- Most experts recommend removal of the IUD if the strings are visible, though this removal has a small chance of miscarriage.
- Leaving the IUD in place increases the risk for miscarriage and possible septic abortion, while removing the IUD decreases these risks.

References

1. Trussell J. Contraceptive failure in the United States. *Contraception* 2011;83:397–404.

2. www.acog.org/-/media/Practice-Bulletins/Committee-on-Practice-Bulletins--Gynecology/Public/pb121.pdf?dmc=1&ts=20170405T1218111260 ACOG Practice Bulletin 59, Reaffirmed 2015.

3. Brahmi D, Steenland MW, Renner RM, Gaffield ME, Curtis KM. Pregnancy outcomes with an IUD in situ: a systematic review. *Contraception* 2012;85(2): 131–9. doi:10.1016/j.contraception.2011.06.010

4. Selected Practice Recommendations for Contraceptive Use, 3nd edn. Geneva, Switzerland: World Health Organization, 2016, pp. 31–32.

5. Moschos Elysia MD and Diane M. Twickler MD, Intrauterine devices in early pregnancy: findings on ultrasound and clinical outcomes. *Am J Obstet Gynecol* 2011–05–01;204(5):427.e1–427.e6.

6. Anteby E, Revel A, Ben-Chetrit A, Rosen B, Tadmor O and Yagel S, Intrauterine device failure: relation to its location within the uterine cavity. *Obstet Gynecol* 1993;81:112–114.

7. Ganer H, Levy A, Ohel I et al. Pregnancy outcome in women with an intrauterine contraceptive device. *Am J Obstet Gynecol* 2009;201:381.e1–381.e5.

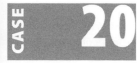

CASE 20

A 30-Year-Old Woman with Irregular Periods (Hypothyroidism)

Scott Graziano

History of Present Illness

A 30-year-old, gravida 2, para 2, woman presents to the office with complaints of a six-month history of irregular menstrual cycles. Cycles occur every six to eight weeks and last for seven days. Her last menstrual period began seven weeks prior to this visit. She denies intermenstrual spotting. Cycles are associated with minimal cramping that is relieved with an occasional over-the-counter ibuprofen. Prior to this history of cycle irregularity, her cycle interval was every 28 days. She reports normal appetite, but review of systems is significant for increased fatigue, dry skin, and a five-pound weight gain over the last six months.

She has no significant past medical or surgical history. She has no drug allergies, and her routine health maintenance is up to date. She reports two uncomplicated vaginal deliveries; last delivery two years prior to this visit. She breastfed her second child for six months. She is currently sexually active with one partner, using condoms for contraception. Her only medication is a multivitamin.

Physical Examination

General appearance	Well developed, well nourished, no discomfort
Vital Signs	
Temperature	37.0°C
Pulse	84 beats/min
Blood pressure	115/78 mmHg
Height	65 inches
Weight	135 pounds
Body mass index	21.6 kg/m^2
Neck	No masses, slightly prominent symmetric thyroid palpable, no lymphadenopathy
Heart	Regular rate and rhythm
Abdomen	Soft, non-tender, no masses
Skin	Dry texture, no discrete lesions, no thickening
Vulva/Vagina	No lesions, physiologic discharge
Cervix	Parous, no lesions noted
Bimanual exam	Anteverted uterus, mobile, normal-sized, non-tender, no adnexal masses

How Would You Evaluate and Manage This Patient?

The patient is presenting with oligomenorrhea accompanied by constitutional complaints of fatigue and weight gain over the same period. The differential diagnosis for this patient includes potential causes of ovulatory dysfunction, such as polycystic ovarian syndrome and thyroid disease. Testing for infectious causes, including *Chlamydia trachomatis*, should be considered. Pregnancy should be excluded routinely.

Laboratory evaluation for the patient was obtained and demonstrated the following findings:

Urine pregnancy test	Negative
Hemoglobin	11.9 g/dL
Chlamydia trachomatis screen	Negative
Thyroid-stimulating hormone	15 mU/L
Reflex free thyroxine (T4)	0.2 ng/dL

The likely diagnosis of primary hypothyroid was confirmed with the elevated thyroid-stimulating hormone (TSH) and decreased T4 levels. She was started on levothyroxine 100 mcg. Upon her follow-up visit to the office six weeks later, she reported resolution of her constitutional symptoms and had normalization of her TSH level.

New Onset Hypothyroidism

While there are many clinical manifestations of primary hypothyroidism, there is significant variability in the presentation, related to the severity of the disease. A thorough review of systems, along with a focused physical examination, may help increase suspicion for hypothyroidism. In addition to menstrual irregularities, women may report fatigue, changes in bowel function, muscle pains, and skin and hair changes. If significantly hypothyroid, physical examination findings may include an enlarged thyroid, delayed deep tendon reflexes, or identified changes in the heart rate and blood pressure. However, a clinical diagnosis alone lacks specificity. Clinicians are encouraged to rely on laboratory confirmation with a TSH level and reflexive testing for T4 levels. Primary hypothyroidism is diagnosed with elevated levels of TSH and concomitant low levels of T4. Over 95 percent of hypothyroidism cases are related to primary disease, and women are five times more likely than men to be diagnosed [1].

Thyroid disease can affect reproductive physiology and lead to changes in menstrual function. Traditionally, hypothyroidism was associated with heavy menstrual bleeding, owing to likely ovulatory dysfunction. Many women may in fact report normal menstrual cycles with hypothyroidism. However, up to 20 percent will report significant changes, with the majority being irregular uterine bleeding [2]. Typical complaints will include changes in the length of bleeding, the cycle interval, and the amount of bleeding that occurs during a cycle. TSH level does not always correlate with the severity of changes with the menstrual cycle.

In women who present with abnormal uterine bleeding, it is reasonable and cost effective to evaluate for thyroid disease. Women may also require additional evaluation based on age and other comorbid conditions. Utilization of the PALM-COEIN classification system is useful in the differential of abnormal uterine bleeding [3]. Pregnancy should be ruled out routinely.

There are three main goals when treating primary hypothyroidism [4]. First is to resolve the patient's clinical signs and symptoms of thyroid disease. Second is to normalize the levels of serum thyrotropin. Finally, overtreatment should be avoided (iatrogenic thyrotoxicosis). Negative effects of overtreatment include atrial fibrillation and osteoporosis. In treating women with hypothyroidism, clinicians should routinely monitor TSH levels. Untreated, as well as undertreated, hypothyroidism can have a significant negative impact on a patient's lipid profile and progression of cardiovascular disease.

There are several different methods to initiating levothyroxine therapy. When TSH is markedly elevated (>10 mU/L), full replacement doses should be considered. The initial dose is based on the patient's weight, using 1.6 mcg/kg of body weight. Clinicians may consider a lower starting dose of 25–50 mcg when the TSH is less elevated, in elderly patients, or in those with significant comorbidities. In cases of significant comorbidity and elderly women, initial therapy should "start low and go slow" to avoid side effects or cardiac events. Additionally, rapid thyroid replacement may accelerate cortisol metabolism,

leading to acute adrenal insufficiency and crisis. While there are limited data, it is recommended that patients avoid taking levothyroxine with most medications and supplements, including calcium carbonate and ferrous sulfate, by utilizing a four-hour separation period between oral ingestion [4].

After therapy has been initiated, it is recommended to reassess TSH in four to six weeks. Gradual increases or decreases may be needed after starting full replacement. Once stable levels have been established, clinicians may consider dose adjustments periodically with aging, changes in body weight, and pregnancy.

Key Teaching Points

- When suspecting hypothyroidism, clinical diagnoses lack specificity, and hence should be confirmed with laboratory testing for TSH and reflexive testing for free thyroxine.
- The goals of hypothyroid therapy are resolution of clinical symptoms, normalization of TSH, and avoidance of overtreatment.
- Untreated and undertreated hypothyroidism have a negative impact on lipid profiles and progression of cardiovascular disease.

References

1. Krassas GE. Thyroid disease and female reproduction. *Fertil Steril* 2000;74:1063–1070.

2. Krassas GE, Pontikides N, Kaltsas TH et al. Disturbances of menstruation in hypothyroidism. *Clin Endocrinol* 1999;50:655–659.

3. American College of Obstetricians and Gynecologists. Diagnosis of abnormal uterine bleeding in reproductive-aged women. Practice Bulletin No. 128. *Obstet Gynecol* 2012;120:197–206.

4. Jonklaas J, Bianco A, Bauer A et al. Guidelines for the treatment of hypothyroidism. *Thyroid* 2014;24:1670–1751.

A 25-Year-Old Woman with Midcycle Spotting

Ann Lee Chang and Tod C. Aeby

History of Present Illness

A 25-year-old nulligravid patient has come to your clinic with a complaint of midcycle spotting. Since menarche at age 14, her cycle length has been 28 days long with 5 days of "heavy" menstrual flow and moderate cramping. Over the past several months, she has developed unpredictable intermenstrual spotting that can happen at any time during the month. As a consequence, she wears light pads on a daily basis. She denies postcoital spotting or bleeding. She denies any change in discharge.

She is sexually active with her fiancé and, though she has used combined oral contraceptive pills in the past, they are currently using condoms for birth control. They plan to marry and start a family in the next few years.

Her past medical history is unremarkable, she is on no medications, and she is in good health. Her cervical cytology screening is up to date and normal.

Physical Examination

General appearance	Well-developed, normal-weight woman in no acute distress

Vital Signs

Temp	36.8°C
Pulse	65 beats/min
BP	111/69 mmHg
Weight	126 lb
Height	64 inches
BMI	21.6 kg/m^2

Abdomen Soft, NT, no masses, no organomegally

Vulva and vagina	Normal external genitalia with a small amount of blood in the vagina
Cervix	Normal appearing, no ectropion or polyp

Bimanual Exam

Uterus	Small, regular, non-tender, and mobile
Adnexa	No palpable mass and non-tender.

Laboratory Analysis

Gonorrhea and Chlamydia PCR negative

Imaging

Transvaginal 3D ultrasound with saline infusion hysterography was obtained, which demonstrated a 1.5 × 2.5 × 1.0 cm endometrial polyp and a narrow uterine septum extending to just above the cervical os.

How Would You Evaluate and Manage This Patient

Regular menstrual cycles with midcycle spotting are consistent with ovulatory bleeding. The differential for midcycle spotting can include uterine and cervical etiologies. Intracavity masses, such as submucosal fibroids and polyps, breakthrough bleeding from combined hormonal contraception, and infections such as endometritis or pelvic inflammatory disease are the more common *uterine* sources of midcycle bleeding. Rare causes include endometrial hyperplasia or malignancy. *Cervical* causes of midcycle bleeding include cervical polyps, cervicitis from sexually transmitted infections such as chlamydia and trichomonas, cervical ectropion, or cancer.

Evaluation for gonorrhea and chlamydia testing was negative. Evaluation for vaginitis was negative for bacterial vaginosis, and trichomonas was also negative.

This patient's symptoms can be explained by the finding of an endometrial polyp. The septum is not likely to be responsible for her complaints as evidenced by the recent onset of bleeding consistent with development of the polyp. After a lengthy discussion of the risks and benefits, the patient elected to have a hysteroscopic polypectomy and concomitant uterine septum resection. (The septum was resected because hysteroscopic resection of the polyp was to be performed.) Recovery was uncomplicated and her midcycle spotting resolved.

Endometrial Polyps

Endometrial polyps are hyperplastic endometrial overgrowths and contain endometrial glands, stroma, and blood vessels. They range in size and can be pedunculated or sessile in shape. PALM-COEIN, the International Federation of Gynecology and Obstetrics (FIGO) classification system of abnormal uterine bleeding (AUB), recognizes endometrial polyps to be among the four most frequent structural causes of abnormal uterine bleeding [1]. Risk factors for developing endometrial polyps include advancing age, increased levels of estrogen, tamoxifen use, and obesity. Polyps are almost always benign; in women of reproductive age, only an estimated 1–3 percent of polyps have endometrial intraepithelial neoplasia, and only 0.5–3 percent are malignant [2].

Endometrial polyps are often asymptomatic, and approximately 10–15 percent of women without abnormal uterine bleeding will have polyps [2]. However, 64–88 percent of women with polyps will experience abnormal uterine bleeding [3]. Abnormal bleeding due to polyps, AUB-P, is usually characterized by heavy menses, irregular menses, postcoital bleeding, and, most frequently, intermenstrual bleeding [4].

On occasion, an endometrial or cervical polyp can be seen protruding from the cervical os, but more often polyps are not prolapsed. If a polyp is suspected, evaluation can be performed with hysteroscopy or pelvic ultrasound. Hysteroscopy, the gold standard, can directly visualize abnormalities in the uterine cavity that can be resected. Pelvic ultrasound (TVUS) is non-invasive and can visualize an abnormal uterine lining suggestive of an intracavitary mass. Increasingly popular is the sonohysterogram, or saline infusion sonogram (SIS), as it can visualize and localize filling defects in the uterine cavity that are suggestive of a polyp (Figure 21.1). All three diagnostic modalities have similar detection rates [3]:

Table 21.1 Endometrial polyp detection rates

	Sensitivity (%)	Specificity (%)	PPV (%)	NPV (%)
TVUS	91	90	85	90
SIS	95	92	95	94
Hysteroscopy	90	93	96	93

Benefits of TVUS include its noninvasive nature. SIS improves accuracy and is overall well tolerated by patients. Both with or without SIS, TVUS includes the ability to evaluate the myometrium and the adnexa, if needed. Hysteroscopy, either in office or in the operating room, offers the most accuracy and allows for the removal of polyps if present. However, it is invasive and can be costlier, especially when performed under anesthesia. Given similar performance, any of the above modalities can be used initially to detect endometrial polyps.

After polyps are diagnosed in a symptomatic patient, they should be removed under hysteroscopic guidance, rather than with blind curettage alone. Hysteroscopy followed by blind polyp removal utilizing a grasping instrument and subsequent hysteroscopy to confirm removal of the polyp can be performed. Alternatively, polyps can be removed under direct visualization using a variety of instruments, including an electrosurgical loop (resectoscope), grasping forceps, microscissors, electric probe, or hysteroscopic morcellator. There is a paucity of data to recommend one modality over another. The majority of women, 75–100 percent, experience improvement of symptoms with removal [5].

Uterine Septum

A uterine septum is a congenital abnormality that is caused by failure of resorption after fusion of the two mullerian ducts. This leads to a wedge-shaped wall that divides the uterine cavity. The degree of separation is variable and can range from a small, clinically insignificant ridge to a complete separation of the uterus into two endometrial cavities. The external surface of the uterus is normal. Occasionally, the septum can extend further, leading to a double cervix and vagina. In general, a uterus with a septum that is less than 1–1.5 cm in length is considered "arcuate," a normal variant and not clinically relevant.

Uterine septa are typically asymptomatic and only become apparent during evaluation for recurrent pregnancy loss, infertility, preterm labor, or malpresentation of a fetus during pregnancy. Not infrequently, they are an incidental finding, as in this patient, and require no treatment. Because uterine septa tend to be asymptomatic, the exact incidence is unknown. The best estimates are that, in the general population, 1–15 women in a thousand will have a uterine septum. The incidence in women with fertility issues has been found to be much higher [6].

While surgical evaluation of the internal and external contours of the uterus is the gold standard for diagnosis (Figure 21.2), modern imaging techniques are equally accurate and less invasive. The external contour of the uterus

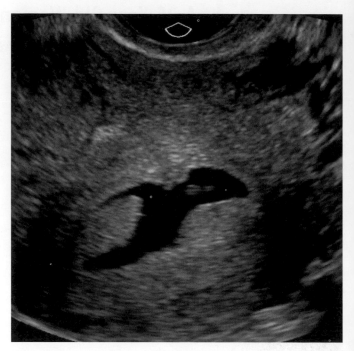

Figure 21.1 Sonohysterogram demonstrating a polyp.

should be assessed to differentiate a bicornuate uterus; hysterosalpingography and hysteroscopy alone are not sufficient. MRI is frequently used for evaluating mullerian anomalies, but its accuracy for diagnosing uterine septa has been called into question (Figure 21.3). Three-dimensional transvaginal ultrasound, with saline infusion hysteroscopy, seems to be the most predictive minimally invasive imaging modality [5].

Some congenital mullerian anomalies are associated with renal abnormalities, but this does not seem to be the case for patients with a uterine septum, and thus imaging of the renal system is unnecessary [6].

There are no randomized studies looking at the role of uterine septa in infertility, recurrent pregnancy loss, or abnormal obstetric outcomes. All published studies are observational and thus at risk for significant bias. Nonetheless, there appears to be good evidence that resection of a septum leads to an improvement in fertility rates, and a decrease in rates of miscarriage, preterm labor, and fetal malpresentation.

In the distant past, uterine septa were resected, at open laparotomy, using various techniques that involved large uterine incisions. With the advent of safe operative hysteroscopy, open procedures have been abandoned. At hysteroscopy, cold scissors, lasers, various electrosurgical cutting instruments, and mechanical morcellators can be used to remove the septum. All techniques have a low rate of complication and there does not exist sufficient evidence for recommending one modality over another [7].

Experts tend to recommend a two-month wait, after surgery, before attempting pregnancy, but there is lack of evidence to guide that recommendation.

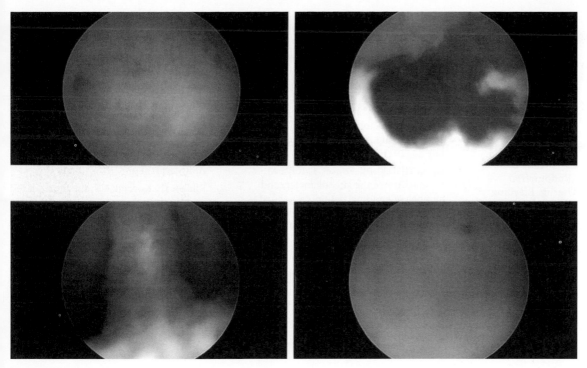

Figure 21.2 Hysteroscopic appearance of a uterine septum.

(a)   (b)

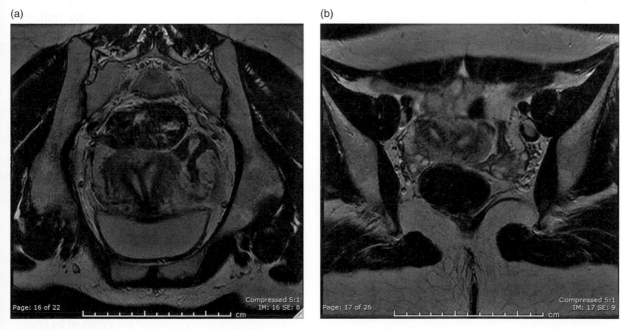

Figure 21.3 MRI of the same patient with a uterine septum.

Key Teaching Points

- Endometrial polyps are a common cause of abnormal uterine bleeding and they are rarely malignant.
- Hysteroscopy and pelvic ultrasound, with or without a saline infusion sonogram, are the best ways to diagnose polyps.
- Polyps should be removed using hysteroscopic guidance.

- Uterine septa are rare and often asymptomatic.
- The presence of a uterine septum has been associated with infertility, early pregnancy loss, fetal growth restriction, preterm birth, placental abruption, and fetal malpresentation.
- The best imaging techniques for diagnosing a septum are MRI or 3-D ultrasound with sonohysterography.

References

1. Munro MG, Critchley HO, Broder MS, Fraser IS, FIGO Working Group on Menstrual Disorders. FIGO classification system (PALM-COEIN) for causes of abnormal uterine bleeding in nongravid women of reproductive age. *Int J Gynaecol Obstet* 2011 April;113 (1):3–13.

2. Clark TJ, Stevenson H. Endometrial Polyps and Abnormal Uterine Bleeding (AUB-P): What is the relationship, how are they diagnosed and how are they treated? *Best Pract Res Clin Obstet Gynaecol* 2017 April;40:89–104. doi: 10.1016/j.bpobgyn.2016.09.005. Epub October 1, 2016.

3. Salim S, Won H, Nesbitt-Hawes E, Campbell N, Abbott J. Diagnosis and management of endometrial polyps: a critical review of the literature. *J Minim Invasive Gynecol* 2011 September–October;18(5): 569–81. doi: 10.1016/j.jmig.2011.05.018. Epub July 23, 2011.

4. Hassa H, Tekin B, Senses T, Kaya M, Karatas A. Are the site, diameter, and number of endometrial polyps related with symptomatology? *Am J Obstet Gynecol* 2006 March;194(3):718–721.

5. Nathani F, Clark TJ. Uterine polypectomy in the management of abnormal uterine bleeding: a systematic review. *J Minim Invasive Gynecol* 2006 July–August;13(4):260–268.

6. Uterine septum: a guideline. *Fertil Steril* 2016 September 1;106(3):530–540. doi: 10.1016/j.fertnstert.2016.05.014. Epub May 25, 2016. Practice Committee of the American Society of Reproductive Medicine. ASRM@asrm.org.

7. Rikken JF, Kowalik CR, Emanuel MH et al. Septum resection for women of reproductive age with a septate uterus. *Cochrane Database Syst Rev* 2017 January 17;1:CD008576. doi: 10.1002/14651858.CD00 8576.pub4.

22 A 25-Year-Old Woman with No IUD String Visible One Year after Placement (IUD in Uterus)

Adrianne Dade

History of Present Illness

A 25-year-old G4P4004 presents to the office for an annual well-woman exam. She reports light menses every 28 days for one day duration. She has no other complaints. She is currently using a levonorgestrel intrauterine device (IUD) for contraception that was placed six weeks postpartum after her last delivery. She has had four uncomplicated pregnancies with normal vaginal deliveries. Her youngest child just completed her first birthday. The patient is sexually active with one partner and reports no problems with sexual intercourse. Cervical cytology screening is current and last reported as negative. She has no other gynecologic complaints.

Her past medical history is negative. She had a hernia repair as a child. Her family history is significant for maternal hypertension. She has no known drug allergies and her social history is negative for alcohol or illicit drug use.

Physical Examination

General appearance	Well-developed, overweight female in no acute distress
Vital Signs	
Temperature	37.0°C
Pulse	65 beats/min
Blood pressure	132/81 mmHg
Respiratory rate	18 breaths/min
Oxygen saturation	98% on room air
BMI	28.6 kg/m^2
Height	67.2 inches
Weight	177 lb
Neck	No masses or lymphadenopathy
Axillae	No masses or lymphadenopathy
Chest	Clear to auscultation
Abdomen	Soft, non-tender, non-distended, normal active bowel sounds, no palpable masses, no hepatosplenomegaly, no fluid wave
External genitalia	Unremarkable, no lesions or lymphadenopathy
Vagina	Normal in appearance, scant discharge
Cervix	No lesions or cervical motion tenderness; no IUD strings visible at the cervical os
Uterus	normal size, mobile, non-tender, no masses
Adnexa	Palpable bilaterally, not enlarged, and non-tender

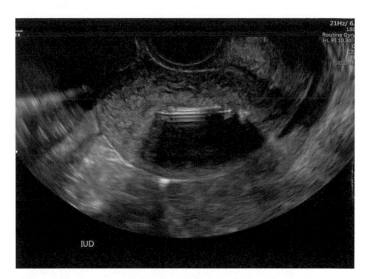

Figure 22.1 Characteristic acoustic shadowing of IUD within the uterine cavity.

Imaging

Pelvic Ultrasound	Uterus 8 × 4.5 × 6 cm with IUD noted at the uterine fundus. Left ovary 3.7 × 2.2 × 2.4 cm with several sub-centimeter follicles. Right ovary not visualized (Figure 22.1)

How Would You Evaluate and Manage This Patient?

IUD strings were not visualized at the cervical os during the exam for this patient. The differential diagnosis for this case includes displaced IUD strings into the cervix or uterus, a displaced IUD versus IUD expulsion. The patient's history of continued light menses is reassuring that the IUD has not been expelled. On exam, the IUD strings were not visible at the cervical os; a cytobrush was used to sweep the endocervical canal in an attempt to draw the IUD strings through the cervical os into the vagina. The IUD strings were not successfully visualized with the cytobrush technique and a transvaginal ultrasound was subsequently performed to identify intrauterine placement and position. On ultrasound, the IUD was visualized in the uterine cavity and is appropriately oriented at the fundus. The patient was counseled about the findings and was instructed to return with any change in menses. Repeat pelvic ultrasonography was planned for a follow-up exam if the IUD strings are not visualized or with reported change of menses.

Misplaced Intrauterine Device

The levonorgestrel intrauterine system and the copper T380A are the two most commonly used IUDs in the United States. The copper T380A IUD, which is wrapped with copper wire around the stem and arms, is approved for ten years and has a failure rate at one year of 0.8 per 100 women. The copper IUD also has ten-year failure rate comparable to that of female sterilization, which is 1.9 per 100 women over ten years. The proposed mechanisms of action include inhibition of sperm migration and viability, change in transport speed of the ovum, and damage to or destruction of the ovum [1]. The most common side effects are increased menstrual bleeding and dysmenorrhea.

The levonorgestrel intrauterine system (52 mg) is FDA approved for five years, but may be effective for up to seven years and releases 20 µg of levonorgestrel daily. It has a failure rate at one year of 0.2 per 100 women. The mechanism of action is similar to that of the copper IUD, but in addition the levonorgestrel intrauterine system causes endometrial suppression and changes the amount and viscosity of cervical mucus. Women may have hormonal side effects such as breast tenderness, nausea, depression, headaches, and cyst formation. Menses can be lighter and less painful [1].

Additional lower dose levonorgestrel devices (13.5 and 19.5 mg) are now available, but they are used less widely than the aforementioned devices.

On follow-up exam after IUD placement, the provider may not see the IUD string(s) protruding from the cervical os during a speculum exam [2]. Often the string is displaced just inside the cervical os. A cytobrush or similar device may be used to sweep the string from the cervical canal through the cervical os into the vagina. If this technique is unsuccessful in visualizing the strings, the uterus should be imaged with ultrasound to determine if the IUD is in the uterus and appropriately placed. The levonorgestrel IUD has a characteristic appearance, with acoustic shadowing between the echogenic proximal and distal ends, whereas copper IUDs are more completely echogenic. The IUD should be visualized as centrally located within the endometrial cavity, with the crossbar in the fundal portion of the endometrial cavity [3]. The distance from the top of the uterine cavity to the IUD should be 3 mm or less [4]. If the IUD is visible on ultrasound and appropriately placed in the uterus near the fundus, then the provider can reassure the patient that the IUD is in the correct position. A 3D transvaginal ultrasound coronal view of the uterus can also be performed to evaluate for an embedded IUD if available (Figure 22.2) [5]. If the patient desires removal of the IUD or it is incorrectly located in the uterus, an attempt to perform removal of the IUD with or without ultrasound guidance can be considered utilizing an IUD hook or other instrumentation in the office setting. Alternatively, IUD removal via operative hysteroscopy can be performed.

If the IUD is not visualized within the uterus on the ultrasound, the patient should be offered back-up pregnancy protection. An anteroposterior and lateral radiograph may then be

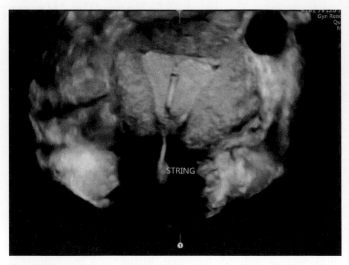

Figure 22.2 IUD visualized utilizing 3D ultrasound.

ordered to determine if the IUD is located within the peritoneal cavity. The levonorgestrel and copper TCu-380A frames contain barium sulfate for radiopacity [6]. If there is no extrauterine IUD on x-ray, then IUD expulsion has been confirmed.

The approximate first-year expulsion rates are commonly quoted as 2–10 percent and vary by IUD type [7]. If the IUD is identified on x-ray, then the patient should be informed that she has had a uterine perforation and she should be counseled regarding the expulsion retrieval via laparoscopy or a laparotomy. The potential for bowel perforation and fistula formation has been reported and should be considered when counseling [8].

According to the World Health Organization (1987), the risk of IUD perforation is 1 per 1,000 [9]. Similarly, in the European Active Surveillance Study on Intrauterine Devices, perforation rates were 1.1 per 1,000 in LNG-IUS and 1.1 per 1,000 in copper IUD users [10]. Of the baseline characteristics, the authors of this study concluded that breastfeeding at time of insertion and a time interval less than 36 weeks from delivery were the strongest risk factors for uterine perforation. Heartwell and Schlesselman found that breastfeeding and not "time since last delivery" increased the risk of perforation [2].

When counseling a patient for contraception after the management of a migrated or expulsed IUD, repeat placement of an IUD is not contraindicated. If an IUD is the preferred contraceptive method of the patient and no other contraindications have emerged further limiting an IUD as a safe option, an IUD may be placed. However, uterine size is an important variable; uterine cavities measuring less than 6 cm may have an increased rate of expulsion. Understandably, patients with IUD migration or expulsion may be reluctant to use an IUD again as a preferred contraceptive agent.

Key Teaching Points

- If IUD strings are not visualized at the time of IUD surveillance, in many cases, a cytobrush can be utilized to sweep the endocervical canal to draw IUD strings into the vagina.

- Transvaginal ultrasound is the best imaging modality to determine IUD placement and position within the uterus.

- An anteroposterior and lateral radiograph should be used to determine if the IUD is located within the peritoneal cavity or has been expulsed when ultrasound fails to identify intrauterine IUD placement.

References

1. American College of Obstetricians and Gynecologists. Long-Acting Reversible Contraception: Implants and Intrauterine Devices. ACOG Practices Bulletin no 121. American College of Obstetricians and Gynecologists, Washington, DC; 2011. Accessed August 5, 2017.

2. Heartwell SF, Schlesselman S. Risk of uterine perforation among users of intrauterine devices. *Obstet Gynecol* 1983;61(1):31–36.

3. Peri N, Graham D, Levine D. Imaging of intrauterine contraceptive devices. *Journal of Ultrasound in Medicine* 2007;26:1389–1401.

4. Boortz HE, Margolis DJ, Ragavendra N, Patel MK, Kadell BM, Migration of intrauterine devices: radiologic findings and implications for patient care. *RadioGraphics* 2012; 32(2):335–352.

5. Benacerraf BR, Shipp TD, Bromley B. Three dimensional ultrasound detection of abnormally located intrauterine contraceptive devices which are a source of pelvic pain and abnormal bleeding. *Ultrasound Obstet Gynecol* 2009;34:110–115.

6. Nowitzki KM, Hoimes ML, Chen B, Zheng LZ, Kim YH. Ultrasonography of intrauterine devices. *Ultrasonography* 2015;34(3):183–194.

7. Madden T, McNicholas C, Zhao Q et al. Association of age and parity with intrauterine device expulsion. *Obstet Gynecol* 2014;124(4):718–726.

8. Uçar MG, Şanlıkan F, Ilhan TT, Göçmen A, Çelik Ç. Management of intra-abdominally translocated contraceptive devices, is surgery the only way to treat this problem? *J Obstet Gynaecol* 2017 May;37 (4):480–486.

9. World Health Organization: Mechanism of action, safety and efficacy of intrauterine devices. Report of a WHO scientific group. Technical Report Series 753. Geneva, WHO Health Organization, 1987, pp 1–91.[9]

10. Heinemann K, Reed S, Moehner S, Do Minh T. Risk of uterine perforation with levonorgestrel – releasing and copper intrauterine devices in the European Active Surveillance Study on Intrauterine Devices. *Contraception* 2015;91:274–279.

A 29-Year-Old HIV-Positive Woman Requesting Oral Contraceptive Pills

Patricia Huguelet

History of Present Illness

A 29-year-old gravida 1, para 1, female presents to the office requesting a refill of her oral contraception. Her medical history is significant for human immunodeficiency virus (HIV), diagnosed three years ago. She reports regular follow-up with the infectious disease clinic and daily compliance with her antiretroviral therapy. She is currently taking two nucleoside reverse transcriptase inhibitors, Zidovudine and Stavudine, and one non-nucleoside reverse transcriptase inhibitor, efavirenz, to manage her HIV. She reports regular monthly withdrawal bleeds and is overall very happy with her current method of contraception. She is in a monogamous, heterosexual relationship and uses condoms regularly as her partner is HIV negative.

Past medical history	HIV – diagnosed three years prior. Compliant with medications
Past surgical history	Cesarean section at term for breech presentation, uncomplicated
Medications	Zidovudine, stavudine, efavirenz, and ethinyl estradiol 0.03 mg/desogestrel 0.15 mg

Physical Examination

General appearance	Healthy-appearing woman, in no apparent distress
Vital Signs	
Temperature	37.1°C
Pulse	72 beats/min
Blood pressure	110/62 mmHg
Respiratory rate	16 breaths/min
Lungs	Clear bilaterally, no rhonchi, rales, or wheezes
Cardiovascular	Regular rate and rhythm, no murmurs
Abdomen	Soft, non-tender, non-distended, no masses
Pelvic	Deferred
Laboratory Studies	
CD4 count	1,200 cells/mm^3
Viral load	undetectable

How Would You Manage the Patient?

Although hormonal contraception is safe and effective in HIV-infected women on multidrug antiretroviral therapy, studies have shown decreased hormonal contraceptive levels in the setting of efavirenz and certain other HIV medications. Therefore, this patient should be counseled on the theoretical decreased efficacy of her hormonal contraception. She should be encouraged to continue with dual therapy, with consistent use of condoms and oral contraception. Alternatively, she may be offered an intrauterine device for improved contraceptive efficacy.

HIV Medications and Oral Contraceptive Pills

Around the world, an estimated 35.3 million people are living with HIV and women comprise nearly half of those infected [1, 2]. While the spread of HIV has slowed, addressing the health needs of women infected with HIV remains a priority. Women living with HIV are often of reproductive age, and many desire and need effective contraception to prevent pregnancy. This is not only essential to the health of the woman but also to her future children. The majority of children acquire HIV through vertical transmission from mother to fetus, so effective contraception is essential [1].

Oral contraceptives, including combined oral contraceptive pills (COCs) and progestin-only pills (POPs), are highly effective methods of contraception, with failure rates of 1 percent with perfect use and 8 percent with typical use [3]. Contraceptive hormones are metabolized by the hepatic cytochrome (CYP) P450 pathway, which is also responsible for the metabolism of many antiretroviral drugs (ARVs). Orally administered contraceptive hormones are subject to extensive first-pass hepatic metabolism. Systemic hormonal contraceptives work by negative feedback inhibition of the hypothalamic-pituitary-ovarian (HPO) axis, with additive effects on cervical mucus and the endometrium. Both exogenous estrogen and progestin suppress the HPO axis. However, most of the contraceptive effects, including ovulation suppression, endometrial thinning, and cervical mucus thickening, are due to progestin and are dose-dependent [1]. Ethinyl estradiol (EE), the estrogenic component of most currently marketed COCs, induces ovulation suppression and is primarily metabolized through the hepatic CYP pathway. Specifically, hydroxylation of EE is catalyzed by the hepatic enzymes CYP3A4 and CYP2C9 [2, 3].

Management of patients with HIV typically involves a combination of ARVs, commonly referred to as highly active antiretroviral therapy (HAART), as monotherapy frequently leads to the development of viral resistance to drug therapy. Typically, a patient will be started on a HAART regimen that includes two nucleoside reverse transcriptase inhibitors (NRTIs) and a protease inhibitor (PI), two NRTIs and a non-nucleoside reverse transcriptase inhibitor (NNRTI), or three NRTIs [1]. Ritonavir, a PI, is rarely used for its own antiretroviral activity, but is used for its inhibitory effect on CYP3A4, the liver enzyme that normally metabolizes PIs. Ritonavir is used to enhance other PIs, thereby improving ARV efficacy.

Since ARVs and contraceptive pills are both metabolized by the CYP system, ARVs could theoretically decrease contraceptive efficacy, leading to unintended pregnancy, or increase levels of the contraceptive method, leading to toxicity. Similarly, hormonal contraceptives could theoretically decrease efficacy of ARVs, leading to increased likelihood of treatment failure, or conversely toxicity. Unfortunately, most evidence regarding hormonal contraception and ARV therapy

Box 23.1 Categories of medical eligibility criteria for contraceptive use

Category	Recommendation
Category 1	Condition for which there is no restriction for use of the contraceptive method
Category 2	Condition for which the advantages of using the method generally outweigh the theoretical or proven risks
Category 3	Condition for which the theoretical or proven risks usually outweigh the advantages of using the method
Category 4	Condition that represents an unacceptable health risk if the contraceptive method is used

Table 23.1 Antiretroviral and contraceptive drug interactions: CDC MEC recommendations

	Progestin-only pills (POPs)	Combined oral contraceptive pills (COCPs)
Nucleoside reverse transcriptase inhibitors (NRTIs)	1	1
Abacavir	1	1
Tenofovir	1	1
Zidovudine	1	1
Lamivudine	1	1
Didanosine	1	1
Emtricitabine	1	1
Stavudine	1	1
Non-nucleoside reverse transcriptase inhibitors (NNRTIs)	2	2
Efavirenz	1	1
Etravirine	1	1
Nevirapine	1	1
Rilpivirine		
Ritonavir-boosted protease inhibitors (PIs)	2	2
Ritonavir-boosted atazanavir	2	2
Ritonavir-boosted darunavir	2	2
Ritonavir-boosted fosamprenavir	1	1
Ritonavir-boosted lopinavir	2	2
Ritonavir-boosted saquinavir	2	2
Ritonavir-boosted tipranavir		
PIs without ritonavir		
Atazanavir	1	2
Fosamprenavir	2	3
Indinavir	1	1
Nelfinavir	2	2
CCR5 co-receptor antagonists	1	1
HIV integrase strand transfer inhibitors	1	1
Fusion inhibitors	1	1

is based on pharmacokinetic studies and secondary analysis, rather than prospective clinical trials assessing pregnancy failure [4]. Given the theoretical concern of drug interactions between hormonal contraception and ARV therapy, as both are metabolized by the CYP pathway, patients must be advised that full efficacy cannot be guaranteed. This is particularly true for estrogen-containing COCs, as estrogen is primarily metabolized through the hepatic CYP pathway.

The Centers for Disease Control (CDC) annually publishes recommendations on the safe use of contraceptive methods for women with various medical conditions [5]. Health-care providers can use the medical eligibility categories (Box 23.1) when assessing the safety of a contraceptive method for a particular patient's medical condition. On an annual basis, the most recent medical literature is reviewed and updates are made to the guidelines. Table 23.1 summarizes the 2016 medical eligibility criteria for HIV-infected women on ARV therapy. Notably the recommendations can be summarized as follows:

- NRTIs do not appear to have significant risk for interactions with oral contraceptive pills.

- Drug interactions exist between POPs/COCs and efavirenz, which may reduce contraceptive hormone levels.
- Drug interactions exist between POPs/COCs and Ritonavir-boosted PIs, as well as certain unboosted PIs, which may reduce contraceptive hormone levels.
- Specific studies of fosamprenavir and COCs demonstrated decreased concentration of fosamprenavir and theoretical decreased *efficacy of the ARV*, resulting in the only Category 3 rating among all ARVs.

An equally important question for providers and patients is whether hormonal contraception affects transmission and progression of HIV and AIDS. Overall, evidence does not support an association between oral contraceptives and risk for HIV acquisition, nor progression of disease [6, 7].

Based on the available evidence, women using oral contraceptive pills should either use an additional contraceptive method or change methods if they are using efavirenz or a boosted PI. In women seeking hormonal contraception using fosamprenavir, the risk of decreased ARV efficacy outweighs the benefit and an alternative contraceptive method should be recommended by healthcare providers. Interactions are not problematic with NRTIs and patients can be reassured of full clinical efficacy with their oral contraceptive method. Additionally, all patients with HIV should be counseled that dual contraception, with the concomitant use of condoms and additional contraception, is the optimal contraceptive strategy to reduce heterosexual transmission of HIV and other sexually transmitted infections, and to minimize the risk of unintended pregnancy [8].

Key Teaching Points

- Contraception is important in order to optimize women's health care and to prevent vertical transmission, the leading cause of HIV acquisition for children.
- Hormonal contraception, including COCs and POPs, generally is considered safe for use by HIV-infected women, including those who use ARV therapy.
- Health-care providers should consider drug-specific interactions between ARV therapy and certain hormonal contraceptives when counseling patients about the best options, particularly when patients are taking efavirenz, ritonavir-boosted PIs, and fosamprenavir.

References

1. Phillips S, Steyn P, Temmerman M. Contraceptive options for women living with HIV. *Best Pract Res Clin Obstet Gynaecol* 2014;**28**: 881–90.

2. Robinson JA, Jamshidi R, Burke AE. Contraception for the HIV-positive woman: a review of interactions between hormonal contraception and antiretroviral therapy. *Infect Dis Obstet Gynecol* 2012;**2012**:1–15.

3. Amy JJ, Tripathi V. Contraception for women: an evidence based overview. *BMJ* 2009;**339**:563–568.

4. Nanda K, Stuart G, Robinson J et al. Drug interactions between hormonal contraceptives and antiretrovirals. *AIDS* 2017;**31**:917–952.

5. Curtis KM, Tepper NK, Jatlaoui TC et al. U.S. medical eligibility criteria for contraceptive use, 2016. *MMWR Recomm Rep* 2016;**65**:1–103.

6. Polis CB, Curtis KM. Use of hormonal contraceptives and HIV acquisition in women: a systematic review of the epidemiological evidence. *The Lancet* 2013;**13**:797–807.

7. Phillips SJ, Polis CB, Curtis KM. The safety of hormonal contraceptives for women living with HIV and their sexual partners. *Contraception* 2016; **93**:11–16.

8. American College of Obstetricians and Gynecologists. Gynecologic care for women and adolescents with human immunodeficiency virus. Practice Bulletin No. 167. *Obstet Gynecol* 2016; **128**:e89–110.

A 42-Year-Old Woman with IUD and *Actinomyces* on Cervical Cytology

Regan N. Theiler

History of Present Illness

A 42-year-old, gravida 3, para 2–0–1–2, woman presents for her routine well-woman visit and the review of systems is without specific complaints. She has a history of copper T380 intrauterine device (IUD) insertion five years prior to presentation. When discussing her reproductive life planning, she states that she and her husband are finished child-bearing. She is satisfied with her IUD and desires to keep her current contraceptive method for several more years. She has been in a monogamous relationship for 12 years and denies concerns for sexually transmitted infection.

Her pap history includes no history of previously abnormal testing with her last screen five years prior to this visit. Her menstrual history is unremarkable, with moderate menstrual bleeding for four to five days every four weeks. She denies intermenstrual bleeding or dysmenorrhea.

She has no significant medical or surgical history. Her pregnancies were uncomplicated.

Physical Examination

General appearance	Well-appearing, appears stated age and no acute distress

Vital Signs

Temp	36.8°C
Pulse	65 beats/min
BP	111/69 mmHg
Weight	134 lb
Height	64 inches
BMI	26 kg/m²
HEENT	Normocephalic, conjunctiva anicteric. Neck without thyromegaly or lymphadenopathy
Cardiovascular	Regular rate and rhythm, no murmurs/rubs/gallops
Pulmonary	Lungs clear bilaterally, normal effort
Abdomen	Soft, non-tender. No masses or surgical scars. Normoactive bowel sounds
Extremities	No edema or clubbing. No calf tenderness

Pelvic

External genitalia	Normal architecture, without lesions
Urethra	Normal meatus, no hypermobility or masses
Bartholin's, Skene's ducts	Normal openings without masses
Vagina	Moist with normal rugae. No abnormal discharge or blood. No cystocele or rectocele
Cervix	Parous without lesions. IUD strings not visualized. No cervical motion tenderness. Liquid cytology/HPV testing was performed
Uterus	Six weeks' size, anteverted, non-tender, and mobile
Adnexa	Non-palpable, non-tender

Laboratory Studies

Liquid-based pap	Negative for intraepithelial lesion or malignancy. Adequate cellularity with endocervical cells seen. *Actinomyces seen on cytology* (Figure 24.1).
HPV testing	Negative for high-risk HPV types

Imaging

Transvaginal ultrasound	Small, anteverted uterus with IUD in normal position in the endometrial cavity. Normal bilateral adnexa and no free fluid in the pelvis.

How Would You Manage This Patient?

The patient has a copper IUD correctly positioned in her uterus, and the device is colonized with *Actinomyces*. On follow-up visit, the patient denies any pelvic pain. She has no unusual vaginal discharge, fever, dyspareunia, or urinary symptoms. She is relieved to know that her IUD is appropriately located in her uterus and prefers to continue her current contraceptive device if it is a safe option for her.

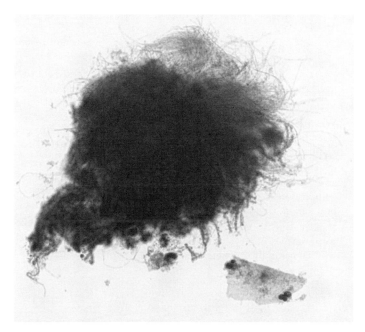

Figure 24.1 *Actinomyces*: Branching clusters of Gram-positive bacilli on liquid-based cervical cytology from a patient with an IUD. Courtesy of Lananh N. Nguyen

Because she is asymptomatic and desires to continue her IUD as her preferred contraceptive method, a plan is made for routine annual follow-up and precautions given to call the office should she develop any pelvic pain or fevers.

Actinomyces Colonization in IUD Users

Detection of *Actinomyces israelii* and other *Actinomyces* species in the cervical and vaginal smears of women with intrauterine contraceptive devices is a phenomenon that has been recognized for decades. Gram-positive bacteria in the *Actinomyces* genus are uniquely recognizable on cytology and Gram stain because of their arrangement of bacilli in branching, filamentous "spider" formations (Figure 24.1). Several species of *Actinomyces* are known to be members of the female genital flora, with *Actinomyces israelii* being the most usual cause of pelvic pathology. *Actinomyces urogenitalis* and other species have been identified in urogenital specimens, and other non-*Actinomyces* organisms can look similar to *Actinomyces* bacilli on pap cytology [1]. Given this heterogeneity of species known to reside in the urogenital tract, the literature often refers to detection of *Actinomyces*-like organisms (ALOs) on cervical cytology [2]. One study has compared rates of ALO detection between liquid-based cytology and conventional smear specimens, with markedly higher detection rates noted in liquid-based cytology specimens [3].

Prevalence of *Actinomyces* colonization increases with duration of IUD use, reaching colonization rates of 25 percent after several years of IUD use in some studies [4, 5]. The finding of *Actinomyces* in pap smears of non-IUD users is exceedingly rare, with most studies reporting 0 percent incidence. IUD-specific genital colonization may be related to formation of biofilms, as has been demonstrated in vitro on the surface of copper-containing devices [6]. Many studies have sought to answer the question of whether specific devices are more prone than others for colonization with ALOs. These studies have found conflicting results, with some suggesting higher colonization of plastic devices and some finding higher colonization rates with copper IUDs. The most consistent finding among these studies has been a correlation between increased colonization rate and longer time of IUD use.

As in the case described above, *Actinomyces* is often diagnosed as an incidental finding during routine cervical cancer screening. Actinomyces on cytology in the absence of other symptoms rarely (0.001 percent) leads to pelvic *Actinomyces*. Treatment with antibiotics and/or removal of the device are/is not recommended [7, 8].

Multiple case reports have described pelvic actinomycosis with tubo-ovarian abscesses and bowel collections mimicking malignant processes [9, 10]. Such cases may be associated with fever and other systemic symptoms and may present with or without acute pelvic inflammatory disease. Cases of pelvic actinomycosis may occur in the presence or absence of an IUD and should be suspected in the setting of complex, disseminated pelvic disease. For patients with symptomatic pelvic actinomycosis, antimicrobial therapy should be initiated. If an IUD is present, it should be removed. *Actinomyces* species are sensitive to penicillin, with the treatment of choice being oral or parenteral ampicillin or amoxicillin/clavulanate for cases of Gram stain confirmed pelvic actinomycosis.

Key Teaching Points

- A finding of *Actinomyces* on screening cervical cytology is associated with the presence of an intrauterine contraceptive device.
- *Actinomyces* colonization of the female genital tract is largely asymptomatic and does not require treatment.
- The IUD may remain in situ in the presence of asymptomatic *Actinomyces* colonization.

References

1. Bhagavan BS, Gupta PK. Genital actinomycosis and intrauterine contraceptive devices. Cytopathologic diagnosis and clinical significance. *Hum Pathol* 1978;**9**(5):567–578.

2. Westhoff C. IUDs and colonization or infection with Actinomyces. *Contraception* 2007;**75**(6 Suppl):S48–50.

3. Cheung ANY et al. Liquid-based cytology and conventional cervical smears: a comparison study in an Asian screening population. *Cancer* 2003;**99**(6):331–335.

4. Kalaichelvan V, Maw AA, Singh K. Actinomyces in cervical smears of women using the intrauterine device in Singapore. *Contraception* 2006;**73**(4):352–355.

5. Merki-Feld GS et al. The incidence of actinomyces-like organisms in Papanicolaou-stained smears of copper- and levonorgestrel-releasing intrauterine devices. *Contraception* 2000;**61**(6):365–368.

6. Carrillo M et al. In vitro Actinomyces israelii biofilm development on IUD copper surfaces. *Contraception* 2010;**81**(3):261–264.

7. American College of Obstetricians and Gynecologists. Long acting reversible contraceptives: implants and intrauterine devices. Practice Bulletin 121. *Obstet Gynecol* 2011;**118**:186–194.

8. American College of Obstetricians and Gynecologists. Clinical challenges of long-acting reversible contraceptive methods. Committee Opinion 672. *Obstet Gynecol* 2016;**129**:e69–77.

9. Muller-Holzner E et al. IUD-associated pelvic actinomycosis: a report of five cases. *Int J Gynecol Pathol* 1995;**14**(1):70–74.

10. Nugteren SK et al. Colitis and lower abdominal mass by Actinomyces israelii in a patient with an IUD. *Neth J Med* 1996;**49**(2):73–76.

A 25-Year-Old Woman with a History of Pulmonary Embolism on OCPs Who Desires Contraception

Hedwige Saint Louis

History of Present Illness

A 25-year-old nulliparous woman presents to the office for contraceptive counseling. She reports regular menstrual cycles of normal duration and flow with her stated last menstrual period three weeks prior to this visit. Her past medical history is significant for a pulmonary embolus diagnosed at age 23, which occurred two months after initiation of combination oral contraceptives. The pulmonary embolus was not associated with trauma, surgery, or other exacerbating events. She was treated initially with Lovenox and transitioned to warfarin, which was discontinued after three months since she had no known risk factors. Her initial evaluation included screenings for antithrombin III, protein C and protein S deficiency, Lupus anticoagulant, Factor V Leiden mutation, and prothrombin mutation due to a family history of a deep vein thrombosis (DVT) that were reported as normal.

The patient is not currently on anticoagulation therapy and review of symptoms is negative for dizziness, dyspnea, calf tenderness, and chest pain. She has been sexually active, using barrier contraceptives inconsistently. She desires a more reliable contraceptive method.

Her past medical history is otherwise unremarkable and her past surgical history is negative. She had negative cervical cytology performed at the time of initiation of oral contraceptives.

She has no known drug allergies, does not smoke, and only drinks socially. Her medications include a vitamin B supplement, fish oil, and a daily multivitamin.

Physical Examination

General appearance	Well-nourished, well-developed young woman, appearing her stated age, in no acute distress, alert, and oriented
Vital Signs	
Temperature	36.1°C
Pulse	72 beats/min
Blood pressure	118/56 mmHg
Respiratory rate	16 breaths/min
Oxygen saturation	100% on room air
Weight	150 lb
Height	5 feet 6 inches
BMI	24.2 kg/m^2
Heart	Regular rate and rhythm
Lungs	Clear to auscultation

How Would You Manage This Patient?

Given this patient's past medical history of pulmonary embolus presumably induced with estrogen exposure in combined oral contraceptive, her options for effective and reliable contraception as advised by the US Medical Education Criteria (US MEC) published by the CDC include

- Copper intrauterine device (first-line option-US MEC 1)
- Progesterone contraceptives (second-line option-US MEC 2) including
  - Levonorgestrel (LNG) intrauterine device
  - Depomedroxyprogesterone acetate (DMPA)
  - Etonorgestrel implant (Nexplanon)
  - Progesterone-only oral contraceptive pill (POP)

Additionally, the patient should be counseled on less effective alternatives such as barrier methods, fertility awareness-based methods, and withdrawal. The limited efficacy of these methods should be discussed, focusing on the patient's increased risk of recurrent thromboembolus in pregnancy should failure occur.

Given her normal menstrual cycle, a nonhormonal agent such as a copper-containing intrauterine device would be the best recommendation for this patient. A copper-containing IUD has a low failure rate and does not have the hormonal agent that could potentiate her risk of a recurrent DVT. If mutually agreed upon, the IUD can be placed without difficulty and the patient educated on the appropriate confirmation of IUD placement. Although a pelvic exam is not mandatory for contraceptive counseling, this patient should be offered STI screening given her history of inconsistent condom use.

If the patient desires same-day placement, STI screening can be performed concomitantly. If there are findings concerning for an active STI at the time of placement, treatment can be initiated and placement delayed for three to four weeks days.

Deep Vein Thrombosis and Combined Hormonal Contraceptives

DVT and pulmonary embolism (PE) affect as many as 900,000 people in the United States [1]. Risk factors for DVT/PE include cigarette smoking, obesity, pregnancy, exposure to estrogen-containing contraceptive and hormone replacement therapy, immobilization, surgery, and trauma. Predisposing genetic factors such as Factor V Leiden mutation have been found in about 5–8 percent of cases. Certain chronic medical illnesses such as congestive heart failure and cancer also predispose to DVT/PE. In women of childbearing age who are not using hormonal contraceptives, the incidence of DVT/PE is about 1 in 10,000. The risk is increased three- to fivefold for women on estrogen-containing hormonal contraceptives and is significantly higher during pregnancy (four- to fivefold), especially in the postpartum period [2, 3].

The link between estrogen-containing oral contraceptives and thromboembolism has been established since the introduction of the oral contraceptive pill (OCP) in 1960 [4]. Epidemiological studies identified both a time- and dose-dependent link between estrogen and the risk of thromboembolism, i.e., the longer the duration of use and the lower the dose of estrogen, the lower the risk of DVT/PE [5]. This evidence spurred the reformulation of the oral contraceptive pill with lower doses of estrogen.

The link between progestogens and DVT/PE has been difficult to demonstrate and an association was not thought to exist until studies comparing third-generation progestogens such as gestodene, drospironone, and desogestrel to second-generation progestogens such as levonorgestrel indicated a slight increased risk of DVT/PE [5, 6].

Estrogen increases DVT/PE risk by increasing the concentration of clotting factors II, VII, X, and XII, factor VIII, and fibrinogen and predisposing the clotting system toward clot formation. Data also indicate that third-generation progestogens increase plasma concentration of factor VII, thus further increasing the risk of DVT/PE. [7].

Based on the CDC's 2016 US Medical Eligibility Criteria (US MEC) for contraceptive use, a history of PE on estrogen-containing oral contraceptives increases the risk for recurrent thromboembolic event [8]. A copper intrauterine device is considered MEC 1, providing a safe, reliable, long-acting reversible contraceptive that will not increase the risk of a thromboembolic event. Progesterone contraceptives, including levonorgestrel intrauterine devices, subdermal implants, depo-medroxyprogesterone injections, and progestin-only pills, are considered acceptable but second-line agents for this patient due to the potential risk of thromboembolism associated with progesterone [8].

Regarding the risk of DVT/PE, the 2016 US MEC for contraceptive use provides the following guidelines [8]:

- Women without risk factors for recurrence of thromboembolic events should be counseled similarly as those with risk factors, with the exception that combined hormonal contraceptives (CHC) are considered US MEC 3, meaning CHC are not recommended unless there are no viable alternatives for the patient.

- For women with acute DVT/PE, whether on anticoagulant therapy or not, both copper-containing IUDs and progesterone-only contraceptives are considered US MEC 2, secondary to the potential risk of increased bleeding that is associated with both categories of these contraceptives.

- Again in these women the risk of recurrence determines whether CHC are considered US MEC 3 or US MEC 4 category.

- In women with a family history of a first-degree relative with DVT/PE but no personal history of thromboembolic event, the copper-containing IUD and progesterone-only contraceptives are considered MEC 1, while CHC are MEC 2 and can be offered as an alternative to the patient.

- For women undergoing major surgery who are facing prolonged immobilization, CHC are considered US MEC 4

and should not be offered due to the significant risk they pose to the patient. Alternative options include the copper-containing IUD (US MEC 1) or progesterone-only contraceptives (US MEC 2). If a patient is having minor surgery or is not anticipating prolonged immobilization after major surgery, she can be offered any method safely, including CHC (MEC2).

Other nonhormonal forms of contraception, including barrier methods, fertility awareness-based methods, and withdrawal, should also be discussed as alternatives for patients presenting with history of deep venous thrombosis or pulmonary embolus. Though less effective, these methods may be more acceptable to the patient and are a better option than not providing any contraception and putting the patient at risk for pregnancy, which is associated with a higher rate of recurrent DVT/PE and concomitant complications. The high failure rate associated with these methods should be discussed.

Key Teaching Points

- Women at increased risk for thromboembolic events, DVT/PE, should be offered effective, reliable contraception since the risk of DVT/PE is greater in pregnancy than while using hormonal contraception.

- The risk of thromboembolic event on estrogen-containing contraceptives is dose- and time-dependent: the longer the duration of use and the lower the dose of estrogen, the lower the risk of thromboembolic event.

- A copper intrauterine device should be considered a first-line contraceptive option for patients with history of a thromboembolic event or who are at increased risk for a thromboembolic event, who are not on anticoagulation therapy, as the most effective nonhormonal contraceptive currently available.

- Women on anticoagulation therapy can be offered LNG IUDs as these contraceptive agents do not seem to pose an increased bleeding risk and may be helpful in managing menorrhagia in these women.

- The US MEC for contraceptive use should be used by providers as a tool to counsel and help women identify the most reliable, effective, and accessible contraceptive option that is acceptable to them through shared decision making. However, respecting patient autonomy, women should be fully informed about *all* their choices, from the most effective to the least effective contraceptive.

- A pelvic exam is not mandatory with contraceptive counseling regardless of the patient's sexual history. Unless the patient has gynecological complaints, a pelvic exam is of low yield. However, the patient should be offered STI testing based on their sexual history and risk factors.

References

1. Center for Disease Control and Prevention. Venous Thromboembolism: Data & Statistics. 2017. www.cdc.gov/ncbddd/dvt/data.html (accessed June 12, 2017.)

2. Pomp ER, Lenselink AM, Rosendaal FR, Doggen CJ. Pregnancy, the postpartum period and prothrombotic defects: risk of venous thrombosis in the MEGA study. *J Thromb Haemost* 2008 April 6;**4**: 632–637.

3. Heit JA, Kobbervig CE, James AH et al. Trends in the incidence of venous thromboembolism during pregnancy or postpartum: a 30-year population-based study. *Ann Intern Med* 2005 November 15. 143(10):697–706.

4. Vandenbroucke Jan P, Rosing Jan, Kitty WM et al. Oral contraceptives and the risk of venous thrombosis. *N Engl J Med* 2001;**344**:1527–1535.

5. Lidegaard O, Lokkegaard E, Svendsen AL, Agger C. Hormonal contraception and risk of venous thromboembolism: national follow-up study. *BMJ* 2009;**339**:b2890.

6. Committee on Gynecologic Practice. ACOG Committee Opinion Number 540: risk of venous thromboembolism among users of drospirenone-containing oral contraceptive pills. *Obstet Gynecol* 2012;**120**:1239–1242.

7. Evidence-Based Medicine Consult. The Mechanism of Oral Contraceptive (Birth Control Pill) Induced Clot or Thrombus Formation (DVT, VTE, PE). 2015. www.ebmconsult.com/articles/oral-contraceptive-clotting-factors-thrombosis-dvt-pe (accessed June 12, 2017).

8. Curtis KM, Tepper NK, Jatlaoui TC et al. U.S. Medical Eligibility Criteria for Contraceptive Use, 2016. *MMWR Recomm Rep* 2016; 65(No. RR-3):1–104.

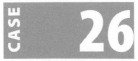

A Pregnant 22-Year-Old Woman Who Desires Long-Acting Postpartum Birth Control (Immediate Postpartum LARC)

Stacey L. Holman

History of Present Illness

A 22-year-old female, gravida 2, para 1, presents for routine prenatal care visit at 24 weeks gestation. Postpartum contraceptive counseling is routinely scheduled in the third trimester in your practice. During counseling, the patient states that she is in a monogamous relationship with her current partner and they do not plan to have another child for several years. She has successfully used oral contraceptives prior to her first pregnancy and during the interpregnancy interval. She is now interested in a method that does not require her to remember to take a daily pill. She plans to breastfeed.

Her gynecologic history is significant only for regular, heavy menses, which have been controlled by combined oral contraceptive pills in the past. She has no history of sexually transmitted infections and cervical cancer screening is up-to-date. She has no medical problems and denies any surgeries. Her last delivery was uncomplicated and she delivered at term. She has no known drug allergies.

Physical Examination

Vital Signs

Temperature	98.6
Heart rate	88 bpm
Blood pressure	125/81
Fetal heart tones	144 bpm
General appearance	Well developed, no acute distress
Abdomen	Gravid, non-tender, fundal height 24 cm

Pelvic (from Initial Obstetric Physical Exam)

Normal external genitalia, normal vagina
without lesion or discharge

Cervix	no lesions
Uterus	16 weeks globular (consistent with gestational age)
Adnexa	non-tender, no masses palpated

Laboratory Studies (from Her Initial Visit at 16 Weeks Gestation)

Pap smear	Negative for intraepithelial lesion or malignancy
Gonorrhea	Negative
Chlamydia	Negative

How Would You Manage This Patient?

During counseling, all options for birth control are reviewed with the patient, including barrier methods, hormonal agents, long-acting reversible contraceptive (LARC) choices (implant and intrauterine device [IUD]), and permanent sterilization. Risks and benefits of immediate versus postpartum forms of LARC placement are discussed with the patient. The patient has no contraindications to immediate postpartum LARC based on the US Medical Eligibility Criteria for Contraceptive Use (US MEC). She is also informed that if a hemorrhage or uterine infection occurs at the time of delivery, she will no longer be a candidate for an IUD.

Through shared decision making, the patient elects for postpartum placement of an IUD immediately following delivery of the placenta. She delivers a term, 7 lb 6 oz female infant and has placement of a levonorgestrel IUD approximately 5 minutes after delivery of the placenta using the manual insertion technique. When following up at her postpartum visit, IUD strings are visualized extending from the cervical os. She is counseled for removal and replacement if desired at the appropriate time interval based on the package insert for the selected device.

Long-Acting Reversible Contraception in the Immediate Postpartum Period

Contraceptive services continue to be critical in the United States as nearly 50 percent of pregnancies are unintended. Highest-risk populations for unintended pregnancy include women of young age (18–24), women of low socioeconomic status, women who cohabitate, and minority groups [1]. According to 2014 data from the Guttmacher Institute, nearly 38 million women in the United States were in need of contraception [2]. Of those women who used contraception (those who were sexually active and able to become pregnant but did not wish to become so), 18 percent had incorrect or inconsistent use of their method. The inconsistent use in this cohort contributed to approximately 40 percent of the total unintended pregnancies [2].

Because LARC methods have the highest effectiveness, continuation rates, and potential to reduce unintended pregnancy [3], the American Congress of Obstetricians and Gynecologists (ACOG) recommends LARCs as first-line contraceptive methods for most women. Postpartum timing of LARC is optimal as many patients are highly motivated to avoid unintended pregnancies, and the location is convenient for both provider and patient. Pregnancy in the postpartum state is a valid concern with studies showing that nearly 45 percent of women have intercourse before the postpartum appointment [4]. With proper prenatal counseling and appropriate patient selection, an IUD or an implant can be offered to most patients in the immediate postpartum period or prior to discharge, respectively.

The statistics above provide supporting evidence for the utilization of immediate postpartum LARC use. While ACOG and the Centers for Disease Control and Prevention (CDC) support immediate postpartum LARC, the timing of placement is not consistent within the indications provided by the

Table 26.1 Postpartum LARC selection as defined by breastfeeding and timing of placement

Condition	Cu-IUD	LNG-IUD	Implant
Immediate postplacental IUD placement:			
Breastfeeding			
<10 minutes after placenta	1	2	-
10 minutes to <4 weeks	2	2	-
Non-breastfeeding			
<10 minutes after placenta	1	1	-
10 minutes to <4 weeks	2	2	-
Postpartum implant placement:			
Breastfeeding			
<21 days	-	-	2
21–29 days	-	-	2
30+ days	-	-	1
Non-breastfeeding			
<21 days	-	-	1
21–29 days	-	-	1
30+ days	-	-	1

Adapted from the CDC U.S. Medical Eligibility Criteria, 2016

manufacturer. It is considered to be an off-label use not approved by the Food and Drug Administration (FDA).

IUD selection for immediate postpartum LARC placement includes the copper-containing IUD, whose mechanisms of action include inhibition of sperm migration and damage to the traveling ovum. This device has FDA approval for ten years of use. The levonorgestrel IUD can also be used, and its mechanisms of action include suppression of the endometrium and changes in viscosity of cervical mucus. There are several commercially available levonorgestrel IUDs available. These include

1. 52 mg – approved for five years (Mirena)
2. 13.5 mg – approved for three years (Skyla)
3. 19.5 mg – approved for five years (Kyleena)
4. 52 mg – approved for four years (Liletta)

Also available is the 68 mg etonogestrel implant which is placed subdermally and has FDA approval for three years of use; however, similar to the IUD, it is not approved for immediate postpartum placement. The mechanism of action for the contraceptive implant is to suppress ovulation by altering the axis between the hypothalamus, pituitary gland, and ovaries. The implant also functions to alter cervical mucus and suppress endometrial activity.

The safety profile for each selected device should be checked with the US MEC from the CDC prior to placement

[5]. Medical comorbidities should also be considered when selecting the appropriate device. In addition, breastfeeding after postpartum LARC placement is considered safe (see Table 26.1).

Counseling regarding postpartum utilization of LARC should include the following:

- Advantages – immediate contraception, convenience, >99 percent efficacy
- Disadvantages – potential for low reimbursement, higher rate of IUD expulsion as compared to interval placement (10–25 percent)
- Contraindications:
  - IUD – intrauterine infection at time of delivery, postpartum hemorrhage, puerperal sepsis, any contraindication by US MEC criteria
  - Implant – any contraindication by US MEC criteria

The etonogestrel implant can be inserted at any time prior to discharge from the hospital by following the standard aseptic technique recommended by the manufacturer.

Placement of an IUD should occur within the first 10 minutes after placental delivery [4, 5]. Formal training in postpartum insertion techniques is recommended and is a requirement in many facilities. Providers must be familiar with postpartum anatomy, obtain consent for placement of the

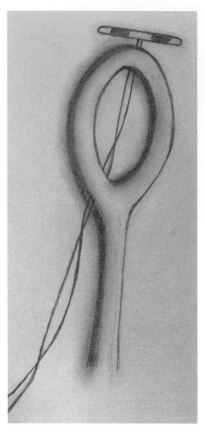

Figure 26.1 Ring forceps technique: horizontal arms within the forceps, strings falling away from the instrument, ratchets of forceps not fully closed. *Illustration courtesy of Amber C. Abney*

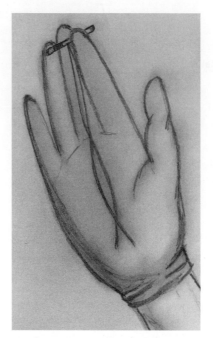

Figure 26.2 Manual insertion technique: vertical arm held between index and middle fingers of dominant hand. *Illustration courtesy of Amber C. Abney*

device, and review the patient's status after delivery to ensure that eligibility criteria are still applicable.

Method of insertion of IUD:

1. The IUD is removed from the inserter and the horizontal arms of the device are grasped gently with ring forceps (see Figure 26.1).
2. After vaginal delivery and removal of the placenta, the IUD is passed through the cervix and placed at the fundus. The abdominal hand can be used to confirm proper placement. Manual placement of the IUD can also be performed (see Figure 26.2).
3. Once proper placement is achieved, the strings are trimmed above the hymen.
4. In a cesarean delivery, once the placenta has been removed and the uterus is hemostatic, the IUD is placed at the fundus manually or with ring forceps. The strings are then gently pushed into the cervix and the hysterotomy is closed.

Routine post-procedure counseling should be performed prior to discharge. Consider ultrasound confirmation if any concerns arise during the procedure. At the time of scheduled postpartum visit, visible string extruding from the cervix should be confirmed. If no string is confirmed, ultrasound should be employed to ensure the presence and proper placement of the device.

Key Teaching Points

- LARC should be considered as a first-line option for most reproductive-age women.
- Breastfeeding is not contraindicated with any method of LARC utilization.
- Postplacental IUD placement should be performed only if there is no evidence of amniotic infection, sepsis, or postpartum hemorrhage.
- Expulsion rates for post-placental IUD are 10–25 percent, and the patient must be made aware of this risk during prenatal contraception counseling.

References

1. Immediate postpartum long-acting reversible contraception. *ACOG Committee Opinion #670*, August 2016.
2. www.guttmacher.org/pubs/fb_contraceptive_serv.html (accessed July 2017)
3. Trussell J. Contraceptive failure in the United States. *Contraception* 2011;83 (5):397–404.
4. Long-acting reversible contraception: implants and intrauterine devices. *ACOG Practice Bulletin #121*, July 2011.
5. www.cdc.gov/reproductivehealth/contraception/mmwr/mec/summary.html (accessed July 2017)

A 33-Year-Old G4P4 Unable to Palpate Implant Desiring Removal

Michael K. Chinn

History of Present Illness

A 33-year-old female, gravida 4, para 4, with a five-month history of utilizing an etonogestrel implant is referred by her primary care provider for implant removal. Her primary care provider noted that the implant was not palpable on his exam. The primary care provider ordered X-rays and confirmed an implant was in the arm (Figure 27.1).

The patient is requesting removal, secondary to menstrual complaints. She has had irregular bleeding and long menses >7 days with her cycles, which are difficult to track. Her last menstrual period began two weeks prior to presentation and has not subsided. She uses both pads and tampons, and will change every 3 hours normally, but has been changing every 1–2 hours for the last 2 days. She also complains of decreased libido. She is requesting removal and a change in contraceptive method. The patient reports never being able to feel the implant and having a very large bruise after placement.

Review of symptoms is negative for any pelvic pain and she reports no recent intercourse due to the bleeding. She denies easy bleeding or bruising and reports normal cycles of four days duration until the implant was placed.

She has no significant past medical or surgical history. She has been married for seven years. She has no allergies to medications. Her only medication is a daily multivitamin.

Physical Examination

Vital Signs

Temperature	37.0°C
Pulse	69 beats/min
Blood pressure	109/63 mmHg
Respiratory rate	16 breaths/min
Height	65 inches
Weight	122 lb
BMI	20.3 kg/m^2
General appearance	Well-developed, well-nourished woman in no apparent distress

Extremity Exam

Thin left arm with minimal subcutaneous fat and unable to palpate implant. Small scar in left arm consistent with implant placement.

Laboratory Studies

Urine pregnancy test	Negative
HB	14.8 g/dL
HCT	43.1%
WBCs	8,300/μL
Platelets	230,000/μl

How Would You Manage This Patient?

The patient has clinical documentation of placement of an implant and a scar consistent with that placement. X-ray

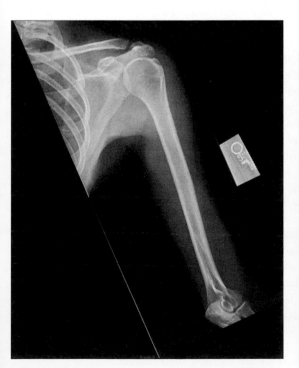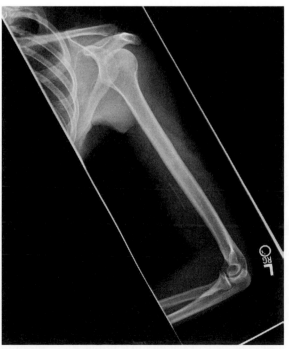

Figure 27.1 Radiology images: X-ray of left upper arm. Implant is barely visible over the distal humerus on the A/P view. In the lateral image implant is clearly seen parallel to the humerus.

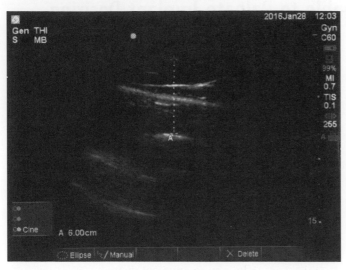

Figure 27.2 Ultrasound image of left arm showing depth of implant.

confirmation by the primary care provider demonstrated implant placement. As the implant was not palpable, ultrasound with a high-frequency probe was used to identify the implant's location and to identify any involvement in critical vascular or nervous structures. The ultrasound probe was placed parallel to the axis of the arm and just above the scar. The implant appeared as hyperechoic and 4 cm in length (Figure 27.2). Removal using the "Pop-out" technique was performed.

The "Pop-out" removal technique was performed by placing a 5–10 mm incision at the end of the implant along the long axis of the implant [1]. The incision was made along the long axis of the implant to allow for extension of the incision if the implant did not pop out or if the implant could not be grasped. With the opposite hand, the index finger was applied to the end of the implant opposite of the incision to push the other end of the implant toward the incision. The implant had a fibrous capsule due to the duration of placement. A mosquito clamp was used to grasp the implant as close to the skin as possible, and due to the fibrous capsule, a scalpel was used on the circular end of the implant to separate the pseudo capsule; a second clamp was then used to grasp the freed implant for removal. After the implant was removed, the skin was reapproximated with a Steri-Strip.

Contraceptive counseling was performed and the patient opted for combined oral contraceptive pills while she is considering another option for long-acting reversible contraception.

Deep Placement of Etonogestrel Implant

Deep insertion of etonogestrel implant is estimated at 1 per 1,000 uses [2]. Placement of an implant deep into the subcutaneous tissue is more common with patients of higher BMI. Placement into muscle can occur with any patient but patients with a low BMI are at higher risk [3]. Confirmation of placement by provider and patient is an essential patient safety step of the placement procedure. The patient's ability to continue to

confirm location is important for confidence in ongoing contraception and to note if migration has occurred. Post procedure, if the provider and the patient cannot confirm placement through palpation, then immediate removal should be considered.

Most deep placements are presumed to result at the time of insertion rather than migration. Deep placement can damage blood vessels, muscle, and nerves. X-rays are essential to identify the presence of a radio-opaque implant when ultrasound imaging is not available. Anterior-posterior view and lateral images are helpful to identify the location of the implant. Ultrasound is essential for successful safe removal of non-palpable implants by identifying the depth of the implant and significant surrounding blood vessels and nerves. Ultrasound may be used for identification and location primarily in experienced hands if a prior radiograph has not been obtained.

Once the location of implant has been confirmed by imaging, then reexamination of the patient with palpitation and/or ultrasound is performed for removal. In a study of referrals to an implant service in the United Kingdom, one-third of the implants were palpable on at least one end and most implants deeper than 3 mm were not palpable [4]. An ultrasound probe with a high-frequency transducer (15–18 MHz) is recommended to identify the implant and other important surrounding structures, such as the blood vessels (brachial artery and vein) and nerves (brachial plexus.)

Once the location of the implant is identified by ultrasound in a patient with a non-palpable implant, a marking pen may be used to indicate the direction of the implant in arm. The skin should be marked with the arm in the same position as the planned removal to avoid misaligning the implant and skin. Supination or pronation of the arm will alter the alignment. Identification of surrounding significant blood vessels, nerves, and muscle will determine which end of the implant is safest to remove. The end of the implant closest to the insertion scar is typically closest to the skin unless migration has occurred. Implant location near significant blood vessels or nerves should warrant consultation with orthopedics or general surgery. Removal of an implant has been described with fluoroscopy guidance [5]. If the implant is unidentifiable on ultrasound, MRI may be indicated to determine the exact location of the implant.

Most deep implants are in the subcutaneous tissue and can be grasped and elevated with mosquito clamps. The "Pop-out" technique recommended by the manufacturer and the Food and Drug Administration is very effective once the implant end is grasped and elevated to the incision. Additionally, a modified "U" technique using a modified vasectomy clamp removal described by Chen and Creinin that was previously recommended for the six-rod implant may be utilized [1]. In this technique, a 5 mm incision is performed on top of the implant and in the same direction. A straight hemostatic clamp is used to bluntly dissect the subcutaneous tissue to the level of the implant. The modified vasectomy clamp is used to bring the implant to the incision for removal.

For implants located in muscle, the fascia surrounding the muscle may need to be excised in order to remove the implant. An assistant to hold skin retractors may be necessary for direct visualization of the muscle fascia.

Due to the difficulty with identification and removal of deeply placed implants, recommendations have been made to create centers for referral and removal [6, 7]. Pillai recommends an experienced professional with knowledge of the anatomy of the upper extremity and access to a high-frequency ultrasound. A standard protocol that includes skin labeling and a minimal volume of at least 12 cases per year is recommended. A musculoskeletal radiologist and a surgeon for complicated cases should be associated with the center. Quality assurance is also a defined essential component and requires the provision of follow-up and education to providers of patients with more frequent deep placements [6].

Key Teaching Points

- Palpation of etonogestrel implant by provider and patient should occur directly after insertion.
- X-ray of the arm with both lateral and anterior-posterior views or ultrasound is recommended to confirm the presence and location of a non-palpable implant.
- Ultrasound with a high-frequency (15–18 MHz) probe is recommended to identify and mark the location of non-palpable implant prior to removal.
- Ultrasound guidance during the procedure to avoid damage to significant surrounding blood vessels and nerves is recommended.
- An implant located in close proximity to critical blood vessels or nerves on imaging should warrant referral to a specialized center or to interventional radiology or surgery for removal.

References

1. Mansour D, Walling M, Glenn D et al. Removal of non-palpable etonogestrel implants. *J Fam Plann Reprod Health Care* April 2014;40:126–132.

2. Mansour D. Nexplanon: what Implanon did next. *J Fam Plann Reprod Health Care* October 2010;36:187–189.

3. Mansour D, Fraser IS, Walling M et al. Methods of accurate localisation of non-palpable subdermal contraceptive implants. *J Fam Plann Reprod Health Care* January 2008;34:9–12.

4. Brown M, Britton J. Neuropathy associated with etonogestrel implant insertion. *Contraception* November 2012;86:591–593.

5. Guiahi M, Tocce K, Teal S, Green T, Rochon P. Removal of Nexplanon implant located in the biceps muscle using a combination of ultrasound and fluoroscopy guidance. *Contraception* December 2014;90(6): 606–608.

6. Pillai M, Cazet AC, Griffiths M. Continuing need for and provision of a service for non-standard implant removal. *J Fam Plann Reprod Health Care* April 2014;40:126–132.

7. Chen, M, Creinin M. Removal of a nonpalpable etonogestrel implant with preprocedure ultrasonography and modified vasectomy clamp. *Obstet Gynecol* November 2015;126(5): 935–938.

A 24-Year-Old Woman with a Contraceptive Implant Placed Three Weeks Ago Presents with Positive Pregnancy Test

Roxanne Jamshidi

History of Present Illness

A 24-year-old woman presents with a positive pregnancy test after missing her period. Her last normal menstrual period began five weeks and four days prior to this presentation. Three weeks prior to this presentation, she had a contraceptive implant placed. The patient reports very mild menstrual like cramping, but no bleeding. She denies nausea, vomiting, fevers, dizziness, discharge, or urinary symptoms. Her last bowel movement was one day ago.

Her past medical history is significant for epilepsy, controlled on anti-seizure medications. She has had no seizure activity for three years. Her past surgical history is significant for tonsillectomy as a child. She is in a long-term monogamous relationship with her boyfriend of three years. She does not smoke and drinks alcohol occasionally. She has no known drug allergies. Her only medication is lamotrigine.

Physical Examination

General appearance	Well-developed, well-appearing woman who appears nervous but comfortable

Vital Signs

Temperature	37.1°C
Pulse	76 beats/min
Blood pressure	115/68 mmHg
Respiratory rate	16 breaths/min
Height	66 inches
Weight	135 lb
BMI	21.8
Abdomen	Soft, non-tender, non-distended, no guarding or rebound
External genitalia	Unremarkable
Vagina	Moist, normal ruggae, no lesions, scant physiologic appearing discharge
Cervix	Nulliparous, no lesions, closed
Uterus	Anteverted, slightly globular, mobile, non-tender
Adnexa	No masses or tenderness bilaterally

Laboratory Studies

Urine pregnancy test	Positive
Beta-hCG	2,025 mIU/mL
Blood group and Rh	A positive
WBCs	9,700/μL
Hgb	11.6 g/dL
Hct	36.0%
Platelet count	293,000/μL
Imaging	Transvaginal ultrasound shows normal uterus with an intrauterine sac but no yolk sac present, normal ovaries bilaterally, no free fluid

How Would You Manage This Patient?

The patient is approximately six weeks pregnant with a contraceptive implant in place. From the timing of her last menstrual period, she most likely had an early luteal phase pregnancy at the time of her implant insertion. Intrauterine pregnancy should be documented; increased ectopic pregnancy risk has been associated with conception in the presence of a progestin-containing contraceptive. In this case, ultrasound was performed and showed the characteristic eccentric location within the uterine cavity and a double decidual sign. However, if there had been uncertainty about the location of the pregnancy, her hCG level could be followed. Repeat ultrasound in a few days should demonstrate the presence of a yolk sac. The patient was counseled about her pregnancy options, and decided to undergo a surgical abortion, which was uncomplicated. Because the contraceptive implant was placed after conception, this pregnancy is not considered a method failure, but rather a mistimed insertion. She was counseled regarding contraceptive options and she decided to maintain the implant for contraception.

Contraceptive Implants and Pregnancy

As with initiation of other contraceptive methods, pregnancy should be excluded prior to insertion of a contraceptive implant. Pregnancy can usually be excluded through a detailed history. According to the Centers for Disease Control and Prevention [1], a health-care provider can be reasonably certain that a woman is not pregnant if any of the following criteria are met:

- ≤7 days since the start of a normal menses
- No sexual intercourse since the start of last normal menses
- Consistent and correct use of a reliable method of contraception
- ≤7 days after a spontaneous or induced abortion
- Within four weeks of delivery
- Exclusively or nearly exclusively breastfeeding, amenorrheic, and less than six months postpartum.

If these criteria are met, a health-care provider can be 99–100 percent assured that the patient is not pregnant (i.e., negative predictive value) prior to insertion of a contraceptive device.

Routine pregnancy tests are not required prior to insertion of a contraceptive implant. However, a health-care provider may use clinical judgment to decide if a pregnancy test is indicated and should be aware of the limitations of the test relative to the timing of last intercourse and recent pregnancy. For example, for a woman with oligomenorrhea who presents desiring an implant, last menses five weeks prior to presentation and last intercourse two weeks prior to presentation, a pregnancy test might be useful. Additionally, emergency contraceptive pills (levonorgestrel or ulipristal) can be recommended if unprotected intercourse occurred within five days of presentation. Although the efficacy of ulipristal theoretically may be decreased by concomitant start of a hormonal implant, the benefit of starting the implant right away is generally considered to outweigh the risk of delaying insertion [1].

The American College of Obstetricians and Gynecologists recommends providing implant insertion on the same day requested if pregnancy can be reasonably excluded [2]. In situations when a health-care provider may be uncertain if a woman is already pregnant, the benefits of immediate placement of the implant generally outweigh the risk of delaying initiation. In those situations where pregnancy cannot be reliably excluded, performing a follow-up pregnancy test two to four weeks after insertion is recommended. Pregnancy outcomes among women who are exposed to combined hormonal contraception in early pregnancy do not have an increased risk of birth defects or adverse pregnancy outcomes [3,4]. Similarly, exposure to etonogestrel early in pregnancy is not expected to have teratogenic effects [4].

For women not using a hormonal method of contraception with a contraceptive implant placed within the first five days of the menstrual cycle, backup contraception is not recommended. Summarized in Table 28.1 are other considerations when backup contraception is not recommended. For women in whom a contraceptive implant is placed outside of the window as described in Table 28.1, pregnancy should be reasonably excluded and a backup method of contraception (e.g., abstinence or a barrier method) is recommended for seven days after insertion.

A medication history should be taken prior to contraceptive implant insertion. Medications and herbal supplements that induce hepatic enzymes, including cytochrome P-450 3A4, may decrease the plasma concentration of progestins and therefore decrease efficacy of the contraceptive implant. For the etonogestrel implant in particular, the following drugs or herbal products induce metabolism of progestin and therefore decrease contraceptive efficacy:

- barbiturates
- bosentan
- carbamazepine
- felbamate
- griseofulvin
- oxcarbazepine
- phenytoin
- rifampin
- St. John's wort
- topiramate

In addition, HIV protease inhibitors and non-nucleoside reverse transcriptase inhibitors may also decrease efficacy of the implant by reducing progestin levels. Patients should be

Table 28.1 Timing of contraceptive implant

Previous contraceptive method or state	Timing of insertion
None	During the first 5 days of menstrual cycle
Combined hormonal contraception	On the same day or the day following the last pill, or removal of the patch or ring
Progestin-only contraceptive pill	Within 24 hours of last pill
Progestin-only injectable contraception	Before next dose is due
Progestin implant or intrauterine system	Same day as removal
First trimester termination of pregnancy or miscarriage	Within 5 days of abortion or miscarriage
Second trimester termination of pregnancy or miscarriage	Within 21–28 days following the abortion or miscarriage
Postpartum	Within 21–28 days of delivery

reminded to inform other health-care providers of their contraceptive agent, so that this history can be utilized in recommended treatment and choice of pharmaceuticals.

When a pregnancy is diagnosed with a contraceptive implant in place, ectopic pregnancy must be excluded. Progestin-only methods of contraception are thought to impact tubal motility and therefore increase the risk of ectopic pregnancy if a contraceptive failure were to occur. Ectopic pregnancies among women using the etonogestrel implant with concomitant use of a cytochrome P-450 hepatic enzyme inducer have been reported. Overall, the contraceptive implant, in particular the etonogestrel implant, is extremely effective. The actual incidence of ectopic pregnancy in patients using the etonogestrel implant is unknown and may not actually be increased [5]. However, because of the possible increased risk, ectopic pregnancy should be ruled out in cases of a contraceptive failure or pregnancy conceived immediately prior to the implant insertion. A history of a previous ectopic pregnancy is not a contraindication to a contraceptive implant.

When an unplanned intrauterine pregnancy is diagnosed concomitantly in a patient using a contraceptive, counseling for pregnancy options should be employed. Although there are no known adverse effects of the implant on pregnancy, the implant should be removed if the patient plans to maintain the pregnancy. If the patient chooses to terminate her pregnancy and the implant was likely placed shortly after conception, the patient may retain the implant as her contraceptive method as the pregnancy was not a contraceptive failure but rather an error in timing of placement.

Patients with a contraceptive failure with the etonogestrel implant who have an early unintended and undesired pregnancy have the option of surgical or medical abortion. Surgical abortion may be preferred if the pregnancy is very early and ectopic pregnancy cannot yet be excluded (e.g., hCG below discriminatory zone, or intrauterine sac only seen and patient prefers to terminate pregnancy right away rather than continuing to follow hCG levels or follow ultrasound findings). Theoretically, the efficacy of medication abortion may be diminished in the presence of a contraceptive implant as the progestin could counteract the effects of mifepristone. However, decreased efficacy was not demonstrated when the etonogestrel implant was placed concomitantly with administration of mifepristone [6]. Thus, a patient with a contraceptive implant desiring medical termination of pregnancy could be offered the standard mifepristone and misoprostol regimen. She should be counseled that the exact effects of the implant on abortion efficacy are unknown.

Key Teaching Points

- A contraceptive implant can be inserted when a health-care provider is reasonably certain that a patient is not already pregnant.
- If recent unprotected intercourse has occurred, emergency contraception should be offered with implant insertion. Patients presenting in the luteal phase can be offered insertion of implant, with counseling that a pregnancy test in two to four weeks is recommended to rule out an early pregnancy.
- If the implant is placed outside the recommended period (see Table 28.1), backup contraception (barrier or abstinence) is recommended for seven days after insertion.
- Once an ectopic pregnancy has been ruled out in a woman who is pregnant with an etonogestrel implant, she should be counseled about her pregnancy options.

References

1. Curtis KM, Jatlaoui TC, Tepper NK et al. U.S. selected practice recommendations for contraceptive use, 2016. *MMWR Recomm Rep* 2016;**65**:1–320.

2. American College of Obstetricians and Gynecologists. Increasing access to contraceptive implants and intrauterine devices to reduce unintended pregnancy. Committee Opinion No. 642. *Obstet Gynecol* 2015;**126**:e44–48.

3. Charlton BM, Molgaard-Nielsen D, Svanstrom H et al. Maternal use of oral contraceptives and risk of birth defects in Denmark: prospective, nationwide cohort study. *BMJ* 2016; **352**:h6712.

4. Curtis KM, Tepper NK, Jatlaoui TC et al. U.S. medical eligibility criteria for contraceptive use, 2016. *MMWR Recomm Rep* 2016;**65**:1–104.

5. Callahan R, Yacobson I, Halpern V, Nanda K. Ectopic pregnancy with use of progestin-only injectables and contraceptive implants: a systematic review. *Contraception* 2015;**92**:514–522.

6. Raymond EG, Waever MA, Tan Y et al. Effect of immediate compared with delayed insertion of etonogestrel implants on medical abortion efficacy and repeat pregnancy: a randomized controlled trial. *Obstet Gynecol* 2016;**127**: 306–312.

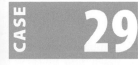

A 32-Year-Old HIV-Positive Woman Requesting IUD

Christy M. Boraas

History of Present Illness

A 32-year-old, gravida 2, para 1-0-1-1, female with past medical history significant for human immunodeficiency virus (HIV) infection presents to clinic for a contraception consultation. She was recently diagnosed and has been taking antiretroviral therapy (ART) for six months. She desires to prevent pregnancy for at least one year. She is interested in a long-acting, reversible contraception (LARC) method, specifically an intrauterine device (IUD). She no longer has a current sexual partner with whom she used condoms (last intercourse six weeks ago), and her last menstrual period was six days ago.

The remainder of her past medical history is unremarkable. Her past surgical history includes a dilation and curettage for missed abortion in the first trimester. She had one term vaginal delivery at age 27 prior to her HIV diagnosis. She has regular menses of four days duration. She is single and reports a four-pack-year smoking history. She has no allergies and her only medications include her three-drug ART regimen.

Physical Examination

General appearance	Well developed, well nourished

Vital Signs

Temperature	37.0°C
Pulse	89 beats/min
Blood pressure	121/79 mmHg
Respiratory rate	18 breaths/min
Height	64 inches
Weight	165 lb
BMI	28.3 kg/m^2
Cardiovascular	Regular rate and rhythm, no murmurs
Pulmonary	Clear to auscultation bilaterally, no crackles or wheezes
Abdomen	Normoactive bowel sounds, soft, non-tender, non-distended
External genitalia	Normal female, no lesions
Cervix	Parous in appearance, no lesions or masses, closed
Uterus	Not enlarged, anteverted, mobile, non-tender
Adnexa	No masses, non-tender

Laboratory Studies

Urine pregnancy test	Negative
CD4 T-cells	500 cells/mm^3
Hb	12.5 g/dL
HIV viral load	<50 copies/mL
Electrolytes and liver function tests	Within normal limits

How Would You Manage This Patient?

This patient is requesting an IUD for LARC. The combination of last intercourse, regular menses, menstrual cycle day 6, and negative urine pregnancy test reliably exclude pregnancy. Her HIV disease is well controlled on ART as evidenced by her undetectable viral load and normal CD4 T-cell count, and she reports no history of tuberculosis.

The patient was counseled about available contraceptive options and she strongly prefers an IUD. Differences between copper IUD and hormonal IUD options were reviewed with the patient. She elected a five-year levonorgestrel IUD that was inserted at her appointment with same-day testing for other sexually transmitted infections (STIs). She was also counseled about dual method use with a barrier method such as a male or female condom for prevention of HIV transmission, cervical neoplasia, and acquisition of STIs from a future partner(s).

HIV-Positive Women and Contraception

Women living with HIV have many options for both desired fertility and contraception. Empowering HIV-positive women to help plan pregnancies is an important component of prevention of perinatal HIV transmission. Providing patient-centered reproductive life planning counseling, including management of HIV during pregnancy and options for contraception, is an important strategy to help women living with HIV optimize their health. To assess a patient's reproductive life goals, asking whether she desires pregnancy in the coming year is an excellent first question.

For HIV-positive women who are not interested in future childbearing, options for sterilization utilizing laparoscopic and hysteroscopic approaches should be reviewed. For any woman who wishes to delay or prevent pregnancy, taking a thorough medical, surgical, obstetrical, gynecological, sexual, and other social history can elicit other health conditions or behaviors that may limit safe use of some contraceptive options. Comorbid conditions such as hypertension, diabetes, and venous thromboembolism should be considered especially for estrogen-containing contraceptive methods. The Centers for Disease Control and Prevention's (CDC) US Medical Eligibility Criteria for Contraceptive Use (US MEC) can provide assistance when trying to select a safe contraceptive method for a patient with particular comorbidity [1]. Close attention should also be paid to the HIV-positive patient's current medications as some antiretroviral medications, most notably efavirenz, can induce the cytochrome p450 pathway and reduce systemic contraceptive progestin exposure and contraceptive efficacy [2]. The patient should also be assessed for history of tuberculosis (TB) as active pelvic TB is a relative contraindication for IUD initiation, and certain TB medications, such as rifampicin, have drug-drug interactions with other available contraceptive methods [3].

To provide patient-centered contraceptive counseling, assessing a patient's contraceptive use history (side effects, both positive and negative) and goals and expectations for use of a new contraceptive method is paramount. Additionally, ensuring patients have evidence-based information regarding available

Table 29.1 US medical eligibility criteria for contraceptive use for HIV infection [1]

Condition	Subcondition	LNG-IUD		Cu-IUD		Implant	Injection	POP	Combined pill, patch, ring
		I	C	I	C				
HIV						1*	1*	1*	1*
	Clinically well receiving ART	1	1	1	1				
	Not clinically well or not receiving ART	2	1	2	1				

1 = Use without restrictions
2 = Advantages generally outweigh risks
I = Initiation, C = Continuation
* Drug-drug interaction
Cu-IUD, copper intra-uterine device; LNG-IUD, levonorgestrel intrauterine device; POP, progestogen-only pill

options is crucial as patients may receive inaccurate information. If a patient is truly undecided about a desired method, many providers advocate consideration of an approach beginning with methods most effective at preventing pregnancy. This conversation can be facilitated by a visual aid chart with tiers based on the efficacy of methods with the most effective (IUDs, implants, and permanent sterilization), the moderately effective (injections, pills, ring, patch, and diaphragm), and the lowest effective methods (condoms, withdrawal, sponge, fertility awareness/calendar-based method, spermicide) listed [4].

For the HIV-positive woman, HIV alone is not a contraindication to the use of any particular method (Table 29.1) and the use of hormonal contraception has not been shown to accelerate HIV disease progression [5]. Assisting an HIV-positive woman make a contraceptive choice should involve shared decision making between the patient and the provider and aim at identification of the method most likely to achieve prevention of pregnancy and other desired positive side effects and minimize potential negative method-associated side effects. For women motivated to use a more user-independent method, LARC including IUDs and contraceptive implants prevents the need to remember to take a pill or return to clinic for injections. LARC methods are very effective and safe, and have low risk of complications. While up-front costs are higher, LARC methods are more cost-effective over time.

IUDs are a great choice for many women living with HIV, given their high effectiveness, continuation, and satisfaction rates, and no known drug-drug interactions with ART medications. Clinically well HIV-positive women have no increased risk of IUD complications or infection compared to HIV uninfected women [6]. IUD use by HIV-positive women is not associated with increased risk for transmission to sexual partners [6]. Women using an IUD who develop AIDS should be monitored for signs and symptoms of pelvic infection. Pelvic inflammatory disease does not necessitate IUD removal unless symptoms persist or worsen despite appropriate therapy [7]. Further counseling regarding potential expected bleeding profiles, Food and Drug Administration (FDA) approved

length of use, and likely reduced risk over time of ascending infections with levonorgestrel IUDs will further help a patient decide between a copper and hormonal (levonorgestrel) IUD.

The copper IUD (ParaGard) is FDA approved for use for 10 years with evidence supporting off-label use up to 12 years. Approximately 0.8 percent of women will experience an unintended pregnancy within the first year of typical use of the copper IUD [8]. Four different levonorgestrel IUDs are currently on the market, three with FDA approval up to five years of use (Mirena, Liletta, and Kyleena) and one with FDA approval up to three years of use (Skyla). Only 0.2 percent of women using the Mirena IUD will experience an unintended pregnancy in the first year of use [8]. The contraceptive implant is another LARC method generally safe and effective for use by HIV-positive women. The etonogestrel implant (Nexplanon) is FDA approved for use for up to three years, with growing evidence of efficacy for up to four years of use. Typical use unintended pregnancy rate in the first year of use is 0.05 percent [8]. Particular attention must be paid to an HIV-positive woman's medication regimen. If she is taking certain medications that are expected to have drug-drug interactions with the implant or other progestin-containing methods, in particular efavirenz, the associated decreased contraceptive efficacy should be included in counseling. Other available hormonal moderately effective methods would include injectable contraceptives (depo-medroxyprogesterone acetate), combined hormonal contraceptives (pill, patch, ring), and progestin-only pills. Each has typical use unintended pregnancy rates between 6 and 9 percent and a host of potential positive and negative side effects to consider for each patient [8].

Other contraceptive considerations somewhat unique to HIV-positive women must include dual use/dual protection and a discussion of potential contraception and ART drug interactions. Dual use of a more effective method of contraception in addition to condoms (male or female) is recommended in order to prevent HIV or other STIs transmission to a sexual partner and acquisition of other STIs. Male condoms are not an ideal first choice for contraception, given their 18 percent typical use failure rate in the first year of use [8]. Spermicides are another contraceptive method that may be used alone but are often used in addition to a barrier method of contraception. The active ingredient in many spermicides is nonoxyl-9, which can increase the risk of both acquisition and transmission of HIV by causing vaginal mucosal irritation and epithelial erosions. Thus, HIV-positive women should be counseled against using spermicides.

Many antiretroviral medications affect hepatic cytochrome p450 enzyme pathways; steroid contraceptives are metabolized by cytochrome p450 enzymes. Therefore, coadministration of systemic hormonal contraceptives and ART can lead to drug-drug interactions that decrease efficacy of systemic hormonal contraceptives. As previously discussed, most concerning is the non-nucleoside reverse transcriptase inhibitor, efavirenz, which may reduce the progestin hormone in serum by over 50 percent and, thus, affect contraceptive efficacy with the greatest concern for the contraceptive implant [2]. Additionally, ritonavir-boosted protease inhibitors are cytochrome p450 inhibitors that increase the serum levels of progestin contraceptive steroid hormone in studies of oral contraceptive pills and implants leading to concerns about increased side effects, though clinical studies have failed to demonstrate such an effect. Conversely, ritonavir-boosted protease inhibitors also decrease the estrogen component of combined contraceptive pills [2]. For women utilizing these medications for ART, a higher dose of ethinyl estradiol may be needed to prevent breakthrough bleeding. The US MEC has a separate condition section on ART. Most oral progestin-containing methods and the implant are US MEC category 2 (advantages of use generally outweigh risks). Counseling regarding these few circumstances more unique to the HIV-positive patient requesting contraception is necessary to help empower a woman to choose her best method.

Key Teaching Points

- Living with HIV is not a contraindication to the use of any particular contraceptive method; however, there are important considerations.
- LARC methods are highly effective and safe for women with HIV to use.
- Interactions exist between the antiretroviral medication, efavirenz, and systemic hormonal contraceptives that may limit contraceptive effectiveness.
- Dual contraceptive method use inclusive of a barrier method (condom) is important for limiting HIV transmission and lowering risk of other STIs.

References

1. Curtis KM, Tepper NK, Jatlaoui TC et al. U.S. medical eligibility criteria for contraceptive use, 2016. *MMWR Recomm Rep* 2016;65(No.RR-3):1–104.

2. Scarsi KK, Darin KM, Chappell C et al. Drug-drug interactions, effectiveness, and safety of hormonal contraceptives in women living with HIV. *Drug Saf* 2016 November;39(11):1053–1072. Review.

3. Haddad LB, Tarleton J, Sheth AN, Ofotokun, I. Contraception for women living with HIV. In: Allen RH and Cwiak CA, eds. *Contraception for the Medically Challenging Patient.* New York, Springer Science+Business Media. 2014; 93–117.

4. The Centers for Disease Control and Prevention. Effectiveness of Family Planning Methods. www.cdc.gov/reproductivehealth/unintendedpregnancy/pdf/contraceptive_methods_508.pdf. (Accessed May 1, 2017.)

5. Phillips SJ, Polis CB, Curtis KM. The safety of hormonal contraceptives for women living with HIV and their sexual partners. *Contraception* 2016 January;93(1):11–16. Review.

6. Tepper NK, Curtis KM, Nanda K, Jamieson DJ. Safety of intrauterine devices among women with HIV: a systematic review. *Contraception* 2016 December;94 (6):713–724. Review.

7. Tepper NK, Steenland MW, Garffield ME et al. Retention of intrauterine devices in women who acquire pelvic inflammatory disease: a systematic review. *Contraception* 2013 May;87(5): 655–660. Review.

8. Hatcher RA, Trussel J, Stewart FH, et al. *Contraceptive Technology, 20th* rev ed. New York, Ardent Media, Inc.; 2011, 791–792.

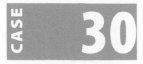

CASE 30

A 23-Year-Old Woman Presents Two Hours after Sexual Assault

Shandhini Raidoo

History of Present Illness

A 23-year-old female, gravida 0, presents as an unscheduled emergency to the office reporting that she was sexually assaulted by an acquaintance the night prior to her presentation. She reports that she was at a party when an acquaintance approached her. They began talking and he led her to a room at the back of the house where he forced her to perform fellatio and penile-vaginal intercourse. She denies any severe physical injury during the assault. She reports that the assailant used a condom initially but removed it prior to ejaculation. She did not lose consciousness at any point during the assault. Immediately following the assault, she told a friend, who suggested that she be evaluated by a physician. She has not changed her clothes or bathed since the assault occurred because her friend advised her that evidence would need to be collected. She has not yet considered whether she would like to press charges against the assailant.

She has no significant past medical history. She has no allergies and does not currently take any medications. She has been sexually active in the past but is not currently using any method of contraception. The first day of her last menstrual period was nine days ago. She denies any tobacco or illicit drug use and consumes alcohol on weekends. She denies any history of childhood sexual abuse or prior sexual assault.

Physical Examination

Vital Signs

Temperature	37.6°C
Blood pressure	110/65
Pulse	85 beats/min
Respiratory rate	16 breaths/min
BMI	22.1
General appearance	Well-appearing anxious woman, tearful, in no acute distress
Cardiovascular	Regular rate and rhythm
Pulmonary	Clear to auscultation bilaterally
Abdomen	Normoactive bowel sounds, soft, non-tender
Extremities	Bruising on bilateral upper arms
Pelvic	Exam deferred to emergency department

How Would You Manage This Patient?

This patient was counseled about the need for a comprehensive evaluation, including collection of a forensic rape kit, and the limited resources available in the office setting to perform this evaluation. She was advised to present to the emergency department where a sexual assault nurse examiner (SANE) was contacted who performed a detailed examination and collected a forensic rape kit of evidence. At the time of the

SANE examination, pregnancy and STI testing were done, and the patient was given a dose of emergency contraception as well as empiric treatment for gonorrhea, chlamydia, and trichomoniasis. She was counseled about the risk for HIV acquisition and offered HIV postexposure prophylaxis. She was offered a referral for mental health counseling services. A follow-up appointment in the office was scheduled in one week.

Sexual Assault

Sexual assault is prevalent and often underreported. Sexual assault may vary from sexual coercion to inappropriate sexual contact to rape, including oral, anal, or vaginal penetration and penetration with an object [1]. Eighteen percent of women report having experienced rape at some point in their lifetime, with the majority of women having experienced rape by a current or former intimate partner or an acquaintance [2]. Fourteen percent of women report experiencing rape by an unknown assailant [2]. State laws may vary in their definitions of assault and rape, and often define these crimes with regard to the victim's relationship to the assailant. Women who experience sexual assault are at risk for unintended pregnancy, STIs, and long-term mental health consequences as a result of the assault [3]. Guidelines for STI testing, empiric treatment, prophylaxis, and follow-up testing are summarized in Table 30.1.

Prompt and sensitive evaluation by an experienced clinician is important in order to minimize the potentially traumatic impact of an examination on the survivor. On initial exam, a detailed objective history of the assault should be taken and the survivor's narrative accurately documented. Physical injuries may range from minor bruises and scratches to more severe lacerations and fractures [1]. Any severe injuries must be addressed rapidly and stabilized. All injuries, including minor ones, should be documented with photographic evidence when possible and included in a forensic rape kit. If a woman contacts a provider prior to presenting to a hospital or emergency room, she should be instructed not to change clothes, bathe, urinate, defecate, eat, drink, or wash her mouth or skin to ensure comprehensive evidence collection [1].

Many hospitals and emergency departments have healthcare professionals, SANEs, or sexual assault forensic examiners, who are specifically trained in the examination of sexual assault survivors. If available, they should be contacted when a survivor presents for evaluation. Sexual assault examiners will conduct a detailed examination and collect a forensic rape kit, samples of clothing, hair, blood, semen, saliva, and other bodily fluids that can be used to identify the assailant and as evidence in the survivor's case. This evidence should be collected and stored even if the survivor is uncertain about pursuing legal action.

A pregnancy test done at the time of the assault will detect a preexisting pregnancy. It is important to assess the survivor's

Table 30.1 Post-sexual assault STI testing and prophylaxis

STI	Testing at initial evaluation	Empiric treatment/ prophylaxis	Follow-up testing
Gonorrhea	NAAT at all sites of penetration	Ceftriaxone 250 mg IM once AND azithromycin 1 g orally once	Not indicated unless survivor has not previously been tested
Chlamydia	NAAT at all sites of penetration	Azithromycin 1 g orally once	Not indicated unless survivor has not previously been tested
Trichomoniasis	Vaginal or urine NAAT, wet mount, or point-of-care DNA probe testing	Metronidazole OR tinidazole 2 g orally once	Not indicated unless survivor has not previously been tested
Syphilis	Serum syphilis testing (RPR, VDRL, or syphilis IgG)	None	• 4–6 weeks • 3 months
Hepatitis B	Serum HBsAg; serum HBsAb if previously vaccinated but immunity not documented	If survivor is unvaccinated and: • Assailant is HBsAg positive: HBIG, initiate hepatitis B vaccine series • Assailant's status is unknown: initiate hepatitis B vaccine series If survivor is vaccinated but immunity is not documented: single booster dose of hepatitis B vaccine	None
HIV	Serum HIV testing	28-day course of postexposure prophylaxis IF survivor is high-risk for having acquired HIV	• 6 weeks • 3 months • 6 months
HPV	None	If survivor is unvaccinated and ≤26 years old: initiate HPV vaccine series	Consider physical exam for anogenital warts 1–2 months after assault

RPR, rapid plasma reagin; VDRL, Venereal Disease Research Laboratory test
Adapted from Workowski and Bolan [4]

risk for pregnancy from the assault, including current contraceptive method and adherence to the method. Emergency contraception should be offered to all survivors who present within 120 hours of a sexual assault incident, and it is recommended that hospitals and emergency departments have emergency contraceptive methods such as levonorgestrel or ulipristral acetate immediately available to provide to survivors in a timely manner [1, 4]. All survivors should be counseled to take a pregnancy test two to three weeks after the sexual assault incident regardless of whether or not they used emergency contraception.

Gonorrhea, chlamydia, and trichomoniasis are the most commonly diagnosed STIs following a sexual assault, and this reflects the high prevalence of these STIs in the population [4]. Nucleic acid amplification testing (NAAT) for gonorrhea and chlamydia should be done at all sites of penetration. If the survivor was unconscious during the assault, oral, anal, and vaginal specimens must be collected. NAAT for trichomoniasis from a vaginal or urine specimen is an important component of comprehensive STI screening. If point-of-care DNA probe testing or wet mount is available, these can also be used to test for trichomoniasis and

bacterial vaginosis, particularly if the survivor has symptoms such as abnormal discharge, itching, or malodor [4].

Despite testing, these results are often negative soon after an assault as concentrations of organisms may be too low to detect immediately following an assault. Empiric treatment is recommended, and is preferable to waiting for results or repeated testing. Empiric treatment for gonorrhea and chlamydia consists of ceftriaxone 250 mg IM once as well as azithromycin 1 g orally once. Empiric treatment for trichomoniasis consists of metronidazole or tinidazole 2 g orally once. If the survivor has recently ingested alcohol, the dose of metronidazole or tinidazole can be given to the survivor to be taken at home rather than under direct observation due to the potential for drug interactions with alcohol and adverse gastrointestinal side effects [4].

Serum testing for HIV is done as part of routine post-assault evaluation. If the assailant is known to be HIV positive, postexposure prophylaxis (PEP) is highly recommended. Nonoccupational PEP guidelines are extrapolated from occupational PEP guidelines, and should be offered if the survivor is determined to be at risk for HIV acquisition and presents within 72 hours of the assault [5]. In addition to the assailant's HIV status, which is often not known to the survivor, risk of HIV acquisition is dependent upon the prevalence of HIV infection in the population, the assailant's risk factors for HIV infection (intravenous drug use, men who have sex with men, etc.), and the circumstances of the assault, such as the presence of mucosal lesions, ejaculation on mucous membranes, and potential exposure to HIV-infected blood [4, 5]. PEP consists of a 28-day course of antiretroviral medications, which can be associated with adverse side effects. Close follow-up is recommended to ensure adherence to regimen and assess for possible side effects. Consultation with an HIV or infectious disease specialist is recommended if PEP is being initiated. Serum HIV testing should be repeated at six weeks, three months, and six months following the assault as seroconversion from an acute HIV infection is likely to be detected within that time period [4].

Serum testing for syphilis should be done at the time of presentation for post-assault evaluation. It is unlikely that a syphilis infection acquired at the time of the recent assault will be detected; therefore, it is necessary to repeat testing in four to six weeks and then at three months. There is no recommended empiric treatment or prophylaxis for syphilis infection.

Serum testing for hepatitis B is also recommended. If the survivor has not been previously vaccinated against hepatitis B, the vaccine series should be initiated at the time of evaluation and appropriate follow-up or referrals should be made to ensure completion of the vaccine series. If the survivor has previously been vaccinated but has not had postvaccination testing to determine immunity, this testing can be done at the time of evaluation and the survivor should also receive a booster dose. In the event that the assailant is known to be HBsAg positive and the survivor has not been vaccinated, the hepatitis B vaccine should be given as well as a dose of hepatitis B immunoglobulin (HBIG) [4]. Follow-up vaccination for series completion should be given at one month and six months after the initial vaccination.

If the survivor has not previously received the human papillomavirus (HPV) vaccination series and is below the age of 26, this should be initiated at the time of initial evaluation. Appropriate follow-up should be scheduled to complete the vaccine series at one month and six months. Only two doses of the HPV vaccine six months apart are necessary for adolescents aged 14 years and younger to develop sufficient immunity [6].

Survivors may be uncertain about their desire to undergo counseling following a sexual assault. Whenever possible, referral to a counselor who is specialized in sexual assault is preferable. Survivors of sexual assault are at risk for post-rape trauma syndrome and post-traumatic stress disorder [1, 3]. Information about pursuing legal action should also be offered during an initial evaluation.

A follow-up appointment may be scheduled within one week. This appointment is an important opportunity to assess for any symptoms of STIs that have developed since the initial assessment or to conduct STI testing if it was not performed at the initial evaluation. A follow-up appointment also presents an opportunity to address any side effects from the STI prophylaxis, successful completion of prophylaxis, and side effects and continuation of PEP if relevant. At a one- to two-month follow-up visit, a detailed examination for anogenital warts can be considered. Additional follow-up for completion of vaccination series, additional serum testing for STIs, and counseling referrals should also be done when appropriate [4].

Key Teaching Points

- Detailed documentation of a survivor's report and examination and collection of a forensic rape kit by a trained clinician are important following a sexual assault.
- Comprehensive STI testing, risk assessment, and empiric treatment for STIs should be offered.
- All sexual assault survivors should be offered emergency contraception due to the risk for pregnancy.

References

1. ACOG Committee Opinion no. 592: Sexual assault. *Obstet Gynecol* 2014;123 (4): 905–909.

2. Black MC, Basile KC, Breiding, MJ et al. *The National Intimate Partner and Sexual Violence Survey (NISVS): 2010 Summary Report.* 2011, National Center for Injury Prevention and Control, Centers for Disease Control and Prevention: Atlanta, GA.

3. *Responding to Intimate Partner Violence and Sexual Violence against Women: WHO Clinical and Policy Guidelines.* 2013: World Health Organization.

4. Workowski KA, and Bolan GA. Sexually transmitted diseases treatment guidelines, 2015. *MMWR Recomm Rep* 2015;**64**(Rr-03):1–137.

5. Ford N, Mayer KH. World health organization guidelines on postexposure prophylaxis for HIV: recommendations for a public health Approach. *Clin Infect Dis* 2015;**60 Suppl 3**: S161–S164.

6. Meites E, Kempe A, and Markowitz LE. Use of a 2-Dose schedule for human papillomavirus vaccination – updated recommendations of the advisory committee on immunization practices. *MMWR Morb Mortal Wkly Rep* 2016;**65** (49):1405–1408.

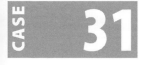

CASE 31

A Woman with a BMI of 40 kg/m² Requests Oral Contraceptive Pills (Efficacy of Contraceptive Methods with Obesity)

Sara Whetstone

History of Present Illness

A 35-year-old woman, gravida 0, presents to her OB/GYN office requesting contraception. She is sexually active with one male partner. She currently uses condoms inconsistently and does not desire pregnancy at this time. She has tried various contraceptives methods in the past and strongly desires oral contraceptive pills.

Her past medical history is notable for class 3 obesity. She has no surgical history. She has no history of cervical dysplasia in the past and is up-to-date with her cervical cancer screening. She has no known drug allergies and does not take any medications. She does not smoke cigarettes; she drinks 2–3 alcoholic drinks per week.

Physical Examination

General appearance
Well-appearing woman in no acute distress

Vital Signs
Blood pressure   112/72 mmHg
Height   63 inches
Weight   228 lb
BMI   40.4 kg/m²
                  Remainder of physical exam deferred

How Would You Manage This Patient?

For a woman seeking contraception, it is the obligation of the obstetrician-gynecologist to provide counseling about all contraceptive methods, including intrauterine devices (IUDs) and implants. Counseling should include (1) information about administration of contraception, (2) contraceptive efficacy, (3) potential side effects and risks, and (4) need for barrier protection for women at risk of sexually transmitted infections.

The US Medical Eligibility Criteria for Contraceptive Use (US MEC) can be utilized to counsel this patient in regard to her request for oral contraceptive pills [1]. For obese women with a BMI > 30 kg/m², combined oral contraceptive pills are assigned a category 2, meaning the advantages of using the method generally outweigh the theoretical or proven risks. Current evidence around the effect of obesity on oral contraceptive efficacy is limited; most studies do not show an increased risk of contraceptive failure in obese women as compared to normal weight women. Among studies that do report a decreased efficacy in obese women compared to normal weight women, the absolute increase in number of pregnancies due to contraceptive failure is small.

Shared decision making is a valuable approach to contraceptive counseling and has been associated with increased patient satisfaction [2]. This model of care occurs when the provider contributes his or her medical expertise and the patient shares her values, goals, and preferences. For this patient, it would be helpful to explore her previous experiences with other contraceptive methods, preferences in method of administration of hormonal contraception, goals around menstrual changes, and acceptable risk of pregnancy. If she selects the combined hormonal pill after shared decision making with her provider, it is reasonable and safe to prescribe oral contraceptive pills to this patient with class 3 obesity.

Due to inconsistent use of barrier contraception, urinary nucleic acid amplification testing (NAAT) for gonorrhea and chlamydia was performed.

Obesity and Hormonal Contraception

Understanding the safety and effectiveness of hormonal contraception for obese women is critical, as approximately one-third of adults are considered obese in the United States. The World Health Organization (WHO) defines obesity as a BMI greater than or equal to 30 kg/m²; obesity is often subdivided into categories to further characterize elevated BMIs (Table 31.1). Overall, obese women are less likely to use contraception or to receive preventive services in comparison to women of normal BMI. Obese women are at higher risk for pregnancy-related complications, including spontaneous abortion, hypertensive disorders of pregnancy, gestational diabetes, venous thromboembolism, postpartum hemorrhage, intrauterine fetal demise, and cesarean delivery. Therefore, access to safe and effective contraception should be a priority for obese women.

The US MEC should be considered when initiating contraception for women with medical comorbidities. Based on the US MEC, combined hormonal contraception (CHC) for obese women is rated as a category 2, the advantages outweighing the theoretical or proven risks [1] (Table 31.2). This categorization stems from the epidemiologic observation that obese women who use combined oral contraceptives (COCs) are more likely

Table 31.1 Weight categories by BMI

Category	BMI (kg/m²)
Underweight	<18.5
Normal weight	18.5–24.9
Overweight	25.0–29.9
Obese	≥30
(a) Class 1 obesity	30.0–34.9
(b) Class 2 obesity	35–39.9
(c) Class 3 obesity	≥40

Table 31.2 US medical eligibility criteria for contraceptive use: obesity (Centers for Disease Control and Prevention, 2016)

Condition	Subcondition	Cu-IUD	LNG-IUD	Implant	DMPA	POP	CHC
Obesity	(a) BMI $\geq$ 30 kg/m2	1	1	1	1	1	2
	(b) Menarche to <18 years and BMI $\geq$ 30 kg/m^2	1	1	1	2	1	2

Notes:
  1: No restriction **2**: Advantages generally outweigh theoretical or proven risks
  3: Theoretical or proven risks generally outweigh benefits **4**: Unacceptable health risk
  Cu-IUD, copper intrauterine device; LNG-IUD, levonorgestrel intrauterine device; Implant, etonogestrel subdermal implant; DMPA, depo medroxyprogesterone acetate; CHC, combined hormonal contraceptives

than obese women who do not use COCs to experience venous thromboembolism (VTE). There is limited information about the effect of CHC and VTE risk in obese women. Irrespective of COC use, obese women are found to have two- to threefold risk of VTE in comparison to normal weight women. No safety data for contraceptive use are available for women with a BMI $\geq$ 40 kg/m^2 [1]. Although the risk of VTE is increased for women with a BMI $\geq$ 30 kg/m^2, the risk of VTE among obese women using contraception is still lower than the risk of VTE among obese women who are pregnant or postpartum.

While the safety of CHC for obese woman with a BMI $\leq$ 39.9 kg/m^2 has been established, the effectiveness of CHC for overweight and obese women has been questioned. Until recently, most clinical trials for contraception excluded women whose body weight was greater than 130 percent of ideal body weight [3]. Importantly, there is no evidence that hormonal contraception is ineffective for obese women. Limited studies suggest that the effectiveness of contraception varies by BMI or body weight and that obese women who use CHC are at increased risk of contraceptive failure and unintended pregnancy [4–6]. The decreased efficacy in hormonal contraception is presumed to result from differences in the pharmacokinetics of steroid hormones affecting drug levels; some examples include a lower maximum serum level of steroid hormone and an increased time to reach steady state in obese women compared to normal weight women. The ultimate question is whether these pharmacokinetic alterations lead to differential risks of contraceptive failure, that is, unintended pregnancy, by BMI.

Most of the available literature on the effect of obesity on hormonal contraception involved COCs. Overall, oral contraceptives are quite effective at preventing pregnancy in women. The data on the efficacy of COCs in obese women, however, are mixed. Most studies show no association between BMI and contraceptive effectiveness; few studies identified an increased risk of contraceptive failure in obese women in comparison to normal weight women [4–6]. While a higher risk of pregnancy in obese women who use COCs was reported in a few studies, the absolute number of unintended pregnancies due to contraceptive failure was quite small. One study estimated that the reported increased risk in contraceptive failure among overweight

women would result in 2–4 extra pregnancies per 100 woman years of COC use among women whose BMI was >27 in comparison to those with a lower BMI [3]. Another study estimated that the failure rate of COCs among women with a BMI $\geq$ 35 would be 4.5 percent, a figure still lower than the typical failure rates for CHC. Most efficacy studies excluded women in the highest BMI categories or failed to report the proportion of women in these categories. Nonetheless, the available evidence suggests that overweight and obese women are at similar or only at slightly higher risk of pregnancy from COC failure compared to women of normal weight [3].

In regard to other contraceptive methods, concern exists for decreased efficacy of the contraceptive patch containing ethinyl estradiol and norelgestromin (EE/NGMN) in obese users. In one study involving pooled analysis of multicenter, open label studies of the patch, the overall failure rate was low; however, 5 of the 15 pregnancies detected in the study occurred among women weighing $\geq$ 90 kg while women with this weight comprised only 3 percent of the study population [5–6]. Pooled data from Phase 3 clinical trials submitted to the US Food and Drug Administration demonstrated that obese women using the patch had an increased risk of contraceptive failure [7]. Although this evidence is limited, it does suggest decreasing efficacy of the EE/NGMN patch with increasing body weight and BMI. For the vaginal ring containing ethinyl estradiol and etonorgestrel (EE/ENG), there are no data comparing effectiveness between obese and non-obese users as large clinical trials excluded obese women. A small study of the EE/ENG ring showed equivalent suppression of follicular development in both normal weight and obese women [8].

Notably, no association was found between BMI and contraceptive failure for depot medroxyprogesterone acetate (DMPA), etonorgestrel (ENG) implant, and the levonorgestrel (LNG) IUD [5]. Interestingly, a small study did show pharmacokinetic differences between obese and normal weight users of DMPA, with obese women having lower median levels of MPA; however, the median levels of MPA for all women, including those with class 3 obesity, exceeded the level needed to prevent ovulation [8]. Both the ENG implant and the LNG IUD have low reported failure rates, which do not vary by BMI. Similar to DMPA, there is some evidence that obese users of the ENG implant compared to normal-weight users had lower serum levels of ENG but again these levels were above the therapeutic threshold needed to suppress ovulation.

In summary, current evidence for contraceptive failure and obesity is limited. Most evidence does not support an increased risk of pregnancy from contraceptive failure for overweight or obese women. Some studies suggest decreased effectiveness of COCs and contraceptive patch in obese women; however, the absolute number of pregnancies predicted to result from contraceptive failure of COCs is small. This risk should be incorporated in a shared decision model with the obese patient as should non-contraceptive benefits of various methods, including the potential to decrease risk for endometrial hyperplasia and cancer.

Key Teaching Points

- There is limited evidence regarding contraceptive efficacy and safety in obese women, as this population has often been excluded from clinical trials, especially women with class 3 obesity.
- Most studies do not show an association between increased BMI and increased risk of contraceptive failure.
- Shared decision making is important to help women choose a method that they will use reliably as the risks of pregnancy and obesity far outweigh the risks of contraceptive use and obesity.
- A woman's contraceptive choice should not be restricted because of her weight or BMI.

References

1. Curtis KM, Tepper NK, Jatlaoui TC et al. U.S. medical eligibility criteria for contraceptive use, 2016. *MMWR Recomm Rep* 2016;65(No 3):1–103.

2. Dehlendorf C, Grumback K, Schmittdiel JA et al. Shared decision making in contraceptive counseling. *Contraception* 2017;95:452–455.

3. Society of Family Planning. Contraceptive considerations in obese women. *Contraception* 2009;80:583–590.

4. Grimes DA, Shields WC. Family planning for obese women: challenges and opportunities. *Contraception* 2005;72:1–4.

5. Lopez LM, Bernholc A, Chen M et al. Hormonal contraceptives for contraception in overweight or obese women. *Cochrane Database Syst Rev* 2016, Issue 8. Art No.: CD008452. DOI: 10.1002/14651858.CD008452.pub4.

6. Dragoman MV, Simmons KB, Paulen ME, Curtis KM. Combined hormonal contraception (CHC) use among obese women and contraceptive effectiveness: a systematic review. *Contraception* 2017;95:117–129.

7. Yamazaki M, Dwyer K, Sobhan M, Davis D et al. Effect of obesity on the effectiveness of hormonal contraceptives: an individual participant data mega-analysis. *Contraception* 2015;92:445–452.

8. Dragoman M, Petrie K, Torgal A, Thomas T, Cremers S, Westhoff CL. Contraceptive vaginal ring effectiveness is maintained during 6 weeks of use: a prospective study of normal BMI and obese women. *Contraception*. 2013 Apr;87(4):432–6.

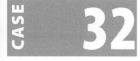

A 41-Year-Old Woman with Bilateral Clear Nipple Discharge (Physiologic Discharge)

Christine Robillard Isaacs

History of Present Illness

A 41-year-old, gravida 2, para 2, presents to your office complaining of bilateral clear nipple discharge experienced intermittently over the last three months. She notices scant amounts of discharge in her sport bra and can evoke discharge with squeezing the areola. The patient denies any breast pain and does not note any masses. Her routine screening mammogram ten months prior was normal.

She has a levonorgestrel-releasing intrauterine system (LNG-IUS) in place for contraception, and her periods stopped a few months after it was initiated. She has no medical problems and has no significant surgical history. Her last pregnancy was five years prior. Her only medication is a daily multivitamin, and she runs approximately 12 miles per week for exercise.

Physical Examination

General appearance	Well-developed, healthy appearing woman
Vital Signs	All within normal limits
Temperature	36.9°C
Pulse	75 beats/min
Blood pressure	105/70 mmHg
Respiratory rate	14 breaths/min
Height	63 inches
Weight	122 lb
BMI	21.6 kg/m^2
HEENT	No focal deficits. Visual fields intact. No palpable thyroid masses.
BREASTS	Symmetric. No skin changes or trauma. No palpable masses or lymphadenopathy. Gentle squeeze/pressure at the base of the areola evokes a minute amount of clear nipple discharge (not bloody) from 2 to 3 ducts bilaterally.
ABDOMEN	Thin, soft, non-tender. No palpable masses.

Laboratory Studies

Urine pregnancy test	Negative
Screening mammogram ten months prior	BI-RADS 1, Negative

How Would You Manage This Patient?

This patient has bilateral clear nipple discharge, which, in most cases, is benign. The findings from the history and physical examination of bilateral, multi-ductal, discharge, which occurs with breast manipulation, support a benign process. While medications can be a common cause of galactorrhea, this patient is only taking a multivitamin. Neurogenic stimulation, either from chronic breast stimulation or from clothing such as a poorly fitting bra, is another possibility, and in this case is likely since she may wear a sports bra that produces significant rubbing during her exercise routine.

A diagnostic mammogram should be obtained given that the patient is over 40 years old. Based on these findings, a breast ultrasound may be considered. A thyroid-stimulating hormone and prolactin levels were obtained and were normal. The patient should be reassured that she has physiologic nipple discharge and should be counseled to avoid provoking nipple stimulation by herself, her partner, or possibly by a poorly fitting sports bra. She was asked to monitor her symptoms for three months with this awareness and return for her well-woman exam. After this counseling and reassurance, the patient embarked on bra resizing. She avoided all personal nipple stimulation and all spontaneous nipple discharge resolved within two months. She should continue with age-appropriate screening mammograms thereafter.

Clear Nipple Discharge

Nipple discharge is the third most common breast issue women experience after breast pain and breast masses [1]. Up to 80 percent of women in their reproductive years can express some fluid from their nipples [2]. Nipple discharge can evoke fear, and, even when benign, can be bothersome to the patient.

Nipple discharge is typically categorized in one of three ways. Normal or benign/physiologic nipple discharge is generally bilateral, multi-ductal, and provoked, as in the patient described earlier. Lactation is also physiologic but is related to pregnancy and the puerperium and may persist for up to one year postpartum or after cessation of breastfeeding. Milky nipple discharge that is outside of pregnancy or occurring more than one year after nursing cessation and is not caused by intrinsic breast disease is defined as galactorrhea. In the case of galactorrhea, elevated levels of prolactin that lead to galactorrhea can be caused by medications, by pituitary gland changes, or by persistent breast stimulation [1]. Pathologic nipple discharge indicates a concerning process within the breast. The discharge is typically spontaneous and unilateral, usually from a single duct opening on the nipple and can be clear, serous, or bloody [3]. While most nipple discharge is caused by benign conditions, up to 15 percent may be associated with an underlying malignancy.

Evaluation of a patient with nipple discharge should therefore start with a history to determine if the nipple discharge is unilateral or bilateral, bloody, or spontaneous or provoked. Non-pathologic nipple discharge is usually bilateral and non-bloody and occurs as a provoked event with breast manipulation and mechanical stimulation of the nipple/duct system. In contrast, spontaneous discharge, which raises concern for pathology, is typically serous, sanguineous, or serosanguineous and produced in larger amounts that can often be noted on the patient's clothing or personal garments.

The patient's age, duration of nipple discharge, pregnancy, and lactation history should be noted [2]. As it is normal for many women to express milky discharge spontaneously or with external pressure up to one year postpartum or after cessation of breastfeeding, in this timing and context, reassurance can be provided. Women under age 40 years with provoked (non-spontaneous) or multi-duct discharge that is not serous or serosanguineous should be educated to stop compression/manipulation of the breast and should be observed. Women 40 years of age or older with the same findings should receive the same guidance but should also have a diagnostic mammogram and ultrasound if not done recently [4].

A review of the patient's current medications should be undertaken, noting those that can inhibit dopamine, such as phenothiazines, antipsychotic drugs, metoclopramide, methyldopa, verapamil, and combined oral contraceptives. These medications are common causes of iatrogenic galactorrhea and, when discontinued, will likely result in alleviation of symptoms [4]. A personal or family history of breast conditions or malignancy of the breast or ovary should be obtained.

Clinical breast examination includes visual inspection of the breasts by having the patient seated with her hands on her waist, noting breast size, symmetry, and skin integrity. The skin over the nipple areolar complex should be examined for lesions or trauma that may mimic nipple discharge. Palpation should be performed to assess for any breast masses or lymphadenopathy. An attempt to reproduce the nipple discharge with gentle pressure at the base of the areola should be performed to provoke symptoms and to determine whether the discharge originates from a single duct or multiple ducts. Discharge originating from a single duct is more concerning of a pathologic process than discharge from multiple ducts. Cytology of nipple discharge has poor sensitivity and specificity and does not add to clinical decision making and should not be performed [2]. The thyroid should also be palpated to determine enlargement or the presence of a palpable mass [2].

A pregnancy test should be obtained even in the setting of highly effective, long-acting, reversible contraception, followed by measurement of a thyroid-stimulating hormone (TSH) and prolactin levels in the context of discharge that is bilateral and/or milky in nature [4]. When TSH or prolactin levels are abnormal, corrective medical management should resolve the nipple discharge. When prolactin levels are in excess of normal, resulting in nipple discharge, and the evaluation does not confirm pregnancy, lactation, or medication side effects, an MRI of the head should be performed to look for a mass lesion (pituitary adenoma) in the hypothalamic-pituitary region.

When appropriate laboratory tests and/or studies are normal and the history and physical examination suggest an otherwise benign, physiologic process, patients should be reassured that this is benign physiologic discharge. Approximately two-thirds of non-lactating women have small amounts of fluid secreted from the nipple with manual expression [2]. Repeated stimulation of the nipple by a woman, her partner, or her clothing can promote nipple discharge; however, the discharge often resolves when the nipple is left alone, so observation is appropriate.

Suspicious/pathologic nipple discharge is often spontaneous (non-provoked), unilateral, and bloody or serosanguineous; arises from a single duct opening; and is persistent. Malignancy is found in 5–15 percent of patients with suspicious/pathologic nipple discharge, so it requires further evaluation [2]. The most common cause of pathologic nipple discharge is a benign papilloma (48%) followed by ductal ectasia (15–20%). The least likely but most significant finding is carcinoma (10–15%) [1]. Women under 30 years of age with a concerning history or clinical exam finding should undergo a breast ultrasound and possible diagnostic mammogram. Women aged 30 years or older should have both a diagnostic mammogram and an ultrasound. Concerning findings should lead to a tissue biopsy in most cases. Ductograms or breast MRI may be considered if initial radiologic findings are uncertain [5].

Key Points

- The evaluation of nipple discharge in nonpregnant patients starts with the clinical history and physical examination.
- Benign/physiologic discharge is typically bilateral and non-bloody, and can be provoked from multiple ducts.
- Laboratory evaluation should include a pregnancy test, followed by TSH and prolactin levels. Breast imaging depends on the clinical presentation and the age of the patient.
- Benign physiologic nipple discharge typically resolves when the nipple is left alone and not stimulated. Observation is thus appropriate.
- Nipple discharge that is persistent, spontaneous, unilateral, uniductal, or bloody suggests possible underlying pathology and requires further evaluation.

References

1. Hussain AN, Policarpio C, Vencent MT. Evaluating nipple discharge, *Obstet Gynecol Surv* 2006 April;**61**(4):278–283.

2. Onstad M, Stuckey A. Benign breast disorders, *Obstet Gynecol Clin N Am* 2013;**49**:459–473.

3. Morrogh M, Park A, Elkin EB, King TA. Lessons learned from 416 cases of nipple discharge of the breast, *Am J Surg* 2010 July;**200**(1):73–80.

4. American College of Obstetricians and Gynecologists' Committee on Practice Bulletins – Gynecology. Practice Bulletin 164 – Diagnosis and management of benign breast disorders, *Obstet Gynecol* 2016 June;**127**(6): e141–156.

5. National Comprehensive Cancer Network. Breast Cancer Screening and Diagnosis. Version 2.2016. NCCN Clinical Practice Guidelines in Oncology. Fort Washington, PA: NCCN; 2016. Available at: www.nccn .org/professionals/physician_gls/pdf/ breast-screening.pdf. Retrieved May 12, 2016.

A 38-Year-Old Woman with New-Onset, Unilateral Bloody Nipple Discharge

Esther Fuchs

History of Present Illness

A 38-year-old nulligravid woman presents to the office with the complaint of nipple discharge. The discharge is present in the left breast only, is bloody, appears spontaneously without nipple stimulation, and is reproducible on application of pressure on the left upper-outer quadrant of the breast. There is no nipple discharge from the right breast. She discovered the discharge for the first time two weeks ago. She has not noticed any breast lump, and denies breast pain, recent trauma, or fevers. She has no previous history of breast problems and no prior pregnancies. Her menarche was at age 14 and she has regular menstrual cycles. She has no medical problems or prior surgeries and is on no medications and has no known drug allergies. She does not smoke, nor use drugs or alcohol. Her family history is negative for cancer.

Physical Examination

General appearance   Alert, no acute distress

Vital Signs

Temperature	36.8 °C
Pulse	95 beats/min
Blood pressure	125/80
Respiratory rate	14 breaths/min
Oxygen saturation	98% on room air
BMI	24

Breast Exam

Inspection	Symmetric breast tissue. No dimpling of the skin. No erythema, swelling or color changes of nipple and skin. Nipples show no retraction, crusting, or ulceration.
Palpation	No masses in all four quadrants bilaterally. On palpation of the left upper outer quadrant, there is discharge of a small sanguineous droplet, reproducible on applying pressure at the periphery of the areola sweeping toward the nipple, possibly involving the area of one duct. No enlarged lymph nodes palpable in the axillary and supraclavicular stations.

Laboratory Studies

Urine pregnancy test Negative

Imaging

Diagnostic mammogram – Cranial caudal images showed an oval mass with circumscribed margins in the subareolar position in the left breast (Figure 33.1)

Left breast ultrasound – oval, circumscribed intraductal mass within a dilated duct in subareolar position (Figure 33.2)

BI-RADS® Category 4 – suspicious, with a recommendation of biopsy and tissue diagnosis

Insertion of Mammogram and Ultrasound images. Courtesy of Dr. D. L. Lam, University of Washington

How Would You Manage This Patient?

This patient has pathologic nipple discharge, since it is unilateral, spontaneous, bloody, and associated with an intraductal mass within a dilated duct on mammogram and ultrasound.

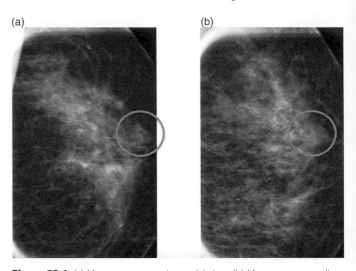

(a)   (b)

Figure 33.1 (a) Mammogram cranio-caudal view. (b) Mammogram medio-lateral view.

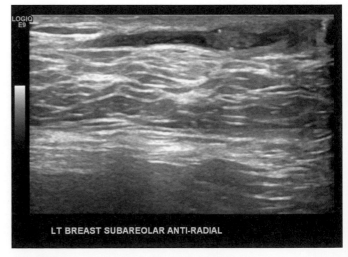

Figure 33.2 Ultrasound: left breast subareolar anti-radial.

A core needle breast biopsy was performed and pathology showed an intraductal papilloma without atypia. A selective duct excision was performed both for diagnosis and therapy to stop the nipple discharge. The final pathology of the excised duct confirmed a benign intraductal papilloma. At her postoperative follow-up visit, the patient presented with a well-healed incision on the breast, and reported that the nipple discharge had disappeared.

Bloody Nipple Discharge

Nipple discharge is the third most common cause for referrals to breast clinics, following breast lumps and pain. It is anxiety provoking for patients. It is important to distinguish if the discharge is benign or suspicious for an underlying pathology such as a papilloma, high-risk lesion, or cancer.

The clinical history is important in assessing risk, including timing of any lactation in the last year; color of the discharge (milky, white, green, brown, gray versus clear, serosanguineous or sanguineous); bilateral or unilateral; multi-ductal or uniductal; persistent, spontaneous, or only present when provoked by stimulation; and whether associated with a mass or enlarged lymph node. Risk factors for breast cancer and any family history that would identify the patient as a candidate for genetic screening should be determined, along with any prior breast procedures.

Bilateral, multi-ductal, non-bloody discharge is usually benign. Bilateral milky discharge outside of pregnancy, postpartum period, and one year after cessation of breastfeeding is called galactorrhea and is not caused by intrinsic breast disease [2, 3]. In contrast, pathologic discharge is usually spontaneous, unilateral, possibly localized to a single duct, and persistent. It can be serous (clear), sanguineous, or serosanguineous. Bloody nipple discharge is associated with a significantly higher risk for breast cancer than non-bloody discharge. One of the strongest risk factors for an underlying malignancy is patient's age, with older patients being much more likely to receive the diagnosis of cancer.

A complete clinical breast examination including axillary, infra-, and supraclavicular areas should be performed to detect any palpable mass. Attempts should be made to provoke the discharge from the nipple by massaging from the periphery of the areola toward the center in a clockwise fashion. The nipple should be inspected for areas of retraction, crusting, scaling, erythema, thickened areas, or ulceration, particularly when patients note bloody stains on their clothing without obvious nipple discharge. Skin findings of scaly, raw, vesicular, or ulcerated lesion associated with bloody discharge can be a sign of Paget's disease of the breast, and require a biopsy of the nipple.

Most cases (65–95 percent) of bloody nipple discharge are benign in origin. However, intraductal hyperplasia or carcinoma (ductal carcinoma in situ [DCIS] or invasive carcinoma) must always be ruled out. Intraductal papillomas, which are wart-like benign tumors that grow from the lining of the breast duct, are the most common diagnosis associated with bloody nipple discharge. Solitary and centrally located papillomas that are close to the duct opening often present with bloody nipple discharge and are less commonly palpable as a mass. They are not usually associated with malignancies on pathology, but there can be atypical cells or DCIS within the papillomas. When intraductal papillomas are multiple and peripheral (sometimes even in both breasts), patients do not typically present with nipple discharge, because the location of the lesions are peripheral and deep. However, patients with multiple papillomas are at higher risk for coexisting breast cancer or development of cancer later in life [3].

The second most common cause of bloody nipple discharge is ductal ectasia (also known as plasma cell mastitis), which is a benign subareolar periductal chronic inflammatory process that is characterized by dilated ducts and can lead to ductal occlusion. It is most often seen in peri- or postmenopausal patients. Duct ectasia identified on mammogram or sonography can have underlying histologic findings such as papilloma or malignancy in about 5 percent of cases [7].

The diagnostic evaluation of nipple discharge depends on the age of the patient. For patients below 30 years of age, initial radiologic evaluation is with ultrasound only, whereas women age 30 and above are initially evaluated by combined imaging of mammogram and ultrasound. The mammogram is helpful to visualize microcalcifications, a sign of DCIS or invasive cancer, as well as to evaluate the entire breast for other areas of concern. If imaging is normal or likely benign, further evaluation with a ductogram or MRI is the next step [1]. If the imaging findings are BIRADS® Category 4 or 5 findings (suspicious or highly suggestive of malignancy), a tissue biopsy is warranted.

A ductogram can help to localize and characterize an intraductal lesion, and can also help with an intraoperative selective excision. It is only possible to locate the affected duct if it demonstrates discharge at the time of study [4]. A ductogram might be the only means to localize and resect the breast lesion associated with the discharge if physical examination and other imaging studies are negative [7].

MRI is emerging as a less invasive alternative to ductography [6]. It has a very high sensitivity for detecting breast cancer (94–100 percent) and a percutaneous MRI-guided core biopsy can be accomplished [4]. MRI, however, has variable specificity and a high false-positive rate.

Most experts do not recommend cytology of nipple discharge, including for the evaluation of bloody nipple discharge, because it is of little complementary value and may even confuse the management [5]. However, there is some controversy and there are some experts who recommend obtaining cytology because it is noninvasive and can have specificity >90 percent if it shows signs of suspected or clear malignancy.

An evaluation with biopsy is needed in the case of a palpable mass or if imaging shows a BI-RADS® Category 4 or 5 lesion [1]. Excision of the affected milk duct is still considered the gold standard for bloody unilateral discharge even in the setting of normal mammogram and ultrasound findings. Selective duct excision is called microdochectomy. A negative core needle biopsy does not guarantee a benign finding on subsequent ductal excision. Previous research has shown that some lesions identified as papilloma on core needle biopsy were upgraded to atypical ductal hyperplasia and DCIS after excision of the duct [8]. Ductoscopy is not currently offered at every center but gaining in popularity. A microendoscope is inserted into the ductal system to directly visualize the lesion. It may contribute to a more accurate resection of intraductal lesions [9] or offer the possibility of intraductal biopsy or resection.

Key Teaching Points

- Benign discharge is usually bilateral, multi-ductal, and non-bloody.
- Pathologic discharge is usually spontaneous, unilateral, possibly localized to a single duct and persistent. It can be serous (clear), sanguineous, or serosanguineous.
- Bloody nipple discharge is associated with a significantly higher risk for breast cancer than non-bloody discharge.

- Patient's age is one of the strongest risk factors for an underlying malignancy, with older patients much more likely to have cancer.
- Initial radiologic evaluation is with ultrasound only for patients below age 30 years, whereas combined imaging of mammogram and ultrasound is recommended for women age 30 and above.
- If imaging is normal or likely benign, further evaluation with a ductogram or MRI is the next step.
- Most experts do not recommend cytology of nipple discharge because it is of little complementary value and may even confuse the management.
- The most common origin of bloody nipple discharge is (benign) intraductal papilloma, followed by ductal ectasia.
- Atypical ductal hyperplasia, DCIS, and invasive carcinoma have to be ruled out.
- Selective duct excision is the gold standard for evaluation and treatment of bloody unilateral, uniductal nipple discharge.

References

1. National Comprehensive Care Network (NCCN) Guidelines. NCCN clinical practice guidelines in oncology: breast cancer screening and diagnosis, Version 1.2016 – July 27, 2016. Available at www .nccn.org/professionals/physician_gls/p df/breast-screening.pdf. Accessed 4/1/ 2017. To view the most recent and complete version of the guideline, go online to NCCN.org

2. ACOG Practice Bulletin #164; June 2016. Diagnosis and Management of Benign Breast Disorders.

3. Pearlman MD, Griffin JL. Benign Breast Disease. Obstet Gynecol. 2010; 116 (3):747–758, September 2010.

4. Patel BK, Falcon S, Drukteinis J. Management of nipple discharge and the associated imaging findings. Am. J. Med. 2015; 128: 353–360.

5. Kooistra BW, Wauters C, Van de Ven S, Strobbe L. The diagnostic value of nipple discharge cytology in 618 consecutive patients. EJSO. 2009; 35: 573–577.

6. Morrogh M, Morris EA, Liberman L et al. The predictive value of ductography and magnetic resonance imaging in the management of nipple discharge. Ann Surg Oncol. 2007;14(12):3369–3377.

7. Cabioglu N, Hunt KK, Singletary SE et al. Surgical decision making and factors determining a diagnosis of breast carcinoma in women presenting with nipple discharge. J Am Coll Surg. 2003;196(3):354.

8. Mercado CL, Hamle-Bena D, Oken SM et al. Papillary lesions of the breast at percutaneous core-needle biopsy. Radiology. 2006; 238: 801–808

9. Moncrief RM, Nayar R, Diaz LK et al. A comparison of ductoscopy-guided and conventional surgical excision in women with spontaneous nipple discharge. Ann Surg. 2005 April; 241(4): 575–581.

A 34-Year-Old Newly Pregnant Woman with a Breast Mass

Asha Bhagsingh Bhalwal and Pamela D. Berens

CASE 34

History of Present Illness

A 34-year-old Hispanic female, gravida 4, para 2, spontaneous abortion 1, was seen for a routine prenatal visit at 23 weeks. She reported noticing a lump in her right breast at around 19 weeks. There was no associated pain, nipple discharge, or trauma. The patient denied any change in the breast size, asymmetry, skin changes, or nipple inversion.

Her past medical history was significant for asthma and a history of chlamydia. Her past surgical history included one cesarean delivery. She breastfed her two other babies. She has never had a breast biopsy. She was married and has previously used Nuvaring, combined oral contraceptive pills, and progesterone-only pills for birth control. She breastfed her other two children without complications. She denied a family history of breast, ovarian, endometrial, or colon cancer. She had no known drug allergies. Her only medication was a daily prenatal vitamin.

Physical Examination

General appearance	Well-developed, well-nourished woman in no apparent distress

Vital Signs

Pulse	80 beats/min
Blood pressure	101/65 mmHg
Body mass index	23 kg/m²
Abdomen	Gravid uterus with fundal height 24 cm
Fetal heart tones	157 beats/min
Breast exam	No skin changes, nipple inversion, or asymmetry seen. 2–3 cm smooth, mobile mass in right lower outer quadrant. No palpable axillary adenopathy.

How Would You Manage This Patient?

The patient has a breast mass in pregnancy, which was detected by breast self-awareness. She is young with no risk factors for breast cancer. She did not have a family history of early onset premenopausal breast cancer, had breastfed her other two babies, and had no history of previous breast biopsy. On physical examination, the breast mass was felt to be regular and mobile, but solid and non-tender, suggestive of a fibroadenoma. A breast ultrasound with possible biopsy was ordered to delineate further characteristics of the mass. Breast ultrasound demonstrated normal left breast and axilla. On the right breast, there was a 2.5 cm × 1.5 cm × 3.2 cm irregular area with an indistinct margin at 7 o'clock 5 cm from the nipple (Figures 34.1–34.3). This irregular area was hypoechoic. There was also a 1.2 cm × 0.6 cm × 1.1 cm lymph node in the right axilla with focal cortical thickening.

Biopsy was performed and pathology indicated malignant invasive ductal carcinoma and ductal carcinoma in situ cribriforming. Hormone receptor testing showed estrogen receptor negative, progesterone receptor negative, and HER2 positive. The patient was counseled on the diagnosis and need to evaluate for distant metastatic disease. To protect the fetus, chest radiograph with shielding, ultrasound of the liver, and MRI of the spine without contrast were performed. These tests showed no evidence of metastatic disease.

She was referred to a breast surgeon and a medical oncologist. The patient opted to continue with pregnancy and had a mastectomy with axillary lymph node dissection. She was stage IIA (T2N0M0) based on her final pathology. She received three cycles of Adriamycin and cyclophosphamide, with one cycle given prior to delivery. She was delivered at 37 weeks gestation, and then completed her treatment with four cycles of Taxotere/Herceptin/Pertuzumab.

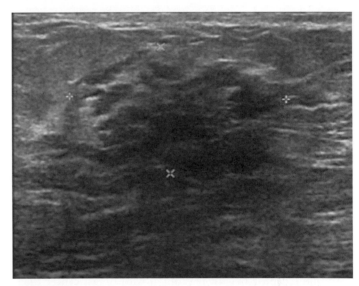

Figure 34.1 Ultrasound image of right breast demonstrating 2.5 × 3.2 × 1.5 cm hypoechoic irregular area.

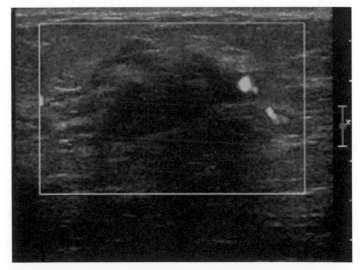

Figure 34.2 Ultrasound of right breast with color flow demonstrating vascularity.

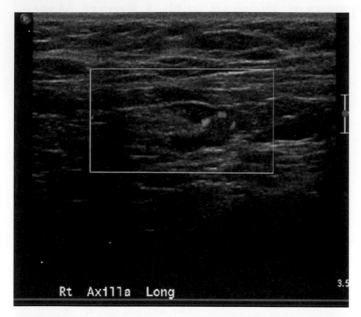

Figure 34.3 Right axilla with 1.2 × 0.6 × 1.2 cm lymph node with focal cortical thickening.

Table 34.1 Breast lesions in pregnancy

Breast lesion	Clinical presentation	Diagnosis
Lactation adenomas	Painless, palpable mass located in the breast periphery	Breast ultrasound Fine needle aspiration
Fibroadenomas	Solid, non-tender masses; firm, mobile, and rubbery in consistency	Breast ultrasound Biopsy
Breast cysts	Painful mobile, fluctuant, or elastic to palpation	Ultrasound to ascertain if simple or complex
Breast infarcts	Associated with fibroadenomas, hamartomas, and lactation adenoma Ill-defined and tender with skin fixation	Core biopsy*

* Fine needle aspiration unlikely to be helpful due to necrosis

Breast Masses in Pregnancy

Pregnancy-associated breast cancer or gestational cancer is usually defined as a breast cancer diagnosed during pregnancy or up to 12 months postpartum. The incidence of pregnancy-associated breast cancer is increasing as more women are postponing pregnancy to their late thirties and forties. Approximately 25 percent of all breast cancer patients are diagnosed during their reproductive years, with a reported incidence of pregnancy-associated breast cancer of 15–35 per 100,000 deliveries [1] and a mean age of 35 years at presentation. Infiltrating ductal carcinoma is the most common histologic type of pregnancy-associated breast cancer, and most are hormone receptor negative. Women with breast cancer diagnosed in pregnancy typically present with more advanced disease, especially in terms of lymph node status, than women who are not pregnant. This may stem from delay in diagnosis or difficulties in tumor detection due to breast engorgement and hypertrophy [3, 4]. Pregnancy-associated breast cancer has poorer prognosis than cancer diagnosed outside of pregnancy. The prognosis may be poorer because of delay in diagnosis and desire to limit radiation exposure to the fetus. Such delay can increase the risk of nodal involvement by 1–2 percent and adversely impact outcome. Survival is the same between pregnant and nonpregnant patients after controlling for age and stage of disease. Because of the more advanced disease at presentation, a high index of suspicion and rapid diagnostic evaluation are warranted.

Pregnancy-associated breast cancers typically present as masses, which may be benign or malignant. A benign mass may be solid or cystic, whereas a malignant mass is typically solid. Breast masses during pregnancy should have the exclusion of carcinoma by the least invasive but most reliable means possible. Breast lesions detected during pregnancy or nursing are not very different from those detected in nonpregnant women. The differential diagnosis of a breast mass in young women includes benign cyst, fibrocystic change, lactation adenoma, fibroadenoma, breast abscess, galactocele, fat necrosis, and malignancy [5]. Breast lesions most likely to develop in pregnant women (Table 34.1) include lactation adenomas, fibroadenomas, breast hamartomas, and axillary breast tissue. The hormone-induced physiological changes occurring in the pregnant breast make diagnosis more difficult.

Solid masses usually warrant biopsy. The clinical presentation of a palpable breast mass is variable. Some masses are detected through breast self-awareness, while others are found on clinical breast examination [6]. Evaluation should include history, breast and axillary exam, diagnostic mammogram, and ultrasound to determine if the mass is cystic or solid [5, 6]. History should include when the mass was first noticed, any change in size, association with trauma, pain, any skin changes, breast asymmetry, and nipple discharge. Galactorrhea is normal in late pregnancy. A patient complaint of a possible breast mass should prompt a thorough breast exam, which should include systematic breast palpation for masses, inspection for skin retraction, and palpation of the axilla and supraclavicular area. The size, shape, location, consistency, mobility, and presence of borders and edges should be noted. The physiologic changes in the breast that accompany pregnancy, including breast enlargement and ductal proliferation, make the physical examination challenging and interpretation of findings more difficult.

Outside of pregnancy, mammography is the first-line diagnostic imaging test in a woman over age 30, with sensitivity of 75–88 percent and specificity of 90–95 percent for detecting cancer. Mammography is not contraindicated in pregnancy, but the sensitivity is reduced by the increased water content, higher density, and loss of contrasting fat in the pregnant or lactating breast [3]. Mammography can be done safely with shielding, with sensitivity of 80 percent [7]. Mammography may provide other information such as calcifications, asymmetric density, axillary lymphadenopathy, and skin and trabecular thickening, which can aid in the diagnosis of malignancy, even if a mass is not detected.

Ultrasound has been reported to be abnormal in up to 100 percent of breast cancers in pregnancy [7]. Ultrasonography is a more dependable diagnostic procedure for pregnant and lactating women with sensitivity of 93–98 percent [2, 3]. It is the first-line imaging test for evaluation of a breast mass in a pregnant woman. Complex echo pattern and posterior acoustic enhancement are common findings in pregnancy-associated breast cancers compared with cancers diagnosed outside of pregnancy [3]. When a suspicious lesion is seen by ultrasound, ultrasound-guided fine needle aspiration cytology or core biopsy should be performed for diagnosis. Core needle biopsy is preferred as it provides tissue for histologic confirmation of invasive disease as well as adequate tissue for hormone receptor and HER2 analysis [8]. Results of these procedures should be interpreted carefully as several cellular morphological changes during pregnancy and lactation can lead to false positive results. If a lactating patient has a palpable mass without abnormality on ultrasound, mammography may be considered to reveal microcalcifications or other suspicious mammographic findings. In this case, once the finding of breast mass was confirmed on exam, rapid evaluation with ultrasound was obtained. Ultrasound showed suspicious findings, which prompted biopsy, confirming the diagnosis of breast cancer.

Lumpectomy, modified radical mastectomy, and axillary dissection can be safely performed during pregnancy. Breast-conserving surgery can be performed in the second trimester of pregnancy with or without neoadjuvant chemotherapy, with radiation therapy delayed until after delivery [8, 9]. The majority of chemotherapy agents used in pregnancy-associated breast cancer can cause teratogenesis, intrauterine growth restriction, fetal deformity, and stillbirth. Risk of teratogenicity is up to 20 percent in the first trimester. Pharmacokinetics of anticancer drugs are altered by the physiological changes in pregnancy, including increased renal blood flow, glomerular filtration rate, and creatinine clearance. There is increased accumulation of drug in the amniotic fluid, with decreased excretion. Drugs such as cyclophosphamide, fluorouracil, and cisplatin are teratogenic in the first trimester, but rarely have adverse effects during the second and third trimesters. Counseling of the pregnant patient with breast cancer should include review of treatment options, which include mastectomy or breast-conserving surgery as well as the use of systemic therapy. Modified radical mastectomy, as performed in this patient, is the most common surgical procedure. Breast-conserving surgery does not appear to have a negative impact on survival. Communication between oncologist and obstetrician is necessary to balance optimal breast cancer treatment with pregnancy outcome.

Key Teaching Points

- Ultrasound is preferred for evaluating breast masses in pregnancy, but mammography can be done safely with shielding.
- Core needle biopsy is the preferred diagnostic test for tissue diagnosis in breast cancer.
- Surgery is the primary treatment of breast cancer in pregnancy. Chemotherapy can be administered safely after the first trimester. Radiotherapy should be reserved for postpartum treatment.

References

1. Andersson TM, Johansson AL, Hsieh CC et al. Increasing incidence of pregnancy-associated breast cancer in Sweden. *Obstet Gynecol* 2009;114:568.

2. Sabate JM, Clotet M, Torruba S et al. Radiologic evaluation of breast disorders related to pregnancy and lactation. *Radiographics* 2007;27 Suppl1:S101.

3. Ann BY, Kim HH, Moon WK et al. Pregnancy- and lactation-associated breast cancer: mammographic and sonographic findings. *J Ultrasound Med* 2003;22(5):491–497.

4. Stensheim H, Moller B, Van Dijk T, Fossa SD. Cause specific survival for women diagnosed with cancer during pregnancy or lactation: a registry based cohort study. *J Clinical Oncol* 2009; 27:45–51.

5. The American College of Obstetricians and Gynecologist. Diagnosis and management of benign breast disorders. Practice Bulletin No.164. *Obstet Gynecol* 2016;127:e141–156.

6. National Comprehensive Cancer Network. Breast cancer screening and diagnosis Version 1. June 2017 www.nccn.org/professionals/physician_gls/pdf/breast-screening.pdf

7. Yang WT, Dryden MJ, Gwyn K et al. Imaging of breast cancer diagnosed and treated with chemotherapy during pregnancy. *Radiology* 2006;239:52–60.

8. National Comprehensive Cancer Network. Clinical Practice Guideline on Breast cancer. Version 2.2017. www.nccn.org/professionals/physician_gls/pdf/breast.pdf

9. Hahn KM, Johnson PH, Gordon N et al. Treatment of pregnant breast cancer patients and outcomes of children exposed to chemotherapy in utero. *Cancer* 2006; 107 (6):1219–1226.

A 29-Year-Old Woman with Lactational Mastitis and Persistent Fevers and Erythema

Pamela D. Berens

History of Present Illness

A 29-year-old women, gravida 1, para 1, complains of persistent fever and breast erythema 48 hours after beginning antibiotic therapy for mastitis. She underwent an uncomplicated vaginal delivery six weeks ago. Initially, she experienced difficulty latching the infant and had nipple trauma with fissuring, which has since healed after working with a lactation consultant and improving the infant's latch. Breastfeeding was going well until the past week when she returned to work outside the home. She has pumped at work every three hours, similar to her baby's feeding schedule. One day prior to symptom onset, she missed a pumping and the breast became engorged. She subsequently developed fever and unilateral breast tenderness. She contacted her obstetrician and was prescribed dicloxicillin 500 mg QID, which she has been taking as directed while continuing to breastfeed. Her symptoms initially improved; however, she has continued to have breast redness and fevers. Her past medical history and surgical history are noncontributory.

Physical Examination

Vital Signs

Temperature	38.7°C
Pulse	92 beats/min
Blood pressure	100/68mm Hg
Respiratory rate	16 breaths/min
Oxygen saturation	100% room air
Height	65 inches
Weight	155 lb
BMI	25.8 kg/m^2

Breasts

Nipples normal bilaterally with no fissuring or trauma

Bilateral galactorrhea

Right breast with no erythema, palpable masses, or axillary adenopathy

Left breast with diffuse erythema in upper outer quadrant with a discrete 3 cm fluctuant mass with overlying erythema in the upper outer quadrant. No palpable axillary adenopathy.

Laboratory Studies

Milk culture collected from left breast

Imaging
Image 1–1. Left breast ultrasound reveals a 3 cm fluid collection, suggestive of a breast abscess (Figure 35.1)

How Would You Manage This Patient?

This patient has a lactational breast abscess, as evidenced by persistent fevers, erythema, and a fluctuant breast mass on

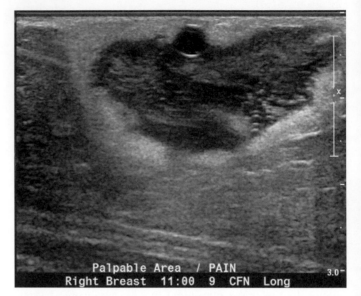

Figure 35.1 Right breast ultrasound showing 3 cm fluid collection consistent with breast abscess.

examination, which was confirmed by ultrasound. As this patient failed to adequately respond to the initial mastitis treatment using dicloxicillin, management includes antibiotic treatment selected to treat the suspected causative organism. The breast abscess was aspirated and drained with ultrasound guidance, and a milk culture from the breast abscess aspirate was sent to guide treatment. While waiting for this culture to return, because of the high likelihood of a drug-resistant causative organism in lactational breast abscesses, antibiotics were changed to cover methicillin-resistant *Staphylococcus aureus* by using sulfamethoxazole 800 mg/trimethoprim 160 mg twice daily for 14 days. The patient was asked to follow up in 48 hours. She remained afebrile after the initial aspiration. Ultrasound was again performed, which showed a small reaccumulation (1.5 cm) of the abscess which was again aspirated. Her antibiotics were continued and she again followed up in 48–72 hours at which time there was no further reaccumulation of fluid to suggest persistence of the abscess. She was clinically improved (the fever was resolved and breast erythema regressed). She was encouraged to continue the full course of antibiotics and to contact the office if any symptoms worsened. The patient was counseled about the importance that the affected breast remain well drained during treatment, by continuing frequent breastfeeding or pumping. In this case, there was no incision near the areola (where breastfeeding would interrupt the wound), so she was able to continue breast emptying through breastfeeding. A lactation consultant reviewed her feeding technique to ensure good latch and a regular feeding/emptying schedule. The patient subsequently followed up in two weeks upon completion of her antibiotics.

She was without complaints and her breast examination was then normal. This patient did not need open incision and drainage of the lactational breast abscess because she responded to serial aspiration and antibiotics. She was able to continue breastfeeding and did not have further difficulties.

Failure of Mastitis to Respond to Initial Antibiotic Therapy

The incidence of lactational mastitis is approximately 9–20 percent. Breast abscesses occur in approximately 3 percent of women with mastitis (or overall 0.4 percent of breastfeeding mothers) [1]. Predisposing factors for breast abscess are similar to mastitis, and include nipple trauma/ fissuring, failure to empty the breast due to engorgement or plugged ducts, primiparity, and history of mastitis with prior lactation. In addition, breast abscesses may result from delayed or inadequate treatment of mastitis [2]. Mastitis typically responds well to therapy with an antibiotic providing coverage for skin organisms such as penicillin-resistant *Staphylococcus* species, *Streptococcus* species, or enteric organisms such as *E. coli*. These antibiotics include dicloxicillin or a cephalosporin and, in patients with severe penicillin allergy, clindamycin (though culture of the breast milk should be considered). In addition, frequent breast emptying is recommended.

Failure of the initial antibiotic therapy to improve symptoms should prompt evaluation of the patient in the office to explore potential reasons. Possibilities include poor compliance with antibiotic administration, resistant organisms, failure to adequately drain the breast, and breast abscess. A detailed breastfeeding history and breast examination should be able to differentiate between these causes. Factors that predispose to infection include nipple trauma, plugged duct, and engorgement. A provider experienced in lactation such as an International Board Certified Lactation Consultant may be of assistance to help reduce these issues. Prior mastitis and/or breast abscess is a risk factor for recurrence of mastitis/ breast abscess (both during the same lactation period and with a future lactation). Recurrent infections in the same location in the breast should prompt a thorough examination to exclude a breast mass. Pregnancy-associated breast cancer is rare but may occur either during pregnancy or during lactation.

Symptoms of mastitis and breast abscess are similar, and include fever, muscle aches, flu-like systemic symptoms, tachycardia, fatigue, breast pain, and erythema. Physical examination should include inspection of the breast for evidence of nipple trauma and erythema, systematic palpation of the breast to evaluate for the presence of a fluctuant mass, and palpation of the axilla for adenopathy. A palpable breast mass discriminates a breast abscess from mastitis. A plugged duct can also present as a tender palpable mass, but fever, systemic symptoms, and overlying breast erythema would not be expected with a plugged duct.

If no discrete mass is identified on examination, a clean catch milk culture should be sent. This may be collected in a midstream fashion into a sterile container through manual breast expression. First, a small initial portion of milk from the affected breast should be expressed and discarded. Next, milk is collected by expression into a sterile container with care taken not to touch the inner aspect of the cup to limit contamination. Alternatively, milk can be collected using a breast pump with sterilized pump parts. Cleansing the nipple prior to collection may limit contamination with skin flora. This culture would not be expected to be sterile but serves to assure the sensitivity of the cultured organism to antibiotic selected. One study on breast abscesses requiring hospital admission in a large urban area found more than 60 percent of abscesses were associated with methicillin-resistant *S. aureus* (MRSA) [3]. Antibiotics covering MRSA while awaiting sensitivities may be prudent.

If a discrete mass is palpable on physical examination, further evaluation with an ultrasound is beneficial. A small superficial, fluctuant breast mass suspicious for a breast abscess (tender and erythematous) may be amenable to aspiration without breast imaging. Deeper or larger suspected abscesses warrant ultrasound to evaluate for size, loculation, and ultrasound guidance during aspiration. This should be performed by a physician familiar with evaluation and management of lactational breast abscesses.

Ultrasound-guided aspiration in addition to oral antibiotics for the initial management of lactational breast abscess is frequently successful and can often avoid more interventional open incision and drainage [3, 7]. Aspirated milk/abscess contents should be sent for culture to assure antibiotic sensitivity, and antibiotics are continued for a typical course of ten days. Techniques to perform aspiration of lactational breast abscesses vary. Ultrasound guidance is helpful in most circumstances. A local anesthetic is used in the skin overlying the abscess and a large bore needle (such as 14–18 gauge) is used for aspiration of the abscess.

Variation surrounds the schedule of ultrasound aspirations from reported case series, with some authors recommending a frequency of every two to three days, while others recommend every four to seven days, with an endpoint of no reaccumulated abscess on imaging [4, 5, 6]. The number of follow-up aspirations until resolution varies between 1 and 4 [4]. One study using ultrasound-guided aspiration found a single aspiration was required in the vast majority of postpartum patients. This researcher used 1 g of dicloxicillin three times daily, aspiration with a 0.8–1.2 mm needle, and a 5.7 French catheter was left in place if the abscess was >3 cm [5]. The catheter remained on average four days in those requiring placement. Other research suggests that lactational breast abscesses larger than 3 cm and <10 cm may benefit from the placement of a drainage catheter, though it remains unclear that a drain improves outcome when compared to serial aspiration. Overall, there is a reported success rate of 82–97 percent for this outpatient and less invasive management method.

The optimal duration of antibiotic therapy has not been adequately studied. A recent systematic review found only two studies meeting criteria and suggested that more research on antibiotics to treat mastitis is needed [8]. Most providers use of 7–10 days of antibiotics for mastitis and 10–14 days for a breast abscess [2]. Hospitalization is required for patients who are clinically unstable, are unable to tolerate oral antibiotics, or have other risk factors for developing sepsis.

Disadvantages of open incision and drainage include a higher likelihood of hospitalization, longer healing time, need for regular dressing changes, and possible prohibition of continued direct breastfeeding if the incision is near the areola and will be disrupted and painful for continued breastfeeding. Additionally, cosmetic results of open incision and drainage on the enlarged lactating breast may not be optimal after involution has occurred. Open incision and drainage techniques such as employing smaller incision size and the use of drains may minimize disadvantages. Incision and drainage of larger, deeper, and peri-areolar lactational breast abscesses and use of packing may increase the risk of milk fistula formation. The overall risk for this complication is low (5–12 percent) [4]. Milk fistula results in milk drainage through the incision during continued lactation. This may be distressing and require occluding the area with something to collect leaked milk until resolution of the fistula or weaning. However, abscesses >10 cm, or those that fail initial management with serial aspiration and antibiotics, may require management with open incision and drainage.

Effective pain management is an important component of treatment. Pain inhibits the milk ejection reflex needed for milk letdown and good breast drainage. Nonsteroidal anti-inflammatory agents such as ibuprofen can be used to treat pain and may also provide benefit as an anti-inflammatory agent. Patients who undergo incision and drainage may require narcotics for adequate pain control.

Continued breast drainage is important in the management of breast abscess. Breastfeeding from the contralateral breast should be continued, and breastfeeding from the affected breast will depend on practical issues related to pain, choice of management (aspiration or incision and drainage), and location of abscess relative to the nipple and drainage site. If direct breastfeeding cannot continue, pumping or manual expression for breast drainage should be employed.

Key Teaching Points

- Failure of the initial antibiotic therapy to improve symptoms should prompt evaluation of the patient in the office to explore potential reasons. Possibilities include poor compliance with antibiotic administration, resistant organisms, failure to adequately drain the breast, and breast abscess.
- Ultrasound-guided aspiration in addition to oral antibiotics for the initial management of lactational breast abscess is frequently successful and can often avoid more interventional open incision and drainage.
- Variation surrounds the schedule of ultrasound aspirations, with some authors recommending a frequency of every two to three days, while others recommend every four to seven days, with an endpoint of no reaccumulated abscess on imaging, and this recommendation is based on expert consensus.
- Continued breast drainage and effective pain management are important in the management of breast abscess.

References

1. Amir LH, Forster D, McLachlan H, Lumley J. Incidence of breast abscess in lactating women: report from an Australian cohort. *BJOG* 2004;**111** (12):1378–1381.

2. Amir LH. Academy of Breastfeeding Medicine Clinical Protocol #4: Mastitis. *Breastfeed Med* 2014;**9** (5):239–243.

3. Berens P, Swaim L, Peterson B. Incidence of methicillin-resistant *Staphylococcus aureus* in postpartum breast abscesses. *Breastfeed Med* 2010;**5** (3):113–115.

4. Irusen H, Rohwer AC, Steyn DW, Young T. Treatments for breast abscesses in breastfeeding women. *Cochrane Database Syst Rev* 2015;(8).

5. Trop I1, Dugas A, David J et al. Breast abscesses: evidence-based algorithms for diagnosis, management, and follow-up. *RadioGraphics* 2011;**31**(6):1683–1699.

6. Christensen AF, Al-Suliman N, Nielson KR et al. Ultrasound-guided drainage of breast abscesses: Results in 151 patients. *Br J Radiol* 2005;**78**:186–188.

7. Ulitzsch D, Nyman MKG, Carlson RA. Breast abscess in lactating women: US-guided treatment. *Radiology* 2004;**232**(3): 904–909.

8. Jahanfar S, Ng CJ, Teng CL. Antibiotics for mastitis in breastfeeding women. *Sao Paulo Med J* 2016 May–June;**134** (3):273.

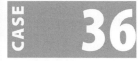

CASE 36

A 45-Year-Old Woman with Unilateral Green Nipple Discharge (Duct Ectasia)

Tricia Camille Yusaf and Katherine Chua

History of Present Illness

The patient is a 45-year-old perimenopausal female who presents to her OB/GYN physician with right breast nipple discharge for the past six months. The discharge is spontaneous and green in color, and a small amount of discharge is noted by the patient on her bra each time she removes her clothing. She also states that the discharge is not bloody. She has no medical problems and no prior surgeries. She had one full-term normal vaginal delivery at 30 years of age and she smokes one pack of cigarettes per day for the last ten years. The patient has no family history of breast cancer and she is currently not taking any medications.

Physical Examination

General appearance	Well developed, well nourished, and in no apparent discomfort

Vital Signs

Temperature	37.0°C
Pulse	88 beats/min
Blood pressure	116/80 mmHg
Respiratory rate	16 breaths/min
Oxygen saturation	100% on room air
BMI	23 kg/m^2
Breast	Symmetric, normal nipple position, everted nipples, and normal skin appearance bilaterally. No palpable masses, no erythema, and no edema. No axillary or clavicular adenopathy. During palpation of the nipple areolar complex of the right breast, a small amount of clear, green discharge was elicited from a single duct located at 3 o'clock.

Laboratory

Urine pregnancy test	Negative
Prolactin	13 ng/mL (Normal)
White blood cell count	9,000/μL

Imaging

Mammogram	Dilated retroareolar ducts with tubular branching structures widest at the nipple and tapering as the ducts proceed into the breast parenchyma. BIRADS-2
Breast ultrasound	Dilated subareolar ducts containing anechoic fluid

How Would You Manage This Patient?

This 45-year-old patient has nipple discharge that is green in color, unilateral, and uniductal, which are characteristics associated with duct ectasia. Duct ectasia is a benign breast disease and a common cause of nipple discharge typically seen in the perimenopausal period. It is an inflammatory process affecting the ducts below the nipple, resulting in dilation of one or more ducts due to poor emptying and stagnation of ductal secretions [1, 2]. Physical examination of the right breast reproduced the discharge and also localized it to uniductal involvement. Ultrasound and mammogram were obtained to confirm the diagnosis of duct ectasia and to further elucidate the patient's risk for breast cancer. Imaging revealed the classic features of duct ectasia, which are enlarged dilated retroareolar ducts that were BIRADS-2 (benign, noncancerous finding). The patient was instructed to use hot compresses and see if there was resolution or persistence of the discharge. At her follow-up appointment in six months, the patient continued to have the nipple discharge and was therefore referred to a breast surgeon. The duct was excised and pathology results confirmed the diagnosis of duct ectasia with mild periductal mastitis. The patient reported complete resolution of the nipple discharge after duct excision was performed.

Management of Women with Spontaneous Nipple Discharge and Management of Mammary Duct Ectasia

Mammary Duct Ectasia

Nipple discharge that is green in color, unilateral, and uniductal are characteristics associated with mammary duct ectasia. Duct ectasia is a benign breast disease and common cause of nipple discharge typically seen in the midlife and beyond (though it can rarely be seen in children). Risk factors include cigarette smoking and parity. It is an inflammatory process affecting the ducts below the nipple, with dilation of one or more ducts due to poor emptying and stagnation of ductal secretions. Patients may present with discharge, a subareolar mass, nipple inversion, noncyclic breast pain, or infection/abscess. On physical examination, there may be nipple inversion and a palpable lump [1, 2]. Ultrasound and mammogram can help make the diagnosis of duct ectasia. Ultrasound often shows anechoic smooth-walled branching structures that taper peripherally. On mammogram, breast ducts wind and twist, and are enlarged (usually greater than 2 mm in diameter), with the ampullary portion of the duct usually greater than 3 mm. Ducts may be filled with fluid or thick secretions and may contain cellular debris [7]. Duct ectasia can be managed expectantly and does not require surgery unless there is a suspicious breast mass or abnormal imaging. Treatment options may include expectant management, warm compresses, antibiotics, or duct excision if nipple discharge is persistent and troublesome to the patient [2]. While mammary duct ectasia itself is not a risk factor for breast cancer, if nipple discharge is associated with a breast mass or is accompanied by abnormal breast imaging, then the presence of a precancerous lesion or breast cancer is still possible and tissue biopsy should be performed [1, 3]. If patients have persistent nipple discharge from duct ectasia, the duct can be excised.

Evaluation of Nipple Discharge

Nipple discharge is a common complaint of approximately 2–5 percent of women visiting health-care providers. The majority of patients will have benign nipple discharge. However, nipple discharge can also be a presenting sign of a papilloma, duct ectasia, a precancerous lesion, or breast cancer [2, 4]. The primary goal of evaluation of patients with a nipple discharge is to differentiate those with a normal (physiologic) nipple discharge, a discharge not associated with cancer or precancerous lesion, from those who have an underlying high-risk precursor lesion or breast cancer [4, 5]. The clinical history and physical findings are helpful in making these distinctions.

A normal or physiological nipple discharge is typically bilateral and nonspontaneous, and involves multiple breast ducts. It is usually white or clear, but can also be yellow or green [4, 6–7]. An abnormal nipple discharge is typically unilateral, uniductal, spontaneous, reproducible on examination, or associated with a breast mass, or occurs in women older than 40 years of age. An abnormal nipple discharge can be serous, sanguineous, or serosanguineous, and the presence of blood is associated with a higher risk of malignancy [2–4, 6–8]. The information in Table 36.1 can be used as a guide to help differentiate between the two types of nipple discharge. The patient in this case had many characteristics associated with an abnormal nipple discharge, as her discharge was unilateral, uniductal, spontaneous, and reproducible.

Lactation and galactorrhea are causes of nipple discharge and are not associated with malignancy. The nipple discharge associated with lactation is caused by the production of breast milk and colostrum. This occurs during pregnancy and can continue for years after delivery and cessation of breastfeeding [2]. Galactorrhea is a nipple discharge that is unrelated to pregnancy or breastfeeding. This discharge typically appears milky, involves both breasts, and involves multiple ducts of the breast tissue. Hyperprolactinemia is a common cause of galactorrhea. Pituitary adenoma, chronic breast stimulation, medications inhibiting dopamine, and medications causing lactotroph stimulation in the brain can all cause hyperprolactinemia [1, 2].

In addition to careful history taking, the physical examination should include careful inspection of the breast contour, skin, nipple, and areola. Palpation of all the breast tissues should be performed including the nipple areolar complex and lymph node tissues [1, 2]. On examination, it is important to try to elicit the discharge from the nipple and identify the involved duct or ducts. Pressure in a clockwise fashion around the nipple areolar complex can help to identify a specific site or duct involved in producing the nipple discharge.

One algorithm for management of women with a spontaneous nipple discharge is described in Figure 36.1. Patients with a physiologic discharge have a low cancer risk and are followed with observation and age-appropriate diagnostic imaging [1, 2, 8–9]. Patients with abnormal discharge undergo ultrasound +/– mammogram (age 30 and older should undergo diagnostic mammogram) [1, 9]. If the

Table 36.1 Characteristics of physiologic and abnormal nipple discharge

	Physiologic (Normal)	Abnormal
Breast involvement	Bilateral	Unilateral
Spontaneity of the discharge	Nonspontaneous	Spontaneous
Number of ducts	Multiple	Single
Discharge color	Milky, green	Serous, serosanguineous, or sanguineous
Differential diagnosis	Breastfeeding, galactorrhea	Intraductal papilloma, duct ectasia, carcinoma

mammogram and ultrasound are normal (BI-RADS 1–3), then the risk of carcinoma is low. Close clinical follow-up with physical examinations and imaging (mammogram +/- ultrasound) is recommended at six months, and if the discharge becomes persistent or recurrent, then duct excision is considered for symptomatic relief and tissue diagnosis for breast cancer screening [2, 3, 7]. Women with an abnormal discharge and abnormal imaging (BI-RADS 4–5) should have a tissue biopsy performed to make a histological diagnosis and rule out cancer [2–3, 6, 10]. Tissue biopsy is also indicated if there is a concurrent breast mass. The patient in this case had ultrasound and mammogram findings consistent with duct ectasia that were BI-RADS 2, and duct excision was performed because she had a persistent nipple discharge.

MRI of the breast can also be considered, and is especially useful in younger women with dense breast tissue that can limit visualization on ultrasound and mammogram. There is limited benefit to cytological evaluation of nipple discharge because the results are unreliable, and a negative cytology does not exclude breast malignancy [1, 8]. The benefits of ductogram and ductoscopy are controversial and they are not widely performed.

Key Teaching Points

- Nipple discharge that is green in color, unilateral, and uniductal are characteristics associated with mammary duct ectasia. It is a benign breast disease and common cause of nipple discharge typically seen in the midlife and beyond.
- Duct ectasia is an inflammatory process affecting the ducts below the nipple, with dilation of one or more ducts due to poor emptying and stagnation of ductal secretions. Patients may present with discharge, a subareolar mass, nipple inversion, noncyclic breast pain, or infection/abscess.
- Ultrasound often shows anechoic smooth-walled branching structures that taper peripherally. On mammogram, breast ducts wind and twist and are enlarged (usually greater than 2 mm in diameter), with the ampullary portion of the duct usually greater than 3 mm.

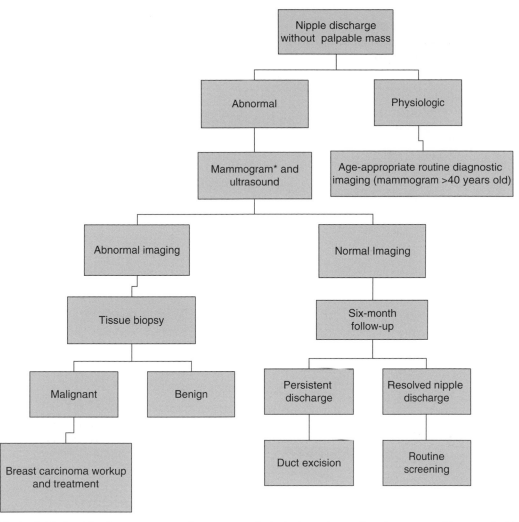

Figure 36.1 Algorithm for management of spontaneous nipple discharge in a nonlactating woman without a palpable mass.
*Women age 30 and older

- Duct ectasia can be managed expectantly and does not require surgery unless there is a suspicious breast mass or abnormal imaging. Duct ectasia itself does not increase the risk for breast cancer.
- Treatment options for duct ectasia may include expectant management, warm compresses, antibiotics, or duct excision if nipple discharge is persistent and troublesome to the patient.
- Nipple discharge is categorized as physiologic (normal) or abnormal.

- A normal or physiologic nipple discharge is generally described as bilateral, nonspontaneous, or multi-ductal.
- An abnormal nipple discharge is generally unilateral, spontaneous, uniductal, reproducible on exam, or associated with a concurrent breast mass. It has a higher risk of association with a precancerous or cancerous lesion.
- If a woman has a nipple discharge with abnormal features, she should be further evaluated for cancer with mammogram, breast ultrasound, and possible breast biopsy.

References

1. Ramalingam K, Srivastava S, Vuthaluru S, Dhar A, Chaudhry R. Duct ectasia and periductal mastitis in Indian women. *Ind J Surg* 2015; 77(3): S957–S962.

2. Gray R, Pockaj B. Current management of nipple discharge. *Breast Disease: Comprehen Manag* 2015;113–119.

3. Sangma M, Panda, K., Dasiah, S. A clinico-pathological study on benign breast disease. *J Clin Diagn Res* 2013;7 (3):503–506.

4. American College of Obstetricians and Gynecologists. Diagnosis and management of benign breast disorders.

Practice Bulletin No. 164. *Obstet Gynecol* 2016;127: e141–e156.

5. Murad TM, Contesso G, Mouriesse H. Nipple discharge from the breast. *Ann Surg* 1982;195:259.

6. Patel B, Falcon S, Drukteinis J. Management of nipple discharge and the associated imaging findings. *Am J Med.* 2015;128(4):353–360.

7. Dietz J. *Nipple Discharge.* Management of Breast Diseases. Springer International Publishing Switzerland 2016. 57–72.

8. Zervoudis S, Latrakis G, Economides P, Polyzos D, Navrozoglou I. Nipple Discharge Screening. *Women's Health.* 2010;6(1): 135–151.

9. NCCN Guidelines Version 2.2016 Breast Cancer Screening and Diagnosis. *National Comprehensive Cancer Network.* 2017;2. BSCR-13.

10. Ferris-James D, Iuanow E, Mehta T, Shaheen R, Slanetz P. Imaging approaches to diagnosis and management of common ductal abnormalities. *Radiographics.* 2012;32(4):1009–1130.

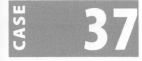
A 35-Year-Old Woman Who Complains of Cyclic Breast Pain (Idiopathic Mastodynia)

Dorota Kowalska

History of Present Illness

A 35-year-old, gravida 2, para 2, presents to the office complaining of bilateral breast pain that is dull and diffuse. Her pain occurs a few days before her menses and improves with the onset of menses. At its worst, her pain inhibits her from completing her daily activities. She is unable to exercise and on most occasions has to stay home from work because wearing a bra is extremely uncomfortable. She reports that she has been experiencing the pain for a few months and is not sure what brought it on. She does not recall any recent trauma to her breasts. She is not breastfeeding, her last delivery was six years ago, and she uses a copper intrauterine device for contraception. She denies any neck, back, or shoulder pain; fever; or chills. She denies any nipple discharge or masses, and has never had a breast biopsy. She does not take oral nonsteroidal anti-inflammatory drugs (NSAIDs) as they upset her stomach, and she tried topical NSAIDs and this did not improve the pain. She is anxious and concerned as her maternal aunt was recently diagnosed with breast cancer at age 55.

She has no medical problems and her surgical history is only significant for a laparoscopic cholecystectomy. She does not smoke or use drugs, and uses alcohol socially. Her only medication is a multivitamin.

Physical Examination

General appearance   Healthy woman in no acute distress

Vital Signs
Temperature   38.1°C
Pulse   87 beats/min
Blood pressure   118/76 mmHg
BMI   27 kg/m^2
Pulmonary   Clear to auscultation bilaterally
Abdomen   Soft, non-tender, no lesions

Breast Exam
Breasts symmetric, no skin retraction or dimpling, no erythema, no ulcerations, no crusting of nipple, no color changes, no palpable axillary or supraclavicular lymph nodes. No breast masses or nipple discharge, non-tender.

Laboratory Studies
Urine pregnancy test Negative

Imaging
Breast ultrasound   No mass lesions in the right or left breast. Bi-Rads Assessment Category:1 (negative)
Mammogram   Normal Bi-Rads assessment category:1 (negative)

Breast Cancer Risk Assessment
Five-year risk
of developing breast cancer   0.03%
Lifetime risk of developing breast cancer   9.2%

How Would You Manage This Patient?

The history of bilateral and diffuse breast pain that is worse in the days prior to the onset of menses and resolves with menses, combined with a normal breast examination, is a classic presentation for cyclic mastodynia. Imaging is not necessary as the pain is diffuse and cyclical, and the physical examination is normal. However, because this patient was extremely concerned about having cancer, a breast ultrasound and a mammography were performed and were normal. She was reassured that this was a benign disorder and asked to keep a menstrual calendar for two months to record the degree of pain she experiences as it relates to her menstrual cycle. She was counseled that some women find elimination of caffeine helpful in reducing symptoms, though this has not proven effective in published trials, and that the evidence for using evening primrose oil and vitamin E is inconclusive. A well-fitting bra to better support her breasts and a sports bra during exercise were advocated.

She returned after two months and reported that supportive garments, caffeine restriction, vitamin E, and primrose oil did very little to relieve her pain. She was still limited by her symptoms, and every month for almost a week she could not perform her daily activities. At this point, options for medical management were offered. She gets stomach upset with NSAIDs, so the patient decided to proceed with Danazol 200 mg daily. The dose was then reduced every two months until 100 mg daily for two weeks of the month was achieved. She continued on the medication for about one year but self-discontinued due to hirsutism. Her mastodynia was resolved at that time.

Breast Pain (Mastodynia, Mastalgia)

Breast pain (mastodynia, mastalgia) is a very common medical symptom, with 47 percent of all breast-related visits due to breast pain [1]. It is classified into three categories: cyclical, noncyclical, and extra mammary (referred pain from outside the breast). Cyclical pain occurs one week prior to menses and tends to resolve with menses. It is the most common category (two-thirds of patients) and is thought to be due to hormonal fluctuations during the late luteal phase of the menstrual cycle. Cyclical pain is often bilateral and worse in the upper outer quadrant of the breast, and pain can refer to the upper arm and axilla. Etiology of cyclical pain is thought to be due to stimulation of ductal elements by estrogen, stromal stimulation by progesterone, and ductal secretion by prolactin. A menstrual calendar can help in differentiating between cyclical and noncyclical pain. Extra mammary pain is referred pain from a source other than the breast. It can include chest wall trauma, costochondritis, rib fractures, herpes zoster, angina, and gastroesophageal reflux.

Mastodynia can range from extremely mild to severe and incapacitating. In most patients with cyclic mastodynia, reassurance is sufficient, but in 10–15 percent of patients, the degree of pain affects their quality of life, and drug treatment is necessary [2]. Patients who decide to start medical therapy typically report their pain to be severe enough that it affects their sexual, physical, social, and school activities.

Initial evaluation should include a thorough history, physical examination, and radiologic evaluation, if indicated. The history should include the duration and location of pain, worsening or improvement of symptoms over time, relationship with the menstrual cycle, if palpable masses are felt, and presence or absence of nipple discharge [3]. A variety of medications can cause breast pain, including hormonal medications, antidepressants, antihypertensives, cardiac medications, and antimicrobial agents. History of recent trauma, infections, or pregnancy/breastfeeding should be discussed as well.

The physical examination should be done in both seated and supine positions. It should start with inspection to evaluate for symmetry, erythema, edema, and skin/nipple retraction. Palpation should include the breast and axillary/supraclavicular lymph nodes, and any palpable concern should be evaluated further by appropriate imaging modality.

Imaging with mammography and ultrasonography in patients with mastodynia and a normal breast examination are generally not valuable, since most patients will have normal imaging [4]. However, some patients may need the reassurance of a negative imaging study, especially if medical therapy will be instituted. A reasonable approach in these situations is a breast ultrasound for women under age 30 without risk factors for breast cancer. For women over age 30, a mammogram and an ultrasound can be performed.

In contrast, breast imaging may be a valuable tool when either focal pain or a palpable abnormality is found on physical examination, and the patient's age and risk for breast cancer can guide evaluation. In patients with focal breast pain and no mass on physical examination, evaluation should include targeted ultrasound in patients younger than 30 and targeted ultrasound and mammography in patients older than 30. If imaging is normal, treatment can be initiated if desired by the patient.

In patients with pain and a palpable mass, ultrasonography is recommended for women under 30, and both ultrasonography and diagnostic mammography should be obtained in women older than 30 years. Calculating a breast cancer risk assessment by using the Breast Cancer Risk Assessment Tool from the National Cancer institute [5], which can be used in women over the age of 35, can also be beneficial to determine the need for genetic counseling referral, enhanced screening, or risk reduction therapies in women who present with breast pain.

For most patients, reassurance is all that is needed. If reassurance does not provide adequate relief, treatment can be initiated. Lifestyle and dietary modifications should be instituted first, as they are simple and have few side effects. Lifestyle modification of using a well-fitting brassiere, support bra with underwire, and sports bra during exercise has been shown to reduce breast pain, especially if the pain is related to movement [6].

There is inconclusive evidence when it comes to the use of nonhormonal drugs such as evening primrose oil and vitamin E. Evening primrose oil contains gamma linoleic acid. The therapeutic dose is 3 g and it contains 240 mg of gammalinoleic. The gamma linoleic acid is thought to improve the plasma fatty acid profiles in women with breast pain as well as change the prostaglandin metabolism [7]. The results, if any, usually take up to four months to be seen, so patients need to be made aware that the effects will not be immediate. Side effects are mild and include abdominal bloating and nausea.

If the pain is related to oral contraceptive or hormone replacement therapy usage, decreasing the dose of oral estrogen or skipping the hormone-free week can be effective. Medication for mastodynia should be reserved for refractory cases that are affecting the patient's quality of life. Danazol is the only FDA-approved drug for treatment of mastodynia. It has many unpleasant side effects; therefore, it is usually used for refractory cases or patients who desire a fast response. Danazol is started at 200 mg daily on the second day of the menstrual cycle and taken daily. The dose can be reduced every two months if symptoms improve and the improvement is maintained. The lowest dose can be 100 mg daily for two weeks out of the month or every other day if the patient is amenorrhoeic. The most common side effect is weight gain and menstrual irregularities, followed by headache, GI upset, hair loss, and hirsutism. A clinically useful response rate was 79 percent in patients treated with Danazol [8, 9]

NSAIDS, including oral or topical, can be considered. Oral NSAIDS are proven to improve breast pain but long-term use can lead to gastrointestinal bleeding and respiratory complications in asthma patients. Topical NSAIDS are thought to have a better safety profile, minimal side effects, and good pain response rates if used for over six months. Some of the topical NSAIDS used in the United States are Aspercreme and Nuprin (which contains salicylate) as well as Flector patch (which contains diclofenac). The response rate is as high as 81 percent [10].

Tamoxifen, which is a synthetic anti-estrogen, can relieve severe breast pain (10 mg daily dosing). Side effects are hot flashes, vaginal dryness, joint pain, and leg cramps. It can also cause blood clots, strokes, and uterine cancer, which is why it is limited in use. The response rates are 71–96 percent [11].

Bromocriptine (a dopamine agonist) decreases prolactin levels. Prolactin causes enlargement of the mammary glands in the breast and stimulation of the glands for milk secretion [12]. Most of the side effects occur at the beginning of treatment and with time tend to subside. The most common side effects are nausea, vomiting, and headaches, followed by postural hypotension, vasospasms, constipation, and abnormal uterine bleeding. Dropout rates are high, as it takes time and effort to ensure dose adjustment [8, 13]. It is started at 1.25 mg at night and increased by 1.25 mg until 2.5 mg twice-daily dose is achieved. It can take two or more weeks to reach the therapeutic dose. Response rate is 54 percent in patients treated with bromocriptine [8].

Some newer drugs include the nonsteroidal selective estrogen reception modulator, Ormeloxifene, which works as anti-estrogen in the uterus and breast. Its only side effect is a prolonged menstrual cycle. Its therapeutic effect was found to be significant, as well as its rapid response: however, more research needs to be conducted [14].

Key Teaching Points

- Cyclic mastodynia (mastalgia, breast pain) is very common, and in most cases, simple reassurance and lifestyle supports such as a supportive bra are all that are needed.
- Ultrasonography and/or mammography are unnecessary unless focal pain or a palpable abnormality is present.
- Mastodynia that interferes with quality of life should be treated with medication.
- Bromocriptine, Danazol, and Tamoxifen all offer significant relief from mastodynia; however, there is no good data on direct comparison between them. Danazol is the only medication that is FDA approved for mastodynia.
- Topical NSAIDs have good response rates and minimal side effects.
- Evening primrose oil appears to be ineffective.
- Breast cancer risk assessment in patients over the age of 35 can help institute risk reduction strategies.

References

1. American College of Obstetricians and Gynecologists. Diagnosis and management of benign breast disorders. Practice bulletin No. 164. *Obstet Gynecol* 2016;127:e141–156.

2. Pye JK, Manse RE, Hughes LE. Clinical experience of drug treatments for mastalgia. Lancet 1985;ii 373–377.

3. American College of Obstetricians and Gynecologists. Breast cancer risk assessment and screening in average-risk women. Practice bulletin No. 179. *Obstet Gynecol* 2017;130:e1–16.

4. Chetlen AL, Lapoor MM, Matts MR. Mastalgia: Imaging work-up appropriateness. *Acad Radiol* 2017 March;24(3):345–349.

5. National Cancer Institute. Breast Cancer Risk Assessment Tool. www.cancer.gov/bcrisktool/.

6. Smith RP, Pruthi S, Fitzpatrick LA. Evaluation and management of breast pain. *Mayo Clini Proc* 2004;79:353. Jacueline Blommers. Evening primrose oil and fish oil for severe chronic mastalgia: A randomized, double-blind, controlled trial. *Am J Obstet Gynecol* 2002;187:1389–1394.

7. Gateley CA, Miers M, MAnscl RE, Hughes LE. Drug treatments for mastalgia: 17 years experience in the Cardiff Mastalgia Clinic. *J R Soc Med* 1992;85:12–15.

8. Harrison BJ, Maddox PR, Mansel RE. Maintenance therapy of cyclical mastalgia with low-dose Danazol. *J R Coll Surg Edinb* 1989; 34:79–81.

9. Colak et al. Efficacy of Topical Nonsteroidal Anti-inflammatory drugs in mastalgia treatment. *J Am College Surg* April 2003;196(4):525–530.

10. Messinis IE, Lolis D. Treatment of premenstrual mastalgia with tamoxifen. *Acta Obstet Gynecol Scand* 1988;67:307–309.

11. Zinger M, McFarland M, Ben-Jonathan N. Prolactin expression and secretion by human breast glandular and adipose tissue explants. *J Clin Endocrin Metabol* February 2003;88 (2):689–696.

12. Fentiman IS, Caleffi M, Hamed H, Chaudary MA. Studies of Tamoxifen in women with mastalgia. *Br J Clin Pract* 1989;43 (suppl 68):34–36.

13. Rathi J, Chawla I, Singh K, Chawla A. Centchroman as first-line treatment for mastalgia: results of an open-labeled single-arm trial. *The Breast J* 2016;22:407–412.

14. Srivastava A, Mansel RE, Arvind N, Prasad K, Dhar A, Chabra A. Evidence-based management of mastalgia: A meta analysis of randomized trials. *Breast* 2007;16:503–512.

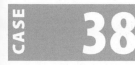

CASE 38 A 22-Year-Old Woman with LSIL on Initial Cervical Cytology

Mark K. Hiraoka

History of Present Illness

A 22-year-old woman presents to discuss management of her initial cervical cytology, which returned as low-grade squamous intraepithelial lesion (LSIL). She has no other complaints.

Her past medical and surgical histories are unremarkable. She is heterosexual, has had a total of two partners, and has been in a new relationship for the past four months. She is using combined oral contraceptive pills as her method of birth control and is happy with them. She is not taking any other medications. She has never received the human papilloma virus (HPV) vaccine. She denies smoking or illicit drug use.

Physical Examination

General appearance	Well-developed, well-nourished woman in no discomfort

Vital Signs

Temperature	37.0°C
Pulse	60 beats/min
Blood pressure	110/72 mmHg
Respiratory rate	16 breaths/min
Height	65 inches
Weight	130 lb
BMI	21.6 kg/m^2
Abdomen	Thin, soft, non-tender, non-distended, no guarding, no rebound
External genitalia	Unremarkable
Vagina	No blood or discharge
Cervix	Nulliparous, closed
Uterus	Anteverted, mobile, normal size, no tenderness on bimanual examination
Adnexa	No masses or tenderness bilaterally

Laboratory Studies

Cervical cytology result	Low-grade squamous intraepithelial lesion
Gonorrhea and chlamydia nucleic acid amplification tests	Negative

How Would You Manage This Patient?

The patient is a young woman with an LSIL cervical cytology result. After discussion with the patient, the patient was managed according to the American Society for Colposcopy and Cervical Pathology (ASCCP) 2012 Updated Consensus Guidelines for the Management of Abnormal Cervical Cancer Screening Tests and Cancer Precursors. Rather than immediate colposcopy, which would have been the preferred choice in older women, she was managed according to the algorithm for women ages 21–24 with either atypical squamous cells of undetermined significance (ASC-US) or LSIL, and was scheduled for repeat cytology alone in 12 months. She received the first dose of the HPV vaccine at this visit, with completion of the series at two and six months. Repeat cytology without HPV co-testing was performed in 12 months, which returned negative for intraepithelial lesion or malignancy. Repeat cytology was recommended in 12 months, with plan to return to routine screening if that test was also normal.

LSIL in Young Adults

HPV Infection

HPV infection is a necessary precursor to cervical dysplasia and cervical cancer. Most HPV infections are transient and spontaneously regress. Persistent HPV infection is associated with the development of cervical dysplasia and cervical cancer. HPV infection is most common in teenagers and young women in their early twenties, with as large as a six- to eightfold increase in HPV prevalence in younger women compared to older women [1]. A number of factors make HPV and its consequences different in this age group from older women. The greatest risk factor for having an incident infection is having a new sexual partner. Younger patients are more likely to have an increased number of sexual partners in a shorter time frame. In adolescence, the cervix is mainly comprised of columnar epithelium, which is slowly replaced by squamous epithelium. This metaplasia is caused by changes in the acidity of the vagina, and possibly by sexual activity. High metaplastic activity makes the younger cervix more susceptible to HPV infection and dysplasia. Age affects the immune response. HPV infections are usually transient, taking an average of only eight months to clear. Younger patients have a stronger immune response, so clearance rates are higher when compared to older adults. These factors result in a high prevalence rate of HPV infection in the setting of tremendously low cervical cancer rates in the younger age groups [2, 3].

LSIL

Management

Based on these differences in the natural history of HPV infection and extremely low risk of cervical cancer in younger patients, LSIL and ASC-US found in patients between the ages of 21 and 24 years are managed differently than in older women (Boxes 38.1 and 38.2). The risk of histologic high-grade intraepithelial lesion (HSIL) (CIN 2 or 3) with LSIL cytology is low enough in young women that colposcopy is not necessary. Clinically significant abnormalities are usually associated with persistent disease. HSIL in this age group does not appear to progress rapidly as evidenced by the low cervical cancer rates in this younger group. This slow progression to cancer in younger women allows management by follow-up cytology, identifying those at risk for significant abnormalities by focusing further evaluation on patients with persistent disease.

> **Box 38.1** ASCCP guidelines for the management of women aged 21–24 years with LSIL [8]
>
> For women with LSIL who are aged 21–24 years, follow-up with cytology at 12-month intervals is recommended. Colposcopy is not recommended. For women with ASC-H or HSIL+ at the 12-month follow-up, colposcopy is recommended. For women with ASC-US or worse at the 24-month follow-up, colposcopy is recommended. For women with two consecutive negative results, return to routine screening is recommended.

> **Box 38.2** ASCCP guidelines for the management of women aged 21–24 years with atypical squamous cells of undetermined significance [8]
>
> **Initial Management**
>
> For women aged 21–24 years with ASC-US, cytology alone at 12-month intervals is preferred, but reflex HPV testing is acceptable. If reflex HPV testing is performed with ASC-US and the HPV result is positive, repeat cytology in 12 months is recommended. Immediate colposcopy or repeat HPV testing is not recommended. If reflex HPV testing is performed and is negative, return for routine screening with cytology alone in three years is recommended.
>
> **Follow-Up**
>
> For women with ASC-US who are aged 21–24 years, follow-up with cytology at 12-month intervals is recommended. Colposcopy is not recommended. For women with ASC-H or HSIL+ (HSIL, atypical glandular cells [AGC], or cancer) at the 12-month follow-up, colposcopy is recommended. For women with ASC-US or worse at the 24-month follow-up, colposcopy is recommended. For women with two consecutive negative results, return to routine screening is recommended.

Unlike older women, an immediate colposcopy following ASC-US or LSIL is explicitly not recommended in younger women. Instead, cytology alone should be repeated in 12 months. If the 12-month follow-up cytology has a higher-grade abnormality (ASC-H, AGC, or HSIL), then colposcopy should be performed. Otherwise, if cytology is negative or again shows a low-grade abnormality (ASC-US or LSIL), cytology alone should be repeated again in 12 months. The patient can be returned to routine screening if both the 12-month and 24-month repeat cytology are negative. If any cytologic abnormalities are present 24 months after the initial abnormal cytology, colposcopy should be performed. Colposcopy is typically performed in patients with a negative 12-month cytology but an abnormal 24-month cytology [8] (Figure 38.1).

HPV testing is not recommended as a reflex test with LSIL because 77 percent of LSIL cytologic specimens are HPV positive [9]. As screening recommendations for women under age 30 do not include co-testing, HPV test results should not be inadvertently available as they sometimes are in older women with LSIL cytology. ASC-US management differs slightly from LSIL management. The preferred approach is similar to LSIL: testing with cytology alone and repeating in 12 months. Management without HPV testing is preferred. However, unlike LSIL, HPV reflex testing is acceptable following ASC-US. If the HPV test is positive, then the recommendation is to repeat cytology at 12 and 24 months. Immediate colposcopy is not recommended. If the HPV test is negative, then the patient can return to routine screening (repeat cytology in three years).

Management of a woman turning 25 during the surveillance period is not explicitly covered in the ASCCP guidelines. If the patient turns 25 years old during the surveillance period, it would be reasonable to complete the surveillance as planned.

Table 38.1 Regression of CIN 2 over time in women ages 21–24 years [11]

Time interval (years)	Regression rate (%)
1	38
2	63
3	68

However, an abnormality detected should be managed per the management guidelines for women 25 and older [8].

In this case, the implications of LSIL cytology and management recommendations were reviewed with the patient. She was counseled that if her cytology at 12 months revealed a higher-grade abnormality, then a colposcopy should be performed at that time. HSIL cytology reveals HSIL histology on biopsy up to 70 percent of the time, which is significantly higher than found with LSIL cytology. Under Lower Anogenital Squamous Terminology nomenclature, cervical HSIL lesions include what were previously termed CIN 2 and CIN 3 [10]. HSIL histology is usually treated by excision or ablation in older women. However, because of high regression rates (Table 38.1) and potential pregnancy-related complications associated with treatment, a conservative approach is permissible for the management of cervical HSIL in patients like this one with fertility concerns. Cervical HSIL (CIN 2) can be followed with cytology and colposcopy at six-month intervals. In this case, her repeat cytology was negative, and she was scheduled to return for repeat cytology in 12 months [8, 11]. Use of HPV vaccine in a woman with abnormal cytology is discussed in detail in Case 44.

Key Teaching Points

- HPV infection is common in adolescents and young adults, while cervical cancer is tremendously rare.

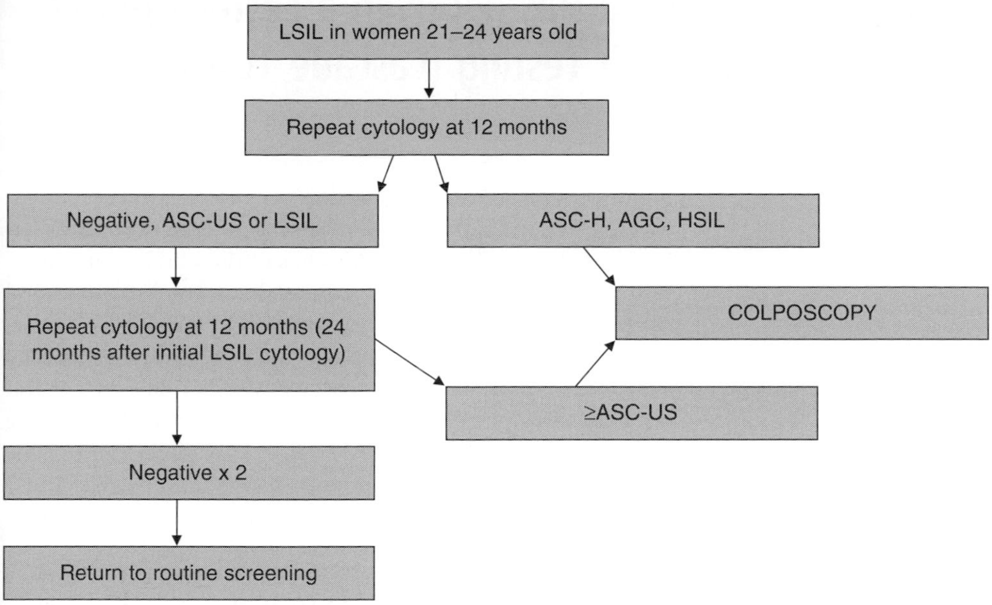

Figure 38.1 Management of LSIL in women 21–24 years old [6].

- HPV infections and abnormal cytology have a higher resolution rate in younger adults than in older women.
- LSIL cytology is managed more conservatively in young adults since regression rates are higher and rates of HSIL histology lower than in older women.
- Women ages 21–24 with LSIL are typically followed with annual cytology without HPV testing. Colposcopy is reserved for women with high-grade abnormalities or low-grade abnormalities that persist for 24 months. Patients can return to routine screening after two consecutive normal cytology results.
- Reflex HPV testing is acceptable with ASC-US cytology. If HPV positive, risk is similar to LSIL, so management is similar.

References

1. Moscicki, A. HPV infections in adolescents. *Disease Markers* 2007;23:229–234.

2. American College of Obstetricians and Gynecologists. Cervical cancer screening and prevention. Practice bulletin No. 168. *Obstet Gynecol* 2016;128:111–130.

3. American College of Obstetricians and Gynecologists. Management of abnormal cervical cancer screening test results and cervical cancer precursors. Practice Bulletin No. 140. *Obstet Gynecol* 2013;122:1338–1367.

4. Katki HA, Schiffman M, Castle PE et al. Benchmarking CIN 3+ risk as the basis for incorporating HPV and Pap cotesting into cervical screening and management guidelines. *J Low Genit Tract Dis* 2013;17 (5 Suppl 1):S28.

5. Benard VB, Watson M, Castle PE, Saraiya M. Cervical carcinoma rates among young females in the United States. *Obstet Gynecol* 2012;120:1117–1123.

6. Cox JT, Schiffman M, Solomon D. Prospective follow-up suggests similar risk of subsequent cervical intraepithelial neoplasia grade 2 or 3 among women with cervical intraepithelial neoplasia grade1 or negative colposcopy and directed biopsy. *Am J Obstet Gynecol* 2003;188:1406–1412.

7. Katki HA1, Schiffman M, Castle PE et al. Five-year risk of CIN 3+ to guide the management of women aged 21 to 24 years. *J Low Genit Tract Dis* 2013;17 (5 Suppl 1): S64–S68.

8. Massad L, Einstein M, Huh W et al. 2012 Updated consensus guidelines for the management of abnormal cervical cancer screening tests and cancer precursors. *J Low Genit Tract Dis* 2013;17 (5 Suppl 1): S1–S2.

9. Arbyn M, Sasieni P, Meijer CJ et al. Chapter 9: Clinical applications of HPV testing : a summary of meta-analyses. *Vaccine* 2006;24 (suppl 3): S78–S89.

10. Waxman AG, Chelmow D, Darragh TM, Lawson H, Moscicki AB. Revised terminology for cervical histopathology and its implications for management of high-grade squamous intraepithelial lesions of the cervix. *Obstet Gynecol* 2012 December;120 (6):1465–1471.

11. Moscicki A, Ma Y, Wibbelsman C et al. Rate of and risks for regression of cervical intraepithelial neoplasia 2 in adolescents and young women. *Obstet Gynecol* 2010;116:1373–1380.

A 25-Year-Old Woman Who Has Received a Letter from an Aunt Recommending Lynch Testing (Cascade Testing)

Jessica M. Kingston

History of Present Illness

A 25-year-old woman presents for annual exam. She provides a letter from her aunt recommending that she undergo testing for Lynch Syndrome. Her mother was diagnosed with endometrial cancer at age 47, her maternal aunt was recently diagnosed with colon cancer at age 48 and tested positive for Lynch Syndrome, and her maternal grandmother had endometrial cancer diagnosed at age 53.

Her past medical and surgical histories are negative. Menarche was at age 12. Menses are normal and regular. She has no history of sexually transmitted infections, has had four lifetime sexual partners, and has been monogamous with a male partner for two years. She uses condoms for contraception. Pap test done three years ago was normal. She has never been pregnant and plans for pregnancy in about five years. She has never smoked, has less than one alcoholic drink per week, and denies substance use. She is an art history graduate student.

Physical Examination

General appearance   Well developed, well nourished

Vital Signs

Temperature	37.0°C
Pulse	76 beats/min
Blood pressure	110/68 mmHg
Respiratory rate	16 breaths/min
Height	63 inches
Weight	142 lb
BMI	25 kg/m^2
Breasts	Symmetric, no skin changes, no palpable masses or axillary lymphadenopathy, no nipple discharge
Abdomen	Thin, soft, non-tender, no masses
External genitalia	Normal female
Vagina	Scant physiologic discharge
Cervix	Nulliparous without lesions
Uterus	Anteverted, mobile, normal size, non-tender
Adnexa	No palpable masses, non-tender
Depression screen	Negative
Laboratory Studies	Pap test negative for intraepithelial lesion, gonorrhea and chlamydia tests negative

How Would You Manage This Patient?

The patient's family history is notable for three relatives with Lynch associated cancers diagnosed at young ages. Her maternal aunt has a Lynch syndrome mutation. Cascade testing (genetic testing for an at-risk individual who has a family member with a known mutation) is indicated. The patient was referred to a cancer genetics specialist, underwent counseling, and chose to be tested. Presence of the MSH2 gene mutation was confirmed. She initiated a combination oral contraceptive pill to reduce her risk for endometrial and ovarian cancers and aspirin 600 mg daily to reduce colorectal cancer risk. Screening colonoscopy was normal, and repeat screening was planned every 1–2 years. Additional screening recommendations included annual clinical breast and pelvic examinations, and starting at age 30–35, endometrial biopsy every 1–2 years. She plans hysterectomy with bilateral salpingoophorectomy by age 40.

Lynch Syndrome and Cascade Testing

Lynch Syndrome

Lynch syndrome is an autosomal dominant cancer syndrome characterized by defects in DNA mismatch repair genes. Colorectal, endometrial, and ovarian cancers are the most common cancers associated with Lynch syndrome. Other primary tumors include gastric, small bowel, hepatobiliary, some types of breast, renal pelvis and ureter, and certain brain and sebaceous skin tumors [1]. The most common mutations involve MLH1, MSH2, MSH6, and PMS2 genes [2].

Population prevalence of Lynch syndrome ranges from 1 in 600 to 1 in 3,000 [1]. Three to five percent of uterine cancer is hereditary, and Lynch accounts for most of these cases [3]. Eight to 13 percent of ovarian cancers are hereditary, and 10–15 percent of these are associated with Lynch syndrome [3], which is also responsible for most hereditary cases of colorectal cancer. A retrospective review of Lynch syndrome families found that in most women with gastrointestinal and gynecologic metachronous cancers, the gynecologic cancer presented 11 years earlier than the gastrointestinal cancer [4].

Risks for colorectal, endometrial, and ovarian cancer in women with Lynch syndrome are much higher compared to risks for sporadic cancers [2], and they also have an earlier age of onset (Table 39.1). Lynch-associated tumors exhibit different biology than sporadic cancers. More than half of Lynch syndrome ovarian cancers are diagnosed as Stage I or II. They are usually non-serous, whereas BRCA-associated tumors are almost always high-grade serous carcinomas. Lynch-associated ovarian cancers may also have a more favorable prognosis [3]. Similar to ovarian cancers, colorectal cancer tends to be diagnosed at earlier stages with fewer distant metastases compared to sporadic cases, with more favorable prognosis. Most Lynch-associated cancer is found in the proximal colon. Studies differ on whether Lynch-associated endometrial cancer has more aggressive histology or less favorable prognosis compared to sporadic cases [1].

Table 39.1 Lynch syndrome cancer lifetime risk and mean age of onset compared to sporadic cancers [1, 2, 3, 8]

	Risk to age 70		Mean age at onset (years)	
	Lynch (%)	Sporadic cases (%)	Lynch	Sporadic cases
Colorectal	18–61	1.7	45	63–72
Endometrium	16–61	2.6	50	60
Ovary	6–14	1.4	42–49	60–65

Table 39.2 Comparison of Amsterdam criteria[5] and revised Bethesda guidelines[6]

Amsterdam II criteria	Revised Bethesda guidelines
Three or more relatives with an associated cancer and one is a first-degree relative of the other two	Colorectal cancer diagnosed in patient age less than 50
Two or more successive generations affected	Presence of synchronous or metachronous Lynch syndrome-associated tumors regardless of age
One or more relatives diagnosed < age 50	Colorectal carcinoma with high microsatellite instability histology in a patient age less than 60
Familial Adenomatous Polyposis should be excluded in those with colorectal cancer	Colorectal cancer diagnosed in one or more first-degree relatives with a Lynch syndrome-associated tumor, with one of the cancers diagnosed age less than 50
Tumors should be verified by pathologic evaluation	Colorectal cancer diagnosed in two or more first-degree or second-degree relatives with Lynch syndrome-associated tumors, regardless of age

Risk Assessment and Testing

Genomic instability in Lynch syndrome is due to a defect in DNA mismatch repair affecting the entire genome, including noncoding single nucleotide and dinucleotide repeats scattered throughout the DNA. Microsatellites are noncoding single nucleotide and dinucleotide repeats. Microsatellite instability is the insertion or deletion of additional nucleotides into or from the microsatellites. Almost all Lynch syndrome tumors exhibit microsatellite instability. Nonhereditary tumors can arise from microsatellite instability, but the mechanism differs, and is due to methylation of the MLH1 promoter.

Testing for Lynch syndrome can be complex, and referral to a cancer genetics specialist is advised. Family history alone can suggest risk for Lynch syndrome. Women with a first-degree relative with endometrial or colorectal cancer diagnosed before age 60 or a pattern of repeated generations affected by Lynch-associated cancers should be referred for genetic counseling [1]. Referral should also be considered if the relative with cancer is a distant relative if few family members reached advanced age, if she has few female relatives, or female family members had hysterectomy or oophorectomy at young ages [1]. Guidelines can help identify at-risk individuals (Table 39.2). The Amsterdam II criteria have sensitivity and specificity for diagnosing Lynch syndrome of 22 percent and 98 percent respectively [5]. If each of the criteria is met, Lynch syndrome should be suspected. The Revised Bethesda Guidelines aim to identify individuals with colorectal cancer who should undergo tumor testing. The sensitivity and specificity of any one of these guidelines are 82 percent and 77 percent respectively [6].

When possible, Lynch syndrome testing should start with tumor tissue from an affected relative. Immunohistochemistry can detect Lynch syndrome mismatch repair genes. Presence or absence of these genes further guides germline testing. Lynch syndrome is excluded if all four mismatch repair proteins are present. However, when family history is suspicious, microsatellite instability testing can be done. If microsatellite instability is absent, Lynch syndrome is excluded. When immunohistochemistry reveals MLH1 protein absence, promoter methylation testing is done. If there is promoter methylation, Lynch syndrome is excluded. If promoter methylation is absent, then unaffected relatives require germline DNA testing. If tumor testing reveals absent MSH2, MSH6, or PMS2,

then targeted germline testing can be done for at-risk relatives. If a tumor from an affected relative is not available, relatives should first be counseled by a cancer genetics specialist, and then undergo testing as appropriate.

Risk Reduction

Women with Lynch syndrome can reduce cancer risk through screening, chemoprevention, and surgery. There are no current proven cost-effective endometrial or ovarian cancer screening strategies for women with Lynch syndrome. National Comprehensive Cancer Network guidelines recommend endometrial sampling every 1–2 years starting at age 30–35 [7, 8]. Transvaginal ultrasound and CA 125 measurements are not useful in screening for Lynch-associated ovarian cancer likely because these tumors are different than BRCA-associated tumors [3]. Screening colonoscopy significantly reduces risk for colorectal carcinoma in Lynch syndrome patients, and is recommended every 1–2 years starting at age 20–25, or 2–5 years before the earliest relative's cancer diagnosis, whichever is earlier [7, 8]. While some breast cancers are included in Lynch syndrome, routine screening is recommended [1].

Chemoprevention for women with Lynch Syndrome further reduces cancer risk. Aspirin 600 mg daily can reduce colorectal cancer risk by up to 63 percent [7]. Participants in the CAPP2 trial taking aspirin also noted reduction in all Lynch-associated cancers [9]. Given the 50 percent reduction in endometrial and ovarian cancers in the general population on combination hormonal contraceptives, it is thought that

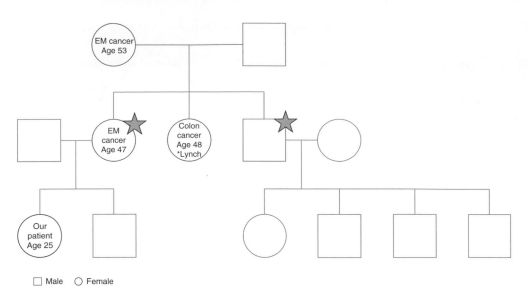

Figure 39.1 Pedigree for our patient's family to illustrate cascade testing. First-degree relatives of maternal aunt (patient's mother and uncle) should be offered testing first.

☐ Male ○ Female

women with Lynch syndrome will also benefit, although studies of affected families are limited [3]. Progestin only medications may also reduce risk for endometrial cancer.

Risk-reducing hysterectomy with bilateral salpingoophorectomy should be offered once childbearing is complete [8, 10]. Surgical approach should be individualized, and colorectal screening should be up to date preoperatively. Gynecologic surgery can be done concurrently for women with Lynch syndrome undergoing surgery for colorectal cancer.

Cascade Testing

Cascade testing is active, targeted genetic testing of at-risk individuals who have a family member with a known mutation. When the exact mutation and its location are known, testing is efficient and less costly. Cascade testing systematically reaches all potentially affected family members to allow identification and cancer prevention while minimizing screening and testing costs. Mutation carriers can benefit from increased surveillance, chemoprevention, and risk-reducing surgery, and those who test negative can follow routine cancer screening guidelines. The estimated cost of testing an individual for all Lynch mutations is $1500–4000 versus $200–500 when the specific mutation is known [11]. When a family member tests positive for Lynch syndrome, all first-degree relatives have a 50 percent chance of having the mutation. Therefore, genetic testing should be offered and begin with all first-degree relatives of the tested patient, and then branch outward [11]. For our patient, her mother and uncle should be offered testing first (Figure 39.1). If her mother tests positive, then our patient should be offered testing. If her uncle tests negative, his children do not need testing. Cascade testing is similarly effective for other autosomal dominant adult onset diseases such as familial hypercholesterolemia and hereditary breast and ovarian cancer.

When discussing Lynch syndrome testing results with an affected patient, The American Medical Association and other authors support protecting patient confidentiality [12]. Patients who test positive for Lynch syndrome should be informed of the risks to their family members, as well as the benefits for family members who undergo testing. The affected family member should be encouraged to disclose this information to all relatives. Physicians should offer to assist with disclosure to other family members, including enlisting the help of a cancer genetics specialist [12]. A multicenter study of 174 affected individuals who underwent Lynch syndrome testing showed that 98 percent disclosed test results to their relatives. As a result, up to three first-degree relatives were tested for Lynch syndrome for each affected individual [13].

Cascade testing confers cost savings and significant public health benefit; however, communication and organizational barriers exist in implementation. Physicians and patients may not understand test results and genetic testing options. Patients may express privacy concerns, fear blame, or may not be in contact with relatives. Other countries employ national cancer registries and public health coordinators to track results, arrange genetic testing, contact relatives, and schedule surveillance exams. Studies and experience gleaned from other countries shows that direct contact of family members by genetic counselors improves testing uptake [11]. Efforts are underway to improve US systems, including the Electronic Medical Records and Genomics (eMERGE) network, part of the National Human Genome Research Institute of the NIH. A secure website developed by genetic counselors at the University of California San Francisco, Kintalk.org, provides Lynch syndrome patients a forum to share results, connect with others, and be updated regarding new research. The site also includes educational videos on genetic counseling and testing for Lynch syndrome. These and other broad-based public health outreach strategies will be necessary to improve the rate of cascade testing for relatives of individuals affected with Lynch syndrome as well as those affected by other autosomal dominant adult onset diseases.

Key Teaching Points

- Women with personal or family history suggestive of Lynch syndrome should be referred to a cancer genetics specialist.
- When possible, Lynch syndrome testing should begin with tumor tissue to yield the most informative results for affected and unaffected relatives.
- Screening for women identified with Lynch syndrome should include endometrial biopsy every 1–2 years starting between age 30–35 and colonoscopy every 1–2 years. starting between age 20–25, or 2–5 years before the earliest cancer diagnosis in the family, whichever is earlier.

- Aspirin 600 mg daily can reduce colorectal cancer risk. Progestin-only treatment or combination oral contraceptives may reduce risk for endometrial and ovarian cancers.
- Cascade testing includes genetic counseling and targeted testing of family members who have a relative diagnosed with diseases caused by autosomal dominant mutations.
- Cascade testing reduces screening and testing costs, and facilitates early identification and disease treatment.
- Cascade testing for Lynch syndrome allows early initiation of measures to reduce cancer risk in affected family members.

References

1. American College of Obstetricians and Gynecologists. Lynch syndrome. Practice bulletin No. 147. *Obstet Gynecol* 2014;124:1042–1054.

2. Barrow E, Hill J, Evans DG. Cancer risk in Lynch syndrome. *Fam Cancer* 2013;12 (2):229–240.

3. Nakamura K, Banno K, Yanokura M et al. Features of ovarian cancer in Lynch syndrome. *Mol Clin Oncol.* 2014;2 (6):909–916.

4. Lu KH, Dinh M, Kohlmann W et al. Gynecologic cancer as a "sentinel cancer" for women with hereditary nonpolyposis colorectal cancer syndrome. *Obstet Gynecol* 2005;105:569–574.

5. Vasen H, Watson P, Mecklin JP, Lynch H. New clinical criteria for hereditary nonpolyposis colorectal cancer (HNPCC, Lynch syndrome) proposed by the International Collaborative Group on HNPCC.

Gastroenterology 1999;116 (6):1453–1456.

6. Umar A, Boland CR, Terdiman JP et al. Revised Bethesda guidelines for hereditary nonpolyposis colorectal cancer (Lynch syndrome) and microsatellite instability. *J Natl Cancer Inst* 2004;96(4):261–268.

7. National Comprehensive Cancer Network Clinical Practice Guidelines in Oncology. Genetic/Familial High-Risk Assessment: Colorectal. Version 1.2017. Available at NCCN.org.

8. Lindor NM, Petersen GM, Hadley DW et al. Recommendations for the care of individuals with an inherited predisposition to Lynch syndrome: a systematic review. *JAMA* 2006;296:1507–1517.

9. Burn J, Gerdes AM, Macrae F et al. CAPP2 Investigators: long-term effect of aspirin on cancer risk in carriers of hereditary colorectal cancer: an analysis from the

CAPP2 randomised controlled trial. *Lancet* 2011;378:2081–2087.

10. Schmeler K, Lynch HT, Chen L et al. Prophylactic surgery to reduce the risk of gynecologic cancers in the Lynch Syndrome. *N Engl J Med* 2006;354:261–269.

11. Hampel H. Genetic counseling and cascade genetic testing in Lynch syndrome. *Fam Cancer* 2016;15:423–427.

12. Stoffel EM, Ford B, Mercado RC et al. Sharing genetic test results in Lynch syndrome: communication with close and distant relatives. *Clin Gastroenterol Hepatol* 2008;6(3):333–338.

13. American Medical Association, Code of Medical Ethics. Opinion E-2.131: Disclosure of Familial Risk in Genetic Testing. www.ama-assn.org/ama/pub/physician-resources/medical-ethics/code-medical-ethics/opinion2131.page. Accessed 11 January 2013.

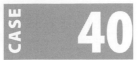

40 A 30-Year-Old Woman with Positive Margins on LEEP for HSIL

Jordan B. Hylton

History of Present Illness

A 30-year-old gravida 1, para 1 woman presents for follow-up after a Loop Electrosurgical Excision Procedure (LEEP) three weeks ago. Her referral Pap showed a high-grade squamous intraepithelial lesion (HSIL) and was human papillomavirus (HPV) positive. Colposcopy performed three weeks prior to the LEEP revealed a small punctate lesion with an area of mosaicism at 6 o'clock. The pathology of the colposcopy directed biopsies showed cervical HSIL. The pathologist commented "cervical intraepithelial neoplasia (CIN) III in the background of CIN II noted at the squamocolumnar junction at 6 o'clock" on her ectocervical biopsy. An endocervical curettage (ECC) performed at the time was read as CIN II. The patient's LEEP procedure was uncomplicated. During the consent discussion before the LEEP, the patient expressed significant concerns regarding impact of the procedure on future child bearing.

She has a history of smoking, but discontinued use following her abnormal colposcopy. She reports first intercourse at age 14. She is currently in a monogamous relationship. She has had regular cervical screening, and all prior tests were normal. She has no significant medical, surgical, or family history. She had chlamydia when she was an adolescent.

Physical Examination

General appearance	Well-appearing obese female in no apparent discomfort. Alert and oriented.

Vital Signs

Temperature	37.2°C
Pulse	88 beats/min
Blood pressure	112/68 mmHg
Respiratory rate	16 breaths/min
Oxygen saturation	99 percent on room air
Abdomen	Soft, nontender, nondistended, no rebound or guarding
External genitalia	Unremarkable, no lymphadenopathy
Vagina	Normal vaginal mucosa
Cervix	Parous cervix with no visible lesions. No friability or bleeding. Site of LEEP procedure healing appropriately.
Uterus	Anteverted, mobile, normal size with no tenderness on bimanual exam.
Adnexa	No abnormalities appreciated on palpation.
Extremities	No tenderness or edema.
Pathology report of LEEP specimen	Foci of HSIL (CIN II/III) as well as extensive background of CIN II extending past ectocervical surgical margin. (Figure)

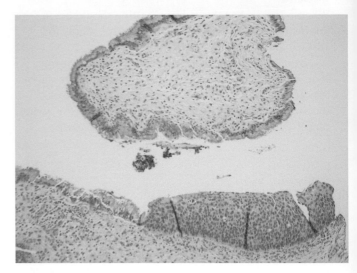

Figure 40.1 Cervical biopsy showing diffuse strong p16 expression in areas of atypical squamous epithelium extending beyond the margin of the LEEP specimen. Image provided by Cora Uram-Tuculescu, MD

How Would You Manage This Patient?

The patient has HSIL present at her LEEP ectocervical specimen margin. She strongly desires optimal outcomes in planned future pregnancies. Her risk factors for cervical dysplasia include her history of smoking and prior sexually transmitted disease. She successfully ceased use of tobacco following her abnormal colposcopy.

She was thoroughly counseled on the risk and benefits of the different management options. The preferred option is cervical cytology with endocervical sampling 4–6 months following her LEEP. Performing a repeat diagnostic excisional procedure was presented as an alternative, acceptable option. Preservation of her future fertility was her main concern, so she chose repeat cytology with ECC in four months. Her findings at that time were notable for HSIL on the endocervical sample. She and her provider chose to proceed with a second LEEP after colposcopy revealed vascular changes at 6 o'clock and pathology notable for normal ECC and cervical HSIL (CIN II-III) on ectocervical biopsy. Pathology of the repeat LEEP specimen showed cervical HSIL (CIN II-III) with clear endocervical and ectocervical margins. She became pregnant six months later. Her pregnancy was uncomplicated and she underwent cesarean delivery at term for active phase arrest. Repeat cotesting was recommended 12 months after her LEEP. This was done during her pregnancy, and both cytology and HPV tests were negative.

Positive Margins at Time of LEEP Procedure

Eighty-four percent of patients undergoing LEEP have negative margins on their pathology specimens, indicating

---

Box 40.1 ASCCP 2012 recommendations for managing positive margins after LEEP

If CIN 2, CIN 3, or CIN 2,3 is identified at the margins of a diagnostic excisional procedure or in an endocervical sample obtained immediately after the procedure, reassessment using cytology with endocervical sampling at 4–6 months after treatment is preferred. Performing a repeat diagnostic excisional procedure is acceptable. Hysterectomy is acceptable if a repeat diagnostic procedure is not feasible.

A repeat diagnostic excisional procedure or hysterectomy is acceptable for women with a histologic diagnosis of recurrent or persistent CIN 2, CIN 3, or CIN 2,3.

From: Massad SL, Einstein MH, Huh WK, et al. 2012 updated Consensus guidelines for the management of abnormal cervical cancer screening tests and cancer precursors. *J Low Genit Tract Dis* 2013; 17: S1–S27.

---

complete excision of their lesions [1]. Following initial excisional treatment, high-grade disease was present in 18 percent of women with incomplete excision compared to 3 percent with complete excision. Most recurrences presented within the first 24 months after the procedure [2]. Women who smoke tobacco (OR = 2.01) or have high-grade Pap tests (OR = 1.96) are more likely to have positive margins at the time of LEEP [3]. Additional risk factors include parity, age, and immunosuppression.

Ensuring complete excision is important to treat any residual high-grade disease and ensure that no cancer is present. In a study assessing the invasive potential of CIN 3, women with adequate treatment had a 0.7 percent risk for developing CIS over 30 years. In women with untreated CIS, 31.3 percent developed cancer within 30 years [4]. Residual dysplasia has been found in up to 63 percent of women with positive endocervical margins who underwent cold knife cone biopsy 4–6 weeks after the initial LEEP [5]. In a gynecologic oncology referral practice, 15.8 percent of women with CIN 3 on ECC at the time of their LEEP procedure had invasive cervical carcinoma on follow-up cold knife conization. Although these numbers were from a specialized referral practice with a high incidence of cancer in the initial specimens, it suggests that positive endocervical margins may be especially concerning [6]. Women who have CIN I on the margin of a LEEP specimen also have a risk of persistent or recurrent cervical dysplasia.

The 2012 American Society for Colposcopy and Cervical Pathology (ASCCP) updated *Consensus guidelines for the management of abnormal cervical cancer screening tests and cancer precursors* provide guidance on the management of positive margins at time of LEEP procedure (Box 40.1) [7]. While they include three options, follow-up, repeat excision, and hysterectomy, they clearly differentiate follow-up to be the preferred option. The ASCCP defines "preferred" as the option that is "the best (or one of the best) when there are multiple options." "Acceptable" means "one of multiple options when there is either data indicating that another approach is superior or when there are no data to favor any single option."

Follow-up is the preferred option because it balances the need to detect residual high-grade disease with minimizing the risk of overtreatment. Most patients with positive margins have no residual disease, and the few that do are unlikely to progress to cancer over the few months prior to reassessment. The low incidence of residual high-grade disease likely reflects a combination of lesions that were fully excised, natural regression of persistent disease,

and ablative cautery past the edge of the specimen at the time of the procedure. Immediate reexcision results in overtreatment for many patients. Most women who undergo immediate reexcision for positive margins had negative endocervical and ectocervical margins on the repeat specimen [8]. Following the repeat excision, 6.1 percent (three patients) had recurrent CIN 3 over a median follow-up time of two years [8]. Immediate reexcision is probably most appropriate in patients at high risk of loss to follow-up or who have completed childbearing. Hysterectomy is of much higher risk than reexcision, and should be reserved for patients where reexcision is not feasible. For most patients, retesting at 4–6 months is the most appropriate management. Choosing one of the alternate "acceptable" options over the preferred option should be reserved for special circumstances and occur only after careful counseling and shared decision making. Either reexcision or hysterectomy is acceptable for women with documented persistent high-grade disease.

The ASCCP guidelines do not have explicit recommendations for women with CIN I at the margins. For these women, a reasonable approach would be to repeat Pap and ECC at 4–6 months. If there is no suspicion for high-grade disease based on these tests, they can be managed as women with CIN I with cotesting at 12 and 24 months. Fifty-two percent of CIN I patients regress and approximately 10 percent progress to high-grade disease within one year. The risk of progression is increased with a prior high-grade lesion, so follow-up is particularly important in women with CIN I margins after LEEP for high-grade disease [9].

The effects of cervical excision procedures on preterm birth are controversial, and clouded by the possibility that CIN itself is a risk factor. Based on limited data, increasing volume or depth of LEEP specimens was not associated with increased risk of preterm birth in a recent meta-analysis [10]. However, these studies generally involved women having a single procedure. Multiple repeat excisions likely lead to cervical structural weakness. Follow-up cervical assessment is particularly appropriate in women with future pregnancy concern as it minimizes the risk of needing multiple excisions. ASCCP has an additional alternative for women with residual high-grade disease who are particularly concerned about pregnancy in the near future (CIN 2, CIN 3, or CIN 2,3 in Special Populations/Young Women) [7]. This algorithm allows observation for up to 12 months using colposcopy and cytology at 6-month intervals, provided colposcopy is adequate. While the ASCCP recommendations use the term "young women," they define "young women" as those women "who after counseling by their clinicians consider risk to future pregnancies from treating cervical abnormalities to outweigh risk for cancer during observation of those abnormalities." They clarify that no specific age threshold is intended [7].

In the case patient, reassessment using cytology with endocervical sampling 4–6 months after the LEEP is most appropriate for her for all the reasons it is generally preferred, and additionally optimizes her fertility plans. The advantages are avoiding invasive procedures, expedited assessment of margin status, and minimization of possible risks associated with future childbearing. Disadvantages to reassessment include delay in treatment of the few women with residual high-grade disease, although this is mitigated by the remote possibility of progression to cancer over the short time frame. Immediate reexcision can be considered in special circumstances like high likelihood of not returning for follow-up.

Key Teaching Points

- If Cervical HSIL (CIN 2 or 3) is identified at the margins of an excisional procedure or endocervical curettage (ECC) performed at the time of the LEEP, cytology, and ECC at 4–6 months is the preferred management.
- In women who have completed childbearing or are not interested in future fertility, reexcision is an acceptable, alternative option. Hysterectomy can be performed if reexcision is not possible.
- Women with CIN 1 at the LEEP margin can be reassessed with Pap and ECC at 4–6 months. If there is no concern for residual disease on these tests, they can be followed with cotesting at 12 and 24 months.
- Women with residual high-grade disease and immediate child-bearing plans can be followed with every six-month Pap and colposcopy for up to two years.
- Reexcision or hysterectomy are acceptable alternatives for women with documented residual high-grade disease after LEEP.

References

1. Duesing N, Schwarz J, Choschzick M et al. Assessment of cervical intraepithelial neoplasia with colposcopic biopsy and efficacy of loop electrosurgical excision procedure. *Arch Gynecol Obstet* 2012;286:1549–1554.

2. Ghaem-Maghami S, Sagi S, Majeed G, Soutter W P. Incomplete excision of cervical intraepithelial neoplasia and risk of treatment failure: a meta-analysis. *Lancet Oncology* 2007;8 (11):985–993.

3. Liss J, Alston M, Krull MB, Mazzoni SE. Predictors of positive margins at time of Loop Electrosurgical Excision Procedure. *J Low Genit Tract Dis* 2017;21 (1):64–66.

4. McCredie MR, Sharples KJ, Paul C et al. Natural history of cervical neoplasia and risk of invasive cancer in women with cervical intraepithelial neoplasia 3: a retrospective cohort study. *Lancet Oncol* 2008;9:425–434.

5. Felix JC, Muderspach LI, Duggan BD, Roman LD. The significance of positive margins in loop electrosurgical cone biopsies. *Obstet Gynecol* 1994;84 (6):996–1000.

6. Temkin SM, Hellmann M, Lee YC, Abulafia O. Dysplastic endocervical curettings: a predictor of cervical squamous cell carcinoma. *Am J Obstet Gynecol* 2007 May;196(5):469. e1–469.e4

7. Massad SL, Einstein MH, Huh WK et al. 2012 updated consensus guidelines for the management of abnormal cervical cancer screening tests and cancer precursors. *J Low Genit Tract Dis* 2013;17: S1–S27.

8. Ayhan A, Boynukalin FK, Guven S et al. Repeat LEEP conization in patients with cervical intraepithelial neoplasia grade 3 and positive ectocervical margins. *Int J Gynaecol Obstet* 2009:105 (1):14–17.

9. Bansal N, Wright JD, Cohen CJ, Herzog TJ. Natural history of low grade cervical intraepithelial lesions. *Anticancer Res* 2008 May–June;28 (3B):1763–1766.

10. Jin G, Lanlan Z, Li C, Dan Z. Pregnancy outcome following loop electrosurgical excision procedure (LEEP) a systematic review and meta-analysis. *Archives of Gynecology and Obstetrics* 2014;289 (1):85–99.

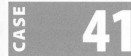

A 32-Year-Old Woman Whose Paternal Aunt and Grandmother Had Ovarian Cancer

Roopina Sangha

A 32-year-old gravida 1, para 1, presents to your office for an annual well-woman exam. She is asymptomatic, having regular menstrual cycles, and is currently using combined oral contraceptive pills (OCPs). Her daughter is three years old, and she would like to have at least one additional child. Review of her family history reveals her paternal grandmother died at age 68 years from ovarian cancer, and she has a paternal aunt who was diagnosed with ovarian cancer at age 49 and recently passed away at age 53. She then becomes tearful and states that her aunt's death has made her fearful of ovarian cancer, and she asks you to order tests to screen for this.

She is African American and has no known Jewish ancestry. She achieved menarche at age 11 years and was 29 years of age when she had her first child. Extensive review of her family history did not reveal any other cancers. Her physical examination, including clinical breast exam, was completely normal.

How Would You Manage This Patient?

This patient has a family history that is suspicious for a hereditary cancer syndrome, particularly a BRCA mutation, given the history of ovarian cancer in two paternal relatives. You inform her that there are currently no recommendations to screen for ovarian cancer in the general population [1, 2]; however, given her family history, there are options for enhanced screening in high-risk individuals. You refer her to a genetic counselor, where she undergoes multigene testing for mutations that are associated with an increased risk for ovarian cancer. Her testing reveals she is a BRCA1 carrier; therefore, she is offered enhanced screening for breast and ovarian cancer as well as medical and surgical risk-reduction options.

She undergoes pelvic ultrasonography and CA-125 screening, which are both negative. Shortly thereafter, she stops her OCPs and is able to achieve pregnancy. At the age of 33, after delivering a healthy baby, she starts annual mammography and breast MRI for enhanced breast cancer screening and restarts OCPs for ovarian cancer risk reduction. In addition, she has yearly pelvic ultrasounds with CA-125 testing to screen for ovarian cancer. At the age of 35, she is certain she has completed childbearing and requests hysterectomy with risk-reducing bilateral salpingo-oophorectomy, which is performed without incident. Following surgery, she is started on estrogen replacement therapy and is considering bilateral mastectomy in the near future.

Hereditary Breast and Ovarian Cancer Syndrome

Hereditary or germline mutations such as BRCA gene mutations are responsible for approximately 10 percent of inherited ovarian cancers and 3–5 percent of inherited breast cancers [3]. BRCA1 and BRCA2 are tumor suppressor genes found on chromosomes 17 and 13, respectively, and are inherited in an autosomal dominant pattern with a 50 percent chance of transmission. The risk of ovarian cancer with BRCA1 is 39–46 percent and 10–27 percent with BRCA2. In addition, women with BRCA mutations have a 45–85 percent lifetime risk of breast cancer [5] and a 2.5-fold higher risk of pancreatic cancer, melanoma, prostate, and gastric cancer [4].

Guidelines have been created for a referral for a genetic risk assessment for women who are at high risk, defined as having a lifetime risk of 20–25 percent or higher based on family and medical history [4]. National Comprehensive Cancer Network (NCCN) guidelines for referral to genetic testing are given in Box 41.1 [1]. In addition to the BRCA mutations, testing for other hereditary cancer syndromes like Lynch syndrome (Mismatch repair genes, MMR), Li Fraumeni Syndrome (TP53 gene), Cowden syndrome, and *PTEN* Hamartoma tumor syndrome (PHTS) should be considered [1]. If at the time of genetic risk assessment, the patient is found to be at high risk for hereditary breast or ovarian cancer, then genetic testing is offered. Previously, step-wise, single-gene testing, starting with BRCA testing, was recommended. Now, however, initial multigene testing is preferred, as single-panel, multigene tests for *BRCA1, BRCA2, CDH1, PTEN, PALB2, CHEK2, ATM,* and *p53* are commercially available at no extra cost to the patient.

Pretest counseling should include a discussion about insurance coverage and the Genetic Information Nondiscrimination Act of 2008, which protects individuals against health and employment discrimination based on genetic information but does not apply to life or disability insurance. Other issues, such as the psychological and familial impact of testing and various outcomes of testing (positive, negative, uninformative, and variants of unknown significance), need to be considered. The impact of these test results, cancer risks associated with various mutations, and options for surveillance, chemoprevention, and risk-reducing surgery should be shared with the patient.

Ideally, genetic testing should begin in the affected family member, as families with a known, specific hereditary cancer gene will benefit most from testing. In cases where the affected family member carries a specific mutation, negative testing for that mutation in relatives confirms the gene has not been passed along, and those individuals are not at increased risk for cancer. In families with a concerning history but no confirmatory genetic testing of the affected family member(s), negative genetic testing does not necessarily mean that patient is not at increased risk. Nonetheless, genetic testing should still be offered to individuals with a concerning family history.

In women who test positive for any gene causing a hereditary breast or ovarian cancer syndrome, like the patient

Box 41.1 Criteria for referral to genetic counseling

Personal history of ovarian cancer
  Personal history of breast cancer and
  - Diagnosis at age 50 years or younger or triple negative at age 60 years or younger
  - Two breast cancer primaries
  - Male breast cancer
  - Known cancer susceptibility mutation within the family
  - A close relative with ovarian or pancreatic cancer at any age
  - A close relative with breast cancer at age 50 or younger
  - Two or more close relatives with breast and/or pancreatic cancer at any age

Personal history of breast, ovarian, or pancreatic cancer diagnosed at any age in a patient with Ashkenazi Jewish ancestry
  First- or second-degree relative with breast cancer at age 45 years or younger
  Close relative (1st, 2nd, or 3rd degree) with:
  - Known BRCA1 or BRCA2 mutation
  - Two breast cancer primaries in one relative,
  - Two relatives with breast cancer (one at or prior to age 50 years)
  - Ovarian cancer
  - Male breast cancer

Family history of three or more of the following cancers (may include separate primary cancers in the same individual):
  - Breast cancer
  - Pancreatic cancer
  - Prostate cancer with a Gleason score of 7 or greater
  - Melanoma
  - Sarcoma
  - Adrenocortical carcinoma
  - Brain tumors
  - Leukemia
  - Colon cancer or diffuse hamartomatous polyps of the GI tract
  - Endometrial cancer
  - Thyroid cancer
  - Kidney cancer

Adapted from The NCCN Guidelines, 2017 [1]

described above, enhanced surveillance and risk-reducing options, including chemoprevention and risk-reducing surgery, should be offered (see summary in Table 41.1). These should involve a shared decision-making model, keeping in mind her plans for future fertility as well as psychological and quality-of-life issues.

The options for breast cancer screening and prevention should be tailored to the patient's wishes after a thorough discussion of risks and benefits. The NCCN has made clear recommendations for cancer screening of women with *BRCA1/2* mutations [1], which include regular, periodic breast self-exams beginning at age 18 years, annual or semiannual clinical breast exams beginning at age 25 years, and annual MRI beginning between ages 25 and 29 years. Women between the ages of 30 and 75 years should undergo annual MRI and mammography.

Risk-reducing options for breast cancer include chemoprevention and risk-reducing surgery. Tamoxifen has been shown to reduce breast cancer risk by 62 percent in BRCA2, but not in BRCA1 mutation carriers, likely due to lower prevalence of estrogen-positive breast cancers in these women [6]. Prophylactic mastectomy offers a 90–95 percent reduction in the risk of developing breast cancer in high-risk women, including those with *BRCA1/2* mutations [4]. There is a trend toward nipple-sparing mastectomy with immediate reconstruction, and there appears to be no significant change in the benefit from a risk-reduction perspective. Risk-reducing bilateral salpingo-oophorectomy (RRSO) offers reduction in the risk of breast cancer of 40–70 percent and should ideally be performed by the age of 35–40 years or after childbearing has been completed. This recommendation is based on data suggesting that 26–34 percent of BRCA2 carriers develop breast cancer by age 50, and maximal benefit of RRSO on breast cancer reduction is gained by earlier removal of ovaries [4]. This protective effect may be lower in BRCA1 mutation carriers; however, RRSO is also recommended for ovarian cancer risk-reduction, as described below.

Current ovarian cancer screening options have not been found to reduce mortality from ovarian cancer; thus, the NCCN leaves this to the discretion of the provider. Acceptable options for enhanced screening in high-risk patients include annual serum CA-125 screening combined with annual or semiannual pelvic examination and transvaginal ultrasonography with color Doppler beginning at age 25–35 years. With regard to chemoprevention, OCP use in BRCA carriers is associated with a 27–54 percent risk reduction for ovarian cancer (OR 0.58, 95 percent CI, 0.46 to 0.73), with a greater benefit seen with prolonged use, albeit with the potential for a slight increase risk of breast cancer (OR 1.21, 95 percent CI 0.93–1.58) [7].

Due to the limitations of ovarian cancer screening, it is recommended that all BRCA mutation carriers strongly consider RRSO. This is recommended by the age of 35–40 years or after childbearing is complete, as was performed in the above patient, since 10–21 percent of BRCA 1 mutation carriers will develop ovarian cancer by the age of 50. RRSO reduces the risk of ovarian cancer by up to 96 percent, with the remaining 4 percent due to ovarian-like cancer of the peritoneum. RRSO in BRCA patients entails pelvic washings and a detailed pathological examination using a specific protocol, as there is a 10 percent chance of occult cancer [4]. Women with mutations in *BRCA2* may choose to delay BSO for a few years, as the age to develop ovarian cancer is typically later in *BRCA2* mutation carriers (only 3 percent by age 50). There has also been recent interest in performing risk-reducing bilateral salpingectomy at age 35–40 years and delaying oophorectomy

Table 41.1 Screening and prevention options for BRCA mutation carriers.

	Breast Cancer	Ovarian Cancer
Screening	• Regular/periodic breast self-exams beginning at age 18 years • Annual or semiannual clinical breast exams beginning at age 25 years • Annual MRI beginning between ages 25–29 years and annual MRI and mammogram from ages 30 to 75	• Annual or semiannual pelvic examination beginning at age 25–35 years • Annual or semiannual transvaginal ultrasound examination with color Doppler beginning at age 25–35 years • Annual serum CA-125 concentration beginning at age 25–35 years
Chemoprevention	• Tamoxifen (for BRCA 2)	• OCPs
Risk-reducing surgery	• Prophylactic bilateral mastectomy (90–95% risk reduction) • RRSO (40–70% risk reduction)	• RRSO (96% risk reduction)

until the time of natural menopause, recognizing that most ovarian cancer is thought to originate in the fallopian tubes. Currently, the SGO states "salpingectomy might be a feasible option, however it does not reduce risk of breast cancer" [8] and NCCN guidelines state "salpingectomy alone is not standard of care outside of clinical trials" [1].

There are no national guidelines around concomitant hysterectomy at the time of RRSO; however, this procedure would reduce the endometrial cancer risk in women on tamoxifen [4], those with BRCA1 (2.6 percent risk of serous uterine cancer) and those who wish to avoid progestin therapy due to concerns of increased risk of breast cancer. For these reasons, concurrent hysterectomy may be offered after a thorough discussion of risks and benefits.

Although RRSO decreases all-cause mortality by 55 percent in BRCA mutation carriers [9], it is associated with significant morbidity in younger women, often with immediate and severe vasomotor and sexual side effects. Osteoporosis, cardiovascular disease, stroke, and cognitive decline contribute to long-term morbidity. In BRCA carriers without a personal history of breast or ovarian cancer, hormone replacement (HRT) with estrogen alone (if patient has undergone hysterectomy) or a combination of estrogen and a progestin is acceptable for short term and does not significantly diminish the protective effects of RRSO [10].

Key Teaching Points

- If family history is suggestive of high risk for hereditary breast/ovarian cancer, then the patient should be referred to genetic counseling, with subsequent testing as indicated.
- BRCA genes are transmitted in an autosomal fashion; therefore, testing of other adult family members should be considered.
- The risk of ovarian cancer with BRCA1 is 39–46 percent and 10–27 percent with BRCA2. In addition, women with BRCA mutations have a 45–85 percent lifetime risk of breast cancer.
- BRCA mutation carriers should be counseled about the recommendations for screening, chemoprevention, and risk-reducing surgery.
- Since ovarian cancer screening has not been shown to reduce mortality, BRCA mutation carriers should strongly consider RRSO between the ages of 35 and 40 or once childbearing is complete.
- Concomitant hysterectomy at the time of RRSO is reasonable and involves discussion around risks and benefits.
- Benefits from RRSO are not negated by using short-term hormone-replacement therapy.

References

1. National Comprehensive Cancer Network. NCCN Clinical Practice Guidelines in Oncology (NCCN Guidelines): Genetic/familial high-risk assessment: breast and ovarian. Version 2.2017. 2016. www.nccn.org /professionals/physician_gls/pdf/genet ics_screening.pdf. (Accessed April 27, 2017).

2. Moyer VA, Force USPST. Risk assessment, genetic counseling, and genetic testing for BRCA-related cancer

in women: U.S. Preventive Services Task Force recommendation statement. *Ann Intern Med* 2014;160:271–281.

3. Couch FJ, Nathanson KL, Offit K. Two decades after BRCA: setting paradigms in personalized cancer care and prevention. *Science* 2014;343:1466.

4. American College of Obstetricians and Gynecologists, ACOG Committee on Practice Bulletins–Gynecology, ACOG Committee on Genetics, Society of

Gynecologic Oncologists. ACOG Practice Bulletin No. 103: Hereditary breast and ovarian cancer syndrome. *Obstet Gynecol* 2009;113: 957–66 (reaffirmed 2015).

5. Lancaster JM, Powell CB, Chen LM, Richardson DL, SGO Clinical Practice Committee. Society of Gynecologic Oncology statement on risk assessment for inherited gynecologic cancer predispositions. *Gynecol Oncol* 2015;136:3–7.

6. King MC, Wieand S, Hale K et al. Tamoxifen and breast cancer incidence among women with inherited mutations in BRCA1 and BRCA2: National Surgical Adjuvant Breast and Bowel Project (NSABP-P1) Breast Cancer Prevention Trial. *JAMA* 2001;286:2251–2256.

7. Moorman PG, Havrilesky LJ, Gierisch JM et al. Oral contraceptives and risk of ovarian cancer and breast cancer among high-risk women: a systematic review and meta-analysis. *J Clin Oncol* 2013;31:4188–4198.

8. Society of Gynecologic Oncology. SGO clinical practice statement: salpingectomy for ovarian cancer prevention. 2013. www.sgo.org/clinical-practice/guidelines/sgo-clinical-practice-statement-salpingectomy-for-ovarian-cancer-prevention/. (Accessed February 18, 2015).

9. Domchek SM, Friebel TM, Singer CF et al. Association of risk-reducing surgery in BRCA1 or BRCA2 mutation carriers with cancer risk and mortality. *JAMA* 2010;304:967–975.

10. Rebbeck TR, Friebel T, Wagner T et al. Effect of short-term hormone replacement therapy on breast cancer risk reduction after bilateral prophylactic oophorectomy in BRCA1 and BRCA2 mutation carriers: the PROSE Study Group. *J Clin Oncol* 2005;23:7804–7810.

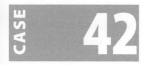
A 23-Year-Old Woman with HSIL on Cervical Cytology

Florencia Greer Polite

History of Present Illness

A 23-year-old woman, gravida 1, SAB 1, presents to your office for her annual exam. Her obstetrical history is significant for a spontaneous abortion at five weeks. Her past gynecologic history is significant only for a remote diagnosis of chlamydia. She received treatment at that time, and subsequent testing for sexually transmitted infections has been negative. She denies a history of cysts or fibroids. She underwent the human papillomavirus (HPV) vaccination at age 17 years and has not had prior cervical cancer screening. She has no prior medical or surgical history. Her only medication is the etonogestrel contraceptive implant, which was placed two years ago, and she has no known allergies. She smokes one pack of cigarettes per day since age 15, drinks about two glasses of beer on the weekends, and denies drug use. She is engaged to be married and plans to have her contraceptive implant removed next year to start a family.

Physical Examination

General appearance	Well-developed, well-nourished, alert, and oriented
Vital Signs	
Temperature	37.5°C
Pulse	80 beats/minute
Blood pressure	120/65 mmHg
Respiratory rate	16 breaths/minute
Height	65 inches
Weight	135 lb
Abdomen	Soft, non-tender, non-distended, no guarding or rebound
External genitalia	Unremarkable
Vagina	No abnormalities
Cervix	Nabothian cyst noted at 6 o'clock, otherwise normal
Uterus	Anteverted, mobile, non-tender
Adnexa	No masses or tenderness

Gonorrhea/chlamydia screening NAATs negative
Cervical cytology returns as high-grade squamous intraepithelial lesion (HSIL)

How Would You Manage This Patient?

This patient is less than 24 years of age and has a high-grade Pap test; therefore, colposcopy is the appropriate next step in her management [1, 2].

The patient was counseled extensively on smoking cessation and advised on the need for colposcopy as the next step in management of her abnormal cervical cytology. Although immediate ("see and treat") Loop Electrosurgical Excision Procedure would be an acceptable option in women aged 25 years and older, it is considered unacceptable in women aged 21–24.

She returned to the office for colposcopy, at which time informed consent and a urine pregnancy test were obtained prior to the procedure. Her colposcopy was adequate, and biopsies were performed and returned as CIN 2 of the ectocervix with a negative endocervical curettage.

She was counseled about the options of observation with colposcopy and cytology at six-month intervals versus excision or ablation of the transformation zone. Based on her nulliparity and desire for childbearing in the near future, she was advised that observation is recommended, provided she was agreeable to return for follow-up. She elected observation, and at her six-month follow-up, she had stopped smoking, her colposcopy showed no lesions, and her Pap returned as negative. Cytology and colposcopy were again negative at her next six-month visit and had negative cotesting a year later. She subsequently returned to routine cervical cancer screening.

HSIL in Young Women

Almost all sexually active women will encounter an infection with the HPV in their lifetimes, and high-risk types of HPV are known to be the causative agent in over 99 percent of cervical cancers. Of these, HPV 16 and 18 are considered the most oncogenic subtypes and together account for almost 75 percent of cervical cancer cases [1, 3]. Fortunately, most HPV infections will resolve spontaneously, causing no untoward outcome. However, persistent HPV infection in women of all ages can lead to high-grade cervical lesions, specifically CIN 2 and 3, which are precursors to cervical cancer. Risk factors known to increase persistence of the HPV infection include smoking, HIV infection, and a compromised immune system. In addition, HPV 16 and 18 are more likely to persist than other subtypes. Young women are most likely to acquire an HPV infection, with a 60 percent prevalence in a two-year period and a cumulative lifetime risk of over 80 percent. Most young immunocompetent women will clear the infection in less than eight months and almost 95 percent will clear the infection to undetectable levels by two years [2].

Colposcopy is the initial management step in young women (aged 21–24 years) with HSIL on cervical cytology, as was done in the above patient. The goal of the colposcopy with biopsy is to aid in diagnosis, exclude invasive carcinoma, and determine the most appropriate next step in management. An adequate colposcopy requires that the entire cervix, transformation zone, and lesion (if present) be visualized. Areas of increased vascularity, acetowhite changes, or mosaicism are concerning for dysplasia and should be noted and biopsied. It is also reasonable to perform random biopsies, particularly if no lesion is visible, as four-quadrant random biopsies have been found to be more sensitive than colposcopically directed biopsies at detecting moderate to severe dysplasia. In patients with high-grade cytology, like the patient described above, an endocervical curettage (ECC) should also be performed, assuming a negative urine pregnancy test. Although pregnancy is not a contraindication to colposcopy with biopsies, it is a contraindication to performing an ECC.

Further management of HSIL cervical cytology will depend on the results from the colposcopic examination. The American Society for Colposcopy and Cervical Pathology (ASCCP) [1] has separate algorithms for special populations, which were endorsed by the American College of Obstetricians and Gynecologists (ACOG) [2], and which apply to this patient. Her HSIL cytology should be evaluated using the ASCCP algorithm for women aged 21–24 with cytologic HSIL, which is strictly age-based. Her high-grade histology should be managed according to their algorithm "Management of young women with biopsy-confirmed cervical intraepithelial neoplasia grade 2,3 (CIN 2,3) in special circumstances." Of note, the ASCCP defines "young women" as "those who after counseling by their clinicians consider risk to future pregnancies from treating cervical abnormalities to outweigh risk for cancer during observation of those abnormalities. No specific age threshold is intended" [1, 2, 4]. This algorithm applies to this patient, not only based on her age, but because of her fertility plans.

Specific recommendations for women aged 21–24 years with HSIL cytology are based on initial biopsy findings and include the following:

No evidence of CIN 2/3 on initial biopsy: surveillance with colposcopy and cervical cytology at six-month intervals for two years:

- If the colposcopy is adequate and the ectocervical and endocervical biopsies are negative or CIN I, the patient should continue to be managed conservatively and return to routine screening at the two-year mark.
- During the two years of surveillance,
  - If the patient has HSIL that persists for 1 year, biopsy is recommended again. If no CIN 2,3 lesion is observed, then observation can continue.
  - If the patient has the appearance of high-grade lesion that develops and persists during this time, biopsy is recommended. If no CIN 2,3 lesion is observed, then observation can continue.
  - If the patient has HSIL cytology that persists for 24 months and biopsy does not reveal a lesion that is CIN 2,3, a diagnostic excisional procedure is recommended.
  - If colposcopy is noted to be inadequate, treatment with a diagnostic excisional procedure is recommended.
  - If CIN 2,3 develops, patients should be managed according the ASCCP guidelines for young women, as outlined below.
  - If CIN 2,3 is evident on endocervical curettage, treatment with excisional procedure is recommended.

CIN 2,3 on initial biopsy may be followed closely or treated using excision or ablation of the transformation zone following the appropriate ASCCP algorithm, depending on immediate fertility plans. Patients should be appropriately counseled, taking into account their plans for fertility. Counseling should include risk for progression of disease and potential impact of cervical treatments on pregnancy. For patients without fertility plans, excision or ablation of the cervical transformation zone is preferred.

For women with immediate childbearing plans, as in the patient described above, observation is appropriate. For those who choose observation, colposcopy and cervical cytology should be repeated at six-month intervals to see if the lesion persists for more than one year.

- In patients who have CIN 2 specified, observation with colposcopy and cytology at six-month intervals is preferred if the colposcopy is adequate.
- In patients who have CIN 3 specified or those who have an inadequate colposcopy, treatment is recommended with either excision or ablation.
- For patients with CIN 2,3 on colposcopic pathology, it is appropriate to offer the patient conservative management with colposcopy/cytology at six-month intervals or treatment with either excision or ablation.
  - For patients who choose conservative management, persistent CIN 2,3 for two years or worsening of colposcopic findings would be an indication to proceed with treatment using excision or ablation of the transformation zone.
  - For patients with negative cytology and a normal colposcopy at two consecutive follow-up visits, cotesting in one year is recommended.
    - If cytology and HPV are negative, cotesting in three years is recommended.
    - If either is abnormal, repeat colposcopy is indicated.

The risks and benefits of treatment must involve an individualized assessment of the potential for resolution or progression of a lesion, the risk of the patient not following up, and the harms of overtreating lesions that will likely resolve, particularly in young patients who have not completed childbearing [4]. Adolescents and young women with CIN 2 appear to be more likely than older women to have resolution of their disease over time. Approximately 65–75 percent of CIN 2 lesions in this age group will resolve within three years [2]. Since young women have the greatest likelihood of resolving their HPV infection, conservative management with colposcopy and cytology at six-month intervals for up to two years, as was done in the above patient with CIN 2, is acceptable and recommended in most cases [1, 2, 4]. In addition, there is inconsistency in the histologic factors that constitute the diagnosis of CIN 2, and there is poor intraobserver reproducibility. Most experts consider CIN 2 to be a mix of true CIN 1 and CIN 3 that could not be differentiated by the pathologist, and the risk of progression of disease with this diagnosis appears to be intermediate [4].

Diagnostic excisional procedures present potential risks to young women considering childbearing, including an increased risk of preterm delivery and the resulting potential neonatal morbidity. Although women with the diagnosis of CIN appear to be at higher risk of preterm delivery compared to women without such history, this risk appears to increase as the volume and depth of tissue removed during excisional procedures increases [2]. In young women, this risk must be considered in the decision-making process, and in general, treatment should be reserved for those at high risk for malignancy or loss to follow-up. In CIN 3 lesions, which have the highest risk of progression to cancer, treatment is recommended regardless of the patient's age or future fertility plans.

Key Teaching Points

- HSIL cervical cytology in women aged 24 years and younger should be managed with colposcopy; an excisional procedure as the initial step is unacceptable in this age group.

- Smoking cessation should be encouraged, as smoking increases the risk that an HPV infection persists and thus increases the risk of subsequent cervical cancer.
- ASCCP algorithms for managing HSIL cytology are age-based, while algorithms for managing high-grade histology depend on the patient's fertility plans.
- Conservative management of HSIL, particularly when no CIN 2,3 is found on initial biopsy, is appropriate when the provider and patient consider risk to future pregnancies from treating cervical abnormalities to outweigh risk for cancer during observation of those abnormalities. For these patients, colposcopy and cytology can be repeated at six-month intervals for a period of up to two years.
- In appropriately counseled women with CIN 2,3 and plans for pregnancy in the near future, either observation at six-month intervals or an excisional or ablative procedure is considered acceptable, assuming that the colposcopy is adequate.
  - In cases where CIN 2 is specified, observation is recommended.
  - In cases where CIN 3 is specified or colposcopy is inadequate, an excisional procedure is recommended.

References

1. Massad LS et al. 2012 updated consensus guidelines for the management of abnormal cervical cancer screening tests and cancer precursors. *J Low Genit Tract Dis* 2013;17:S1.
2. ACOG Practice Bulletin Number 140, Management of abnormal cervical cancer screening test results and cervical cancer precursors, December 2013.
3. ACOG Practice Bulletin Number 168, Cervical cancer screening and prevention, October 2016.
4. Waxman AG, Chelmow D, Darragh TM, Lawson H, Moscicki A-B. Revised terminology for cervical histopathology and its implications for management of high-grade squamous intraepithelial lesions of the cervix. *Obstet Gynecol* 2012;120(6):1465–1471.

A 35-Year-Old Woman with a Strong Family History of Breast Cancer Not Linked to BRCA Mutation

Natalie A. Bowersox

History of Present Illness

A 35-year-old woman, gravida 3, para 2, presents for a well-woman visit. She reports regular periods that began at age 13. She has a Mirena IUD for contraception. Her first pregnancy was at age 25 and she completed childbearing at age 30. She has not had any breast biopsies in the past. She recently found out that her 45-year-old sister has breast cancer. She reports that her mother and her maternal grandmother were diagnosed with breast cancer in their 50s and 70s, respectively. Her sister underwent BRCA testing, which was negative. She would like to know what her risks are and what screening she should have.

She has no other medical problems and has never had surgery. She takes no medications and has no allergies. She denies smoking and using substances or drugs. She has occasional wine with dinner. Family history is otherwise unremarkable. She is not aware of family members with any other cancers.

Physical Examination

General appearance Well-developed, well-nourished woman in no apparent distress

Vital Signs

Temperature	36.5°C
Pulse	70 beats/min
Blood pressure	110/72 mmHg
Body Mass Index	27 kg/m^2
Breast	Visibly symmetric. No masses, skin changes, nipple discharge, tenderness, or enlarged axillary nodes bilaterally
Abdomen	Soft, non-tender, non-distended

Pelvic Exam

External genitalia	Normal appearing
Vagina	Pink and without lesions
Cervix	Normal appearing
Bimanual exam	No midline masses or tenderness, no adnexal masses or tenderness

How Would You Manage This Patient?

This patient clearly has a strong family history for breast cancer and is concerned about her own risk being elevated. Further family history was obtained and did not include any other first- or second-degree relatives with cancer. Her overall risk was assessed with the Gail model [1]. Using the Gail model, her lifetime risk of breast cancer was 31.3 percent and her five-year risk was 1 percent. Despite testing indicating that the familial cancer is not BRCA-related, this patient's lifetime risk of breast cancer is increased. She was referred to a genetic counselor. She was encouraged to stay active, with 30–45 minutes of aerobic exercise each day, and to limit her alcohol intake to less than 1

drink per day. She was advised to follow the National Comprehensive Cancer Network (NCCN) recommendations [2], which include a clinical breast exam every 6–12 months, practicing breast self-awareness, and annual MRI and mammography. You review with her their revised recommendations to "consider" tomosynthesis, and decide you will order it if mammography reveals dense breasts. Given her age and risk, tomosynthesis can be performed after discussion with the patient, but it is not specifically recommended at this time. She was advised to begin the screening immediately as she is within ten years of the age when her sister was diagnosed. Her family history should be reassessed every 5–10 years. She was counseled about the risks and benefits of risk-reducing agents such as tamoxifen or raloxifene. Since her five-year risk according to the Gail model is <1.7 percent, tamoxifen was not recommended at this time [2]. Her risk should be reassessed periodically and chemoprophylaxis readdressed if her risk assessment increases. This patient, with careful counseling, could consider risk-reducing mastectomy as she has a family history that makes her high risk. A risk-reducing bilateral salpingo-oopherectomy would not be indicated as she is not a BRCA carrier [2].

High-Risk Breast Cancer Screening

Breast cancer is the most common malignancy diagnosed in women, accounting for 30 percent of all new cases of cancer diagnosed in women each year [3]. Risk factors include female sex, age, reproductive history, genetic predisposition, history of chest radiation, prior history of breast hyperplasia, carcinoma in situ or cancer, and modifiable risks like exercise, obesity, and alcohol consumption. The incidence of breast cancer increases with increasing age, with a lifetime risk of about 12 percent or a 1 in 8 chance by age 85 [3]. Women who begin menarche before age 12 or who go through menopause after age 55 have an increased risk, as do women who are nulliparous, have their first birth after the age of 30, or never breastfed a child [4]. A personal history of radiation therapy to the chest, especially between the ages of 10 and 30, increases a woman's lifetime risk. This risk is highest in those who received radiation during adolescence. History of atypical hyperplasia, carcinoma in situ, or invasive cancer is associated with an increased risk of invasive cancer in the future. The majority of breast cancers are sporadic; however, 5–10 percent are hereditary, with BRCA 1 and 2 gene mutations accounting for about 30 percent [5]. There are other less common inherited mutations, which include Li-Fraumeni cancer syndrome (mutation of TP53), Cowden syndrome (mutation of PTEN and CDHI), and Peutz-Jeghers syndrome (mutation of STK11).

Screening recommendations are different between low- and high-risk women, and risk-reducing strategies are available for women at high risk. Women should be routinely assessed for breast cancer risk. It is important to identify women with a genetic predisposition for breast cancer as these patients benefit from referral for genetic counseling and possibly genetic testing. History should include age at menarche and menopause, reproductive history, recent use of hormonal contraception or hormone therapy, prior chest radiation therapy, and prior abnormal breast biopsies. Family history should include ethnicity and history of breast, ovarian, and prostate cancer in first-degree (sisters, brothers, parents) and second-degree relatives. History should include the age at diagnosis of these cancers in family members and any other cancers that may have occurred in the family.

Women whose initial history is suggestive of elevated risk should undergo formal risk assessment. There are several models available to determine whether a woman is at elevated risk including Gail, Tyrer-Cuzick, Claus, BRCAPRO, and BODACEA. The NCI Breast Cancer Risk Assessment Tool or Gail model gives lifetime and five-year risk estimates, which take into account the patient's age, age at first period, age at first live birth, breast cancer in first-degree relatives, and personal history of breast biopsies. This test can be completed in 1–2 minutes and is available at www.cancer.gov/bcrisktool [1]. This model has been validated in Caucasians and modified for African American and Hispanic populations. The Gail model is not as useful if there is a strong family history in non-first-degree relatives or a family history of cancers other than breast cancer [3]. The Tyrer–Cuzick model (www.cms-trials.org/riskevaluator) includes family history, age of onset of cancers, height, weight, reproductive history, hormone use, and history of atypical breast biopsies. The Claus, BRCAPRO, and BODACEA incorporate hereditary and familial factors. If the five-year risk assessment is greater than or equal to 1.7 percent or the lifetime risk is greater than 20 percent, the patient is considered high risk (NCCN Breast cancer screening).

Unlike in average risk women, where recommendations for clinical breast examination have changed, NCCN recommends clinical breast exam every 6–12 months in high-risk women. Like average-risk women, women at high risk should be counseled to be familiar with their breasts (breast self-awareness) and be encouraged to report any changes to their provider [6].

According to the NCCN Guidelines, mammography should begin (Table 43.1):

- The earlier of age 25–30 or 10 years younger than the age of diagnosis of premenopausal breast cancer in their youngest affected relative in women with a lifetime risk of greater than 20 percent
- Eight to ten years after mantle radiation in women who received mantle radiation between ages 10 and 30 (but not before age 25)
- Any time at or after age 35 in women with 5-year Gail model risk ≥1.7 percent

Tomosynthesis, a newer imaging modality for the breast, allows a three-dimensional view of the breast using x-ray and improves cancer detection and reduce false positive callback rates. NCCN has revised their guidelines to recommend

annual digital mammography and consideration of tomosynthesis to begin ten years prior to the youngest family member's age at diagnosis but not before age 30. The dose of radiation is doubled from tomosynthesis. Currently, the NCCN recommendations about tomosynthesis are vague, suggesting "consideration," but not making more specific

Table 43.1 Breast cancer screening and diagnosis

Risk factors	Screening/Follow-up
Women with lifetime risk >20% as defined by models largely dependent on family history	• Clinical encounter every 6–12 months to begin when identified as increased risk • Referral to genetic counseling • Annual screening mammogram to begin 10 years prior to age of diagnosis in youngest family member, not less than age 30. Consider tomosynthesis. • Recommend annual breast MRI to begin 10 years prior to age of diagnosis in youngest family member, not less than age 25. • Consider risk-reduction strategies • Breast awareness
Women ≥35 years with 5-year Gail model risk of invasive breast cancer ≥1.7%	• Clinical encounter every 6–12 mo to begin when identified as increased risk by Gail model • Annual screening mammogram to begin when identified as increased risk by Gail model. Consider tomosynthesis. • Consider risk-reduction strategies • Breast awareness
Prior thoracic radiation therapy (RT) (e.g., mantle irradiation) between ages 10 and 30 years old.	• Age <25 years: Annual clinical encounter beginning 8–10 years after RT and Breast awareness • Age ≥25 years: • Clinical encounter every 6–12 mo to begin 8–10 years after RT • Annual screening mammogram 8–10 years after RT but not prior to age 25. • Annual MRI to begin 8–10 years after RT but not less than age 25 years, and breast awareness • Consider tomosynthesis

recommendations [6]. One possible application might be if dense breast tissue is noted on mammography.

MRI has a higher sensitivity than mammogram, but is expensive and should be reserved for women who are at high risk. The increased sensitivity with MRI is most notable in women with dense breast tissue. The overall sensitivity of mammogram alone in high-risk women is 39 percent, and that of mammogram and MRI combined is 94 percent. When ultrasound and mammogram were combined, the sensitivity was 52 percent [4]. Mammogram and contrast-enhanced MRI are the recommended combination for high-risk women. The NCCN Guidelines recommend screening MRI in women with BRCA1 gene mutation and their untested first-degree relatives, women with history of chest radiation between 10 and 30 years of age, other genetic syndromes that would predispose to breast cancer, and women with a lifetime risk >20 percent [2]. Breast ultrasound should be reserved for women who cannot undergo MRI. There is not currently sufficient evidence to recommend thermography, breast-specific gamma imaging, positron emission mammography, or optical imaging [2]. Annual screening mammogram and MRI should begin ten years before youngest family member diagnosed (not earlier than age 30 for mammogram and age 25 for MRI), and referral to genetic counseling should be given (Table 43.1). If a patient appears to fall into more than one high-risk category, the more rigorous recommendation should be followed.

There is inconsistent evidence regarding lifestyle modifications and risk reduction; however, these changes can lead to better health overall. The American Cancer Society recommends maintaining a healthy weight with a BMI within the range of 18.5 to 25.0 kg/m^2, eating a balanced diet, and 150 minutes of moderate intensity exercise or 75 minutes of vigorous activity weekly, which may reduce risk by 25 percent [7]. The consumption of alcoholic beverages has been linked to increased risk for several cancers, including breast. This risk increases 7–9 percent for each additional daily drink [2,8]. They recommend less than 1 drink per day (1 ounce of liquor, 6 ounces of wine, or 8 ounces of beer) [7]. Obesity, especially in the postmenopausal patient, has been associated with an increased risk of breast cancer in seven prospective cohort studies, which showed an excess risk of 12 percent in overweight and 25 percent in obese women. While the risk-reduction benefits seen with these lifestyle modifications are modest, they have minimal risk, are low cost, and will allow motivated women to make positive change [7]. Breastfeeding has been shown in several studies to reduce the relative risk of breast cancer [2].

Chemoprevention has been shown to reduce the incidence of breast cancers in high-risk women. Risk-reducing agents include tamoxifen, raloxifene, exemestane, and anastrozole. Tamoxifen can be recommended to healthy pre- and postmenopausal women ≥35 years old with a life expectancy ≥10 years and who have a ≥1.7 percent five-year risk as determined by the Gail model or a history of LCIS. The NCCN Breast Cancer Risk Reduction Panel recommends tamoxifen at a dose of 20 mg/day. Tamoxifen, a selective estrogen receptor modulator, has been shown to reduce risk of breast cancer by 49 percent when given for five years [2]. The data for tamoxifen use for patients with a history of chest radiation and BRCA mutations are limited. Tamoxifen should not be used in women who have not completed childbearing. Side effects include menopausal symptoms, endometrial cancer risk, risk of thromboembolic events, and arthralgias, so patients should be monitored closely [2]. Raloxifene and aromatase inhibitors are not recommended for use in premenopausal women, but can be used in postmenopausal women.

Risk-reduction surgery includes bilateral mastectomy and bilateral salpingo-oopherectomy (RRSO). Mastectomy can be discussed with women who have a genetic predisposition for breast cancer, a strong family history, or a history of thoracic radiation treatment at age <30. This has been shown to reduce risk of developing breast cancer by 90 percent or more [2]. If a patient chooses this approach, annual exams of the chest and reconstructed breast should continue. RRSO can be recommended to women with known or suspected BRCA 1 and 2 mutations. This decision should be reached with the patient and a multidisciplinary team, which should include a breast surgeon and genetic counselor [2].

Key Teaching Points

- Risk assessment for breast cancer is a key component of any well-woman exam. This should include a family history including first- and second-degree relatives with any cancers, age at onset, and ethnicity.
- Woman who may be high-risk should be assessed with a risk assessment tool. The NCI Breast Cancer Risk Assessment Tool or Gail model gives lifetime and five-year risk estimates and is commonly used.
- A woman is considered high-risk for breast cancer if she has a family history suggestive of a familial breast or ovarian cancer, a first-degree relative who has tested positive for a gene mutation like BRCA, a history of chest radiation between the ages of 10–30, a five-year risk ≥1.7 percent or a lifetime risk of >20 percent according to a risk model, or a personal history of breast cancer or hyperplasia.
- Women who are high-risk should be referred for genetic counseling and possibly genetic testing.
- High-risk women should have increased surveillance, including a clinical breast exam every 6–12 months, breast self-awareness counseling, and annual mammogram and MRI beginning ten years prior to the age of the youngest relative's diagnosis, but not earlier than age 30 for mammogram and age 25 for MRI. Tomosynthesis may be considered.
- Chemoprevention has been shown to reduce the incidence of breast cancers in high-risk women.

References

1. National Cancer Institute: Breast Cancer Risk Assessment Tool. [Online] accessed 7/16/2017 2008. www.cancer.goy/bcrisktool/.
2. National Comprehensive Cancer Network. *NCCN Guidelines Version 1.2017 Breast Cancer Risk Reduction.* [Online] July 16, 2017. www.nccn.org/professionals/physicians_gls/pdf/breast_risk.pdf.
3. American College of Obstetricians and Gynecologists. Breast cancer risk assessment and screening in average-risk women. Practice bulletin No. 179. *Obstet Gynecol* 2017;130: e1–e16.
4. Bevers, T. Clinical management of the patient at increased or high risk. [book auth.] Copeland E, Bland K. *Breast: Comprehensive Management of Benign and Malignant Disease. 4th Edition.* s.l.: Saunders Elsevier, 2009, pp. 1381–1392.
5. Heisey R, Carrol J. Identification and management of women with a family history of breast cancer: practical guide for clinicians. *Can Fam Physician* October 2016;10:799–803.
6. National Comprehensive Cancer Network. *NCCN Guidelines Version 1.2017 Breast Cancer Screening and Diagnosis.* [Online] July 17, 2017. www.nccn.org/professionals/physician_gls/pdf/breast-screening.pdf.
7. Kushi LH, Doyle C, McCullough M et al. and The American Cancer Society 2010 Nutrition and Physical Activity Guidelines Advisory Committee, American Cancer Society guidelines on nutrition and physical activity for cancer prevention. *CA: Cancer J Clin.* 2012;62:30–67. doi:10.3322/caac.20140
8. Rosenberg L, Weber R, Sjoberg D, Vickers A. Impact of self-reported data on the acquistion of multi-generational family history and lifestyle factors among women seen in high-risk breast screening program: a focus on modifiable risk factors and genetic referral. *Breast Cancer Res Treat* 2017;162:275–282.

A 25-Year-Old Woman with LSIL Desiring HPV Vaccination

Christine Conageski

History of Present Illness

A 25-year-old gravida 1, para 0, woman presents for scheduled colposcopy. Her Pap test was reported as low-grade squamous intraepithelial neoplasia (LSIL). This was her first abnormal Pap test. She is currently in a mutually monogamous relationship and reports four lifetime sexual partners. Although she has no complaints today, she has questions regarding her Pap test and requests administration of the human papillomavirus (HPV) vaccine.

She has no medical problems. Prior surgeries include only a dilation and curettage for a missed abortion. She denies any history of smoking and she takes no medications. She is using combined oral contraceptive pills for birth control. She has not been vaccinated against HPV.

Physical Examination

General appearance	Well-developed, age appropriate female in no apparent distress

Vital Signs

Temperature	37.6°C
Pulse	76 beats/min
Blood pressure	110/62 mmHg
Height	64 inches
Weight	135 lb
BMI	23.2 kg/m^2
External genitalia	Normal female external genitalia
Vagina	Normal vaginal mucosa without discharge
Cervix	Nulliparous-appearing cervix. No lesions. Application of dilute (3–5 percent) acetic acid revealed a small area of thin acetowhitening at 5 o'clock without any significant vascularity. Lesion 5 mm in size, involving less than one quadrant of the cervix.
Uterus	Anteverted, small, and mobile. Non-tender.
Adnexa	No adnexal fullness or tenderness.

Laboratory Studies

Urine pregnancy test	Negative
Pap test	LSIL

How Would You Manage This Patient?

The patient has an LSIL Pap test and desires HPV vaccination. She presented to clinic for scheduled colposcopy as recommended by the 2012 American Society for the Study of Cervical Pathology and Colposcopy (ASCCP) Consensus guidelines [1]. Her colposcopy showed no high-grade features. A single biopsy of the acetowhite lesion was performed and pathology showed only cervical LSIL (cervical intraepithelial neoplasia

[CIN] 1). The patient was counseled that although the vaccine would not prevent the HPV she already acquired, it would protect from other high-risk HPV types and possible risk of reinfection in the future. After counseling, she opted to proceed with vaccination and was administered the first dose. She was scheduled to receive additional doses two and eight months later and to return for repeat cotesting in one year.

HPV Disorders

HPV is the most common sexually transmitted infection in the United States. Currently, 79 million Americans are infected with HPV, and over 14 million men and women become newly infected each year. HPV is so common that over 75 percent of sexually active men and women will acquire at least one type of HPV in their lifetime [2]. It is easily transmitted, most commonly through direct genital contact, but extragenital and fomite transmission have been described. HPV prevalence varies by age and is highest for 25- to 29-year-old women and decreases with age [3].

HPV is a double-stranded DNA virus that infects epithelial cells and can induce a variety of benign and malignant tumors resulting in anogenital cancers (cervix, vulva, vagina, penis, and anus), oropharyngeal cancers, and genital warts. There are over 150 identified HPV types, approximately 15 of which are oncogenic (high-risk). HPV 16 and 18 are the most significant of the high-risk types with high rates of persistence and carcinogenicity [4] (Figure 44.1). Together, HPV 16 and 18 account for 64 percent of all invasive HPV-associated cancers (65 percent for females and 63 percent for males) and 70 percent of squamous cell carcinomas of the cervix. 50–60 percent of high-grade cervical neoplasias are attributable to HPV 16 or 18 [5]. Other important high-risk types include HPV 31, 33, 35, 45, and 58, which are responsible for an additional 15 percent of HPV-associated cervical cancers (Figure 44.2).

There are currently no treatments for HPV infections, but most cervical cancers are preventable with regular screening and appropriate management of abnormal test results. Treatments are associated with risks, including pain, bleeding, psychologic stress, cost, and pregnancy complications. Only 80.7 percent of women report up-to-date cervical cancer screening. There are over 12,000 new cervical cancers annually in the United States [6]. There are no accepted screening strategies for other HPV-associated cancers, which affect over 19,000 men and women every year. Primary HPV prevention strategies such as vaccination, therefore, are critical.

The US Food and Drug Administration has approved three vaccines for the prevention of HPV infections. These vaccines cover 2, 4, or 9 HPV types. As of late 2016, the only commercially produced HPV vaccine in the United States is the 9-valent vaccine (9vHPV), approved in 2014. This vaccine covers the two most common and oncogenic high-risk HPV types, 16 and 18, as well as the next five most common high-risk types (HPV 31, 33, 35, 45, and 58). It also offers coverage

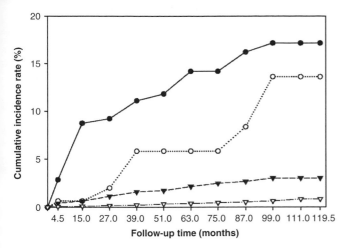

Figure 44.1 Cumulative incidence of cervical intraepithelial neoplasia grade 3 and cancer (≥CIN3) over a 10-year period. HPV 16 (closed circles), HPV18 (open circles), non-HPV16/18 oncogenic types (closed triangles), oncogenic HPV negative (open triangles). From [4] with permission

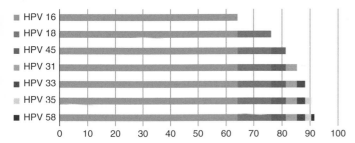

Figure 44.2 Prevalence of HPV Types in women less than 34 years of age with squamous cell carcinoma of the cervix. Data from [5]

for HPV 6 and 11, two low-risk types responsible for over 90 percent of genital warts.

The vaccine is currently licensed for both females and males starting at age 9 through 26 years of age. The Advisory Committee for Immunization Practices (ACIP) recommends routine HPV vaccination for girls and boys at 11–12 years of age as part of the routine adolescent immunization schedule. The vaccine can be given to males and females aged 13 through 26 years not vaccinated previously. For girls and boys who receive their first dose of the HPV vaccine before 15 years of age, only two doses are needed. The second dose should be given 6–12 months after the first. If the interval between the two doses is less than five months, a third dose is recommended. If females or males receive their first dose at 15 years of age or older, three doses are needed, with the second dose one to two months after the first dose and the third six months after the first dose [7] (Table 44.1).

For greatest effectiveness, boys and girls should be vaccinated before initiation of sexual intercourse. Within three years of initial sexual activity (median age 15.6 years), 48 percent of women will have evidence of cervical HPV infection [8]. In a vaccine-naïve population, phase III clinical trials of 4vHPV demonstrated 99 percent antibody response to all four HPV vaccine types regardless of age, sex, race/ethnicity, country of origin, smoking status, or BMI and high efficacy

Table 44.1 ACIP HPV vaccine recommendations

	Routine vaccination	Catch-up vaccination
Girls	Age 11 or 12 years 2 doses	Ages 13 through 26 years 3 doses
Boys	Age 11 or 12 years 2 doses	Ages 13 through 21 years 3 doses Males ages 22 through 26 may be vaccinated
Special populations	HPV vaccination is recommended through age 26 years for men who have sex with men and for immunocompromised persons (including those with HIV)	

Table 44.2 Efficacy in vaccine-naïve women for prevention of HPV-associated disease among females (combined 4vHPV and 9vHPV data)

Vaccine-related endpoint type	Vaccine efficacy	
	%	(95% Confidence interval)
CIN 2/3 or AIS		
HPV 6, 11, 16, 18	98.2	(93.8–99.8)
HPV 16	97.6	(91.1–99.7)
HPV 18	100	(86.6–100.0)
HPV 31, 33, 45, 52, 58	96.3	(79.5–99.8)
VIN/VAIN 2/3		
HPV 6, 11, 16, 18	100.0	(82.6–100.0)
HPV 16	100.0	(76.5–100.0)
HPV 18	100.0	(86.6–100.0)
HPV 31, 33, 45, 52, 58 *CIN2+, VIN2/3, VaIN2/3	96.7	(80.9–99.8)

Source: Markowitz LE, Dunne EF, Saraiya M et al. Human papillomavirus vaccination: recommendations of the Advisory Committee on Immunization Practices (ACIP). MMWR Recomm Rep. 2014;63(RR–05):1–30.

rates for the prevention of high-grade HPV lesions. Vaccination produced antibody titers higher than those from natural infection with HPV. Comparing 9vHPV to 4vHPV, a phase III trial demonstrated noninferior efficacy for HPV 6, 11, 16, and 18, and high efficacy for prevention of ≥CIN2, vulvar intraepithelial neoplasia (VIN) grade 2 or 3, and vaginal intraepithelial neoplasia (VAIN) grade 2 or 3 caused by HPV 31, 33, 45, 52, and 58 [9] (Table 44.2).

Vaccination is recommended regardless of sexual behavior, prior HPV exposure, or history of HPV-associated precancerous lesions. In phase III efficacy trials, the vaccine demonstrated no efficacy for progression of disease or impact on HPV clearance in females with HPV DNA detected at enrollment. The vaccine, however, did demonstrate 100 percent effectiveness at preventing high-grade lesions attributable to types not already acquired [9]. Natural HPV infection does not always elicit a measurable immune response. In a subgroup analysis of women enrolled in phase III trials who were HPV DNA negative, but seropositive (previous infection), prophylactic vaccination demonstrated significant efficacy in preventing reinfection and reactivation [8].

The vaccine is both safe and effective. There have been over 75 million doses of the HPV vaccine distributed in the United States since 2006. Most common side effects are mild, including redness and swelling at the injection site. Studies have shown no increased risks of significant adverse events such as autoimmune disorders, venous thromboembolisms, complex regional pain syndromes, or postural orthostatic tachycardia syndrome [10]. There is a higher incidence of injection-site adverse reactions with the 9vHPV compared with the 4vHPV, specifically increased erythema, and induration at the vaccination site.

This patient has been appropriately screened for cervical disease with cytology alone, which showed LSIL, indicating an acquired HPV infection. In the ASC-US LSIL Triage Study, 77 percent of women with LSIL were HPV-positive. LSIL represents a transient HPV infection and low risk of cervical cancer, but 27.6 percent of women with LSIL had CIN 2+ either on biopsies obtained at the initial colposcopic evaluation or during follow-up over the subsequent two years. For these reasons, the 2012 ASCCP guidelines recommend that women aged 25–29 years of age with an LSIL Pap result be evaluated with colposcopy without using HPV triage [1]. This patient was managed per the ASCCP 2012 guidelines, with colposcopic evaluation of her LSIL Pap test result. Her colposcopic findings and histology confirmed low-grade disease. Low-grade disease can be safely followed. Risk of progression is so small that a repeat co-test in one year is adequate assessment. Despite her HPV infection, she received the 9vHPV (3 doses), which should prevent secondary infections with other high-risk HPV types and decrease risk of reinfection or reactivation with the type she already acquired.

Key Teaching Points

1. HPV infection is common in the United States and is associated with anogenital cancers (cervix, vulva, vagina, penis, and anus), oropharyngeal cancers, and genital warts.
2. Primary prevention of HPV with vaccination is highly effective and safe for both females and males.
3. Women with prior evidence of HPV infection still benefit from vaccination to protect against other types of HPV not already acquired and reinfection or reactivation of already acquired HPV types.

References

1. Massad LS, Einstein MH, Huh WK et al. 2012 updated consensus guidelines for the management of abnormal cervical cancer screening tests and cancer precursors. *J Low Genit Tract Dis* 2013;17 (5 Suppl 1): S1–S27.

2. American College of Obstetricians and Gynecologists. Human papillomavirus vaccination. Committee Opinion No. 704. *Obstet Gynecol* 2017; 129: e173–e178.

3. Markowitz LE, Hariri S, Lin C et al. Reduction in human papillomavirus (HPV) prevalence among young women following HPV vaccine introduction in the United States, National health and nutrition examination surveys, 2003–2010. *J Infect Dis* 2013;208(3):385–393.

4. Khan MJ, Castle PE, Lorincz AT et al. The elevated 10-year risk of cervical precancer and cancer in women with human papillomavirus (HPV) type 16 or 18 and the possible utility of type-specific HPV testing in clinical practice. *J Natl Cancer Inst* 2005;97 (14):1072–1079.

5. Munoz N, Bosch FX, de Sanjose S et al. Epidemiologic classification of human papillomavirus types associated with cervical cancer. *N Engl J Med* 2003;348 (6):518–527.

6. Viens LJ, Henley SJ, Watson M et al. Human papillomavirus-associated cancers – United States, 2008–2012. *MMWR Morb Mortal Wkly Rep* 2016;65 (26):661–666.

7. Meites E, Kempe A, Markowitz LE. Use of a 2-dose schedule for human papillomavirus vaccination – updated recommendations of the advisory committee on immunization practices.

MMWR Morb Mortal Wkly Rep 2016;65 (49):1405–1408.

8. Olsson SE, Kjaer SK, Sigurdsson K et al. Evaluation of quadrivalent HPV 6/11/ 16/18 vaccine efficacy against cervical and anogenital disease in subjects with serological evidence of prior vaccine type HPV infection. *Hum Vaccin* 2009;5(10):696–704.

9. Markowitz LE, Dunne EF, Saraiya M et al. Human papillomavirus vaccination: recommendations of the Advisory Committee on Immunization Practices (ACIP). *MMWR Recomm Rep* 2014;63(RR–05):1–30.

10. Vichnin M, Bonanni P, Klein NP et al. An overview of quadrivalent human papillomavirus vaccine safety: 2006 to 2015. *Pediatr Infect Dis J* 2015;34 (9):983–991.

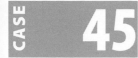

A 55-Year-Old Woman with a White, Itchy Lesion on the Vulva (Lichen Sclerosus)

Nancy D. Gaba

History of Present Illness

A 55-year-old woman, gravida 2 para 2 presents to your office with itching and an intermittent painful burning sensation of the vulva. These symptoms have persisted for six months, and have gotten progressively worse. She tried an over-the-counter remedy containing benzocaine and aloe with limited improvement. She was seen by her internist on two occasions. She was treated with terconazole and later fluconazole for vaginal yeast; however, neither significantly improved her symptoms. She has noted that intercourse has become increasingly uncomfortable, and tried water-based lubricants with limited improvement. The symptoms are worst at night. She denies any vaginal bleeding, spotting, or abnormal discharge.

Her past medical history is significant for hypothyroidism, which is well controlled with medication. She has had two vaginal deliveries after uncomplicated pregnancies.

Physical Examination

General appearance	Well-developed, well-nourished Caucasian woman in mild discomfort

Vital Signs

Temperature	37.0°C
Pulse	92 beats/min
Blood pressure	110/72 mmHg
Height	65 inches
Weight	130 lb
BMI	21.6 kg/m^2
Heent	Oropharynx without lesions, thyroid non-enlarged and without masses
Abdomen	Thin, soft, non-tender, non-distended, no masses
Skin	No lesions

External Genitalia

Vulva	Moderate atrophy with white, cigarette-paper plaques especially around the labia minora and coalescing around the anus. Thick 1.25-cm white plaque seen in the posterior fourchette. Absence of labia minora is noted. The clitoris is concealed.
Vagina	Stenotic and tender introitus with slightly flattened rugae. No lesions.
Cervix	Parous, no lesions, non-tender
Uterus	Anteverted, mobile, normal size, non-tender
Adnexa	No masses, non-tender
Anus	No lesions

How Would You Manage This Patient?

The most likely diagnosis is vulvar lichen sclerosus (LS). A careful analysis of history should consider the possibility of contact dermatitis, a common cause of similar symptoms. Common irritants, such as soaps, detergents, feminine hygiene products, and non-cotton underwear, should be eliminated. Vulvar hygiene should be emphasized. Many women with vulvar symptoms overuse products such as feminine hygiene wipes, which should be avoided. The examiner should inspect the oropharynx for aphthous ulcers. These, and other extragenital manifestations, are present in up to 50 percent of patients with lichen planus and may help in clarifying the differential diagnosis [1]. The thyroid should be palpated, as LS is believed to have an autoimmune origin. Up to 34 percent of women with LS will also have another autoimmune disorder, including thyroiditis, alopecia, pernicious anemia, or vitiligo [1]. The initial examination should include a vaginal pH, and microscopy utilizing potassium hydroxide and saline. Cultures for candida may be performed if indicated. A punch biopsy of the vulva, using a Keyes punch or a similar tool, should be performed under local anesthesia during this visit. This will confirm the diagnosis and exclude other benign as well as malignant skin conditions. Treatment with clobetasol ointment should be initiated once the diagnosis is confirmed. The patient should be re-examined at three and six months to assess response to treatment as well as progression of symptoms.

Lichen Sclerosus

LS is a chronic inflammatory skin condition, which is believed to have an autoimmune component [2]. Other proposed etiologies for this condition include infection with *borrelia burgdorferei*; however, this is controversial [1]. This disorder, first described in 1887, has also been called vulvar dystrophy and lichen sclerosus et atrophicus. Most commonly, LS is diagnosed in the fifth or sixth decades of life, but can also be seen in prepubertal girls. In prepubertal cases, it is best to avoid vulvar biopsy if possible, to reduce trauma. Otherwise the evaluation, management, and follow-up are similar to that recommended for older women.

Prepubertal girls account for approximately 7–15 percent of cases of LS [3].

A complete physical examination should be performed when LS is suspected. Examination of the oropharynx will help exclude lichen planus, which is sometimes confused with LS. Careful inspection of the vulva may also help clarify the diagnosis. Patients with contact dermatitis often exhibit significant thickening (lichenification) of the affected skin, and evidence of scratching may be seen. Lichenification is the result of what is known as the "itch-scratch cycle." Infectious

Table 45.1 Differential diagnosis for white vulvar patch

Acute Conditions	Chronic Conditions
Fungus (candida)	Contact dermatitis
Contact dermatitis	Lichen sclerosus
Scabies infestation	Lichen simplex chronicus
Molluscum contagiosum	Lichen planus
HPV infection	Psoriasis/Eczema
	Atrophy
	Vulvar cancer
	HPV infection

Data from ACOG Practice Bulletin #93 [2]

Box 45.1 Vulvar hygiene

Pearls for Vulvar Hygiene

Avoid gels, scented bath products, cleansing wipes, and perfumed soaps

Used water-based creams/ointments on the vulva

Avoid washcloths which are too harsh on sensitive vulvar tissue

Dab gently to dry the vulva, or use a hairdryer on a cool setting

Avoid tightfitting pants

Change sweaty clothes immediately after exercise

Wear white, cotton underwear, avoid thongs

Avoid scented detergents and consider a second rinse cycle to remove residual detergent

Avoid underwear whenever possible to avoid friction and aid drying of the vulva

Data from ACOG Practice Bulletin #93 [2]

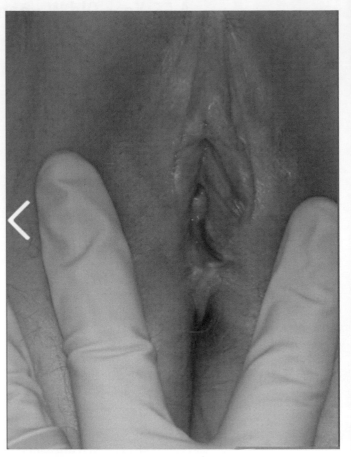

Figure 45.1 Typical presentation of lichen sclerosus. Note hypopigmentation, loss of architecture, and scarring of the introitus. Reproduced from the website http://cvvd.org/conditions/lichen-sclerosus with permission of Dr Andrew Goldstein. Accessed on 5/1/2017

etiologies should also be excluded. The complete differential diagnosis that should be considered in women with the presentation described above is seen in Table 45.1.

Whenever vulvar skin disorders are detected, patients should be counseled regarding proper vulvar hygiene. Box 45.1 contains information regarding key counseling pearls.

The typical appearance of the vulva in a patient with LS can be seen in Figure 45.1, which shows white vulvar plaques that are coalescing lesions. There may be areas of purpura, excoriation, or erosion. Architectural changes of the vulva are common, including partial or complete resorption of the labia minora, scarring of the clitoral hood, and narrowing of the introitus [4].

Vulvar biopsies should be sent to a pathologist with expertise in vulvar skin disorders. Characteristic histologic features include hyperkeratosis of the epidermis, epidermal atrophy, loss of rete ridges, homogenization of the collagen of the upper dermis [4], dense bands of lymphocytic infiltrates, and vasculitic processes [5]. Although many practitioners make the diagnosis of vulvar LS

based on history and clinical presentation, it is imperative that a vulvar biopsy be performed to confirm the diagnosis, especially in cases where a discrete lesion is seen. It should be noted that up to 6 percent of women with vulvar LS develop squamous cell carcinoma of the vulva. In fact, in one study 36 percent of patients with vulvar squamous cell carcinoma had coexisting or synchronous LS at the time of diagnosis [6], suggesting that even more careful follow-up than the standard annual examination recommended by ACOG may be warranted.

Therapy for LS is lengthy, and sometimes indefinite. Although no cure for LS exists, the symptoms can be controlled if appropriate treatment is initiated before destructive or permanent scarring occurs. Since the etiology of LS is likely autoimmune, it is not surprising that the current gold-standard for initial treatment of LS is ultrapotent topical corticosteroid therapy, with agents such as clobetasol or halobetasol. Ointments are generally better than creams, as they are absorbed more readily, and are less irritating due to a base gentler to sensitive skin. It has been reported that the majority of patients (96 percent) will become either symptom-free or will have partial response to this treatment. Older patients are less likely to achieve complete remission [5]. The ideal treatment regimen has yet to be determined. Most experts recommend once or twice daily application of ultrapotent steroid ointment for at least four weeks, and up to three months [2]. Although somewhat controversial, it is generally believed that this therapy reduces the risk of malignant transformation. Long-term use of corticosteroids can have significant side effects and other complications. These include severe atrophy, infection, thickening of the skin, and even adrenal insufficiency [4]. For this reason, other therapies have also been studied.

A Cochrane review found no benefit from topical testosterone, dihydrotestosterone, and progesterone, and these should not be utilized. The immune-modulator pimecrolimus was found to be as effective as clobetasol in relieving itching and burning pain, but may be less effective in achieving visible improvement [7]. Pimecrolimus and tacrolimus are nonsteroidal immunomodulators when applied topically. The mechanism of action involves blockage of calcineurin, inhibiting the production of interleukin-2, interferon, and other cytokines. This leads to the suppression of T-cells and other inflammatory cells. Tacrolimus is lipophilic and penetrates skin easily, but unlike corticosteroids will not cause thinning of the skin [8]. Calcineurin inhibitors are significantly more expensive than corticosteroids. A theoretical concern is the risk of malignant transformation due to immune suppression, and although there are case reports of rapid tumor progression this has not been borne out in the literature [9].

Another promising agent is Human Fibroblast Lysate cream, obtained from cultured human fetal fibroblasts. The proposed mechanism of action is anti-inflammatory cytokines, including interleukin 1 receptor agonists, and growth factors, such as VEGF. In a randomized, placebo-controlled trial this therapy was shown to reduce vulvar symptoms; however, the results were not statistically significantly different from placebo. Further study of this agent is warranted [4].

Photodynamic therapy is another promising option for treatment of LS. A combination of 8-methoxypsoralen cream and UVA light led to significant reduction in pruritus. In separate studies UVA1 has also been reported to decrease symptoms and improve physical findings, as has the combination of 5-aminolevulinic acid and the argon laser. Limited studies have been done and more studies are indicated before this type of therapy could be considered as an alternative to standard therapy [9].

Emollient therapy, with petrolatum, mineral oil, or lanolin, has been shown to help control symptoms after a course of steroids or immune modulators has been completed [9].

Surgical therapy is sometimes utilized to correct anatomic abnormalities such as labial adhesions. Surgical treatment of LS is reserved for cases with poor response to medical therapies, and in some cases to prevent the development of malignancy. Surgical options include vulvectomy, cryosurgery, and laser ablation. Empirical vulvectomy is not indicated, however, there is some evidence that skinning vulvectomy may help prevent cancer in patients with mixed dystrophy, since these patients are at higher risk of malignant transformation. Recurrence rates are high with this therapy as well [10].

Summary

The patient should be offered clobetasol therapy after a confirmatory biopsy, and follow-up examinations should be conducted at three and six months to assess for improvement. Topical estrogen may be offered as an adjunctive therapy for atrophy. Emollients can be initiated once symptoms have improved or resolved. New lesions should be biopsied to rule out malignancy.

Key Teaching Points

- Any hypopigmented vulvar lesion should be biopsied, and LS suspected.
- LS is associated with a 4–6 percent rate of progression to squamous cell carcinoma. Patients with LS should have a thorough examination of the vulva at least annually.
- Topical treatment with an ultrapotent steroid ointment is the first-line therapy for LS.
- Immune modulators are as effective in treating LS as steroids.
- Hormonal therapies, such as testosterone or progesterone, have not been shown to be effective in treating LS.

References

1. Kellogg Spadt S, Kusturiss E. Vulvar dermatoses: a primer for the sexual medicine clinician. *Sex Med Rev* 2015;3:126–136.

2. American College of Obstetricians and Gynecologists. ACOG Practice Bulletin No. 93: 2008 (reaffirmed 2016).

3. Bercaw-Pratt JL, Boardman LA, Simms-Cendan JS. Clinical recommendation: pediatric LS. *J Pediatr Adolesc Gynecol* 2014;27:111–116

4. Goldstein AT, Burrows LJ et al. Safety and efficacy of human fibroblast lysate cream for vulvar LS: a randomized placebo-controlled trial. *Acta Derm Venereol* 2015;95:847–849.

5. Broddick B, Belkin Z, Goldstein AT. Influence of treatments on prognosis for vulvar LS: facts and controversies. *Clin Dermatol* 2013;31:780–786.

6. Davick JJ, Samuelson M et al. The prevalence of LS in patients with vulvar squamous cell carcinoma. *Int J Gynecol Path* 2016;00:1–5.

7. Chi CC, Kirtschig G, Baldo M et al. Topical interventions for genital lichen sclerosus. *Cochrane Database Syst Rev.* 2011;12:CD008240.

8. Strittmatter HJ, Hengge UR, Blecken SR. Calcineurin antagonists in vulvar LS. *Arch Gynecol Obstet* 2006;274:266–270.

9. Fistarol SK, Itin PH. Diagnosis and treatment of LS. *Am J Clin Dermatol* 2013;14:27–47.

10. Abramov Y, Elchalal et al. Surgical treatment of vulvar LS: a review. *Obstet Gynecol Survey* 1996;53(3):193–199.

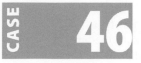

A 55-Year-Old Woman with a New Wart (Vulvar High-Grade Squamous Intraepithelial Lesions)

Diana Curran

History of Present Illness

A 55-year-old nulliparous woman presents to the office for her annual exam complaining of a new lesion on her vulva. She reports that she first noticed a bump over the last couple of weeks. She reports that the lesion is irregular and rough to the touch and is located near her urethra. She denies any pain or associated bleeding with the lesion. She is otherwise healthy.

Her last cervical cancer screening was reported as normal at age 48. Her past medical history includes menopause at age 52; she has no medical problems nor has she had any surgery. She is on no medications. She denies any medication allergies but does report a latex allergy. She is an automotive engineer, denies smoking, and drinks seven alcoholic beverages weekly. She divorced at age 53. She reports a new male sexual partner for the last six months.

Physical Examination

Temperature	36.7 C
Pulse	75 beats/min
Blood pressure	128/65 mmHg
BMI	32 kg/m²
Ht	5′ 6″
Weight	186 lb

General appearance	Well-appearing Caucasian female in no apparent distress
	Abdomen soft, non-tender, no rebound tenderness, guarding or masses
Pelvic Exam	
Vulva/Vagina	Right labium majus has an irregular appearing lesion (see Figure 46.1). Normal vaginal discharge. Postmenopausal atrophy noted.
Cervix	Normal appearing, pale
Uterus	Anteverted, small, regular
Adnexa	No adnexal tenderness or mass

There are no pertinent laboratory findings.

How Would You Evaluate and Manage This Patient?

This irregular appearing lesion requires biopsy. In addition, colposcopy of the vulva was performed to better visualize and document the extent of the lesion and to rule out additional pathology. Punch biopsy was performed after injecting 1 percent lidocaine with epinephrine. The biopsy returns as high-grade squamous intraepithelial lesion (HSIL) (previously called vulvar intraepithelial neoplasia-usual type). Treatment of HSIL of the vulva for this patient would include additional wide local excision if there was risk of occult invasion by punch

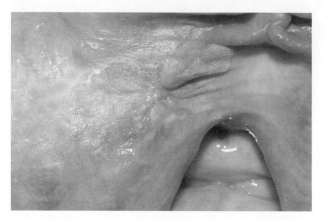

Figure 46.1 High-grade squamous intraepithelial lesion of vulva.

biopsy or ablative therapy if no risk of occult invasion was noted on biopsy. If sensitive or important structures lie within the scope of the lesion, consultation with a vulvar specialist would be recommended.

Pap smear and high-risk HPV screening of the cervix is also performed during the exam consistent with current ASCCP screening guidelines and to rule out concomitant cervical disease. Testing for other sexually transmitted infections was performed.

Vulvar HSIL and Condyloma Accuminata

Vulvar HSIL is associated with high-risk HPV types (i.e., 16, 18, 31, 33, 45) and is considered a precancerous lesion. Vulvar HSIL related to HPV has recently been reported to be more common in women under 50 years. Common symptoms include itching, burning, soreness of the vulva, or painful intercourse. Discoloration of the vulvar skin can also occur.

The International Society for the Study of Vulvovaginal Disease (ISSVD) updated the terminology for vulvar intraepithelial neoplasia in 2015 (Box 46.1)[1] [2]. The ISSVD adopted the 2014 WHO (World Health Organization) Classification of Tumors of the Vulva that divides lesions into squamous cell tumors and precursors that include squamous intraepithelial lesions (SILs), subdivided into LSIL (low-grade SIL), HSIL (high-grade SIL), and differentiated-type VIN (DVIN). What previously was called usual or undifferentiated VIN is now included in HSIL [3].

Treatment of HSIL of the vulva varies depending on the location of the disease. Wide local excision (margins of 0.5 to 1 cm) is preferred in hair-bearing areas or in cases where occult invasion is of concern as may be suggested from the punch biopsy [4]. CO₂ laser is ideal for non–hair-bearing areas, which requires a 2 mm depth. Laser should not be performed on the hair-bearing areas as the depth required to ensure eradication

Box 46.1 Epithelial tumors

SILs

LSIL

HSIL

Differentiated-type VIN

Squamous Cell Carcinoma

Keratinizing

Non-keratinizing

Basaloid

Warty

Verrucous

Basal Cell Carcinoma

Benign Squamous Lesions

Condyloma acuminatum

Vestibular papilloma

Seborrheic keratosis

SIL, squamous intraepithelial lesion; LSIL, low-grade SIL; HSIL, high-grade SIL; VN, vulvar intraepithelial neoplasa.

From Bornstein J, Bogliatto F, Haefner HK et al. Consensus Statement: The 2015 International Society for the Study of Vulvovaginal Disease (ISSVD) Terminology of Vulvar Squamous Intraepithelial Lesions. *Obstet Gynecol.* 127(2): 264–268, February 2016.

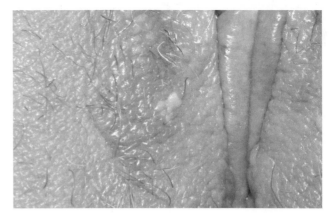

Figure 46.2 White condyloma on vulva.

around the follicles is 3–4 mm in depth and would be painful and disfiguring. An alternative treatment for HSIL of the vulva is the use of topical imquimod (off label use). Topical imiquimod is particularly useful when HSIL is found on the clitoris or urethral meatus.

Recurrence rates for HSIL of the vulva can range from 9 to 50 percent, thus ongoing surveillance is important. Initially, patients should be examined at 6 and 12 months after initial diagnosis and excision/ablation. If no lesions are seen, then annual examination is appropriate [5].

Condyloma accuminata would be classified as benign squamous lesions in the aforementioned classification of the ISVVD [1]. If a vulvar biopsy is performed and returns as condyloma accuminata or anogenital warts (AGWs), the clinical suspicion of a low-risk HPV lesion is confirmed. Ninety percent of condyloma accuminata are caused by HPV 6 and 11 [6,7]. HPV genital infections are the most common STD in the world. Over 50 percent of the sexual population is infected with HPV at some point in time. Recurrence rates for condyloma accuminata have not been clearly delineated but can be common. AGWs are highly contagious – an HPV negative sexual partner has a 65 percent risk of developing an AGW three weeks to eight months after contact with an infected partner. If there is a suspicion of immunosuppression in the patient, further evaluation may be warranted. In patients where condyloma is newly diagnosed, other STI screening tests, including HIV, should be considered.

For lesions with the appearance of typical condyloma accuminata in premenopausal women, biopsy is not warranted (see Figure 46.2). When treatment is indicated, in-office treatments can be administered or self-application treatments at home can be prescribed.

Trichloroacetic acid (TCA) can be applied immediately in the office. Other in-office treatments include cryotherapy, podophyllin, interferon, and sinecatechins (green tea extract) [6]. Alternatively, if the patient does not wish to return for multiple applications of topicals, excision or CO_2 laser with local anesthesia can be performed. At home self-application treatments include Podofilox and imiquimod cream, which are applied topically [7]. Indications for biopsy in the premenopausal state include lesions that do not respond to therapy, the disease worsens during therapy, the lesion becomes atypical, or the patient has compromised immunity.

Extensive lesions may require surgical excision in addition to ablation and can be co-treated with topical medications to decrease the volume of excision. Cotreatment with topical agents, such as imiquimod, can also be used to decrease recurrence rates [8].

Key Teaching Points

- Vulvar lesions in postmenopausal women and atypical vulvar lesions in women under 50 require biopsy.
- HSIL diagnosed on vulvar biopsy with concern for occult invasion requires wide local excision or ablative therapy depending on concern for occult invasion.
- Recurrence of HSIL is common; thus, ongoing disease requires surveillance, initially every six months and then annually thereafter.

- Benign condylomas are amenable to multiple treatments. Imiquimod and podofilox may be successfully administered at home.

- Extensive condylomas can be treated with a combination of topical medication and excision or laser.

References

1. Bornstein J, Bogliatto F, Haefner HK et al. Consensus statement: the 2015 International Society for the Study of Vulvovaginal Disease (ISSVD) terminology of vulvar squamous intraepithelial lesions. *Obstet Gynecol* 2016;127:264–268.

2. The International Society for the Study of Vulvovaginal Disease: www.issvd.org/ Accessed July 29, 2017.

3. Bornstein et al. 2015 ISSVD, ISSWSH and IPPS consensus terminology and classification of persistent vulvar pain and vulvodynia. *Obstet Gynecol* 2016;127:745–751.

4. Lawrie TA, Nordin A, Chakrabarti M et al. Medical and surgical interventions for the treatment of usual-type vulval intraepithelial neoplasia (Review). Cochrane Library, September 2015. Accessed 28 July, 2017.

5. Committee opinion No 675: management of vulvar intraepithelial neoplasia, *Obstet Gynecol*, October 2016;128(4): e178–e182. [See also Committee Opinion No. 675: Management of Vulvar Intraepithelial Neoplasia: Correction, *Obstet Gynecol*, January 2017;29(1): 209.]

6. Thurgar E, Barton S, Karner C, Edwards SJ. Clinical effectiveness and cost-effectiveness of interventions for the treatment of anogenital warts: systematic review and economic evaluation. *Health Technol Assess* 2016;20(24).

7. www.cdc.gov/std/treatment/2010/geni tal-warts.htm. Accessed August 5, 2017.

8. Patel H, Wagner M, Singhal P, Kothari S. Systematic review of the incidence and prevalence of genital warts. *BMC Infect Dis* 2013;13:39.
Acknowledgment: special thanks to Dr. Hope Haefner for providing excellent photos and editorial advice.

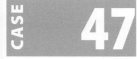

CASE 47

A 25-Year-Old Woman with Perineal Pain and Inability to Have Intercourse (Vestibulodynia)

Vanessa M. Barnabei

History of Present Illness

A 25-year-old G0 female is referred for evaluation and management of pain with intercourse. She reports a one-year history of severe dyspareunia that began when she became sexually active with her husband, who has been her only partner. She has never been able to use tampons because of pain with attempted insertion. She rates her initial pain as 10 out of 10 and describes it as most prominent with penile insertion and dissipating somewhat with continued coitus. She also reports burning pain following intercourse that may last for a few hours. Her symptoms were significantly interfering with her marriage, so her primary gynecologist offered a trial of topical lidocaine 5 percent cream and topical estrogen cream. The lidocaine has improved the insertion pain to a 6 out of 10, but she still has significant discomfort with intercourse and postcoital burning.

The patient's past medical history is positive only for irritable bowel syndrome. She recently stopped her oral contraceptive pills. Her current medications include prenatal vitamins, Colace, hyoscyamine, and topical lidocaine and estrogen creams.

Physical Examination

General appearance	Patient is a well-developed, well-nourished female in no acute distress, appearing her stated age.

Vital Signs

Height	155 cm
Weight	62 kg
Blood pressure	100/60 mmHg
Abdomen	Soft, thin, mildly diffusely tender without masses, guarding, or rebound
External genitalia	Anatomically normal female external genitalia, no suspicious lesions, cotton swab testing confirmed point tenderness of vaginal vestibule lateral to the hymen at 1, 11, 4, and 8 o'clock with slight erythema
Vagina	Normal, non-tender, no discharge
Bladder	Normal
Cervix	Normal
Uterus	Anteverted, small, mobile, non-tender
Adnexa	No masses or tenderness; pelvic floor non-tender

How Would You Manage This Patient?

This patient has primary, localized, provoked vestibulodynia, previously referred to as vulvar vestibulitis, which was confirmed on cotton swab testing. Fungal cultures were obtained and were negative. According to Freidrich's criteria [1], initially described in 1987, this patient's symptoms and physical exam are pathognomonic for this condition. These criteria include (1) severe pain on vestibular touch or attempted vaginal entry; (2) tenderness to pressure localized within the vulvar vestibule; and (3) no evidence of physical findings except for varying degrees of erythema.

The patient was instructed on vulvar care measures and was thoroughly counseled about the treatment options. Although she had a partial response to topical lidocaine, she found the precoital application to be intrusive and non-spontaneous. She elected a trial of oral lamotrigine 25 mg daily, which was titrated up by 25 mg each week to a dose of 100 mg daily. She reported some improvement at her three-month follow-up and is considering the addition of physical therapy with biofeedback.

Vulvodynia and Vestibulodynia

Vestibulodynia is a subset of idiopathic vulvodynia, which is now considered a chronic pain disorder. To make the diagnosis of idiopathic vulvodynia, a patient must have vulvar pain of at least three months' duration in the absence of other identifiable pathology. The International Society for the Study of Vulvovaginal Disease (ISSVD) released updated terminology guidelines in April 2016 [2]. These were reiterated in a subsequent combined ACOG/ASSCP Committee Opinion from 2016 [3].

According to the ISSVD, vulvodynia classification can be broken down into four major areas:

1. Onset – primary, as in this patient, or secondary, occurring after the onset of sexual activity;
2. Location – localized, generalized, or mixed;
3. Timing – provoked, spontaneous, or mixed; and
4. Temporal pattern of pain (constant, intermittent, etc.).

The prevalence of vulvodynia is about 8–16 percent of the female population and affects women of all age and ethnic groups [4]. Localized, provoked vestibulodynia refers to a subset of vulvodynia in which the pain is localized to the vaginal opening or vestibule when the area is provoked by pressure. Provoked vestibulodynia accounts for about 80 percent of idiopathic vulvodynia cases and is more common in reproductive-age women.

The cause of vulvodynia is not known and likely heterogeneous. Studies examining pathophysiology and histopathology have shown results such as peripheral nerve proliferation, alterations in local immune factors, and chronic inflammatory changes [5]. Some women, like the patient described above, will have pain from their first attempt at tampon insertion or penile penetration. For women with secondary vestibulodynia, the onset of pain may be linked temporally to a specific trigger or event, such as a severe candida vulvovaginitis. For most women, however, the onset is more insidious. Vulvodynia can cause significant distress and relationship difficulties because of the impact on sexual function. Many studies have documented a significant association between vulvodynia and

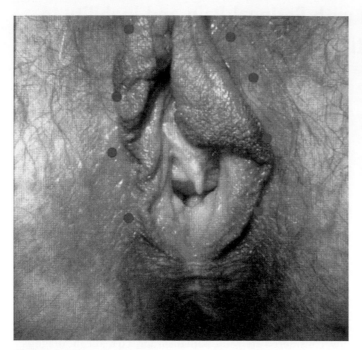

Figure 47.1 Generalized, unprovoked vulvodynia

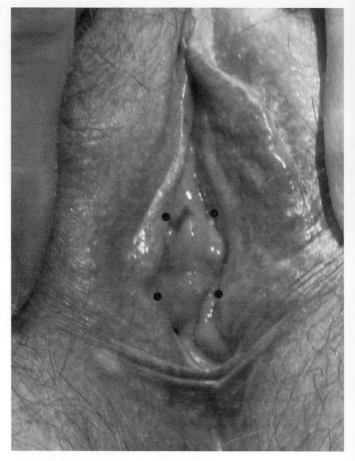

Figure 47.2 Localized, provoked vestibulodynia

other chronic pain conditions, such as interstitial cystitis, fibromyalgia, and irritable bowel syndrome [6]. Depression and anxiety are also common comorbid conditions.

The evaluation of a woman with complaints of vulvar pain should include a thorough medical, obstetrical, and gynecologic history. The American College of Obstetricians and Gynecologists' 2016 Committee Opinion outlines an assessment and treatment algorithm that is helpful in the work-up of persistent vulvar pain [3]. The history should include assessment of urinary tract symptoms, a sexual history, validated sexual distress scale, review of musculoskeletal symptoms, and history of physical or sexual abuse. The external genital exam should be approached systematically, first inspecting the vulva for any lesions, discolorations, or other abnormalities that could be contributing to the patient's symptoms. The standard for assessing tenderness is the use of a cotton swab test. This involves lightly touching the vulva in a consistent pattern, starting with the most lateral aspects and working medially, quantifying patient's pain response at each area on a ten-point Likert scale. A yeast culture should be obtained in women who report pain and/or burning on cotton swab testing, and those who test positive should be treated with an antifungal. The vagina should be assessed for signs of infection or inflammation as well as for vaginal wall and pelvic floor tenderness. In addition, it is important to assess for involuntary contraction of the vaginal and pelvic floor muscles, as the presence of vaginismus would modify the management approach. In the absence of abnormal physical exam findings, vulvar biopsy is not useful.

Evaluation and Treatment Algorithm

Figure 47.1 shows the distribution of pain in women with generalized vulvodynia and Figure 47.2 shows the distribution in women with provoked vestibulodynia. With provoked, localized vestibulodynia, tenderness is usually concentrated around the openings of the minor vestibular glands, which are located medial to Hart's line and lateral to the hymenal ring (Figure 47.3), as well as the posterior fourchette.

Management of symptoms in women with vulvodynia, whether generalized or localized, is challenging. No single treatment option is successful for all women, and response to treatment can take weeks. Randomized controlled trials are rare, and expert opinion and trial-and-error have been the mainstay of therapy choice. Evidence quality in large systematic reviews is almost uniformly low [7,8]. Historical therapeutic options have been tricyclic antidepressants and surgical excision (the latter only indicated for localized vestibulodynia). The association of vulvodynia with other neuropathic pain disorders has led to therapeutic options that have been successful in the treatment of other chronic pain syndromes.

The general approach to treatment should be from least to most invasive. Therapy must be individualized, taking into account the patient's treatment goals, previous therapies, concurrent medical and/or behavioral health conditions, and tolerance to potential side effects. Because most of these women are in significant distress, they want relief as quickly as possible. It is critical to discuss with each patient that good-quality evidence for most of the recommended therapeutics is lacking, that response may take weeks, and that her response to any therapy will be difficult to predict. The initial therapeutic

Table 47.1 Oral pain modulators

Agent	Dose	Side effects	Comments
Amitriptyline	Start 10 mg qhs Increase by 10 mg every 3–4 weeks to maximum of 150 mg	Drowsiness, constipation, dry mouth	Many women cannot tolerate therapeutic dose; decrease in elderly women
Venlafaxine	Start 37.5 mg, increase to 75 mg after 2 weeks; maximum dose 150 mg	Headache, nausea, drowsiness, anorexia, insomnia	May be useful in women with mood disorder or anxiety disorder
Duloxetine	Start 20 mg bid, increase to 30 mg bid after 1 week	Same as venlafaxine	Same as venlafaxine
Gabapentin	Start at 300 mg hs, increase gradually in divided doses to maximum dose of 2700 mg	Dizziness, somnolence, fatigue, weight gain, tremor	May take weeks to reach therapeutic dose
Pregabalin	Start 50 mg, may increase to 75–300 mg gradually in divided doses	Same as gabapentin	More rapid onset than gabapentin but side effects may limit use
Lamotrigine	Start at 25 mg, increase by 25 mg weekly to 100 mg	Dizziness, headache, nausea, diplopia	

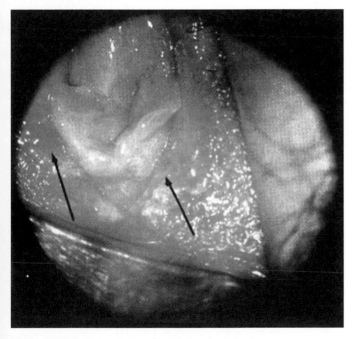

Figure 47.3 Erythema at sites of vestibular gland openings.

choice should be tried for a minimum of 8–12 weeks unless it is not tolerated. Narcotic pain medications should be avoided.

The initial step is good vulvar hygiene, with emphasis on avoidance of irritants such as chemicals, inks, dyes, and perfumes. Topical medications are low risk and can improve symptoms, as topical lidocaine did for our patient; however, they may not provide complete relief. When prescribing topical therapy, an ointment should be chosen over a cream, as ointments tend to have fewer chemical irritants and are better tolerated. Compounded topical antidepressant therapy, mixed with other medications such as baclofen, gabapentin, or doxepin, in a water-soluble, non-irritating base, can provide improvement of symptoms. A commonly used regimen is gabapentin 6 percent, baclofen 2 percent, and amitriptyline 2 percent applied two to four times daily. Although these topical regimens do not cause systemic side effects, some women report burning with initial use.

Cognitive behavioral therapy has been found to be effective at decreasing pain scores and improving overall sexual functioning [9]. Pelvic floor physical therapy (PT) with biofeedback is safe and has been successful for the treatment of both generalized and localized vulvodynia [10]. This may consist of myofascial release, stretching, and strengthening of the pelvic floor muscles, electrical stimulation, and behavioral modification using biofeedback techniques. PT is necessary for women with concurrent vaginismus and can be combined with graduated vaginal dilator use. Referral to a sex therapist may also be beneficial.

Neuropathic pain modulators that act centrally show great promise for the relief of vulvodynia, although clinical trial data for these medications on this disorder are lacking [11,12]. Table 47.1 shows oral pain modulators with recommended dosing and potential side effects. All of these should be tapered gradually before discontinuation, and most are contraindicated in pregnancy. In addition, caution is advised in elderly women, and doses should be adjusted accordingly.

Surgical excision of the vulvar vestibule with advancement and re-approximation of the vaginal mucosa has a 75 percent success rate. However, it can lead to bleeding and scar formation, requires two to six weeks of recovery, and is generally reserved for cases in which medical therapy fails.

Newer therapeutic options on the horizon include transcutaneous electrical nerve stimulation using a vaginal probe [13], pulsed radiofrequency treatment [14], and sacral neuromodulation [15], which has been used to treat recalcitrant urinary tract conditions such as overactive bladder and urinary incontinence.

Key Points

1. Vulvodynia is a diagnosis of exclusion, where vulvar pain is present despite a negative work-up and a normal exam.
2. Vulvodynia is a heterogeneous condition of unknown etiology; therefore, management can be challenging.
3. Initial management includes vulvar care measures and topical therapy, with the addition of oral medications, PT, counseling, and other measures as necessary; choice of therapy relies on expert opinion and trial and error.
4. Surgical treatment of provoked vestibulodynia has good success rates but should be reserved for medical treatment failures.

References

1. Friedrich Jr., EG, Vulvar vestibulitis syndrome. *J Reprod Med* 1987;32:110–114.

2. Bornstein J, Goldstein AT, Stockdale CK, Bergeron S et al. 2015 ISSSVD, ISSWSH, and IPPS consensus terminology and classification of persistent vulvar pain and vulvodynia. *J Lower Gen Tract Dis* 2016;20:126–130.

3. Persistent Vulvar Pain. Committee Opinion 673. American College of Obstetricians and Gynecologists. *Obstet Gynecol* 2016;128:278–284.

4. Reed BD, Legocki LJ, Plegue MA et al. Factors associated with vulvodynia incidence. *Obstet Gynecol* 2014;123:225–232.

5. Chalmers KJ, Madden VJ, Hutchinson MR, Moseley GL. Local and systemic inflammation in localized, provoked vestibulodynia. A systematic review. *Obstet Gynecol* 2016;128:337–347.

6. Arnold LD, Bachmann GA, Rosen R, Kelly S, Rhoads GG. Vulvodynia. characteristics and associations with comorbidities and quality of life. *Obstet Gynecol* 2006;107:617–624.

7. Andrews JC. Vulvodynia interventions-systematic review and evidence grading. *Obstet Gynecol Survey* 2011;66:299–315.

8. De Andres J, Sanchis-Lopez N, Asensio-Samper JM et al. Vulvodynia – an evidenced-based literature review and proposed treatment algorithm. *Pain Prac* 2016;16:204–236.

9. Bergeron S, Khalife S, Glazer HI, Binik YM. Surgical and behavioral treatments for vestibulodynia: two-and-one-half year follow-up and predictors of outcome. *Obstet Gynecol* 2008;111:159–166.

10. Goldfinger C, Pukall CF, Gentilcore-Saulnier E, McLean L, Chamberlain S. A prospective study of pelvic floor physical therapy-pain and psychosexual outcomes in provoked vestibulodynia. *J Sex Med* 2009;6:1955–1968.

11. Leo, RJ. A systematic review of the utility of anticonvulsant pharmacotherapy in the treatment of vulvodynia pain. *J Sex Med* 2013;10:2000–2008.

12. Leo RJ, Dewani S. A systematic review of the utility of řantidepressant pharmacotherapy in the treatment of vulvodynia pain. *J Sex Med* 2013;10:2497–2505.

13. Murina F, Bianco V, Radici G et al. Transcutaneous electrical nerve stimulation to treat vestibulodynia: a randomized controlled trial. *BJOG* 2008;115:1165–1170.

14. Kestřánek J, Špaček J et al. Radiofrequency therapy for severe idiopathic vulvodynia. *J Lower Genit Tract Dis* 2013;17: e1–e4.

15. Ramsay LB, Wright JB, Fischer JR. Sacral neuromodulation in the treatment of vulvar vestibulitis syndrome. *Obstet Gynecol* 2009;114:487–489.

A 30-Year-Old Woman with New Vulvar Lesions (Condyloma Accuminata)

Christopher Maguire

History of Present Illness

A 30-year-old female, gravida 2, para 2, presents to the office with the complaint of "bumps" in the vulvar area. The patient first noticed the lesions two to three months ago. Over this period of time, the lesions have not changed and are not painful; however, she has sought evaluation due to their persistence. She denies any prior history of similar lesions. The patient has no other related gynecologic, gastrointestinal, or urinary complaints. She reports menses every 27–29 days, with 3 to 4 days of moderate flow and without significant pain or cramping. The patient is sexually active and admits to several current partners.

The patient's past medical history is negative for any illness or disease. Her surgical history is significant only for a postpartum tubal ligation. She has not undergone a gynecologic exam or cervical cancer screening in the last six years. Socially, the patient smokes one pack of cigarettes per day and drinks alcohol only occasionally.

Physical Examination

General appearance	Well-developed, well-nourished female in no acute distress.

Vital Signs

Temperature	37.0°C
Pulse	72 beats/minute
Blood pressure	125/68 mmHg
Respiratory rate	16 breaths/minute
Height	65 inches
Weight	130 lb
BMI	21.6 kg/m²
Abdomen	Soft, non-tender, non-distended, no mass
External genitalia	Raised exophytic lesions confined to the perineum and perianal region. 0.5–1 cm in length. Slightly darker than surrounding skin. Non-tender. No erythema.
Vagina	Normal appearing mucosa without lesion
Cervix	Parous without lesions. No cervical motion tenderness.
Uterus	Anteverted, mobile, non-tender. Normal size and shape.
Adnexa	Free of tenderness or mass

How Would You Manage This Patient?

This patient has a classic case of condyloma accuminata, the diagnosis of which is made by direct observation of the characteristic lesions. She was offered screening for other sexually transmitted infections (STIs) and was counseled about treatment options for her genital warts. She desired self-administered therapy and was given a prescription for 5 percent imiquomod cream. She was instructed to apply the cream three times per week at bedtime and to wash it off in the morning, and she was advised to return in three months for reassessment. In addition, she was counseled about smoking cessation, and since she has not had cervical cancer screening in the past six years, it was recommended she undergo well-woman examination and cervical cancer screening at that time.

Her STI screening was negative. At her three-month follow-up, she reported complete resolution of her lesions, and cervical cytology and high-risk HPV screening were performed and were negative.

Condyloma Accuminata (Genital Warts)

Condylomata acuminata represent the most common visible Human Papillomavirus (HPV) induced lesion of the female genital tract. Other terms used to describe this condition include genital warts, anogential warts, or venereal warts. In the United States, it is estimated that 75 percent of sexually active adults have been infected with at least one genital HPV subtype [1]. HPV-6 and/or HPV-11 are found in approximately 90 percent of cases of genital warts, and coinfection with other subtypes is common. Of those who develop visible lesions, the median time from infection to detectable warts has been reported to be 2.9 months [2], and almost all genital HPV infection is acquired via sexual contact.

Risk factors related to development of genital warts include sexual activity, immunosuppression, and smoking. The risk associated with sexual activity is increased with greater numbers of sexual partners and earlier age of sexual debut. The risk of warts increases directly as the number of cigarettes smoked per day and pack year history increases. In addition, immunocompromised states can lead to development of larger lesions and a greater incidence of treatment failures.

The diagnosis of genital warts is typically made by direct observation of the characteristic lesions. The gross appearance may vary and can include flat, cauliflower, plaque-like, verrucous, fungating, dome-shaped, lobulated, filiform, or cerebriform lesions. These lesions are usually skin-colored or slightly hyper- or hypopigmented; however, they may also be brown, violaceous, or erythematous. The extent of lesions can vary widely from minimal 2–3 millimeter papules to extensive exophytic masses covering the entire perineum. Anatomic sites affected include the vulva, perianal region, vagina, cervix, and urethra [5]. The relative incidence based on specific site varies by author. Importantly, genital warts typically present with multiple warts and can be found in more than one anatomic site at presentation. Therefore, a thorough exam of the lower genital tract is warranted when warts are found. In addition, patients diagnosed with genital warts should be offered screening for other STIs in accordance with the CDC guidelines.

When there is uncertainty of the diagnosis or the lesions appear atypical, biopsy should be performed. Biopsy is also recommended when lesions do not respond as expected to therapy, appear to worsen during therapy, or in patients who suffer from immunocompromised states [3].

The primary goal of therapy is to eradicate the visible warts and improve any related symptoms. Regarding the causative agent, HPV, there is no evidence indicating that currently available treatment modalities eradicate or affect the natural history of HPV infection [7]. There are several options that may be used to treat the patient in the above scenario, and there is no definite evidence that one method is superior to another. Factors that may help guide a specific choice would include cost, patient preferences, contraindications, and expected length of therapy. Clinically, the extent and the location of disease and whether or not the patient is pregnant can also influence management [4].

Observation should be considered in those with small, asymptomatic warts, as spontaneous resolution has been reported. It is estimated that approximately one-third of ano-genital warts regress without treatment within four months [6].

For patients desiring treatment, specific therapeutic options can be divided into topical agents or surgical methods. There are several topical therapies that can be applied by the patient and others that require a clinician to apply. The recommended options are summarized in Box 48.1 and are further described below. The cost, efficacy, and recurrence rates vary by specific therapy and should be considered in decision-making (Table 48.1).

Patient-applied methods offer the advantages of fewer clinic visits and the ability to treat in the privacy of one's home. It is important that patients are provided with detailed instructions on use and are able to access all lesions to be treated. Follow-up several weeks after initiation of treatment is recommended to assess questions, side effects, and the response to the therapy.

Imiquimod cream is an immune modulator that works to increase interferon and other cytokines. It is applied directly to the lesions three times per week and washed off with soap and water 6–10 hours after application. It may be used for up to 16 weeks. Possible side effects include local redness, irritation, ulceration, or induration, and although data are limited, it is not contraindicated in pregnancy.

Podofilox is available in gel or solution form and treats warts by inhibiting cell mitosis. It is applied twice daily for three days, followed by four days of no therapy, and treatment can be repeated weekly for up to four weeks. No more than 10 cm² total wart area should be treated, and no more than 0.5 ml of Podofilox should be used in a given day. Local irritation and mild pain are sometimes noted after Podofilox treatment, and its safety in pregnancy has not been established.

Sinecatechins (15 percent ointment) is an immune-modulating agent made from green tea extract. The exact mechanism is unknown, but it appears to have some antioxidant activity and should only be used in immunocompetent patients. The ointment is applied three times per day, for a maximum of 16 weeks. Patients should apply a 0.5-cm strand of ointment to each wart, ensuring complete coverage and leaving a thin layer on the warts. It is not to be washed off

---

Box 48.1 Treatment of external genital warts

Patient applied

1. **Podofilox 0.5% solution or gel.** Apply solution with a cotton swab or gel with finger to visible warts BID For 3 days, followed by 4 days of no therapy. Cycle can be repeated for a total of four cycles if necessary.
2. **Imiquimod 5% cream.** Apply with finger at bedtime, three times a week for up to 16 weeks; wash off in morning; might weaken condoms or diaphragms
3. **Sinecatechins 15% ointment.** Apply three times a day; might weaken condoms or diaphragms

Provider-administered

1. **Cryotherapy with** liquid nitrogen or cyroprobe. Repeat every 1–2 weeks
2. **TCA or BCA 80%–90% solution.** Repeat weekly if necessary
3. **Surgical removal** by tangential scissor excision, tangential shave excision, curretage, laser, or electrosurgery

Alternative regimens (less data available regarding efficacy and side effects)

1. Podophyllin resin
2. Intralesional interferon
3. Photodynamic therapy
4. Topical cidofovir

Adapted from 2015 Centers for Disease Control Recommendations [11]

---

after use, and sexual activity should be avoided during use [8]. Common side effects include pain, induration, vesicular rash, redness, burning, and ulceration, and its safety in pregnancy is unknown.

Trichloroacetic acid and bichloroacetic acid cause a chemical destruction of proteins and are not contraindicated during pregnancy [4]. Due to their low viscosity, they can spread quickly and affect neighboring normal tissue; therefore, it is important to apply these in sparing amounts and allow to dry prior to having the patient sit up. If burning or pain develop, baking soda will neutralize the acid. Preemptively applying a moisture barrier around the warts, like zinc oxide or petroleum jelly, may help prevent local burning.

Cryotherapy with liquid nitrogen causes destruction of warts by means of thermal-induced cytolysis. This mode of therapy can be used on single or multiple warts and is most effective for small warts [9]. The liquid nitrogen is typically applied with a cryoprobe, cotton bud, or fine spray using two freeze-thaw cycles of 10–30 seconds. A small margin of normal skin should be included within the application. Most patients will require one to two treatments per week for an average of four to six weeks. Pain during and after treatment is common; therefore, some providers will use local anesthesia to reduce patient discomfort. Blistering after treatment can also occur.

In patients with large-volume disease or those who want immediate results, topically applied therapies are often not considered first-line due to the expected time required for

Table 48.1 Efficacy and recurrence rates for treatment of genital warts

Therapy	Efficacy (%)	Recurrance rate (%)	Relative cost
Podofilox	45–88	0–60	+
Imiquimod	37–98	13–19	++
Cryotherapy	63–88	21–39	++
Trichloracetic acid	81	36	++
Electrodesiccation	35–94	11–22	+++
Excision	89–93	29	+++
Laser	23–40	95	++++

response. Although large lesions may resolve spontaneously or respond to topical therapies, these patients may be best managed with surgical methods.

Surgical excision may be accomplished using a laser, electrocautery, scalpel or scissors, and the depth of incision should be limited to the upper dermis [11]. It is recommended by some to surgically shave the condyloma and then apply thermal injury to the virus at the base of the lesion [2]. Alternatively, warts can be desiccated using electrocautery and left to fall off or removed by curetting. Clearance rates with electrocautery are similar to surgical excision (94–100 percent), but recurrence is still possible [10]. When extensive or bulky lesions are encountered, general anesthesia may be required. Regardless of the surgical method chosen, care should be taken to control the depth of excision to reduce possible scarring and minimize bleeding. With all the surgical methods, bleeding is typically easily controlled with cautery, and suturing is rarely needed.

Key Teaching Points

- Genital warts are caused by the HPV virus and are typically diagnosed by visual inspection. Biopsy should be obtained when there is doubt of the diagnosis or if response to therapy is inadequate.
- Observation may be considered in asymptomatic patients, as up to one-third of genital warts will resolve without treatment.
- Multiple treatments exist and include self-applied and provider-applied therapies. There is no definite evidence that one method is superior to another; therefore, patients should be involved in the decision-making process.
- The subsequent HPV behavior and natural history after treatment of genital warts remain unknown.
- Recurrence rates vary widely among the recommended treatment options, and no current therapy is 100 percent curative.

References

1. Patel H, Wagner M, Singhal P, Kothari S. Systemic review of the incidence and prevalence of genital warts. *BCM Infect Dis* 2013;13:39.

2. Division of STD Prevention (1999). Prevention of genital HPV infection and sequelae: report of an external consultants' meeting. Atlanta, GA: Centers for Disease Control and Prevention www.cdc.gov/std/hpv/hpvsupplement99.pdf

3. Centers for Disease Control and Prevention. 2015 Sexually Transmitted Diseases Treatment Guidelines: Anogenital Warts.

4. Katz VL, Lobo RA, Lentz GM, Gershenson DM. Comprehensive gynecology. 5th edn. Philadelphia: Mosby Elsevier. c2007. Chapter 22, *General Gynecology*: pp. 576–78.

5. Hoffman BL, Schorg JO, Bradshaw DK et al. eds. *Williams Gynecology*, 3e New York, NY: McGraw-Hill. 2016. Chapter 3, Gynecologic Infection.

6. Yanofsky VR, Patel RV, Goldenberg G. Genital warts: a comprehensive review. *J Clin Aesthet Dermatol* 2012;5:25.

7. Sweet RL, Gibbs RS. Infectious diseases of the female genital tract. 4th edn. Philadelphia: Lippincott Williams & Wilkins; c2002. Chapter 7, *Sexually Transmitted Diseases*: pp. 155–65.

8. www.accessdata.fda.gov/drugsatfda_docs/label/2007/021902s002lbl.pdf

9. Gross G. Clinical aspects and therapy of anogenital warts and papillomavirus-associated lesions. *Hautarzt* 2001;52:6.

10. Lacey CJ, Woodhall SC, Wikstrom A, Ross J. 2012 European guideline for the management of anogenital warts. *J Eur Acad Dermatol Venereol* 2013;27:e263.

11. Workowski Ka, Bolan GA, Centers for Disease Control and Prevention. Sexually transmitted diseases treatment guidelines, 2015. MMWR Recomm Rep 2015;64:1.

A 50-Year-Old Woman with Lichen Sclerosus, Fused Labia, and UTIs

Dawn Palaszewski

History of Present Illness

A 50-year-old woman presents to her gynecologist's office for follow-up of lichen sclerosus She was diagnosed with this condition approximately three months ago by signs and symptoms confirmed by vulvar biopsy. Labial adhesions were noted at that time. She used clobetasol ointment daily, which she was prescribed, with improvement of vulvar irritation and itching. Three days prior to this visit, she was seen by her primary care physician for dysuria and diagnosed with a urinary tract infection. She has had three urinary tract infections in the last six months. She currently reports that dysuria is resolved and further denies fevers, chills, abdominal pain, back pain, nausea, vomiting, or vaginal discharge.

She is postmenopausal for approximately 18 months. Her past medical history is significant for recurrent urinary tract infections and hyperlipidemia. Prior surgeries include a cesarean section and cholecystectomy. She is divorced and has not been sexually active for the past few years. She has no known drug allergies. Her medications include clobetasol ointment, Nitrofurantoin, Lipitor, and a probiotic.

Physical Examination

General appearance	Well-developed, well-nourished woman with no acute distress.

Vital Signs

Temperature	37.0°C
Pulse	80 beats/min
Blood pressure	125/70 mmHg
Respiratory rate	16 breaths/min
Oxygen saturation	100 percent on room air
Height	64 inches
Weight	180 lb
BMI	31
Abdomen	Soft, non-tender
External genitalia	Mild hypopigmentation of the labia bilaterally. Labia minora almost entirely fused in the midline. Atrophic urethra visualized. Speculum was not inserted vaginally due to small size of opening (see Figure 49.1).

How Would You Manage This Patient?

The patient has complications of vulvar lichen sclerosus Topical corticosteroids have helped to control the symptoms of the disease but she has persistent scarring and distortion of labial architecture with labial adhesions now contributing to recurrent urinary tract infections. Due to concern for urethral obstruction and recurrent urinary infections, the decision was made to proceed with sharp dissection of labial adhesions. The dissection was done in

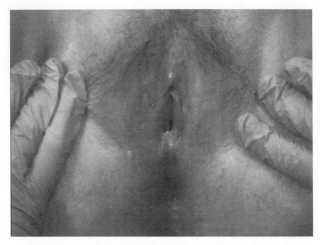

Figure 49.1 Lichen sclerosus Partial fusion of labia.

the outpatient surgical setting using both blunt dissection and Metzenbaum scissors along the adhesion line until the labia were completely separated. The incised edges were then reapproximated with interrupted delayed absorbable suture. Postoperatively, the patient was instructed on continued postoperative use of clobetasol propionate 0.05 percent ointment at night starting three days after surgery. Additionally, manual massage with an emollient such as petroleum jelly three times daily on the suture lines and surrounding areas was suggested [1,2]. Patient had a normal postoperative course with resolution of symptoms.

Complications of Vulvar Lichen Sclerosus

Vulvar lichen sclerosus is associated with several complications.

Malignancy is a potential complication of vulvar lichen sclerosus Squamous cell carcinoma is the most common malignancy. Verrucous carcinoma, basal cell carcinoma, and melanoma also have been associated. The lifelong magnitude of this risk is about 5 percent or less [3]. Vulvar intraepithelial neoplasia or cancer is the most common reason for vulvectomy in patients with lichen sclerosus.

Severe adhesions and scarring from vulvar lichen sclerosus can lead to functional limitations and disfigurement. Some women may have narrowing of the introitus leading to problems with dyspareunia and/or difficulties with micturation. Lysis of adhesions of the labia minora may be required with sharp dissection. For introital narrowing, one may attempt a simple Fenton's median perineotomy where an incision is made at the vaginal entrance vertically toward the rectum and then sutured horizontally (see Figure 49.2) [4]. Alternatively, a modified Fenton's procedure, vulvoperineoplasty, may be performed, in which part of the posterior wall of the vagina is undermined and then advanced to reconstruct a new introitus (see Figure 49.3) [4].

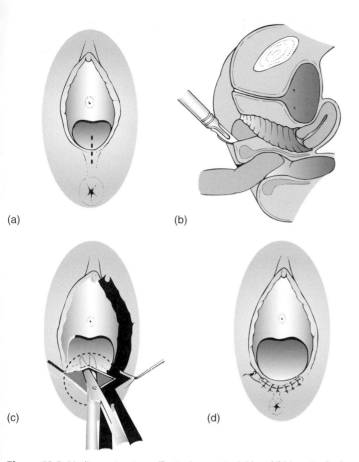

Figure 49.2 Median perineotomy (Fenton's operation). (a) and (b) Longitudinal incision running from the hymenal ring to the perineal skin and cutting into the perineal body; (c) undermining the vaginal wall and perineal skin; (d) transverse suturing. From [4], used with permission.

Women who have any chronic genital disorder will often lose their interest in sexual activity, leading to problems with sexual dysfunction. It is important to be aware of these problems and offer appropriate referral [3].

Vestibulodynia and vulvodynia can occur when the patient remains symptomatic despite clinical improvement or resolution of skin lesions. This neuropathic pain will not respond to topical corticosteroids, and treatment must be aimed at the eradication of the neuronal sensitization. Xylocaine 5 percent ointment should be tried first, progressing to amitriptyline or gabapentin in unresponsive cases [3].

Another potential complication is a pseudocyst of the clitoris. Adhesions of the clitoral hood may result in a seal over the clitoris with keratinous debris building up underneath the hood, forming a painful pseudocyst. Treatment for this problem requires release of adhesions sharply to free the hood from the glans [5].

Surgery is rarely needed for lichen sclerosus Surgical treatment should be used exclusively for malignancy and postinflammatory sequelae as noted above. Ideally, surgery is deferred until the disease is well controlled with medication. Additionally, the use of topical or injected corticosteroids should be considered following surgery. Manual massage can also be utilized to separate adhesions. Vaginal dilators may be required following surgery, the largest size tolerated, with lubricant and lidocaine if very painful. Several weeks after surgery the frequency of topical corticosteroid application, massage, and dilation can slowly be reduced to a maintenance regimen of twice weekly. Recurrence of adhesions is high in patients with lichen sclerosus who have required surgical treatment, even extensive surgery [5].

Recalcitrant Disease

The appropriate initial treatment for lichen sclerosus is a topical high-potency corticosteroid, clobetasol propionate 0.05 percent ointment twice a day for one month then once daily for two months is a recommended treatment strategy. Local corticosteroid treatment is highly effective; potential causes of corticosteroid failure should be carefully considered before resorting to a trial of an alternative drug. Anti-itching and vulvar care measures should be utilized in addition to topical corticosteroids. The cessation of scratching is very important. Cool compresses, oral hydroxyzine, keeping fingernails trimmed to minimize trauma to the skin, and skin moisturizers such as petroleum jelly are helpful adjuncts. Healthy vulvar hygiene practices include avoiding scented soaps or shampoos, scented detergents, synthetic underwear, jeans or tight pants, panty liners, bubble bath, baby wipes, and douches. Once scarring has occurred, it is not reversible by any medical therapy and surgery may be required.

Noncompliance can be an issue. Evaluate for proper use of the medication (right place, right amount, right frequency). Superinfection with *Staphylococcus*, *Streptococcus*, or *Candida* may occur and also require treatment. Thickened hypertrophic plaques may respond poorly to topical corticosteroids and require injection of triamcinolone directly into the involved site. A regimen that may be considered is the injection of bupivacaine (0.25–0.5 percent) and triamcinolone up to 40 mg injected with a 30-gauge needle every four weeks. Triamcinolone is drawn up first then diluted with the amount of bupivacaine needed to cover the surface area affected. Rarely more than three treatments are required [5].

In recalcitrant cases, a biopsy should be considered to reconfirm the diagnosis. Malignancy (in particular, squamous cell carcinoma) is an ever-important consideration. Lichen sclerosus can mimic other scarring diseases, especially lichen planus. Other vulvar diseases such as psoriasis, allergic contact dermatitis, lupus, Behcet's, irritant dermatitis, bullous pemphigoid, and pemphigus may appear similar to erosive lichen sclerosus [5]. Obtaining a diagnostic biopsy may be difficult in patients with subtle disease. However, these patients often have pain and burning symptoms rather than itching. They may respond to the addition of topical 5 percent lidocaine and/or a low-dose tricyclic antidepressant in the evening, 10–25 mg nightly initially [5].

Menopausal symptoms, such as vulvovaginal atrophy, may be present and the affected patient would benefit from estrogen treatment. Allergy to the topical corticosteroid product may also cause poor treatment response. In patients affected by the steroid vehicle, mixing the corticosteroid in Aquaphor can alleviate irritation [5]. If the lichen sclerosus is successfully treated by appearance, but the patient is still symptomatic, she may have developed a secondary sensory problem (vulvodynia) which requires treatment such as Xylocaine ointment, amitriptyline, or gabapentin.

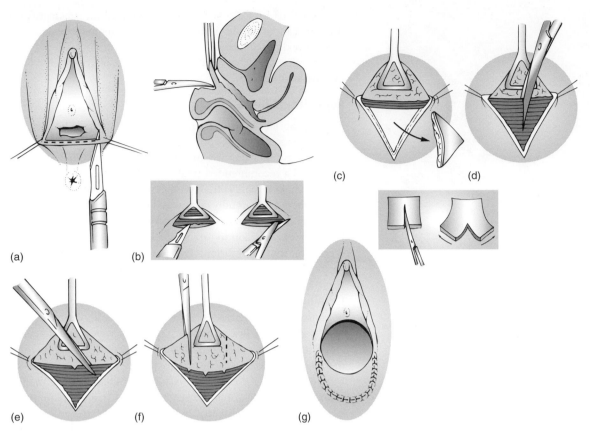

Figure 49.3 Vulvoperineoplasty. (a) Mucocutaneous incision; (b) dissection of the posterior vaginal wall; (c) excision of a triangular patch of perineal skin; (d and e) radial incision of the fibrous perineal body to reduce its height; (f) individualization of a vaginal flap; (g) the vaginal flap is drawn down, making a cover for the perineal defect, and sutured. From [4], used with permission.

If the patient's disease is recalcitrant to the aforementioned treatments, topical calcineurin inhibitors, such as pimecrolimus or tacrolimus ointment, appear to have efficacy for vulvar lichen sclerosus These agents seem to induce less dermal atrophy though long-term safety aspects need further study, thus they should be considered a second-line treatment. Other therapies including topical and oral retinoids, oral cyclosporine, intravenous methotrexate, UVA1 phototherapy, photodynamic therapy, focal ultrasound, CO_2 laser, topical progesterone, topical testosterone, oral antibiotics such as penicillin and cephalosporins, and stem cell transplants combined with platelet-rich plasma have shown some utility [6]. Factors such as limited efficacy data, inconvenience of treatment, and associated adverse effects make these less favorable options. These therapies may be considered for refractory disease.

Key Teaching Points

- Complications of lichen sclerosus include malignancy, severe adhesions and scarring, dyspareunia, difficulty with micturation, sexual dysfunction, dysesthesia such as vulvodynia, and pseudocyst of the clitoris.
- Surgery is rarely needed for lichen sclerosus and should be used exclusively for malignancy and/or complications of postinflammatory adhesions/scarring.
- Local corticosteroid treatment is highly effective; potential causes of corticosteroid failure should be carefully considered before resorting to a trial of an alternative drug.
- Topical calcineurin inhibitors, such as pimecrolimus or tacrolimus ointment, appear to have efficacy for vulvar lichen sclerosus and should be considered a second-line treatment.

References

1. Sideri M et al. Topical testosterone in the treatment of vulvar lichen sclerosus. *Int J Gynecol Obstet* 1994;46:53–56.

2. Simonart T et al. Vulvar lichen sclerosus: effect of maintenance treatment with a moisturizer on the course of the disease. *Menopause* 2008;15(1):74–77.

3. Neill SM et al. Guidelines for the management of lichen sclerosus. *Br J Dermatol* 2002;147:640–649.

4. Paniel BJ, Rouzier R. Surgical procedures in benign vulval disease. In: Neill S, Lewis F, eds. *Ridley's The Vulva.* Wiley-Blackwell. 2009;228–234.

5. Smith Y, Haefner, H. Vulvar lichen sclerosus: pathophysiology and treatment. *Am J Clin Dermatol* 2004;**5**(2):117.

6. Kirtschig G et al. Evidence-based (S3) guideline on (anogenital) lichen sclerosus. *JEADV* 2015;**29**: e1–e43.

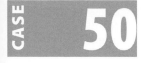

A 25-Year-Old Woman with Recurrent *Candida* Vaginitis

Kimberly Carter

History of Present Illness

A 25-year-old female presents to the office with complaints vulvar itching, burning, and thick white discharge for three days. She states that she had a similar episode four weeks prior to this visit and she self-treated with over-the-counter (OTC) medication. The OTC treatment provided some relief for a few days. Her menses then occurred and her symptoms completely subsided after menses. Seven months prior to the visit, she was seen in the office for similar symptoms, wet mount showed abundant hyphae, and she was treated with one 150 mg dose of oral fluconazole. She states that she self-medicated with OTC medication successfully, another time, between these episodes. She reports that she has used OTC "anti-yeast wipes" and takes lactobacillus for burning and itching relief on and off for the last four months. She complains that she has similar symptoms every month right before the onset of menses which resolves after menses.

The patient is nulliparous. She reports using barrier contraception exclusively. Her past medical and surgical history are negative for significant or chronic illness or surgery. She takes no medications. She has not taken a course of antibiotics for any illness in the last year.

Physical Examination

General appearance	Well-developed, well-nourished woman with no acute distress. Ambulating normally.

Vital Signs

Temperature	37.0°C
Pulse	80 beats/min
Blood pressure	125/70 mmHg
Respiratory rate	16 breaths/min
Oxygen saturation	100 percent on room air
Height	5'3"
Weight	147 lb
BMI	26
Abdomen	Soft, non-tender

Female GU

External genitalia	Mild erythema on bilateral labia minora. Small fissures are noted at the posterior vaginal forchette.
Vagina	Moist mucosa and abnormal thick white discharge; erythematous mucosa
Cervix	Normal appearance, no tenderness or mass
Adnexa	Non-palpable, non-tender

Laboratory

Vaginal pH	4

Wet prep:

WBC	Rare
Hyphae	Abundant
Clue cells	Rare
Trichomonas	Absent
Parabasal cells	Absent

How Would You Evaluate and Manage This Patient?

This patient has symptoms and laboratory confirmation of recurrent vulvovaginal candidiasis (RVVC). RVVC is defined as four or more infections within 12 months. Yeast cultures should be obtained at the time of exam in conjunction with the sample for microscopy as microscopy alone does not demonstrate the presence of yeast in up to 50 percent of patients who have yeast on culture. The culture allows for further diagnostic capabilities in speciating the yeast and in determining sensitivity or resistance to azole therapies.

For immediate symptomatic relief, pending culture results, a topical zinc ointment should be recommended such as a diaper rash cream. This may be applied externally to areas of irritation. Intercourse is permitted during treatment but may be poorly tolerated. Additionally, the patient is evaluated for metabolic and immunosuppressive etiologies for RVVC including a hemoglobin A1 C or fasting glucose and HIV antibody testing where appropriate. Testing for immunocompromise is normal/negative. Yeast culture returns as *Candida albicans* and is resistant to fluconazole. This patient is treated with compounded 600 mg boric acid suppositories nightly for two weeks and then weekly thereafter for six months with resolution of her symptoms.

Recurrent Vulvovaginal Candidiasis (RVVC)

The most common pathogen for yeast infection in general is *C. albicans* (65.6%), followed by *C. glabrata* (11.1%), *C. tropicalis* (6.9%), and *C. parapsilosis* (6.1%) [1]. *C. glabrata* and other non-*albicans Candida* species are observed in 10–20 percent of women with RVVC. Concern for increasing prevalence of *C. glabrata* and RVVC is related to increased use of OTC medications and the short treatment courses of antifungal medications. Additionally, empiric treatment with azoles is not recommended in RVVC as a large number of non-albicans-resistant species are primary pathogens.

RVVC is a common problem. It is estimated that 10 percent of all women will experience RVVC by age 25 and it is more common in African American women [2]. Recent studies point to endogenous reinfection as a cause; this includes colonization of the mouth and transmission through oral sex. Possible triggers for RVVC include (A) diabetes, particularly if it is poorly controlled, (B) use of antibiotics, especially if broad spectrum antibiotics, (C) increased estrogen levels such as oral contraceptive use and pregnancy, (D) immunosuppression such as HIV or use of immunosuppressive medications, and (E) contraceptive devices such as Nuvaring, vaginal sponges, and intrauterine devices. Data are inconsistent but

Box 50.1 Differential of vulvar pruritus

Irritant Dermatitis
- Topical anesthetics (e.g., benzocaine found in OTC antifungal treatments); Chlorhexidine (found in K-Y Jelly); Latex (found in condoms); topical antifungal medications (imadazoles and nystatin); topical antibiotics (Neomycin); perfumes (found in scented panty liners, soaps, and tampons); preservatives such as propylene glycol (in creams, toilet paper, hygiene products and nail polish); spermicides; bubble bath, shampoo, nylon underwear, sweat, urine, talcum powder, douches; Nuvaring; semen; hair dyes; tea tree oil

Infectious
- Candidasis; Herpes simplex virus; Human papilloma virus; Molluscum Contagiosum, Bacterial Vaginosis; Bacterial (*Streptococcus, Staphlococcus, Enterobacter, E. coli*), *Trichomonas vaginalis, Neisseria gonorrhea, Chlamydia trachomatis*, scabies, lice, Enterobiasis

Dermatitis/Inflammatory disorders of the skin and mucosa
- Allergic Contact Dermatitis; Atopic Dermatitis; Seborrheic Dermatitis; Intertrigo (friction); Psoriasis; Lichen Sclerosus et Atrophicus; Lichen Simplex Chronicus; Lichen Planus; Plasma cell vulvitis; Dermatographism

Malignancies
- Extramammary Paget's disease; Vulvar Intraepithelial Neoplasia, Syringomas, Basal cell carinoma

Other
- Diabetes, obesity, poor hygiene, psychogenic (depression); atrophic vaginitis

there is suggestion these contraceptive agents may be colonized and act as a source for reinfection [3, 4, 5].

Studies regarding the optimal evaluation of RVVC are conclusive only in that a combination of microscopy, culture, or PCR should be utilized in evaluation. Due to limited sensitivity of yeast culture, if cultures are negative and suspicion remains high for *Candida*, then PCR should be considered. If cultures and PCR are negative, then alternative diagnosis should be considered, including vulvar dystrophies, vulvodynia, and contact dermatitis. The use and overuse of OTC antifungal treatments can lead to contact dermatitis, which should be considered in the differential if the evaluation is otherwise negative (see Box 50.1).

Importantly, as many as 7 percent of women who are thought to have RVVC on exam have an underdiagnosed entity known as cytolytic vaginitis (CV) or Doderlein's cytolysis [6]. CV occurs due to lactobacillus overgrowth, which results in lysis of vaginal epithelial cells. The signs and symptoms of CV are similar to those of RVVC. The diagnostic criteria for CV include:

- Negative culture and/or PCR for *Candida*.

- An increase in number of *Lactobacilli* on wet prep.
- A paucity of white blood cells on wet prep.
- Evidence of cytolysis on the wet prep.
- The presence of discharge.
- pH between 3.5 and 4.5.

When culture or PCR confirm RVVC, treatment regimens for RVVC as recommended by both CDC and 2016 Update by the Infectious Diseases Society of America are presented below [4, 7].

Albicans Species
Fluconazole 150 mg every 72 hours × 3 doses then once a week for six months (as long as there are no liver lab abnormalities) (strong recommendation; high-quality evidence), or

Topical azole 10–14 days followed by fluconazole 150 mg weekly for six months (strong recommendation; high-quality evidence).

If reoccurrence occurs on this regime, then fluconazole resistance should be considered.

Non-*albicans* Species or Allergy or Resistance to Fluconazole
Compounded boric acid intravaginal 600 mg capsule once daily at night for two weeks followed by weekly suppression for six months (strong recommendation; low-quality evidence).

Nystatin intravaginal suppositories, 100,000 units daily for 14 days followed by weekly suppression for six months (strong recommendation; low-quality evidence).

Compounded flucytosine cream – 17 percent flucytosine cream alone or in combination with 3 percent AmB cream (5 grams) administered daily for 14 days followed by weekly suppression for six months (weak recommendation; low-quality evidence).

Topical gentian violet – use this to paint the affected area for 10–14 days followed by weekly suppression for six months (weak recommendation, low-quality evidence).

Other recommendations for treatment include the following:

- Address risk factors for recurrent yeast such as management of diabetes (if present), immunosuppressive condition (HIV, cancer).
- Change to a lower estrogen dose of oral contraception.
- Cease using saliva or lubrication during sexual intercourse.
- Discontinue/change birth control if non-*albicans* yeast is present and a contraceptive ring is used as some evidence demonstrates adherence of *Candida* to the device [8] (weak recommendations, low-quality evidence).
- Alternative medicine such as garlic, tea tree oil, placing yogurt in the vagina or orally, or placing capsules with live lactobacillus have been studied, but they are not found to be effective in treatment and prevention of RVVC and therefore are not recommended [9, 10].

Key Teaching Points
1. In cases of RVVC, culture to demonstrate presence of yeast and subspeciation of the pathogen is imperative.

2. The majority of women with recurrent yeast do *not* have underlying conditions that would predispose them to repetitive infection such as diabetes or HIV. However, testing for predisposing factors for RVVC may be indicated.

3. Use of lactobacillus while taking antibiotics does not prevent postantibiotic vulvovaginitis, nor does it aid women with RVVC [9].

4. Other conditions mimic RVVC (such as CV and Contact Dermatitis) and should be considered in the differential.

References

1. Pfaller MA, Diekema DJ, Gibbs DL et al. Results from the ARTEMIS DISK Global antifungal surveillance study, 1997 to 2005: an 8.5-year analysis of susceptibilities of candida species and other yeast species to fluconazole and voriconazole determined by CLSI standardized disk diffusion testing. *J. Clin. Microbiol* 2007;45:1735–1745.

2. Foxman B, Muraglia R, Dietz JP, Sobel JD, Wagner J. Prevalence of recurrent vulvovaginal candidiasis in 5 European countries and the United States: results from an internet panel survey.

3. Camacho DP, Consolaro ME, Patussi EV et al. Vaginal yeast adherence to the combined contraceptive vaginal ring (CCVR). *Contraception* 2007 December;76(6):439–443.

4. 2015 STD Treatment guidelines: Diseases characterized by vaginal discharge vulvovaginal candidiasis, Centers for Disease Control andPrevention. www.cdc.gov/std/tg2015/candidiasis.htm Accessed August 2017.

5. Reed BD, Zazove P, Pierson CL, Gorenflo DW, Horrocks J. Candida transmission and sexual behaviors as risks for a repeat episode of candida vulvovaginitis. *J Womens Health (Larchmt)* 2003;12(10):979.

6. Cerikcioglu N, Beksac MS. Cytolytic vaginosis; misdiagnosed as candidal vaginitis. *Infect Dis Obstet Gynecol* 2004;12:13–16.

7. Pappas PG, Kauffman CA, Andes DR et al. Clinical Practice Guideline for the Management of Candidiasis: 2016 Update by the Infectious Diseases Society of America. www.ncbi.nlm.nih.gov/pmc/articles/PMC4725385/ Accessed August 2017.

8. Vazquez JA, Sobel JD, Demitriou R et al. Karyotyping of Candida albicans isolates obtained longitudinally in women with recurrent vulvovaginal candidiasis. *J Infect Dis* 1994 Dec;170(6):1566–1569.

9. Lopez JEM. Candidiasis (vulvovaginal). Systematic review 815. BMJ Clinical Evidence. http://clinicalevidence.bmj.com/x/systematic-review/0815/overview.html. Accessed August 2017.

10. Van Kessel K, Assef N, Marrazzo J, Eckert L. Common complementary and alternative therapies for yeast vaginitis and bacterial vaginosis: a systematic review. *Obstet Gynecol Surv.* 2003;58(5):351–358.

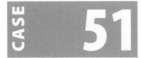

A 35-Year-Old Woman Complaining of a "Knot" in the Vulva (Bartholin's Cyst)

D. Scott Wiersma

History of Present Illness

A 35-year-old, gravida 2, para 1011, presents to the office with a five-day history of a "knot" in the vulva. The knot has grown in size becoming more painful, especially when seated, prompting an urgent visit to the clinic. She reports that the mass is right-sided, and has increased to the size of a small egg. Review of symptoms is negative for bleeding, discharge, fever, or chills. She reports that she has never had anything similar.

She reports no significant medical or surgical history. Obstetric and gynecologic history is significant for an uncomplicated term delivery and a first-trimester pregnancy loss, and no history of sexually transmitted infections or abnormal cervical cytology screening. The patient is married and monogamous.

Physical Examination

General appearance	Well-developed, well-nourished woman in no discomfort, who is alert and oriented
Vital Signs	
Temperature	36.9°C
Pulse	82 beats/min
Blood pressure	116/72 mmHg
Respiratory rate	16 breaths/min
Oxygen saturation	100% on room air
Height	5'3"
Weight	126 lb
BMI	25.6 kg/m^2
Abdomen	Soft, non-tender, non-distended without peritoneal signs
External genitalia	Clean shaven vulva with fluctuant 3 cm diameter moderately tender mass in right posterior vestibule bulging the posterior right labia majora. There is no surrounding erythema or induration.
Vagina	No other masses, no discharge
Cervix	Unable to insert speculum due to her discomfort
Uterus	Normal size, retroverted, mobile, non-tender
Adnexa	Non-tender without mass

Laboratory Studies
Urine pregnancy test Negative

How Would You Manage This Patient?

The patient has a symptomatic Bartholin's gland cyst. The diagnosis is made primarily by the location of the mass in the postero-lateral vestibule. The mass appears to be a cyst rather than an abscess as there is no surrounding edema, induration, or erythema, and tenderness is less pronounced.

The diagnosis of a Bartholin's cyst was explained and the options for treatment reviewed including expectant management, incision and drainage (I&D), marsupialization, placement of a Word catheter, and excision. The patient opted for I&D with placement of a Word catheter. Local anesthesia was accomplished by injecting 1 percent lidocaine using a 27-gauge needle over the surface of the fluctuant mass just inside the hymen. The cyst was incised with a 0.5–1.0 cm incision, drained and irrigated, and the Word catheter was placed uneventfully. The patient was contacted three days after the visit to confirm resolution/reduction of the mass and improvement in her symptoms, and a follow-up appointment was scheduled in one month for removal of the Word catheter.

Uncomplicated Bartholin's Cyst

The greater, or major, vestibular glands described by Caspar Bartholin the Younger in 1677 are located deep to the posterior labia majora. They are 5 mm in diameter and normally are not palpable. The duct of Bartholin's gland (not Bartholin's duct which drains the sublingual salivary gland) is about 25 mm in length and lined by transitional epithelium. It drains via a small opening that is seldom visible just outside the hymen at 5 and 7 o'clock in the posterior vestibule. The Bartholin gland secretes mucus, which can dilate an obstructed duct, forming a cyst or abscess. Two percent of women will have a Bartholin's cyst or abscess during their lifetime, most often occurring during reproductive years.

Successful treatments to treat a Bartholin's cyst or abscess create a new tract/duct to allow continued drainage via marsupialization or Word catheter placement or eradication of mucus production by sclerosing or completely excising the gland. Simple I&D of a Bartholin's gland cyst is not the favored approach for treatment as the cyst will often recur. This approach will usually give immediate relief; however, once the incision heals the still obstructed duct will again fill with mucus.

The differential diagnosis of a Bartholin's cyst may include other vulvar masses. Vulvar abscesses contain purulent material but unlike a Bartholin's abscess are not an epithelium-lined natural cavity and thus are amenable to simple drainage by I&D as the tissues heal completely and there is no persisting cavity.

Diagnosis of Bartholin's cyst or abscess is made by physical exam. A Bartholin's cyst or abscess will be found in the normal anatomic location of the duct. With a finger in the vagina and thumb external (over the posterior labia majora at 5 or 7 o'clock), the cyst (i.e., dilated duct) should be palpable between the thumb and the finger with little or no normal tissue between the mass and the mucosa of the posterior vestibule.

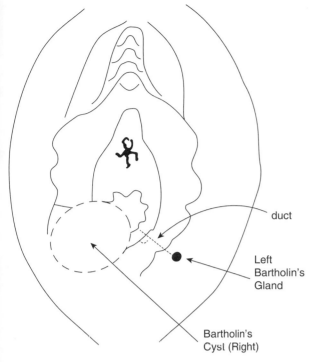

Figure 51.1 Diagram of normal Bartholin's gland and duct anatomy on patient's left with a Bartholin's cyst on the patient's right. Note the location of the gland deep to the posterior labia majora and course of the duct as it runs toward the posterior vestibule.

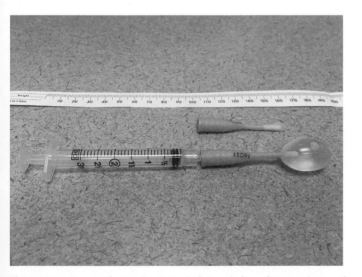

Figure 51.2 Picture of a Word catheter before and after inflation with 3 cc of saline.

A large Bartholin's abscess may extend anteriorly up the labia majora. Swelling extending anteriorly is sometimes associated with edema rather than abscess.

A Bartholin's cyst is differentiated from a Bartholin's abscess by physical exam. The cyst is a fluctuant mass of variable tenderness that has no surrounding erythema, induration, or edema. When small, it is often asymptomatic and does not require treatment. The Bartholin's abscess will be exquisitely tender with surrounding erythema, warmth, induration, or edema. The overlying mucosa may be thinning and peeling

where the abscess is pointing or already draining. A minority of patients can have systemic symptoms with fever, chills, and malaise or even sepsis.

Treatment is not indicated for asymptomatic Bartholin's cysts. Options for treating Bartholin abscesses and symptomatic cysts are Word catheter placement, marsupialization, or complete excision of the mass and gland [1]. While simple I&D may provide immediate relief, its success is limited by frequent cyst recurrence.

A randomized control trial (RCT) of Word catheter fistulization in the office versus marsupialization in the OR found the one-year recurrence rate to be equal, about 10 percent [2]. The Word catheter group reported more pain during the procedure but less analgesic use the day after the procedure. Given the assumed savings in cost and time with an office procedure, the Word catheter will often be preferred. (Marsupialization can also be performed in the office.) Others have found recurrence rates as high as 25 percent.

I&D followed by ablation of the duct wall and gland with laser or silver nitrate may also be employed. An RCT of marsupialization versus silver nitrate application found similar recurrence rates of about 25 percent [3]. The cyst wall was opened, a 5 mm × 5 mm piece of silver nitrate inserted, and then the cyst wall alone (separate from vulvar skin) was closed with suture. The skin edges were left open. The patient returned in three days when the sutures were pulled removing the coagulated cyst wall.

Procedure: Word Catheter placement

The Bartholin cyst is stabilized with one hand and an area for incision selected inside or as close to the hymen as possible. The area is cleansed with Betadine and injected with local anesthetic. After a 5–8 mm stab incision is made, the cyst can be drained and irrigated before inserting the catheter. Alternatively, the Word catheter can be inserted immediately after incision, before the contents have drained and the cavity collapses. This technique may be more likely to result in catheter placement well within the cyst cavity than completely expressing the contents and then trying to insert the catheter. Once in place, the balloon is inflated with 3–5 cc of saline. The remaining end of the catheter can be tucked into the vagina for patient comfort. The Word catheter should remain in place long enough for a new tract to fistulize, four to six weeks. [1] To prevent the Word catheter from falling out prematurely, a smaller incision can be made, the balloon inflated larger (up to 5 cc), and a smaller needle may be used to inject the saline into the catheter (fewer leaks); saline rather than air is used to fill the balloon or place a suture to close the incision around the catheter. Similarly, after initial drainage of the cyst or abscess, one may utilize a unilateral, ipsilateral pudendal block for additional anesthesia.

Marsupialization can be performed in the office setting or an operating room.

A new duct is formed from everting the cyst wall of the dilated duct. The opening must be large enough (allows insertion of a fingertip) so that, despite healing and constriction, a small patent duct will remain. An elliptical or round 1.5 cm diameter piece of vestibular mucosa is typically excised.

159

The cyst wall is incised and contents drained. The cyst walls are then everted and sutured to the mucosal edges with interrupted absorbable suture. Removing the elliptical piece of mucosa helps to hold the suture line apart and keep the new duct open.

Success of treatment will depend on cyst/abscess size. Criteria for successful marsupialization or Word catheter placement depends on cyst size (minimally 2–3 cm) and fluctuance (ensure no solid mass). If aforementioned criteria are not met, the patient can apply warm moist compresses for two or three days (with antibiotics if an abscess is suspected) and then return for reevaluation.

Recurrence is not uncommon after all treatments. Repeat Word catheter placement or marsupialization may be employed. Ultimately, excision may be required but bears greater risks of infection, bleeding, hematoma, disfigurement, and dyspareunia (1).

Bartholin gland cancers are more prevalent in older women. It was historically recommended that women over 40 with Bartholin abscesses and cysts undergo complete excision. However, given that primary Bartholin gland cancer is rare, with an incidence as low as 1/1,000,000 woman-years in post-menopausal women [4], treatment of the postmenopausal woman should proceed similar to that of a premenopausal woman with the exception that cyst wall biopsy should be performed with treatment. After drainage, if resolution of the cyst/abscess does not occur or any palpable firm or fixed mass is palpated, excision may be warranted. Primary excision is recommended if neoplasm is suspected.

Periprocedural antibiotics are not required for Bartholin cyst management. Bartholin abscesses are polymicrobia infections; however, many will respond to drainage alone (Word catheter, marsupialization). MRSA is now reported in more than half of vulvar abscesses [5]. MRSA has also been reported in Bartholin abscesses [6]. Given these findings, cultures should be collected and when indicated appropriate antibiotics tailored to the pathogen. Complicated abscesses which should be treated with antibiotics primarily in addition to drainage include pregnancy, patients with concomitant systemic symptoms, immunocompromised patients, abscesses associated with extensive cellulitis, infections which cannot be drained, those who fail drainage alone, and those treated with excision. Trimethoprim-sulfamethoxazole, 800 mg/160 mg, one tablet by mouth twice daily for seven days will provide adequate coverage for the most organisms involved in Bartholin abscesses including MRSA.

References

1. Wechter ME, Wu JM, Marzano D, Haefner H. Management of Bartholin duct cysts and abscesses: A systematic review. *Obstet Gynecol Surv* 2009;64:395–404.

2. Kroese JA, van der Velde M, Morssink LP et al. Word catheter and marsupialization in women with a cyst or abscess of the Bartholin gland (WoMan-trial): a randomised clinical trial. *BJOG* 2017;124:243–249.

3. Ozdegirmenci O, Kayikcioglu F, Haberal A. Prospective randomized study of marsupialization versus silver nitrate application in the management of Bartholin gland cysts and abscesses. *J Minim Invasive Gynecol* 2009;16:149–152.

4. Visco AG, del Priore G. Postmenopausal Bartholin gland enlargement: A hospital-based cancer risk assessment. *Obstet Gynecol* 1996;87:286–290.

5. Wood S. Clinical manifestations and therapeutic management of vulvar cellulitis and abscess: methicillin-resistant *Staphylococcus aureus*, necrotizing fasciitis, Bartholin abscess, Crohn disease of the vulva, hidradenitis suppurativa. *Clin Obstet Gynecol* 2015;58:503–511.

6. Sherer D, Dalloul M, Salameh G, Abulafia O. Methicillin-resistant *Staphylococcus aureus* bacteremia and chorioamnionitis after recurrent marsupialization of a Bartholin abscess. *Obstet Gynecol* 2009;114 (2):471–472.

A Couple with Medicaid and No Conception after Two Years (Cost-Conscious Infertility Evaluation)

Merielle Stephens

History of Present Illness

A 32-year-old nulligravid woman presents to your office with her husband for infertility. They have been trying to conceive for two years without success, despite having intercourse two to three times per week. They have not sought care until now because their insurance does not cover infertility services and they are concerned about the cost of care.

The patient reports menarche at age 14, with fairly regular menses as an adolescent and young adult, but does report she would skip a menstrual cycle one or two times per year. She started on oral contraceptives at age 22 years. Since stopping her birth control pills two years ago, she reports bleeding every 45–60 days that lasts for 3–10 days. She notes moliminal symptoms prior to about half of those bleeding episodes and denies significant dysmenorrhea or dyspareunia. She also reports a gradual increase in her weight in the past five years as well as increasing fatigue. She denies unusual headaches, hirsutism, galactorrhea, heat or cold intolerance, diarrhea, or constipation. She has no history of sexually transmitted diseases, pelvic inflammatory disease, or abnormal pap smears, and her co-testing was negative two years ago.

Her medical and surgical histories are otherwise unremarkable. She denies family history of infertility or premature ovarian insufficiency. She drinks one alcoholic beverage on the weekends and does not smoke. She works part-time as a teacher. She does not regularly exercise but walks 15 minutes to and from work. She has no allergies and is taking prenatal vitamins. Her last menstrual period was five weeks ago.

Her husband is 34 years old and has not fathered any children. He has no significant medical or surgical history and takes no medications. He works at a construction company and smokes about two to four cigarettes per week and drinks less than two alcoholic beverages per week.

Physical Examination

Vital Signs
Body mass index	29 kg/m^2
Blood pressure	126/84 mmHg
General	Alert, oriented
Skin	No rashes, skin changes, or acne
Breasts	No lymphadenopathy, no masses or nipple discharge
Neck	Thyroid without masses
Chest	Heart regular rate and rhythm, lungs are clear to auscultation
Abdomen	Soft, non-tender, no hepatosplenomegaly, no masses appreciated

Pelvic
Normal external female genitalia

Vagina normally developed, physiologic discharge

Cervix without lesions

Mobile, normal-sized anteverted uterus

Adnexae non-tender and without masses

Urine pregnancy test   Negative

How Would You Manage This Patient?

Traditionally, patients with infertility should have a workup that includes an assessment of ovulatory function, a semen analysis, and an assessment of tubal patency.

This patient has a clinical history suggestive of ovulatory dysfunction; therefore, a thyroid-stimulating hormone (TSH) and prolactin were ordered to evaluate for underlying causes. It was recommended that her husband have a semen analysis to rule out male factor as a cause. Assessment of tubal patency with a hysterosalpingogram (HSG) was discussed; however, since the patient has no risk factors for tubal disease, and cost was a significant concern to the patient and her husband, it was decided to hold off on that, pending the remainder of her workup.

Her labs revealed a normal prolactin, an elevated TSH at 8.2 IU/mL, and a low free T4 of 0.5 ng/mL, consistent with a diagnosis of hypothyroidism. The semen analysis was normal. She was started on levothyroxine and counseled regarding weight loss for overall improvement of her health. She and her husband were also counseled on smoking cessation and limiting alcohol use. After six months, she lost 25 lb, her TSH had normalized, and she reported resumption of regular menses. She conceived three months later.

Cost-Conscious Infertility Evaluation

Diagnostic evaluation for causes of infertility is indicated after 12 months of regular unprotected intercourse when the female partner is under 35 years of age and after six months if the female partner is 35 years or age or older. Eighty-five to ninety percent of apparently normal couples will conceive in the first 12 months [1]. Evaluation is warranted earlier if the couple suffers conditions known to limit fertility such as advanced endometriosis, oligomenorrhea or amenorrhea, known or suspected uterine or tubal disease, or suspected male subfertility. Evaluation and treatment should occur immediately in women over 40 years of age [2].

Ovulatory dysfunction is one of the most common findings in infertile women; therefore, ovulatory status needs to be assessed in each patient. Often, a thorough menstrual history is all that is needed. A patient with monthly menses and moliminal symptoms is considered ovulatory, while those with amenorrhea or oligomenorrhea are unlikely to be ovulating regularly. For those patients in whom ovulatory status is unclear, further testing would be indicated. A simple option is to obtain a midluteal progesterone. This should be scheduled for a week prior to anticipated menses, which would be dependent on the individual patient's cycle length. A progesterone level >3 ng/mL indicates ovulation. Another option is to have the patient use an ovulation predictor kit [5]. It is important to stress to the couple that the color change indicates the luteinizing hormone (LH) surge, which precedes ovulation by 24–48 hours. Intercourse is recommended the day of the LH surge or the following day. Ovulation predictor kits can vary in price but typically cost anywhere from $10 to $50 for a month's supply, whereas a single progesterone level would be around $ 50–$100 if paid out of pocket.

Ovulatory dysfunction, if identified, warrants further investigation to determine a possible etiology and guide treatment. Without going into a thorough discussion, it is similarly important to identify a structured and basic evaluation of oligomenorrhea (<9 cycles / year) or amenorrhea. A TSH and prolactin should be obtained to rule out thyroid disorders and hyperprolactinemia. If these are normal, it would be reasonable to order a serum follicle-stimulating hormone (FSH), particularly if there is concern for primary ovarian insufficiency. These tests are close to $100 each. Polycystic ovarian syndrome is often considered in this evaluation and should be further investigated, especially if the patient reports symptoms of hyperandrogenism such as hirsutism and acne [8].

It is estimated that approximately 25–35 percent of couples suffer male factor infertility [1,3]. Formal recommendations are for a complete medical history of the male partner and at least one semen analysis. There is a great deal of intraindividual variation in the test, and a repeat semen analysis to confirm an abnormality can be useful. As the provider ordering the semen analysis, one should counsel the male partner that the test should be performed after 2–5 days of abstinence. Ideally, the specimen is collected by masturbation at the laboratory in which the testing is performed. The specimen can also be collected in a specialized condom and brought to the lab within an hour [4]. The out-of-pocket costs for a semen analysis are typically equivalent to that of the individual blood tests (~$100). When cost is a significant concern, a home semen analysis kit can be purchased in drug stores or online for $30–$50, and these have a reported accuracy of >98%. Despite its inherent limitations, many providers consider semen analysis an important step prior to moving forward with the treatment of the female partner, given the relatively high prevalence of male factor infertility. On the other hand, couples in which the male partner is healthy, is without risk factors, and has fathered a child in the past may choose to forgo semen analysis initially.

Testing for tubal patency is also a conventional part of an initial infertility evaluation. The most commonly performed test is the HSG due to it being both diagnostic and possibly therapeutic, as there is evidence of increased pregnancy rates following HSG [6]. In addition to showing both proximal and distal tubal occlusion, HSG can detect salpingitis isthmica nodosa and intracavitary abnormalities, such as submucosal fibroids and mullerian anomalies which can affect fertility. Often, further studies are indicated if the HSG is abnormal, such as a pelvic ultrasound to assess fibroids, a 3-D pelvic ultrasound or MRI to further characterize a mullerian anomaly, or even laparoscopy. In a patient in whom laparoscopy is planned, for example those in whom there is concern for endometriosis, a chromopertubation can be performed at the time of surgery, obviating the need for HSG [5]. Unfortunately, the cost of an HSG can be prohibitively high, ranging between $400 and $7,000, depending on the institution. In this case, in the absence of risk factors, it is possible that this test would be of limited value. It may be appropriate to address a finding of ovulatory dysfunction initially and proceed with HSG if the subfertility persists.

The American College of Obstetrics and Gynecology and the American Society for Reproductive Medicine suggest ovarian reserve testing on women over the age of 35 years who present for fertility evaluation as well as others with increased risk of decreased reserve, such as those with a history of cancer or medical problems treated with gonadotoxic therapy, surgery to the ovaries, or pelvic radiation [7]. It is inferred that ovarian reserve testing should not be performed as initial screening in all patients who present with inability to conceive. There are multiple tests for decreased ovarian reserve. The most appropriate initial tests are a basal ("day 3") FSH and estradiol. Elevated FSH of 10–20 IU/L is associated with poor response to ovarian stimulation. Estradiol is often added to the FSH to confirm the value of the FSH. An elevated estradiol (>80pg/mL) can suppress a rising FSH and result in a false negative FSH if it is evaluated alone. An alternative ovarian reserve test is a single measure of the anti-Mullerian hormone (AMH), which reflects the size of the primordial follicle pool. The benefit of this test is that it can be drawn at any time during the menstrual cycle as it has shown little intercycle and intracycle variability [7]. Additionally, the AMH, which costs approximately $100, is less expensive than the FSH and estradiol together (~$200), suggesting this may be the more ideal test when cost is a concern.

Features of the history or physical exam concerning for endometriosis are often identified. Treatment of endometriosis implants with ablation or resection, even in early disease, can improve pregnancy rates [9]. Likewise, the diagnosis of endometriosis will dictate infertility treatment options and is therefore important to make. While surgical evaluation should be performed in women with symptoms concerning for endometriosis or other pelvic / peritoneal pathology, diagnostic laparoscopy for asymptomatic women as part of a standard evaluation is of low yield and should not be a first step [5,9].

Key Points

- Diagnostic evaluation should be performed after 12 months of inability to conceive in patients <35 years of age, after six months in patients age 35 years or older or with obvious risk factors, and immediately in women over age 40 years.

- Ovulatory status should be assessed in every patient and can frequently be done with history alone. Further laboratory testing should be dictated by these findings.
- Semen analysis, HSG, and ovarian reserve testing can be performed in a stepwise fashion, targeting the most likely potential etiologies identified on history and physical exam first, with further workup only if infertility persists.
- Ovarian reserve testing need not be performed on every patient but limited to those >35 years or with significant risk factors for decreased ovarian reserve.
- Diagnostic laparoscopy may be indicated for patients in whom endometriosis or other peritoneal pathology is suggested by history or exam, but should not be performed on all patients.

References

1. Fritz MA, Speroff L. Clinical Gynecologic Endocrinology and Infertility. 8th Edition. Philadelphia: LWW; 2011. 1137, 1156p.

2. The American College of Obstetricians and Gynecologists Committee on Gynecologic Practice, The Practice Committee of the American Society for Reproductive Medicine. Committee Opinion No 589: Female age-related fertility decline. *Obstet Gynecol* 2014;**123**:719–721.

3. Hull MG, Glazener CM, Kelly NJ et al. Population study of causes, treatment and outcome of infertility. *Br Med J* 1985;**291**:1693–1697.

4. Practice Committee of the American Society of Reproductive Medicine. Diagnostic evaluation of the infertile male: a committee opinion. *Fertil Steril* 2015;**103**(3): e18–e25.

5. Practice Committee of the American Society of Reproductive Medicine. Diagnostic evaluation of the infertile female: a committee opinion. *Fertil Steril* 2015;**103**(6): e44–50.

6. Mohiyiddeen L, Hardiman A, Fitzgerald C et al. Tubal flushing for subfertility. *Cochrane Database Syst Rev* 2015; **1**(5) CD003718.

7. The American College of Obstetricians and Gynecologists Committee on Gynecologic Practice. Committee Opinion No 618: Ovarian Reserve Testing. *Obstet Gynecol* 2015;**125**: 268–273.

8. The Practice Committee of the American Society for Reproductive Medicine. Current evaluation of amenorrhea. *Fertil Steril* **200**;86(4): s148–s155.

9. The Practice Committee of the American Society for Reproductive Medicine. Endometriosis and infertility: a committee opinion. *Fertil Steril* 2012; **98**(3):591–598.

A 33-Year-Old Woman with Infertility (Bilateral Hydrosalpinx)

Elizabeth E. Puscheck

History of Present Illness

A 33-year-old woman, gravida 0, para 0, presents with her husband for an infertility evaluation after trying to conceive for 18 months without success. Her husband has not fathered a pregnancy before. She has a history of regular menstrual cycles and has used ovulation predictor kits, which turn positive around cycle days 14–16. They time intercourse appropriately. Her family medicine physician had ordered thyroid-stimulating hormone (TSH), prolactin, follicle-stimulating hormone (FSH), and semen analysis, which were normal.

Her past gynecologic history is notable for chlamydia infection three years ago and pelvic inflammatory disease (PID) with a gonorrhea infection ten years ago. She and her partner were treated. Her cervical cancer screening tests have been normal and her last one was six months ago. She and her husband are otherwise healthy and deny smoking, alcohol, or drug use. She is taking prenatal vitamins. The patient and her husband's family histories were unremarkable for any significant medical or genetic disorders.

To complete her infertility evaluation, she had a hysterosalpingogram (HSG) ordered with doxycycline prophylaxis, given her history of PID.

Physical Exam

General appearance	Well-developed, well-nourished woman in no discomfort
Vital Signs	
Temperature	37.6°C
Pulse	80 bpm
Blood pressure	110/60 mmHg
Respiratory rate	18 respirations/min
Height	5 feet 4 inches
Weight	150 lb
BMI	25.7 kg/m^2
Abdomen	Soft, not tender, not distended, no guarding, no rebound
External genitalia	Unremarkable
Vagina	White and clear discharge with stretchy clear mucus
Cervix	Nulliparous. No bleeding or discharge. Small amount of ectropion noted. No cervical motion tenderness
Uterus	Anteverted, mobile, normal size, no tenderness
Adnexa	Fullness noted bilaterally. No tenderness

Laboratory Tests

Gonorrhea and chlamydia nucleic acid amplification tests negative

Imaging

Hysterosalpingogram	Normal uterine cavity and bilateral hydrosalpinges. No tubal spill (Figure 53.1).
Pelvic ultrasound	Hypoechoic tubular cysts with an incomplete septum consistent with bilateral hydrosalpinges (Figure 53.2).

How Would You Manage This Patient?

This patient has bilateral hydrosalpinges noted on HSG (Figure 53.1) and pelvic ultrasound (Figure 53.2). These hydrosalpinges are large and no mucosal folds are visible. It is unlikely that surgical repair would result in functional tubes. The couple was counseled regarding the imaging findings, including the impact of these large hydrosalpinges on their fertility and the options available. Recommendation was made to remove the tubes or ligate them laparoscopically, and then proceed with in vitro fertilization (IVF) to maximize the chance of pregnancy.

Tubal Factor Infertility

Tubal disease accounts for approximately 25–40 percent of female factor infertility [1–4]. Over 50 percent of tubal disease is due to salpingitis [1]. Salpingitis typically results from sexually transmitted pelvic infections causing PID. Other causes of tubal occlusion include peritonitis, inflammatory changes from endometriosis, appendicitis, Crohn's disease, or ulcerative colitis, and adhesions or damage from other pelvic surgeries including ectopic pregnancy, ovarian cystectomies, abdominal myomectomy, or multiple laparotomies.

Tubal factor infertility may be due to occlusion of the tubes either proximally or distally. The tubes are traditionally evaluated during the initial infertility workup with a HSG or saline infusion sonohysterogram with agitated saline or ultrasound contrast (use of the latter is off FDA label). The reliability of these tests is quite good for confirming patency. Proximal tubal

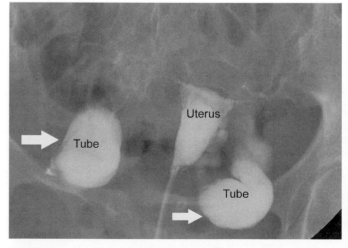

Figure 53.1 Hysterosalpingogram. The white arrows point to the white oblong, tubular structures on each side of the x-ray, which are bilateral hydrosalpinges.

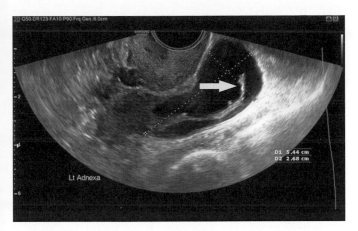

Figure 53.2 Ultrasound of hydrosalpinx. The white arrow points to an incomplete septum in a thin-walled fluid-filled serpiginous tubal shaped structure, which are ultrasound characteristic findings for hydrosalpinx.

obstruction may not be as reliably detected as distal. Repeating an HSG to reevaluate fallopian tubes with suspected proximal occlusion a month later demonstrates tubal patency in about 60 percent of cases [1]. Uterine spasm can make the fallopian tubes appear occluded on HSG. The proximal fallopian tube has a very small diameter at the cornual portion where it traverses through the myometrium. The spasm may not be present on repeat testing. Alternatively, minor debris within the tube may have been partially cleared during the initial HSG. Proximal tubal occlusion can be treated with tubal cannulation with a coaxial system either during fluoroscopy in the radiology suite or intraoperatively with combined laparoscopy and hysteroscopic tubal cannulation. Tubal cannulation has 60–95 percent success in resolving the obstruction with about 50 percent of patients conceiving and one-third re-occluding [1]. Tubal perforation is reported in 3–11 percent of cases but has no clinical consequences. Occasionally, correcting a proximal tubal occlusion will reveal an additional distal tube occlusion, which has a poor prognosis.

Mid- and distal tubal occlusions are not due to spasm since there is minimal muscle surrounding the tube and no myometrial tissue. The diameter of the mid- and distal tube is larger than the proximal tube. Laparoscopy with chromopertubation performed under general anesthesia is considered the gold standard to assess for tubal patency. Distal tubal obstruction occurs with hydrosalpinges. A hydrosalpinx is a dilated, sterile serous fluid-filled fallopian tube. On HSG, a hydrosalpinx appears as a collection of contrast material in an oblong or tubular structure with blunted, rounded ends. Hydrosalpinges may also be detected on 2D ultrasound, saline infusion sonohysterogram, or transvaginal hydrolaparoscopy with chromopertubation [1].

Hydrosalpinges appear to have negative impact on fertility beyond simply obstructing the tubes, and patients undergoing IVF with untreated hydrosalpinges have a 50 percent reduction in pregnancy rates [1, 2]. In a meta-analysis of 11 studies with more than 6,700 IVF cycles, women with untreated hydrosalpinges not only had a 49 percent reduction in pregnancy rates, but also had a two- to threefold increase in miscarriage rates

when compared to controls with tubal factor infertility without hydrosalpinges [10]. The reduced pregnancy rate may be caused by fluid from the hydrosalpinx passing into the uterine cavity, where it may be embryotoxic, may flush the embryo out of the uterine cavity, or may impair uterine receptivity.

Treatment for Hydrosalpinges

Four randomized controlled trials demonstrated that in women with bilateral hydrosalpinges, bilateral laparoscopic salpingectomy improved pregnancy rates over untreated subjects. Three of these trials showed improvement in both ongoing pregnancy and live birth rates [8]. The Cochrane Database review similarly reports improved pregnancy rates when laparoscopic salpingectomy or ligation (tubal occlusion) is performed prior to IVF [7]. Studies are less clear as to whether women with a unilateral hydrosalpinx should undergo a salpingectomy. The American Society of Reproductive Medicine Practice Committee Opinion concluded that unilateral salpingectomy for unilateral hydrosalpinx improves IVF pregnancy rates and recommends unilateral salpingectomy for unilateral hydrosalpinx. It concluded that the spontaneous pregnancy rate is 88 percent within five to six months of surgery with no ectopic pregnancies, but the duration of improved fertility may be as long as three years [1].

Hydrosalpinges are usually removed by laparoscopic salpingectomy. Most commonly, electrocautery is used to separate the tube from the uterus. The tube is excised along the mesosalpinx as close as possible to the tube to avoid compromising the vasculature within the mesosalpinx, which also supplies the ovary. The tube should be excised in its entirety. If there are significant pelvic adhesions or other technical obstacles to salpingectomy, it is reasonable to ligate the tubes at the junction of the tube and uterus, which will block seepage of fluid into the uterine cavity. Some advocate creating large fenestrations in the tube to allow for leakage of the tubal fluid into the abdominal cavity to prevent further distension of the tube and possible future pelvic pain [1].

Ovarian reserve after salpingectomy has been studied. A meta-analysis of 12 retrospective and 6 prospective studies included 1,482 patients with 657 having undergone salpingectomy and 825 not [6]. Their findings showed no difference in estradiol levels, total gonadotropin used in stimulation, or the number of oocytes retrieved. One randomized trial found that use of bipolar cautery was associated with lower ovarian volumes and antral follicle counts, but mechanical clips did not have this effect [1]. Several studies showed no compromise of ovarian reserve with laparoscopic tubal ligation done with bipolar cautery [1]. Carefully performed salpingectomy or ligation does not appear to have a significant impact on ovarian reserve in patients undergoing IVF.

Alternative Approaches

Occasionally, there are situations when laparoscopy may be contraindicated or an abdominal approach may need to be avoided due to concerns for operative morbidity like severe pelvic adhesions. In these situations, alternatives include hysteroscopic tubal occlusion or ultrasound-guided aspiration of the hydrosalpinx. Hysteroscopic tubal occlusion may be performed with an Essure device. Use of Essure to occlude the proximal end of the tube with hydrosalpinx was first reported in 2005 and resulted in a successful pregnancy. Since that time, there have been several studies showing improved pregnancy rates with hysteroscopic proximal tubal occlusion (38.6 percent pregnancy rate and 27.9 percent live birth rates) [2]. Typically, IVF is delayed 3–6 months after the Essure is placed to allow inflammation to resolve and proximal occlusion to be complete. Only 17 percent of coils are completely encapsulated with adhesions within 1 year and 25 percent within 3.5 years [1]. The uterine cavity is often not evaluated between tubal occlusion and performing IVF, so it is unknown if waiting until the adhesions wall off the proximal tubal occlusion coils improves pregnancy rates. Increased incidence of miscarriage and accumulation of uterine fluid has been reported [3].

Ultrasound-guided aspiration of the hydrosalpinx is typically performed at the time of oocyte aspiration. In some patients, the tubal fluid does not recur after aspiration. Others reaccumulate either early or late. Women with tubes that do not reaccumulate fluid or where the fluid returns late (two or more weeks after aspiration) have similar pregnancy rates to those who have had a salpingectomy [6, 9]. Those with rapid reaccumulation of fluid or fluid that collects in the uterine cavity prior to the embryo transfer did not conceive [6, 9].

Patients with mild hydrosalpinx (<3 cm), minimal or no filmy adnexal adhesions, and normal-appearing endosalpinx with preserved mucosal folds on HSG are considered good prognosis. These women will have better pregnancy rates with IVF than women with more significant tubal disease. Tubal repair surgery, such as laparoscopic neosalpingostomy or fimbrioplasty, may be effective. These techniques focus on opening the tube at the fimbrial end, everting the fimbria, and securing them with suture or electrocautery on the tubal serosa [1]. Pregnancy rates are lower after tubal surgery than IVF [5]. Surgery will delay conception and is associated with twice the ectopic pregnancy rate of IVF. In a randomized trial, there were no differences between laparotomy and laparoscopy for pregnancy or ectopic pregnancy rates. Consequently, laparoscopic approaches are recommended. After tubal reconstruction, the pregnancy rate is about 35 percent within one year and 58 percent in two years. The ectopic pregnancy rate is 3.9–5.0 percent. In women with poor prognosis or combined proximal and distal tubal occlusion, the pregnancy rate is 0–22 percent and ectopic rate is 0–17 percent [1]. Tuboplasty is not appropriate for poor prognosis patients or women with combined proximal and distal occlusion.

Key Points

- Salpingectomy is recommended before IVF and gonadotropin therapy for women with bilateral hydrosalpinges. There appears to be no significant impact on ovarian reserve.
- The data are more limited for women with unilateral hydrosalpinx, but salpingectomy is generally performed.
- Alternative approaches such as hysteroscopic proximal tubal occlusion and ultrasound-guided hydrosalpinx aspiration appear to have better pregnancy rates than no treatment, but not as good as salpingectomy or ligation prior to assisted reproductive technologies (ART).
- In good prognosis cases, tuboplasty can be considered, but it appears to have lower success rates and higher ectopic rates than IVF. Tuboplasty should not be performed in women with significant tubal disease.

References

1. The Practice Committee of the American Society of Reproductive Medicine. Role of tubal surgery in the era of assisted reproductive technology: a committee opinion. *Fertil Steril* 2015;103: e37–e43.

2. Arora P, Arora RS, and Cahill D. Essure for management of hydrosalpinx prior to in vitro fertilization – a systematic review and pooled analysis. *BJOG* 2014;121:527–536.

3. Barbosa MW, Sotiriadis A, Papatheodorou SI et al. High miscarriage rate in women treated with Essure for hydrosalpinx before embryo transfer: a systematic review and meta-analysis. *Ultrasound Obstet Gynecol* 2016;48:556–565.

4. Tulandi T, Akkour K. Role of reproductive surgery in the era of assisted reproductive technology. *Best Pract Res Clin Obst Gynaecol* 2012;26:747–755.

5. Zeyneloglu HB, Arici A, Olive DL. Adverse effects of hydrosalpinx on pregnancy rates after in vitro fertilization-embryo transfer. *Fertil Steril* 1998;70:492–499.

6. Noventa M, Gizzo S, Saccardi C et al. Salpingectomy before assisted reproductive technologies: a systematic literature review. *J Ovarian Res* 2016;9:74.

7. Johnson N, Van Voorst S, Sowter MC, Strandell A, Mol BW. Surgical treatment for tubal disease in women due to undergo in vitro fertilization. *Cochran Database Syst Rev* 2010;1;CD002125

8. Yoon SH, Lee JY, Kim S et al. Does salpingectomy have a deleterious impact on ovarian response in in vitro fertilization cycles? *Fertil Steril* 2016;106:1083–1092.

9. Fouda U, Sayed A, Abdelmoty H, Elsetohy KA. Ultrasound guided aspiration of hydrosalpinx fluid versus salpingectomy in the management of patients with ultrasound visible hydrosalpinx undergoing IVF-ET: a randomized controlled trial. *BMC Women's Health* 2015;15:21.

10. Omurtag K, Grindler N, Roehl KA et al. How member of the society for reproductive endocrinology and infertility and society of reproductive surgeons evaluate, define, and manage hydrosalpinges. *Fertil Steril* 2012;97:1095–1100.

A 26-Year-Old Woman with Irregular Menses and Infertility

Helen Dunnington

History of Present Illness

A 26-year-old, gravida 0, presents to clinic to discuss her fertility. She and her husband have been trying to conceive for the past year, and she has not yet become pregnant. She reports her cycles have always been irregular, coming every 30 to 90 days and lasting about 7 days. Her last menstrual period was eight weeks ago. Although they have been actively trying for one year, they have not used any contraception since their wedding two years ago. She denies any pelvic pain or dyspareunia. She reports some dark hair around her nipples and on her lower abdomen.

She has no past medical or surgical history. She has never used hormonal contraception and has no history of sexually transmitted infections. Her family history includes a mother with type 2 diabetes mellitus. Her only mediation is a prenatal vitamin, and she has no allergies. She works as an elementary school teacher, has never smoked or used recreational drugs, and drinks a rare glass of wine. Her husband has never fathered any other pregnancies.

Physical Exam

General appearance | Well-developed, well-nourished, over-weight woman in no acute distress

Vital Signs

Temperature	98.6°F
Pulse	85 beats/min
Blood pressure	130/70 mmHg
Respiratory rate	18 breaths/min
Oxygen saturation	100% on room air
Height	63 inches
Weight	155 lb
BMI	27.5 kg/m^2
HEENT	Rare dark hairs on chin
Neck	No thyromegaly
Chest	Breasts without masses, tenderness, or nipple discharge bilaterally. Rare dark hairs around nipple
Abdomen	Mild dark hair midline lower abdomen, normoactive bowel sounds, soft, non-tender, non-distended, no masses
Pelvic exam	Normal external female genitalia. Vagina normal without discharge. Cervix nulliparous, non-friable, no discharge. Uterus anteverted, mobile, normal size, non-tender. Adnexa without masses, fullness, or tenderness bilaterally.

Laboratory Studies

Urine pregnancy test Negative

Thyroid-stimulating hormone, prolactin, 17-hydroxyprogesterone, fasting lipids normal Free testosterone 4 pg/mL, total testosterone 40 ng/dL Hemoglobin A1c 5.7%, two-hour glucose tolerance: fasting 100 mg/dL, two-hour 135 mg/dL

Pelvic ultrasound Uterus normal size with 6 mm endometrial thickness. Ovaries with increased volume with prominent stroma and multiple peripheral follicles suggestive of polycystic ovarian syndrome (see Figure 54.1).

How Would You Manage This Patient?

This patient has primary infertility with a clinical picture consistent with polycystic ovary syndrome (PCOS). Laboratory evaluation eliminated other causes of oligomenorrhea such as thyroid disorders or hyperprolactinemia, and her testosterone levels and glucose tolerance were on the higher end of normal, which is common in PCOS. Her ultrasound findings also support the diagnosis of PCOS, with increased ovarian volume and multiple peripheral follicles.

Given her desire to become pregnant, the patient underwent hysterosalpingogram and semen analysis to rule out tubal, uterine, and male factor causes of infertility that may be present in addition to her anovulation. Both of these tests were normal. After discussing lifestyle modifications and medical management options and their associated risks, the patient desired a trial of clomiphene citrate (or clomiphene). A withdrawal bleed was induced with medroxyprogesterone 5 mg orally for five days. She then took clomiphene, 50 mg daily on cycle days 5 through 9. An ovulation predictor kit confirmed ovulation. On her third cycle with clomiphene, she ovulated and had a positive pregnancy test two weeks later. She subsequently scheduled a visit to begin prenatal care.

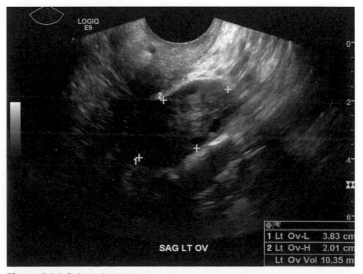

Figure 54.1 Polycystic ovary.

PCOS and Infertility

Approximately 12 percent of reproductive-age women in the United States have difficulty becoming pregnant. For married reproductive-age women in the United States, there is about a 6 percent infertility rate [1]. An essential component to fertility is normal ovulatory function, and ovulatory dysfunction accounts for up to 40 percent of female infertility. The most common cause of female infertility is PCOS. While evaluation for infertility is typically recommended after at least twelve months of unprotected intercourse, earlier evaluation is reasonable after six months of trying to conceive in women who are age 35 years and older or in those with oligomenorrhea or other evidence of anovulation [2].

When ovulatory dysfunction is suspected as the cause of infertility, the evaluation may be more focused. A complete menstrual history may be all that is needed to identify this cause. Ovulatory cycles are regular and predictable. They should occur about every 21–35 days with consistent flow patterns and associated symptoms. In women with oligomenorrhea, typically no specific diagnostic test is required to establish the diagnosis of anovulation. Some tests available to determine ovulation include basal body temperature monitoring, urinary luteinizing hormone detection, serum progesterone levels one week prior to anticipated cycle, or serial transvaginal ultrasounds monitoring follicular changes [2]. It is prudent to evaluate anovulatory women for other factors contributing to infertility in a stepwise approach. Before beginning treatment, one should assess for abnormal thyroid function and hyperprolactinemia. If first-line therapies are unsuccessful in achieving pregnancy, it is recommended to check for tubal patency (via hysterosalpingogram), and male factor infertility (via semen analysis) prior to starting second-line therapies [3]. The hysterosalpingogram is more expensive, uncomfortable, and low yield in someone without risk factors for tubal infertility compared to a few cycles of clomiphene.

While not part of the diagnostic criteria, many women with PCOS are obese. Preconception counseling for these women should emphasize lifestyle modifications that may improve their chances of spontaneous conception. Diet, exercise, or addition of pharmacologic weight loss agents resulting in as little as a 5 percent reduction in body weight have been shown to improve ovulatory function. Weight loss appears to reduce circulating androgen levels and thus can lead to return of ovulation and resumption of spontaneous menses [4]. While weight loss may help some women, many will still need ovulation induction.

Ovulation induction for women with PCOS can be stratified into first- and second-line treatment options, as outlined in Table 54.1.

Clomiphene, a selective estrogen receptor modulator, has been the traditional first-line ovulation induction agent. It acts as an estrogen receptor antagonist in the hypothalamus, thus stimulating gonadotropin-releasing hormone and follicle-stimulating hormone (FSH) production, and also increases circulating sex hormone binding globulin levels. The starting dose is 50 mg per day for 5 days and can be increased by 50 mg per day to a maximum of 150 mg per day. Half of women who conceive with clomiphene do so at the 50 mg dose, and most pregnancies occur

Table 54.1 Fertility treatments for women with PCOS

Preconception	Lifestyle modifications	Recommended dose
First line	Clomiphene citrate (with or without metformin)	50 mg/d cycle days 5–9, increase by 50 mg/d to maximum dose 150 mg/d
	Letrozole	2.5 mg/d cycle days 5–9, maximum dose 7.5 mg/d
Second line	Gonadotropins (FSH, hMG)	Start 50–70 i.u./d, increase by 25–37.5 i.u./d after 14d
	HCG	5000 u. with 17 mm follicle, hold if ≥3 14 mm follicles
	Laparoscopic ovarian drilling	
Treatment failure	In vitro fertilization	

within the first 6 ovulatory cycles. There is a 5–10 percent risk of twin pregnancies with clomiphene, but the risk of higher-order multiples is less than 1 percent [5]. Hot flashes are a common side effect. Not all women will ovulate with clomiphene; obese women are particularly less likely to respond [3].

There may be a role for adjuvant treatments with clomiphene. Metformin is a biguanide used to treat type 2 diabetes. It has been shown to decrease circulating androgen levels, likely through ovarian effects, with resulting improvement in ovulation [5]. Metformin alone, however, compared to clomiphene alone has significantly lower pregnancy and live birth rates. There are data to support the use of metformin with clomiphene, especially in obese PCOS patients, as there are increased ovulation and clinical pregnancy rates when used in combination [6]. The recommended dosing is between 1,500 mg and 2,550 mg per day in divided doses; however, gastrointestinal side effects may limit its use.

An alternative first-line option is off-label use of letrozole, an aromatase inhibitor. Its mechanism of action in ovulation induction is through a decrease in peripherally produced estrogens, such as estrone, resulting in an increase in FSH and thus follicular development. Proposed benefits of letrozole over clomiphene include a shorter half-life, lower rates of recruitment and ovulation of multiple follicles, and less anti-estrogenic effect on the endometrium, resulting in higher implantation and live birth rates and lower multiple pregnancy rates [4,5]. There has been some question of the safety of letrozole use due to possible increased risk of congenital anomalies; however, anomaly rates have been shown to be comparable to those with clomiphene, other methods of ovulation induction, or in vitro fertilization (IVF). The dosing schedule for letrozole is similar to that of clomiphene, with medication taken for five days during the follicular phase. Dosing starts at 2.5 mg per day with a maximum daily dose of 7.5 mg. There is some evidence that letrozole is more effective than clomiphene for ovulation induction in obese

PCOS women with anovulatory infertility, resulting in a significantly higher live birth rate; therefore, letrozole should be considered first line in these women [7,8]. In addition, letrozole may be useful in patients who fail to respond to clomiphene, as it has been found to effectively induce ovulation in 50–80 percent of these women [8].

If ovulation is not achieved within six to nine months of first-line therapies, it is reasonable to offer second-line therapies. Gonadotropins are an appropriate second-line therapy in women with PCOS who fail first-line options. Higher rates of monofollicular development and lower risk of ovarian hyperstimulation syndrome can be achieved with low-dose regimens of gonadotropins while still achieving high rates of ovulation. Either recombinant FSH or menopausal gonadotropins (hMG) can be used with similar outcomes. Dosing regimens should start at 50–70 i.u. and only be increased by 25–37.5 i.u. if there is no response after 14 days. Follicular development should be monitored by ultrasound, and ovulation triggered with a single injection of human chorionic gonadotropin (hCG) 5,000 units when there is a follicle of at least 17 mm in largest diameter. If three or more follicles larger than 14 mm in diameter exist, hCG should not be administered [7]. The first cycle of therapy may be prolonged while the optimal dose is identified.

An alternative second-line therapy is laparoscopic ovarian drilling. Women who are appropriate for ovarian drilling may include those who have persistently elevated luteinizing hormone, require laparoscopic evaluation of the pelvis, or are unable to attend the intensive monitoring necessary for gonadotropins [7]. One proposed mechanism of action is that the destruction of androgen-producing cells in the follicles and interstitial ovary leads to lower androgen and inhibin concentrations, thus allowing an increase in FSH and follicular development [9]. Compared to gonadotropins, there are lower rates of multiple pregnancy and decreased short-term costs. Effects may be temporary and additional therapy may be necessary with clomiphene or gonadotropins. Risks include those of laparoscopic surgery such as risks of anesthesia, injury to surrounding structures, and development of pelvic adhesions.

If ovulation is not achieved with second-line therapies, the next step is IVF. In addition, IVF becomes a reasonable option for women who achieve ovulatory cycles by any of the above mechanisms, but are unable to become pregnant after six to nine cycles.

Key Teaching Points

- PCOS is the most common cause of infertility, accounting for approximately 80 percent of anovulatory infertility, which itself accounts for 40 percent of all infertility.
- Infertile women with PCOS should be evaluated for other factors contributing to infertility by assessing for thyroid function, hyperprolactinemia, tubal patency (via hysterosalpingogram), and male factor infertility (via semen analysis).
- Initial management for obese women with PCOS should start with lifestyle modifications, including diet and exercise.
- First-line medical therapies for ovulation induction are clomiphene or letrozole.
- If ovulation is not achieved within 6–9 months of ovulation induction, second-line therapies, including gonadotropins or ovarian drilling, should be offered.
- IVF is the final management step when ovulation does not occur with second-line therapies or pregnancy is not achieved after six to nine ovulatory cycles using first- or second-line therapies.

References

1. Centers for Disease Control and Prevention. Infertility FAQs. Available at www.cdc.gov/reproductivehealth/infertility/index.htm. (Accessed April 13, 2017).

2. American Society for Reproductive Medicine. Diagnostic evaluation of the infertile female: a committee opinion. *Fertil Steril* 2015;**103**(6): e44–e50.

3. American Society for Reproductive Medicine. Use of exogenous gonadotropins in anovulatory women: a technical bulletin. *Fertil Steril* 2008;**90** (s3): s7–s12.

4. American College of Obstetrics and Gynecology. Polycystic ovary syndrome. Practice Bulletin 108. *Obstet Gynecol* 2009;**114**: 936–49.

5. Legro RS. Ovulation induction in polycystic ovary syndrome: current options. *Best Pract Res Clin Obstet Gynaecol* 2016;**37**: 152–59.

6. Tang T, Lord JM, Norman RJ, Yasmin E, Balen AH. Insulin-sensitising drugs (metformin, rosiglitazone, pioglitazone, D-chiro-inositol) for women with polycystic ovary syndrome, oligo amenorrhoea and subfertility (Review) *Cochrane Database of Systematic Reviews* 2012, Issue 5. Art. No.: CD003053. DOI: 10.1002/14651858.CD003053.pub5.

7. Baleh AH, Morley LC, Misso M et al. The management of anovulatory infertility in women when polycyctic ovary syndrome: an analysis of the evidence to support the development of global WHO guidance. *Hum Reprod Update* 2016;**22** (6):687–708.

8. American College of Obstetricians and Gynecologists. Aromatase inhibitors in gynecologic practice. Committee Opinion No. 663. *Obstet Gynecol* 2016;**127**: e170–e174.

9. Petersen KB, Pedersen NG, Pedersen AT, Lauritsen MP, Freiesleben NC. Mono-ovulation in women with polycystic ovary syndrome: a clinical review on ovulation induction. *Reprod BioMed Online* 2016;**32**:563–583.

A 32-Year-Old Woman with a 3 cm Endometrioma and Infertility

Michael T. Breen

History of Present Illness

A 32-year-old woman, gravida 0, para 0, is referred for consultation regarding difficulty conceiving. She and her partner have been attempting conception for 13 months. The patient reports regular every 28-day painful menstrual cycles since menarche at age 13. She reports her cycles have become more painful. Usually, her dysmenorrhea is relieved with nonsteroidal anti-inflammatory medications. However, while still happening occasionally, she is more frequently absent from work during menses due to pain. She denies a history of sexually transmitted infections and prior pelvic surgery. Her partner has no children. The referring provider initiated an evaluation and sent you results of a normal semen analysis demonstrating normal morphology, hysterosalpingogram demonstrating bilateral tubal patency and normal endometrial morphology, and day 21 progesterone consistent with ovulation. Pelvic ultrasonography showed a 6.8 cm retroverted uterus with a 3.4 cm left complex ovarian cyst with a "ground glass" background and one thin septation suggestive of an endometrioma (Figure 55.1). The patient previously used barrier contraception and withdrawal. She used oral contraceptives for a brief interval, but discontinued them due to side effects.

On review of symptoms, she reports positional dyspareunia. She denies dyschezia or other gastrointestinal symptoms. The patient has no significant medical problems and has never had surgery. She takes no medications other than a prenatal vitamin with folic acid and nonsteroidal anti-inflammatory drugs during her menses. She does not smoke, drink, or use illicit substances. She has no allergies. She denies any significant family history. Vaccinations are up to date. Cystic fibrosis carrier testing and HIV tests were negative. She is immune to rubella and varicella.

Physical Examination

Vital Signs

Height	167 cm (5 ft 5 in.)
Weight	62 kg (136 lb)
BMI	22.2 kg/m²
BP	132/78 mmHg
Pulse	71 bpm
Breasts	Symmetric. No masses or nipple discharge
Abdomen	Thin, soft, non-tender, no mass, no organomegaly

Female Genitalia

- Vulva and vagina unremarkable. Physiologic discharge
- Cervix Normal appearance, no lesion, and no cervical motion tenderness
- Adnexa/Parametria Right fullness with mild tenderness to palpation

How Would You Manage This Patient?

The patient's initial evaluation excludes male factor infertility and tubal or uterine etiology and confirms the patient ovulates. The patient's history is suggestive of endometriosis, which is confirmed by ultrasonography. Given the finding of a 3 cm endometrioma, the patient has at least Stage III or greater disease. The patient is counseled that her infertility is likely related to the presence of the endometrioma/endometriosis and about its effects on ovarian function. Anti-Mullerian hormone (AMH) was obtained and was found decreased, providing further support that the suspected mass is an endometrioma.

She was counseled that she will likely need to undergo assisted reproduction to conceive. As the endometrioma was less than 4 cm in size, she was counseled that options included proceeding directly to a reproductive endocrinologist for assisted reproductive support such as in vitro fertilization (IVF) or undergoing laparoscopy to excise the endometrioma and associated endometriosis prior to a referral for assisted reproductive techniques. She was counseled that because her endometrioma was small, there is no increased fertility with excision prior to assisted reproduction and that the decision to proceed with surgical intervention should be related to potential benefits of reduction in pain symptoms, decreased progression of endometriosis, quantifying the extent of her disease, ruling out the rare chance of occult malignancy, and facilitating oocyte retrieval. She was counseled about the risks of surgery prior to assisted reproduction, which include surgical trauma and complications, the economic impact of the procedure, and decreased ovarian reserve related to removing the endometrioma from the remaining ovarian tissue.

The patient chose surgery because of her cyclic pain and absenteeism. She underwent laparoscopic ovarian cystectomy

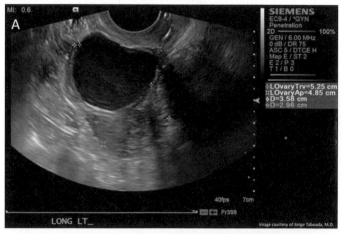

Typical sonographic features of an endometrioma (outlined by + calipers on image A) include hypoechoic, homogenous "low-level" echoes without evidence of vascularity (image B)

Figure 55.1 Ultrasound image of left ovary. 3 × 3.6 cm endometrioma noted. Characteristic features include the hypoechoic, homogenous low-level echoes that are outlined by the calipers.

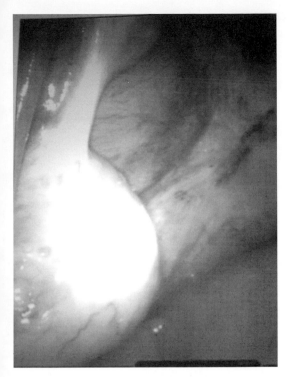

Figure 55.2 Findings at the time of laparoscopy. Note cystic mass in ovary and endometriotic implants in cul de sac (to right of image).

with complete resection. Additional small implants noted in the posterior cul de sac were excised (Figure 55.2). Bipolar cautery was avoided during the excision. Pathology confirmed a benign endometrioma. After recovery, the patient underwent IVF and became pregnant during the second cycle.

Endometriomas and Infertility

Endometriosis is estimated to be present in 6–10 percent of women of child-bearing age, 30–50 percent of women with infertility, and over 70 percent of women with chronic pelvic pain. There appears to be a genetic component [1]. Endometriosis requires histologic confirmation for definitive diagnosis, but the laparoscopic appearance is characteristic and allows for staging based on visual inspection at the time of surgery. Staging endometriosis allows the clinician to quantify the disease burden and potential distortion in anatomy caused by the endometriosis and cyclic bleeding. Stage has not been found to be correlated with measures of pain or infertility [2]. Endometriomas are a form of endometriosis and are pseudoencapsulated ovarian cysts filled with hemosiderin-laden macrophages, which are present in the ovarian stroma. Endometriomas occur in up to 44 percent of women with endometriosis [3]. Endometriomas may be asymptomatic or associated with intermittent or continuous pelvic pain and dyspareunia [5].

Endometriomas have a classic appearance on ultrasound [6]. This appearance includes low-level echogenicity in smooth-walled cysts and a ground glass appearance. These ultrasound findings have a sensitivity of .93 and specificity of .96 for the diagnosis of endometriomas. Multiple locules, hyperechogenic wall foci, combined cystic and solid lesions, and purely solid

lesions have all been described [10]. MRI can be used to further differentiate an endometrioma from a cystic teratoma or hemorrhagic cyst when diagnosis is difficult on ultrasound [4]. Cysts with classic endometrioma findings that appear stable may be followed conservatively while fertility treatments and pregnancy are achieved. If serial evaluation with ultrasound shows significant growth or change in appearance, surgical intervention may be warranted [7].

Symptomatic endometriomas are generally surgically excised. Excision is difficult, but preferred over drainage and pseudocyst wall obliteration [8]. The dense adherence of the pseudocapsule to ovarian stroma makes it difficult to remove all the endometriotic tissues. Postoperative recurrence has been described in up to 29 percent of endometrioma resections [10]. Endometriomas have been rarely associated with endometrioid tumors of the ovary as well as clear cell adenocarcinoma of the ovary [6].

Women with endometriomas have lower AMH levels, indicating decreased ovarian reserve and diminished fertility [9]. Removal of an endometrioma further diminishes AMH levels, presumably from ovarian trauma and damage to the ovarian cortex during the procedure. Removal does not negatively impact success with assisted reproductive technology. Current evidence suggests ovarian cystectomy does not improve reproductive outcomes in women with endometriomas. Women undergoing IVF/intracytoplasmic sperm injection after resection of endometrioma show similar implantation and clinical pregnancy rates compared to women with endometriomas that were not resected [7]. The indications for removal of endometriomas <4 cm are primarily related to pain treatment, confirmation of an endometrioma when the differential is unclear, decreased recurrence of endometriosis, and related symptoms. Potential harms of surgical excision include surgical risks, costs, and potential for decreased ovarian reserve [7, 8, 9]. Among women undergoing assisted reproduction after surgery, success rates are improved when excision of the endometrioma is performed compared to drainage or ablation of the cyst wall [1]. Medical therapies administered before or after surgery have not been found to improve fertility rates and should not be used as they delay assisted reproduction and pregnancy. Medical therapy alone with gonadotropin-releasing hormone agonists, continuous contraceptive pills, or danazol has not been found to enhance fertility in women with endometriomas. Evidence for the use of aromatase inhibitors is limited [9].

Key Teaching Points

- Endometriomas are frequently found in women with endometriosis. They may be asymptomatic or associated with pelvic pain and infertility.
- Endometriomas have a classic characteristic appearance on ultrasound.
- Endometriomas have been associated with diminished ovarian reserve and infertility.
- Excision of small endometriomas prior to undergoing assisted reproductive technologies does not improve success.

- Surgical excision has been associated with further decrease in ovarian reserve as measured by AMH level, but this does not decrease success rates with IVF.

- Ovarian cystectomy is indicated for improvement in symptoms or if the diagnosis of the mass is not clear on imaging.

References

1. Leyland N, Casper R, Laberge P, Singh SS. Endometriosis: diagnosis and management. *J Obstet Gynaecol Canada* 2010;32(7): S1–S32.

2. Ziegler D, Borghese B, Chapron C. Endometriosis and infertility: pathophysiology and management. *Lancet* 2010;376:730–734.

3. Benshcop L, Farquhar C, Vander Poel N, Heineman MJ. Interventions for women with endometrioma prior to assisted reproductive technology. *Cochrane Database Syst Rev*2010;CD008571.

4. Borrelli GM, de Mattos LA, Andres MP et al. Role of imaging tools for the diagnosis of borderline ovarian tumors: a systematic review and meta-analysis. *J Minim Invasive Gynecol* 2017;24:353–363.

5. Vercellini P. Introduction: management of endometriosis: moving toward a problem-oriented and patient-centered approach. *Fertil Steril* 2015;104 (4):761–763.

6. Tajima A, Suzuki C, Kikuchi I et al. Efficacy of the echo pattern classification of ovarian tumors 2000 in conjunction with transvaginal ultrasonography for diagnosis of ovarian masses. *J Med Ultrason* 2016;43:249–255.

7. Johnston EB, Link MH. Controversies in the management of endometrioma: to cure sometimes, to treat often, to comfort always? *Clin Obstet Gynecol* 2015;58(4):754–764.

8. American College of Obstetricians and Gynecologists. Management of endometriosis. Practice bulletin No. 114. *Obstet Gynecol* 2010;116:223–236.

9. Practice Committee of the American Society for Reproductive Medicine. Treatment of pelvic pain associated with endometriosis: a committee opinion. *Fertil Steril* 2014;101 (4):927–935.

10. Levine D, Brown DL, Andreotti RF et al. Management of asymptomatic ovarian and other adnexal cysts imaged at US: Society of Radiologists in ultrasound consensus conference statement. *Radiology* 2010;256(3):943–954.

A 32-Year-Old Woman with Recurrent Pregnancy Loss

Debra A. Taubel

History of Present Illness

A 32-year-old female, gravida 3, SAB 3, para 0, comes to the office for evaluation after three consecutive early pregnancy losses. Her first pregnancy was an anembryonic gestation diagnosed at eight weeks, her second an early embryonic demise diagnosed at eight weeks, and the most recent pregnancy ended in spontaneous abortion at seven weeks. She has had no difficulty conceiving. Her husband was her partner for all three pregnancies. She had early prenatal care for the first two pregnancies. Her initial prenatal visit for the third pregnancy was scheduled several days after the miscarriage.

She is in good health and takes no medications on a regular basis. She reports that her periods are every month and last 4–5 days with minimal dysmenorrhea. Her last menstrual period was three weeks ago. She has never had surgery other than for managing her early pregnancy losses and is up-to-date on her health-care maintenance. She has no knowledge of any family history of inherited diseases, and her mother and sister have never had pregnancy loss or fertility issues. She denies smoking, alcohol use, or use of illicit substances. She works full time as a financial analyst. She has had one lifetime male partner, her husband, who is also in good health and is unaware of any family history of inherited diseases or pregnancy loss.

Physical Examination

General appearance	Well-developed, well-nourished woman with appropriate affect

Vital Signs

Blood pressure	112/78 mmHg
Heart rate	76 beats/min
Height	64 inches
Weight	155 lb
BMI	26.6 kg/m^2
Neck	Supple, no thyromegaly, no lymphadenopathy
Chest	Clear to auscultation bilaterally
Heart	Regular rate and rhythm; no murmurs, gallops, or rubs
Breasts	Symmetric, no inverted nipples, no masses palpated, no skin changes, no lymphadenopathy
Abdomen	Soft, non-tender, no masses
External genitalia	Normal female, no lesions
Vagina	Mucosa intact, no abnormalities, physiologic discharge present
Cervix	Nulliparous os, no discharge or lesions, no cervical motion tenderness
Uterus	Small, anteverted, non-tender, mobile
Adnexa	Non-tender, no masses
Rectovaginal	No masses, non-tender
In-office testing	Urine pregnancy test negative

How Would You Manage This Patient?

With three early pregnancy losses, this patient meets diagnostic criteria for recurrent pregnancy loss. A complete history of each loss was obtained. While history alone can be inaccurate, this patient had received prenatal care and had documentation to confirm that her losses were true pregnancy losses and not inadequately diagnosed episodes of abnormal bleeding. History and review of systems did not reveal symptoms or signs of underlying medical illness, particularly autoimmune disease or inherited disorders. History obtained from the partner did not suggest inherited paternal disorders. Her employment does not include teratogen exposure. Tests for common causes of recurrent pregnancy loss were ordered, including cytogenetic analysis of both parents, screening for antiphospholipid syndrome with lupus anticoagulant, anticardiolipin antibodies, and anti-β2-glycoprotein, and screening for endocrine abnormalities with prolactin, thyroid-stimulating hormone (TSH), and hemoglobin A1c. A sonohysterogram was ordered to rule out structural abnormalities of the uterus. All testing was normal, which is estimated to occur in 50 percent or more of couples diagnosed and evaluated for recurrent pregnancy loss [1]. Reassurance was provided, and the couple had a successful pregnancy with a term delivery 18 months later.

Recurrent Pregnancy Loss

The traditionally accepted definition of recurrent pregnancy loss is a history of three consecutive spontaneous pregnancy losses with or without a previous successful pregnancy. The American Society of Reproductive Medicine has amended the definition to two losses for the initiation of clinical evaluation and possible treatment. Pregnancy loss is relatively common, occurring in up to 25 percent of recognized pregnancies. It is estimated that fewer than 5 percent of couples will have two consecutive pregnancy losses and 1 percent of couples will have three [1].

The differential diagnosis of recurrent early pregnancy loss includes genetic abnormalities, antiphospholipid syndrome, inherited thrombophilias, hormonal and structural abnormalities, and smoking, caffeine, or alcohol use (Table 56.1). The majority of nonrecurrent early pregnancy losses are due to sporadic genetic abnormalities in the setting of normal parental karyotypes. These abnormalities are more common as maternal age increases due to reduction in oocyte number and quality. As the number of early pregnancy losses increases, the probability of sporadic genetic causes decreases [1]. A balanced translocation in either parent can lead to recurrent pregnancy loss and is estimated to account for 2–5 percent of recurrent pregnancy loss [1]. The risk of spontaneous abortion is directly related to the amount and content of the genetic material in the translocation and can be identified by parental karyotyping [2]. Despite the theoretical ability of preimplantation genetic diagnosis to detect chromosomal abnormalities in embryos, it has not been shown to increase live birth rates when compared to conservative management. Currently, there is no recommendation for screening with preimplantation genetic diagnosis [1].

Antiphospholipid antibody syndrome has been associated with early and recurrent pregnancy loss. It is present in approximately 15 percent of patients with recurrent pregnancy loss, and in only 2 percent of patients with normal obstetrical histories. The antibodies are thought to interfere with early placentation and development of vascular structures necessary for normal fetal growth. It is diagnosed by testing for the presence of anticardiolipin antibodies, lupus anticoagulant, and anti-β2-glycoprotein. Testing should be considered in patients who have a history of three or more first-trimester losses, one or more miscarriages of a morphologically normal fetus at ten weeks or later, or one or more second-trimester spontaneous pregnancy losses that cannot be attributed to another cause [2]. The diagnosis of antiphospholipid antibody syndrome requires two positive tests at least 12 weeks apart [2]. The use of low-dose aspirin with low-molecular-weight heparin or traditional heparin in patients with documented antiphospholipid syndrome resulted in live birth rates of approximately 75 percent [1].

Inherited thrombophilias, including Factor V Leiden, decreased Protein S or Protein C activity, antithrombin III deficiency, and prothrombin gene mutation have been theorized to be associated with pregnancy loss, specifically in the second trimester [2]. There has been no conclusive evidence that inherited thrombophilias cause first-trimester or recurrent pregnancy loss, so testing is not recommended [1].

Diabetes and insulin resistance, thyroid dysfunction, and hyperprolactinemia have been implicated in recurrent pregnancy loss. Uncontrolled diabetes in early pregnancy results in fetal wastage and fetal malformations [2]. There is some association of pregnancy loss with insulin resistance in the setting of mild blood glucose elevation [2]. The metabolic syndrome and its persistent associated hyperinflammatory state have been suggested to be a contributor to early pregnancy loss, but this has not been proven. Hypothyroidism has been associated with early miscarriage with or without the presence of antithyroid antibodies [1]. Elevated prolactin can interfere with successful implantation and maintenance of the corpus luteum in the first trimester [1]. Live birth rates are increased with normalization of prolactin by the administration of a dopamine agonist such as bromocriptine or cabergoline, which are considered safe in pregnancy.

Structural uterine abnormalities can cause recurrent pregnancy loss, although reported incidences vary. Septate uteri have the highest association, but other anomalies such as arcuate uteri have also been implicated. Fibroids tend not to be a cause of miscarriage unless in a truly submucosal location. An initial evaluation of uterine anatomy with ultrasound is effective and relatively noninvasive. Additional imaging with sonohysterogram or hysterosalpingogram can be performed if a cavity defect is suspected. Septum resection by hysteroscopy has been shown in several studies to improve the live birth rate for those patients with previous losses [1].

Lifestyle choices, particularly tobacco, alcohol, and substance use, may contribute. Cigarette smoking and alcohol intake are associated with an increased risk of miscarriage. These are modifiable risk factors that also have implications for decreasing pregnancy risk and long-term health [2]. Alcohol use of 3–5 drinks per week has been shown to increase the risk of fetal loss [1]. Excessive caffeine intake, typically greater than three cups of coffee per day, is also associated with an increased risk of miscarriage [1]. Even if not the primary cause, modification may help with the success of other interventions.

Production of adequate progesterone by the corpus luteum is necessary until approximately 12 weeks. Deficiencies of endogenous hormone production, termed luteal phase deficiency, have been hypothesized as a cause of recurrent pregnancy loss. Supplementation with exogenous progesterone has not been shown to improve outcomes in women with recurrent pregnancy loss, and testing for luteal phase deficiency is not recommended [3].

Evaluation begins with history, which needs to be obtained carefully, as recurrent pregnancy loss often provokes stress and anxiety in the patient and the partner. Information should be obtained on each pregnancy and its outcome. Records should be obtained whenever possible, as patient history alone may be inaccurate. Documentation of pregnancy loss by ultrasound or histology is preferred, and cytogenetic results should be reviewed [1]. This will frequently require obtaining records from multiple institutions. Difficulty conceiving should be noted, as should whether the partner has had any pregnancies with another female, assessment for possible exposure to teratogens, and family history of autoimmune disease. Patients should be asked about smoking and alcohol and caffeine intake. Review of systems should obtain information about potential autoimmune disease, thyroid disease, or diabetes.

A complete physical exam should be performed and recommended preventative care should be up-to-date. Initial testing should include karyotype of both parents, pelvic sonogram, serum testing for TSH, prolactin, lupus anticoagulant, anticardiolipin antibody, and anti-β2-glycoprotein antibody. Other testing can be considered if results are inconclusive or if indicated by patient history (Table 56.2). These tests may be done in a staged manner, with diagnoses suggested by history tested for first, or lower cost tests done first in patients with limited or no insurance coverage. No couple should be considered to have unexplained recurrent pregnancy loss until the evaluation is complete.

If testing reveals a specific cause, appropriate management should be initiated (Table 56.1). Patients should be counseled to stop smoking and alcohol consumption and reduce or eliminate caffeine. Many patients, like this one, will have no clear cause identified [1]. When the workup reveals no direct cause for recurrent pregnancy loss, discussion of the findings and reassurance for both parents are important. It is estimated that 50 percent of couples will have no identified cause for their recurrent pregnancy loss. Over 60 percent of these couples will have a live birth in the five years following the diagnosis. This percentage is

Table 56.1 Potentially treatable causes of recurrent pregnancy loss

Condition	Testing	Treatment
Antiphospholipid syndrome	Lupus anticoagulant, anti-cardiolipin antibodies, anti-beta2-glycoprotein	Heparin +/− low-dose aspirin
Inherited Thrombophilias	Protein S/C activity, factor V Leiden, antithrombin III, prothrombin gene mutation	Heparin +/− low-dose aspirin
Diabetes mellitus/insulin resistance	Hemoglobin A1 c, fasting blood glucose	Glycemic control
thyroid disease	TSH	Normalization of thyroid hormone level
Hyperprolactinemia	Prolactin level	Dopamine agonist
Structural uterine abnormality	Ultrasound, sonohysterogram, or hysterosalpingogram	Surgical correction of defect
Smoking, caffeine, alcohol use	History	Counseling

Table 56.2 Testing in recurrent pregnancy loss

Potential cause	Initial evaluation	Secondary evaluation
Anatomic	Pelvic sonogram	Sonohysterogram, hysterosalpingogram, MRI
Genetic	Karyotype (both parents)	
Hormonal	TSH, prolactin	Hemoglobin A1 c
Immunologic	Lupus anticoagulant, anticardiolipin antibody, anti-β2-glycoprotein antibody	
Thrombophilic*	None	Factor V Leiden, prothrombin gene, protein C, protein S, homocysteine, antithrombin III

* Link to recurrent pregnancy loss theorized, but not supported by evidence. Testing not part of usual recommendations.

higher in younger mothers and lower in women over 40 [4]. Success rates are higher in couples who have no difficulty conceiving, and for women who experience miscarriage at a later stage in the pregnancy [5]. Presentation of the data showing that more than 50 percent of couples will have a successful pregnancy with conservative management and observation should be included in the counseling, as was done with this patient.

Key Teaching Points

- Recurrent pregnancy loss affects approximately 1 percent of couples who desire conception.
- Causes of recurrent pregnancy loss include balanced translocations, antiphospholipid syndrome, diabetes,

thyroid disease, elevated prolactin, uterine abnormalities, and smoking and alcohol.

- Initial evaluation should include genetic analysis of the parents, screening for uterine structural abnormalities, hormonal evaluation (thyroid, prolactin, insulin resistance/diabetes), and immunologic causes (antiphospholipid antibody syndrome testing).
- There is no benefit to progesterone supplementation.
- The majority of couples with recurrent pregnancy loss will have no clear cause of pregnancy loss. The five-year live birth rate for couples with recurrent pregnancy loss with or without treatment is over 60 percent. Maternal age is the strongest predictor of future successful pregnancy.

References

1. The Practice Committee of the American Society for Reproductive Medicine. Evaluation and treatment of recurrent pregnancy loss: a committee opinion. *Fertil Steril* 2012;98:1103–1111.

2. Royal College of Obstetricians and Gynaecologists, Scientific Advisory Committee, Guideline No. 17. The investigation and treatment of couples with recurrent miscarriage. 2011. www.rcog.org.uk/globalassets/documents/guidelines/gtg_17.pdf

3. Coomarasamy A, Williams H, Truchanowicz E et al. A randomized trial of progesterone in women with recurrent miscarriage. *NEJM* 2015;373:2141–2148.

4. Lund M, Kamper-Jorgensen M, Nielsen HS et al. Prognosis for live birth in women with recurrent miscarriage. *Obstet Gynecol* 2012;119:37–43.

5. Kling C, Magez J, Hedderich J et al. Two-year outcome after recurrent first trimester miscarriages: prognostic value of the past obstetric history. *Arch Gynecol Obstet* 2016;293:1113–1123.

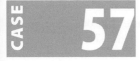

CASE 57 A Couple Planning Pregnancy Who Have Just Returned from Brazil (Zika Virus)

Michael Nix

History of Present Illness

A 26-year-old female, gravida 0, presents to your office with her male spouse for advice about becoming pregnant. They were married two months ago and have recently returned from a two-week honeymoon in Rio de Janeiro, Brazil. They desire to become pregnant as soon as possible.

She has no significant past medical history, past surgical history, or social history. Their family genetic screening history reveals no increased risk.

She notes a history of "pink eye" that developed approximately one week ago and has since resolved. She states that she felt like she had a low-grade fever during the last half of her trip, but was uncertain because they spent most of the time in their jungle bungalow. She states that she and her husband both developed a "heat rash" during their trip that resolved after leaving the jungle and returning to their hotel in the city.

She denies recent history of nausea, vomiting, diarrhea, joint pain, bloody stools, epistaxis, bleeding gums, hematuria, cough, and sore throat.

She has predictable menses coming every 27–28 days and lasting 4–5 days since menarche at age 14. Her last menstrual period was 26 days ago.

She was previously using combined oral contraception pills, but stopped them with her last cycle.

Physical Examination

General appearance	Well-developed, well-nourished woman in no discomfort. Alert and oriented

Vital Signs

Temperature	37.1°C
Pulse	76 bpm
Blood pressure	116/62 mm Hg
Respiratory rate	16 breaths/min
BMI	24.5 kg/m^2
HEENT	Normocephalic, atraumatic head with non-injected and anicteric sclera
Cardiovascular	Regular rate and rhythm, no edema
Pulmonary	Clear to auscultation bilaterally, no crackles or wheezes
Abdomen	Soft, non-tender, no rebound or guarding. No hepatosplenomegaly. Liver edge is non-tender
Skin	No rash, no jaundice, no petechiae
Laboratory:	Urine HCG Negative.

How Would You Manage This Patient?

The patient and her husband have traveled to an area endemic with Zika virus and demonstrate symptomatology consistent with Zika virus infection (conjunctivitis, rash, and subjective

fever), with symptom onset within the last two weeks. Testing for Zika RNA by nucleic acid test (NAT) was performed on urine and serum for both the patient and her partner and results were negative for infection. Subsequent testing for Zika virus immune globulin M (IgM) was then performed on the patient and her partner at a follow-up visit two weeks later. The patient's Zika virus IgM testing was negative for infection, but her partner had a positive titer for Zika virus IgM, which was confirmed with plaque reduction neutralization test (PRNT). Additional testing for dengue and chikungunya IgM was also performed on both partners, and resulted negative for infection.

The patient and her partner were informed of their results, the risks of congenital infection with Zika virus, and the possible methods of transmission. They were advised to continue to use barrier methods for vaginal, anal, or oral intercourse and to avoid conception for three months following the day they left Brazil, which was the last day they were exposed to Zika infection.

Zika Virus

Zika virus is an arthropod-borne virus that is transmitted by mosquitoes of the genus *Aedes*. Zika virus belongs to the genus *Flavivirus*, which also contains dengue virus, yellow fever virus, and West Nile virus. It is named after the Ugandan forest where it was first isolated in 1947.

Human infection with Zika was detected as early as 1952 in Uganda and Tanzania and spread throughout equatorial Africa and Asia. The first major recognized outbreak occurred in Micronesia in 2007, when more than 70 percent of the population was infected. Other outbreaks followed in French Polynesia in 2013–2014. Zika was first detected in the Western hemisphere on Easter Island in 2014 with subsequent infections detected in Brazil in May of 2015. By 2017, mosquito-borne disease had spread to include most countries of Central and South America, the Caribbean islands, and locations within the United States (Texas and Florida).

The Zika virus is commonly transmitted through the bite of an infected *Aedes* mosquito. Additional methods of transmission include vertical transmission from mother to fetus, sexual transmission, laboratory exposure, blood transfusion, and organ transplantation. The virus has been isolated in most body fluids (blood, urine, semen, saliva, female genital tract secretions, amniotic fluid, cerebrospinal fluid, and breast milk) and may be present in semen and cervical mucous even after it has disappeared from the blood. Although the virus has been isolated in breast milk, transmission through breastfeeding has not been documented and the risks of transmission and infection in the newborn are outweighed by the benefits of breastfeeding [1].

Infection with Zika virus is frequently not recognized in the adult population. When it occurs, symptoms appear after a 2- to 14-day incubation period and resolve within 2–7 days. They are mild and typically include low-grade fever, maculopapular rash, arthralgia, and non-purulent conjunctivitis. Less common complaints are myalgia, headache, abdominal pain, nausea, and diarrhea.

In October of 2015, a spike in the number of cases of congenital microcephaly in Brazil was reported to the World Health Organization (WHO). These increases correlated with an outbreak of infection with the Zika virus. Review of outbreaks in French Polynesia in 2013 and 2014 showed a similar correlation. The international science community turned its focus to Zika and the evidence around the infection grew, and continues to grow to this date. The virus has been shown to be able to infect neural stem cells and attenuate their growth [2]. This facilitates the explanation for the devastating effects on the developing neurologic system of infected fetuses.

The WHO, the Centers for Disease Control and Prevention (CDC), and other scientific groups now recognize that Zika virus is a cause of microcephaly [3]. Additional sequelae have also been described, and congenital Zika syndrome has been characterized with the five following features:

- Severe microcephaly with partially collapsed skull
- Thin cerebral cortices with subcortical calcifications
- Macular scarring and focal pigmentary retinal mottling
- Congenital contractures (e.g., club foot)
- Marked early hypertonia and symptoms of extrapyramidal involvement [4]

Other adverse effects noted during pregnancy include fetal loss, intrauterine growth restriction, and hydrops fetalis.

The risk of vertical transmission occurs throughout pregnancy, with the greatest effects on the fetus occurring with infection in the first and second trimesters. The risk of birth defects in fetuses with in utero exposure to Zika appears to be low, but those estimations are confounded by a lack of standard definitions as well as difficulty ascertaining maternal infection rates. The overall risk for adverse outcomes during pregnancies demonstrating maternal infection is also not clearly delineated.

Several countries that have experienced Zika outbreaks have reported increases in cases of Guillain–Barré Syndrome (GBS). Current CDC and WHO research suggests that there is a strong correlation between Zika and GBS, but only a small proportion of people with recent Zika infection get GBS [5, 6]. Other long-term neurologic sequelae have been reported, but have not been substantiated [7].

Testing for the presence of Zika infection can be performed by NATs or detection of Zika IgM. NATs may be used on urine or serum to demonstrate the presence of Zika virus RNA early in the course of illness. If an NAT is positive for Zika virus RNA, infection is confirmed and no further testing is necessary. If the NAT is negative, infection is not excluded and the serum serologic testing for Zika IgM should be performed. The time interval for Zika IgM levels to be detectable is variable. Zika IgM is typically detectable around four days after infection and remains detectable in the serum for 12 weeks. Because of the possibility of persistent IgM positivity, one cannot always reliably distinguish between an infection that occurred during the current pregnancy and one that occurred before the current pregnancy [8]. Zika virus serology may be falsely positive due to infection with other flaviviruses, so positive or equivocal IgM testing should be confirmed with a PRNT. For specimens collected from 7 days to 12 weeks after the onset of symptoms or last exposure, a negative IgM antibody result to Zika rules out recent infection with the virus. Testing is available through the CDC and most state health departments, as well as some commercial laboratories. Care providers should become familiar with where and what type of testing is available in their area [8, 9, 10].

Recommendations for testing, the type of testing performed, and the interpretation of results depend on the presence or absence of symptoms, whether the patient is pregnant or not, and the timing of the clinical presentation or exposure. The CDC recommendations are updated periodically and can be found on its website: www.CDC.gov/zika [11, 12]. The CDC recommends that Zika virus testing be performed on all men and women with Zika virus exposure and symptoms consistent with Zika virus [13]. The CDC previously recommended testing on all women who have been exposed to Zika virus during their pregnancy, regardless of symptomatology [11]. Because of emerging evidence that IgM test results may persist positive past 12 weeks after infection, as of the date of this publication, the CDC recommends that asymptomatic pregnant women who have recent exposure *but without possible ongoing exposure* not receive routine Zika virus testing [8]. Risk of exposures includes travel to an area with active Zika or having unprotected intercourse (vaginal, oral, or anal) with a partner who has recently traveled to an area with Zika. Patients who have been exposed to Zika virus should be screened for the symptoms typically associated with Zika infection. If a patient has experienced fever, rash, arthralgia, or conjunctivitis, he or she may be exhibiting symptoms of Zika disease. The symptoms of Zika are similar to other flavivirus infections, so providers should consider testing for dengue and chikungunya in those patients who have symptoms of infection but whose Zika NAT is negative [8].

There is no known cure for Zika virus infection. If a woman planning pregnancy has been exposed to Zika virus, she should either wait for a sufficient time for the virus to clear from her bloodstream or have serologic testing performed. If the testing is positive, or if no testing is performed, she should be advised to wait for eight weeks after the last possible exposure (if asymptomatic) or after the onset of symptoms (if symptomatic). Zika virus RNA can be detected in semen when it is no longer detectable in blood, so even if serologic testing of a male is negative, the chance of transmission through semen still exists. The ability to culture Zika virus from semen is not widely available, so couples who are planning pregnancy should be counseled to avoid conception for at least *three months* after the last possible exposure or symptoms onset. Couples should be advised to use barrier methods of contraception during vaginal, anal, and oral sex during this time period in order to prevent transmitting the virus to their sexual partners. These may be used in conjunction with more effective methods of contraception to avoid pregnancy [14].

Based on what is known from similar viruses, an infection with Zika virus likely provides individual protection from reinfection with Zika. This may account for the delayed association between Zika and congenital microcephaly. The populations where Zika has been endemic for years may exhibit immunity to infection by the time they enter child-bearing years, thus demonstrating a lower prevalence of microcephaly. There currently is no vaccine to prevent Zika infection, but pharmaceutical companies and the scientific community are actively researching the development of a vaccine [15].

Preconception counseling for all patients should include a discussion of their travel plans, including an overview of the areas that are endemic for Zika. Women and/or their partners who are planning pregnancy should be advised to avoid travel to Zika endemic areas if possible. If a woman or her partner travels to a Zika endemic area, the best method to avoid infection is to prevent mosquito bites. The use of Environmental Protection Agency (EPA)–registered insect repellents is proven to be a safe and effective method for avoiding mosquito bites, even for pregnant and breastfeeding women. Other methods include wearing long-sleeved shirts and long pants, wearing permethrin-treated clothing, using screens on windows and doors to keep mosquitoes outside, using air-conditioning or a mosquito bed net, and emptying collections of standing water that may provide a hatchery site for mosquito eggs [16].

The evidence behind Zika virus and the effects of its infection in humans is growing, as is the area where Zika is endemic. Health-care providers should use up-to-date resources such as the CDC, the American Congress of Obstetricians and Gynecologists, and the WHO to keep abreast of the growing scientific knowledge about Zika transmission and disease [17, 18, 7].

Key Teaching Points

- Zika virus has been associated with congenital microcephaly and other neurologic sequelae in fetuses and newborns with in utero exposure to Zika.
- The most common symptoms of infection in the adult population include:
  - Low-grade fever
  - Maculopapular rash
  - Arthralgia
  - Non-purulent conjunctivitis

- Patients planning on conceiving should be educated about the method of transmission of Zika virus, the risks of Zika infection to pregnancy, and methods to avoid transmission.
- Women who have positive testing for Zika virus or who have been exposed to Zika virus and have not been tested should be advised to wait for at least eight weeks after symptom onset (if symptomatic) or last exposure to the virus (if asymptomatic) prior to attempting conception.
- Men who have been exposed to Zika virus should be advised to wait for at least three months after symptom onset (if symptomatic) or last exposure to the virus (if asymptomatic) prior to attempting to get their partner pregnant. During this time, barrier methods of contraception should be used during intercourse to prevent transmitting the virus to their sexual partners.
- Because of the rapidly expanding body of evidence on Zika virus infection, health-care providers should use up-to-date resources such as the CDC, the American Congress of Obstetricians and Gynecologists, and the WHO to stay informed on how to screen, diagnose, and counsel patients on the disease.

References

1. World Health Organization. [Online]; 2017 [cited April 26, 2017]. Available from: www.who.int/elena/titles/zika_breastfeeding/en/.

2. Tang H, Hammack C, Ogden SC et al. Zika virus infects human cortical neural progenitors and attenuates their growth. *Cell Stem Cell* 2016 March;4:587–590.

3. Rasmussen Sonja A et al. Zika virus and birth defects – reviewing the evidence for causality. *N Engl J Med* 2016;1981–1987.

4. Moore Cynthia et al. Characterizing the pattern of anomalies in congenital Zika syndrome for pediatric clinicians. *JAMA Pediatrics* 2016;171:288–295.

5. Centers for Disease Control and Prevention. Zika and Guillain-Barre Syndrome. [Online]. [cited April 26, 2017]. Available from: www.cdc.gov/zika/healtheffects/gbs-qa.html.

6. World Health Organization. [Online]; 2016 [cited April 26, 2017]. Available from: www.who.int/mediacentre/factsheets/guillain-barre-syndrome/en/.

7. World Health Organization. [Online]; 2016 [cited April 19, 2017]. Available from: www.who.int/mediacentre/factsheets/zika/en/.

8. Centers for Disease Control and Prevention. [Online]; 2017 [cited April 26, 2017]. Available from: www.cdc.gov/zika/hc-providers/types-of-tests.html.

9. Centers for Disease Control and Prevention. [Online]; 2016 [cited April 26, 2017]. Available from: www.cdc.gov/mmwr/volumes/65/wr/mm6521e1.htm.

10. Centers for Disease Control and Prevention. [Online]; 2016 [cited April 26, 2017]. Available from: www.cdc.gov/zika/laboratories/lab-guidance.html.

11. Centers for Disease Control and Prevention. [Online]; 2016 [cited June 27, 2017]. Available from: www.cdc.gov/zika/pdfs/when-to-test-zika.pdf.

12. Centers for Disease Control and Prevention. [Online]; 2017 [cited June 27, 2017]. Available from: www.cdc.gov/zika/pdfs/testing_algorithm.pdf.

13. Centers for Disease Control and Prevention. [Online]; 2017 [cited April 26, 2017]. Available from: www.cdc.gov/zika/hc-providers/women-reproductive-age.html.

14. Centers for Disease Control and Prevention. [Online]; 2017 [cited April 26, 2017]. Available from: www.cdc.gov/zika/hc-providers/reproductive-age/patient-counseling.html.

15. WHO. World Health Organization. [Online]; 2017 [cited April 26, 2017]. Available from: www.who.int/immunization/research/development/zika/en/.

16. Centers for Disease Control and Prevention. [Online]; 2017 [cited April 26, 2017]. Available from: www.cdc.gov/zika/prevention/prevent-mosquito-bites.html.

17. The American Congress of Obstetricians and Gynecologists. [Online]. [cited April 19, 2017]. Available from: www.acog.org/About-ACOG/ACOG-Departments/Zika-Virus.

18. Centers for Disease Control and Prevention. [Online]; 2017 [cited April 26, 2017]. Available from: www.cdc .gov/zika/.

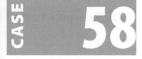

CASE 58

A 26-Year-Old Woman with a History of Depression Planning Pregnancy

Jonathan Schaffir

History of Present Illness

A 26-year-old nulligravida presents to her gynecologist for preconception counseling. She has no significant medical history other than a history of mental illness. At the age of 18, she was diagnosed with major depressive disorder after she was hospitalized for ingesting a large amount of acetaminophen. She had no medical sequelae from the overdose, and received psychiatric care during the admission. She was successfully treated with a combination of psychotherapy and pharmacotherapy. She experienced a relapse three years later when she discontinued her medication, and was again hospitalized for severe depressive symptoms. She was again successfully treated and maintained on pharmacotherapy.

She currently takes 40 mg of citalopram daily, which is prescribed by her family practitioner, and she sees a therapist once monthly. In the last three years, her mood has been stable and she is symptom-free. Earlier this year, she married her partner of two years. She is excited to start a family and is planning to discontinue her oral contraceptive in hope of conceiving soon.

She has no gynecological complaints and notes regular menstrual periods each month. She has been monogamous with her current partner for the past two years and has no history of sexually transmitted diseases. Aside from her citalopram and combination oral contraceptive, her only other medication is a multivitamin. She used to smoke one pack per day, but quit soon after her marriage. She denies any illicit substance use and drinks one to two alcoholic drinks most weekends. Neither she nor her husband has a family history of mental retardation, genetic disorders, or birth defects.

Physical Examination

General appearance   Well kempt, with appropriate affect

Vital Signs

Pulse	80 beats/min
Blood pressure	100/60 mmHg
Height	65 inches
Weight	130 lb
BMI	21.6 kg/m^2
HEENT	No thyromegaly or thyroid nodules present
Neurological exam	No motor or sensory deficits, no tremor or gait disturbance
Extremities	Multiple old linear scars on upper thighs bilaterally consistent with cutting
Genitourinary	Normal pelvic examination with nontender anteverted uterus, nulliparous cervix, and no adnexal masses

Laboratory Studies

TSH	1.82
Urine toxicology	Negative

Rubella and varicella titers consistent with immunity

How Would You Manage This Patient?

This woman has a history of severe depression with relapse and is now in remission for over a year on a selective serotonin reuptake inhibitor (SSRI). Given that she is feeling well with stable mood, this would be an appropriate time to conceive, with a lower risk for relapse during pregnancy. However, she is still at risk for relapse of depression, which could result in significant incapacity that would put both her health and that of her fetus at risk.

Her physician has a frank discussion with her about the risks and benefits of continuing antidepressant medication in the preconception period and in pregnancy. They discuss the possible effects of the use of SSRIs during pregnancy on the fetus and on the neonate after delivery, as well as the potential harms of being depressed while pregnant. After considering the multiple factors involved, she decides to continue using citalopram. Shortly afterward, she returns to the office for prenatal care newly pregnant. Her physician reviews her interval mood and health status and confirms that she is doing well on her present dose. Over the course of her pregnancy, he continues to assess her mood and well-being at each visit, and also encourages her to renew contact with her psychotherapist when she is feeling depressed. After she delivers a healthy full-term infant, he counsels her about signs of postpartum exacerbation to look out for, and arranges a postpartum visit to screen for such change.

Preconception Counseling for Women with a History of Depression

Depression is one of the most common disorders that clinicians who counsel women preconceptionally are likely to encounter. Twenty percent of women will experience an episode of major depressive disorder during their lifetimes, and the most common age of onset is between 20 and 40 years, the prime age for bearing children [1]. Many more women will experience minor episodes of depressed mood or reactive affective disorders that are not as severe as the experience described in the case, but who are nonetheless prescribed antidepressant medication. In the United States, 13 percent of women are exposed to an SSRI in the first trimester [2].

Counseling women with a history of major depression who are planning pregnancy is complex. The medical literature is conflicting and recommendations are difficult to generalize. Counseling and treatment are further complicated by the stigma attached to mental health issues. Providers may not recognize the gravity of the effects of depression in pregnancy and not give it the same consideration as treatment for other chronic illness such as hypertension or diabetes. Family members also fail to recognize the importance of treatment and may not be supportive of a patient's decision. The result is that women seeking treatment for depression in pregnancy may feel guilty or ashamed during a highly vulnerable time [3].

The decision to initiate or continue treatment for depression in the preconception period and in pregnancy involves balancing risks of untreated disease and relapse with risks of medical treatment. Enumerating the effects of depression on pregnancy is difficult due to conflicting reports that are confounded by factors associated with mental health issues such as poor prenatal care, drug and alcohol abuse, and the wide variation in symptom severity. In a meta-analysis of 29 prospective studies that specifically examined the effects of antenatal depression on birth outcomes, both preterm birth and low birth weight were significantly associated with depression [4]. Another review and meta-analysis analyzed a wider assortment of outcomes and included subgroup analyses to assess the effects of potential confounders. This review identified a 37 percent increase in risk for depressed women to deliver preterm relative to nondepressed women, though the association with low birth weight was not significant [5].

Although these studies failed to show significant risks of other birth outcomes, they do not account for many other adverse effects that depressed mood may have on the mother and the infant. Women who discontinue antidepressant medication during pregnancy have a 68 percent chance of relapsing depression, compared with 26 percent of women who continue antidepressant medication. Depression may lead to less compliance in prenatal care and less investment in the care of pregnancy, which may lead to unhealthy practices such as substance abuse and poor nutrition. When depression continues into the postpartum period, there may be downstream effects on the infant, including delayed cognitive and linguistic skills and impaired emotional development. In its most severe form, maternal depression can lead to suicide [1]. Although suicide in pregnancy is rare, it accounts for 20 percent of postpartum deaths [6].

These risks must be balanced with the risk of using antidepressant medication in the preconception period and in pregnancy. The most commonly prescribed medications for treatment of depression are the SSRIs, a medication class for which there is the greatest amount of research on use in pregnancy. Although studies have linked their use in early pregnancy to an increased rate of miscarriage, this risk is no greater than that of depressed women who discontinue treatment prior to conception [2]. Observational studies have suggested a link between SSRI use and a variety of adverse effects, including preeclampsia, postpartum hemorrhage, perinatal death, and neonatal seizures [7]. However, the absolute increase in risk for these events was small, and the studies showed only associations that may have been confounded by other factors in prescribing these medications. Multiple large cohort studies have demonstrated that SSRIs are not associated with congenital malformations. The possible exception is paroxetine, which has been linked to an increased risk of cardiac anomalies in first-trimester exposure in some studies. Some,

but not all, studies have also shown an increased risk of persistent pulmonary hypertension in newborns whose mothers use SSRIs in late pregnancy. Infants born to mothers who use SSRIs in pregnancy commonly display a neonatal adaptation syndrome characterized by tremors, jitteriness, and irritability. These symptoms usually resolve within days, and there appears to be no impact of SSRI use on long-term neurological development [8].

Other classes of medication may also be considered. Tricyclic antidepressants have not been shown to increase the rate of structural malformations, though they can cause a temporary withdrawal syndrome in infants similar to that seen with SSRIs. Dosage for these medications usually needs to increase in the second half of pregnancy due to increased plasma volume and metabolism. Atypical antidepressants such as bupropion, mirtazapine, and trazodone have not been extensively studied in pregnancy, and there is limited information available about their effects in pregnancy [1].

Non-pharmacologic treatment for depression in the preconception period and in pregnancy may be effective in selected women. Both interpersonal psychotherapy and cognitive-behavioral therapy have been demonstrated to be helpful for women with mild to moderate depression. Wellness strategies such as stress reduction and exercise promotion may be helpful, and mind–body modalities such as relaxation and yoga have limited evidence of successful treatment in mild depression.

Counseling and management should also take into consideration that relapse is affected by the interval since the prior episode of depression and its severity. Women who have experienced more severe depression symptoms when not taking medication are more likely to relapse with discontinuation. Prior response to treatment is important, as success with any agent is highly individualized. Consequently, there is no single agent or dose that is considered preferable or recommended at the time of conception. Switching from a drug of known efficacy to one of unknown efficacy is not recommended, because it may increase the rate of relapse since there is no proven benefit in safety profile of one agent over another [9]. The patient's own opinions about how well she is able to cope without pharmacological intervention are also important.

In 2009, the American College of Obstetricians and Gynecologists and the American Psychiatric Association convened a panel of experts to develop best practices for counseling women about managing depression in pregnancy [10]. They suggest that women with mild to moderate depression should preferentially be offered non-pharmacologic therapy, and those on antidepressant medication may consider weaning prior to conception. Women with a recent exacerbation of symptoms should consider waiting to conceive until they achieve 6–12 months of stability. The panel considered it acceptable for women to continue medication if they have a history of severe or recurrent depression, poor prior response to psychotherapy alone, or a strong desire to continue medication.

Some mental health professionals have advocated the use of decision aids that involve the individual patient's input and

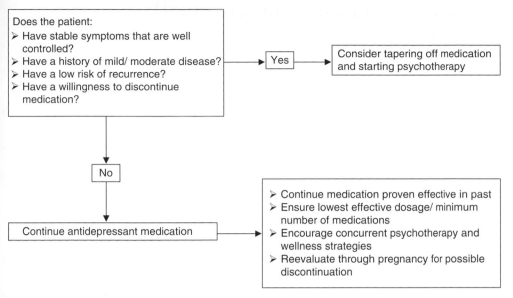

Figure 58.1 An algorithm to aid in counseling patients about treatment for depression during pregnancy.

desires. Such tools explain the risks and benefits of treatment and provide the patient with a stepwise assessment to help them decide what is most important to them. A particularly helpful example, which is currently undergoing clinical trials, is available at Healthwise.net [11]. Figure 58.1 illustrates a simple algorithm for counseling patients about medication use during pregnancy.

It is important to recognize that a patient's needs and priorities may change over the course of the preconception time and during pregnancy. Regular follow-up assessments are important to gauge the effect of treatment, screen for worsening symptoms, and evaluate the need for adjustments in therapy. Such assessments may be made by the primary obstetrical provider or by a mental health professional depending on the patient's needs and preferences and the provider's comfort level.

Key Teaching Points

- Untreated depression may have significant adverse effects on pregnancy, including preterm birth, substance abuse, poor nutrition, and suicide.
- Antidepressant medication is not generally considered teratogenic, but SSRIs are associated with increased risks of persistent pulmonary hypertension and neonatal adaptation syndrome.
- Psychotherapy without medication is preferable and can be an effective treatment for women with mild to moderate depression.
- Women with severe or recurrent depression, poor prior response to psychotherapy alone, or a strong desire to continue medication may be encouraged to continue medication to treat depression during the preconception period and in pregnancy.

References

1. Muzik M, Marcus SM, Heringhausen JE, Flynn H. When depression complicates childbearing: guidelines for screening and treatment during antenatal and postpartum obstetric care. *Obstet Gynecol Clin N Am* 2009;36:771–788.

2. Andersen JT, Andersen NL, Horwitz H, Poulsen HE, Jimenez-Solem E. Exposure to selective serotonin reuptake inhibitors in early pregnancy and the risk of miscarriage. *Obstet Gynecol* 2014;124:655–661.

3. Meltzer-Brody S. Treating perinatal depression: risks and stigma. *Obstet Gynecol* 2014;124:653–654.

4. Grote NK, Bridge JA, Gavin AR et al. A meta-analysis of depression during pregnancy and the risk of preterm birth, low birth weight, and intrauterine growth retardation. *Arch Gen Psychiatry* 2010;67:1012–1024.

5. Grigoriadis S, VonderPorten EH, Mamisashvili L et al. The impact of maternal depression during pregnancy on perinatal outcomes: a systematic review and meta-analysis. *J Clin Psychiatry* 2013;74: e321–e341.

6. Gentile S. Suicidal mothers. *J Inj Violence Res* 2011;3:90–97.

7. O'Connor E, Rossom RC, Henninger M, Groom HC, Burda BU. Primary care screening for and treatment of depression in pregnant and postpartum women: evidence report and systematic review for the US Preventive Services Task Force. *JAMA* 2016;315:388–406.

8. Susser LC, Sansone SA, Hermann AD. Selective serotonin reuptake inhibitors for depression in pregnancy. *Am J Obstet Gynecol* 2016;215:722–730.

9. Vigod SN, Brown S, Wilson CA, Howard LM. Depression in pregnancy. *BMJ* 2016;352:i1547.

10. Yonkers KA, Wisner KL, Stewart DE et al. The management of depression during pregnancy: a report from the American Psychiatric Association and the American College of Obstetricians and Gynecologists. *Obstet Gynecol* 2009;114:703–713.

11. Healthwise. Depression: Should I Take Antidepressants While I'm Pregnant? 2015. https://decisionaid .ohri.ca/AZsumm.php?ID=1161 (Accessed April 17, 2017.)

A 25-Year-Old Woman with a History of DVT Presents for Preconception Counseling

Erica Oberman

History of Present Illness

A 25-year-old, gravida 0, presents to your office for preconception counseling with a history of deep vein thrombosis (DVT) one year ago that developed related to a long airline flight while she was taking oral contraceptives. The patient reports that after a flight from Dubai to New York, she noted some pain and swelling in her left calf. She presented to a local emergency room and was found to have a left-leg deep venous thrombosis. She was told that her thrombus extended from her "lower to mid-thigh," but she does not have any records with her today. She reports that she was treated with low-molecular-weight heparin and then transitioned to warfarin for a total of six months. After this, she was started on the progesterone-only pill for birth control. She then moved to a different state and has had no further follow-up until now.

She reports menarche at 12 years of age, regular periods every 28 days, lasting 3–4 days at a time. She denies any history of dysmenorrhea. She has no other past medical or surgical history and no drug allergies and is on a prenatal vitamin. She recently stopped the progesterone-only birth control pill and is currently using condoms for contraception and would like to conceive in six months. Her family history is unremarkable. Two weeks ago, she had a consultation with a hematologist who ordered laboratory studies.

Physical Examination

Vital Signs

Temperature	37.2°C
Pulse	87 beats/min
Blood pressure	110/75
Height	5'8
Weight	132 lb
BMI	20 kg/m^2
General appearance	Well-developed, well-nourished woman in no acute distress

Laboratory Studies

WBC	7.85
Hgb	14.2
Ht	40.8
Platelets	212
Factor V Leiden mutation	Negative
Factor V Leiden activity	109
Prothrombin 20210A Variant	Negative
Antithrombin III Activity	94%
Protein C antigen	65%
Protein S total antigen	110%
Prothrombin time	9.9
INR	1.0
Cardiolipin Ab Quant	

IgG <15	
IgM <12.5	
IgA <12	
Beta-2-glucoprotein:	
IgG <9	
IgM <9	
IgA <9	
Dilute Russel Viper Venom Time	Negative

How Would You Manage This Patient?

In this patient with a personal history of a thrombotic event one year ago, additional medical and family history was taken focusing on any known history of a thrombophilia as well as her family history to determine if she had any first-degree relatives with a thrombotic episode prior to 50 years of age. Since the patient's thrombosis was a year ago and she is no longer on anticoagulation, laboratory screening was performed to rule out an inheritable thrombophilia (Factor V Leiden mutation, Prothrombin G20210A mutation, and Protein C, Protein S, and Antithrombin deficiencies) as well as antiphospholipid syndrome (lupus anticoagulant, anticardiolipin antibody, and anti-beta-2 glycoprotein I). Most laboratory studies to evaluate a patient with thrombosis should be done at least six weeks after the thromboembolic event, and should not be done during pregnancy and/or while on anticoagulation therapy. Antiphospholipid studies are an exception and are valid during pregnancy and can be done any time. The patient's laboratory studies were all within normal limits.

Because she had a history of a DVT while on estrogen-containing oral contraceptives, she was counseled that she should be started on a prophylactic dose of enoxaparin 40 mg a day (low-molecular-weight heparin [LMWH]) during her pregnancy. Prophylactic dosing during pregnancy is weight based. As the patient gets closer to delivery, she has the option of starting an unfractionated heparin (UFH) either one month prior to her due date or 24 hours prior to a scheduled induction of labor. Postpartum anticoagulation would be started 6 hours after a vaginal delivery and 12 hours after a cesarean section. The patient was counseled that she will need a prophylactic dose of enoxaparin 40 mg/day postpartum for six weeks.

Preconception Counseling and History of Deep Vein Thrombosis

Thromboembolic disease is the leading cause of maternal death in the United States, with 9 percent of maternal deaths (1.1 deaths per 100,000 deliveries) caused by a venous thromboembolus, including pulmonary embolus [1]. The physiologic and anatomic changes in pregnancy put a patient at a four- to

Box 59.1 Recommended thromboprophylaxis for pregnancies complicated by inherited thrombophilias

Clinical scenario	Antepartum management	Postpartum management
Low-risk thrombophilia[†] without previous VTE	Surveillance without therapy or prophylactic LMWH or UFH anticoagulation	Surveillance without anticoagulation therapy or postpartum anticoagulation therapy if the patient has additional risks factors[‡]
Low-risk thrombophilia[†] with a single previous episode of VTE – Not receiving long-term anticoagulation therapy	Prophylactic or intermediate-dose LMWH/UFH or surveillance without anticoagulation therapy	Postpartum anticoagulation therapy or intermediate-dose LMWH/UFH
High-risk thrombophilia[§] without previous VTE	Prophylactic LMWH or UFH	Postpartum anticoagulation therapy
High-risk thrombophilia[§] with a single previous episode of VTE – Not receiving long-term anticoagulation therapy	Prophylactic, intermediate-dose, or adjusted-dose LMWH/UFH regimen	Postpartum anticoagulation therapy or intermediate or adjusted-dose LMWH/UFH for 6 weeks (therapy level should be at least as high as antepartum treatment)
No thrombophilia with previous single episode of VTE associated with transient risk factor that is no longer present – Excludes pregnancy or estrogen-related risk factor	Surveillance without anticoagulation therapy	Postpartum anticoagulation therapy‖
No thrombophilia with previous single episode of VTE associated with transient risk factor that was pregnancy- or estrogen-related	Prophylactic-dose LMWH or UFH‖	Postpartum anticoagulation therapy
No thrombophilia with previous single episode of VTE without an associated risk factor (idiopathic) – Not receiving long-term anticoagulation therapy	Prophylactic-dose LMWH or UFH‖	Postpartum anticoagulation therapy
Thrombophilia or no thrombophilia with two or more episodes of VTE – Not receiving long-term anticoagulation therapy	Prophylactic or therapeutic-dose LMWH or prophylactic or therapeutic-dose UFH	Postpartum anticoagulation therapy or therapeutic-dose LMWH/UFH for 6 weeks
Thrombophilia or no thrombophilia with two or more episodes of VTE – Receiving long-term anticoagulation therapy	Therapeutic-dose LMWH or UFH	Resumption of long-term anticoagulation therapy

Abbreviations: LMWH, low molecular weight heparin; UFH, unfractionated heparin; VTE, venous thromboembolism.
*Postpartum treatment levels should be greater or equal to antepartum treatment. Treatment of acute VTE and management of antiphospholipid syndrome are addressed in other practice bulletins.
[†]Low-risk thrombophilia: factor V Leiden heterozygous; prothrombin *G20210A* heterozygous; protein C or protein S deficiency.
[‡]First-degree relative with a history of a thrombotic episode before age 50 years, or other major thrombotic risk factors (e.g., obesity, prolonged immobility).
[§]High-risk thrombophilia: antithrombin deficiency; double heterozygous for prothrombin *G20210A* mutation and factor V Leiden; factor V Leiden homozygous or prothrombin *G20210A* mutation homozygous.
‖Surveillance without anticoagulation is supported as an alternative approach by some experts.
Reprinted with permission from Inherited thrombophilias in pregnancy. ACOG Practice Bulletin No. 138. American College of Obstetricians and Gynecologists. *Obestet Gynecol* 2013;122:706–717.

fivefold increased risk of thromboembolism [1]. Physiologic changes include an increase in clotting potential, a decrease in anticoagulant activity, and decreased fibrinolytic activity [2]. Anatomic changes caused by the growth of the gravid uterus and its compression of the pelvic veins and inferior vena cava can lead to stasis in the lower extremities.

Assessing risk for venous thromboembolism (VTE) prior to pregnancy is essential for planning anticoagulation therapy in the antenatal and postpartum periods. One of the most important risk factors for VTE in pregnancy is a personal history of thrombosis, as 15–25 percent of cases of VTE are a repeat event. Women should be evaluated for an inherited thrombophilia if they have a personal history of VTE with a nonrecurrent risk factor, such as surgery, a fracture, or prolonged immobilization. Any patient with a first-degree relative with a history of a high-risk thrombophilia should also be screened [3]. Patients with a diagnosis of an inherited thrombophilia are at higher risk for a thromboembolism [3].

Table 59.1 Recommended anticoagulation regimens for pregnancy

		Prophylactic	Intermediate	Therapeutic
Low molecular weight heparin	Enoxaparin	40 mg SC once daily	40 mg SC once daily, increase as pregnancy progress to 1 mg/kg daily	1 mg/kg every 12 hours
	Dalteparin	5000 units SC once daily	5000 units SC every 12 hours	200 units/kg every 12 hours
Unfractionated heparin		1st trimester: 5,000–7,500 units every 12 hours. Second trimester: 7,500 to 10,000 units every 12 hours. 3rd trimester 10,000 units every 12 hours, unless the aPTT is elevated.		Dose patient every 12 hours to keep aPTT 1.5 to 2.5 times control six hours after injection.

Testing should be done at least six weeks after a thrombotic event and should not be done during pregnancy, while on anticoagulation therapy, or on hormonal contraception [3]. Fluctuating values of Protein S binding protein during pregnancy makes it an unreliable test that should not be tested in pregnancy [3].

Anticoagulation therapeutic regimens are based on the diagnosis of a high- or low-risk thrombophilia and whether the patient has a personal history of DVT. High-risk thrombophilias include antithrombin deficiency, double heterozygous for prothrombin G20210A mutation, factor V Leiden homozygous, or prothrombin G20210A mutation homozygous. Low-risk thrombophilias are Factor V Leiden heterozygous, prothrombin G20210A heterozygous, and protein C or S deficiencies. Depending upon the risk profile, patients are then treated with either prophylactic, intermediate, or therapeutic anticoagulation and should remain on therapy until six weeks postpartum (Box 59.1) [4].

The recommendations for DVT prophylaxis in pregnancy are based upon case series and expert opinions. In general, the recommendation for low-risk patients (patients with a low-risk thrombophilia without history of previous VTE) is either no anticoagulation therapy or prophylactic LMWH or UFH. The recommendation remains the same for low-risk patients in the postpartum period, unless they have additional risk factors to consider (first-degree relative with history of a thrombotic event prior to 50 years of age, obesity, prolonged immobility). Patients with high-risk thrombophilias and/or other high-risk

factors for thrombosis may need intermediate or therapeutic anticoagulation (Box 59.1).

The prophylactic dose of enoxaparin (LMWH) is 40 mg SC once daily. The intermediate dose is 40 mg SC every 12 hours. The therapeutic dose is 1 mg/kg every 12 hours (Box 59.1).

Key Teaching Points

- The physiologic and anatomic changes in pregnancy put a patient at a four- to fivefold increased risk of thromboembolism.
- The most important individual risk factor for DVT in pregnancy is a personal history of thrombosis.
- A patient with a personal history of thrombosis or with a first-degree relative with a high-risk thrombosis should be screened for an inherited or acquired thrombophilia. Specific testing includes Factor V Leiden mutation, prothrombin G20210A mutation, protein C and protein S and antithrombin deficiency, lupus anticoagulant, anticardiolipin antibody, and anti-beta-2 glycoprotein.
- Testing should be done at least six weeks after a thrombotic event and should not be done during pregnancy, while on anti-coagulation therapy, or on hormonal contraception.
- Antenatal and postpartum anticoagulation therapy depends on the history of thromboembolism, presence of a high-risk thrombophilia, and additional individual risk factors.

References

1. James AH, Jamison MG, Brancazio LR, Myers ER. Venous thromboembolism during pregnancy and the postpartum period: incidence, risk factors and mortality. *Am J Obstet Gynecol* 2006: 194;1311–1315.
2. Breeme KA. Hemostatic changes in pregnancy. *Best Pract Res Clin Haematology* 2003;16:153–168.
3. American College of Obstetricians and Gynecologists. Inherited thrombophilias in pregnancy. Practice bulletin no. 138 September 2013;122(3):706–717.
4. American College of Obstetricians and Gynecologists. Thromboembolism in pregnancy. Practice bulletin no. 196 *Obstet Gynecol* September 2018;132: e1–17.
5. Bates SM, Greer IA, Pabinger I, Sofaer S, Hirsch J. Venous thromboembolism thrombophilia, antithrombotic therapy and pregnancy: American College of Chest Physicians evidence based clinical practice guidelines. 8th edition. American College of Chest Physicians. *Chest* 2008;133: 844S–886S.

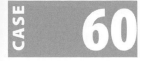

CASE 60

A 25-Year-Old Ashkenazi Jewish Woman Who Desires Pregnancy

Jessica C. Arluck

History of Present Illness

A 25-year-old, gravida 0, para 0, presents to your office for her well-woman examination. She is excited to tell you that she recently became engaged. You asked her if and when she is interested in getting pregnant. She said she would like to try to get pregnant about a year after her wedding. Her mother has told her that because she is of Ashkenazi Jewish descent she "needs to get tested." Her past medical history and surgical history are negative. She has a history of regular menses and is sexually active in a mutually monogamous heterosexual relationship. She uses levonorgestrel intrauterine device (IUD) for contraception and has no complaints. She has never had any sexually transmitted infections and has had normal pap smears. On occasion, she will take ibuprofen for cramps or headaches but otherwise does not take any prescribed or over-the-counter medications, vitamins, or herbal supplements. She is up-to-date on her immunizations. She does not smoke or use illicit drugs, and drinks wine when she goes out to dinner. She has a desk job. To keep in shape, she runs 12 miles per week. She feels safe at home and in her relationship. Her physical exam shows a BMI of 22 and normal vital signs. The rest of her physical exam is unremarkable.

How Would You Manage This Patient?

The next step is to counsel the patient about being healthy prior to pregnancy. It is important for her to continue her current healthy habits (such as exercising and not smoking) before and during her pregnancy, and explain that no amount of alcohol is known to be safe in pregnancy. Next, you discuss the benefits of taking 400 mcg of folic acid daily for at least one month prior to removing her IUD, which decreases her risk of having an infant with neural tube defects [1]. Finally, you have a discussion regarding genetic carrier screening for Ashkenazi Jewish patients. You counsel your patient about the availability of the Ashkenazi Jewish panel, which currently can screen for 19 specific diseases associated specifically with those of Ashkenazi Jewish descent, versus an expanded ethnic panel. Your patient agreed to have the specific Ashkenazi Jewish panel testing. The test results inform you that she is a carrier for Gaucher Disease. You counsel your patient about this disease and to have her partner tested, even though he is not of Ashkenazi Jewish descent. He screens negative. It is important to inform this couple that their offspring will not have Gaucher Disease, but their future progeny may be a potential carrier.

Genetic Preconception Counseling

Preconception counseling is important to optimize a patient's/couple's health and reduce or eliminate risk before conception as well as to give information regarding issues that affect them on an individual level. Providing preconception counseling is vital to allow time for information gathering or to enact changes that can positively affect a future pregnancy [2]. Asking a patient at each touch point "When do you want to be pregnant?" allows for this preparatory discussion. This also allows for intendedness of pregnancy. Approximately 50 percent of pregnancies in the United States are unintended, and therefore family planning and contraception are important discussions with each visit for reproductive-age women.

Once a woman or a couple have made the decision to consider pregnancy, a thorough history allows the preconception conversation to be tailored to specific issues. The American Academy of Pediatrics and the American College of Obstetrics and Gynecology (ACOG) recommend that eight different areas be evaluated:

1. Reproductive awareness
2. Environmental toxins and teratogens
3. Nutrition and folic acid
4. Genetics
5. Substance abuse, including tobacco and alcohol
6. Medical conditions and medications
7. Infectious diseases and vaccinations
8. Psychosocial issues including screening for intimate partner violence [3]

Genetic screening and evaluation of risks in the preconception time allow for nondirective conversations that may affect pregnancy decisions. Preconception planning allows for adequate time to receive test results and obtain follow-up testing, and also allows an opportunity for the couple to make decisions regarding assisted reproductive technologies and preimplantation genetic diagnosis.

The background population risk for a major birth defect or genetic problem is 2–5 percent. There are specific genetic disorders that are more prevalent in the Ashkenazi Jewish population. Ashkenazi Jews, those whose background are from Central and Eastern Europe, make up more than 80 percent of the American Jewish population. Historically, marriage between first cousins was common in Eastern European Jewish communities. The other two Jewish groups include Sephardic, from Spain, and Mizrahi, from the Middle East and Northern Africa. Individuals from these Jewish groups do not share the same genetic risk as individuals of Ashkenazi Jewish ancestry as they are more genetically diverse and do not have genetic disorders that are of ethnic Jewish origin.

The Ashkenazi Jewish genetic disorders are single-gene autosomal recessive in nature. If both members of the couple are carriers for the same disease, then every time they conceive, the chance of having an affected offspring is 25 percent.

The offspring also has a 50 percent chance of being just a carrier and there is a 25 percent chance of the offspring not being affected and not being a carrier. Currently, there are 19 different diseases that can be screened specifically in the Ashkenazi Jewish population. These diseases can occur at a higher prevalence in this population (e.g., Tay Sachs disease) or occur almost exclusively in Ashkenazi Jews (e.g., Familial Dysautonomia). If only one partner is of Ashkenazi Jewish descent, meaning that they have one grandparent who is Ashkenazi Jewish, then that person should be offered screening first. Once the carrier status is determined, the partner should be screened. This is called sequential screening. If timing is important, then simultaneous screening of both partners can be done.

When a patient is found to be a carrier, her partner should then be screened for the specific disease for which she is a carrier. The risk that the infant will be affected is significantly reduced, but not zero. There is a residual risk that although the parent tested negative, he may still be a carrier as he could have a mutation not screened for by the test. The residual risk is different for each disease and ethnic group. For example, screening tests for Gaucher Disease have a 96 percent carrier detection rate. The carrier frequency would then change from 1 in 13 before screening to 1 in 301 if the patient screened negative.

Given that there are 19 conditions recommended, there is a 1 in 3 to a 1 in 4 chance that any one individual of Ashkenazi Jewish descent will test positive for at least one of the conditions. Detection rate and carrier frequency are not as well known in non-Jewish populations (except for Tay Sachs disease and cystic fibrosis). This may make it difficult to determine the couple's numerical risk of having a child with one of these other disorders, especially if the partner is unavailable or chooses not to get screened.

There are a number of screening tests available commercially. Many companies now have expanded ethnic carrier screening for pan-ethnic screening. Through advances in technology and efficiencies in sequencing, many conditions can be looked for simultaneously. Some of the screening kits can assess for over 250 different conditions. Many of these conditions are not currently recommended for screening by any medical society. Some conditions may have variable presentations and population risks may be unknown [4]. As the technology continues to improve, this number will likely expand. One benefit of pan-ethnic screening is that many individuals do not know their ethnic background or are unsure, going back one or more generations. Also many in America's "melting pot" society are multiethnic or multiracial. There are home tests being marketed directly to consumers for home testing without the guidance of a physician or a genetic counselor.

The costs of these tests have decreased over time, with many costing several hundred dollars, compared to thousands of dollars only a few years ago. Many patients may now be able to afford these tests paying out of pocket. It is still important to advise patients to check with their insurance carrier about coverage.

It is important to counsel a patient that when using expanded carrier screening that has over 100 diseases, it is likely that an individual will be positive for at least 1–3 of these conditions. Genetic counseling should be offered for the couple after testing is back if both are found to be carriers of a genetic condition. It is also important to counsel a patient on potential negative consequences of testing. Genetic information is protected by the 2008 Genetic Information Nondiscrimination Act, which prohibits health insurers from denying coverage based on genetic predispositions, and employers cannot use genetic information in their hiring, firing, or promotion practices. This, however, does not apply to other types of insurance, such as life or disability [5].

Currently, ACOG recommends offering genetic screening to those of Ashkenazi Jewish descent for Canavan disease, Familial Dysautonomia, Tay Sachs disease, spinal muscular atrophy, and cystic fibrosis (the last two are recommended for everyone considering pregnancy). However, there are some experts who recommend a more complete list be offered, including Bloom syndrome, Familial hyperinsulinism, Fanconi Anemia C, Gaucher Disease, Glycogen Storage Disease type 1, Joubert Syndrome 2, Maple Syrup Urine Disease, Mucolipidosis Type IV, Niemann-Pick Disease, Usher Syndrome, and Walker Warburg syndrome.

ACOG stated in March of 2017 that genetic screening should be offered to any woman considering pregnancy and that acceptable screening strategies be based either on risk alone or by offering expanded carrier/pan-ethnic screening [5]. It is important to have pre- and post-test counseling. Pretest counseling needs to include risks and limitations in addition to the benefits of the testing. It is not practical to discuss each individual condition, but literature should be available about specific conditions as requested by patients. Discussion should include that risks may not be calculable, especially if one partner is of a different ethnicity. Screening does not preclude neonatal testing (such as newborn screening), and conversely, neonatal testing does not eliminate the need to screen a woman considering another pregnancy who has not been screened [6].

Cost can be a factor for some; so, a patient should be encouraged to check into her insurance coverage. Some companies/organizations have reduced cost of testing for those without insurance coverage. However, cost should not be a factor in offering screening testing. After discussing screening testing, any patient may refuse testing. It is important to have genetic counseling available both before testing, if desired, and after the testing results are available to review them and offer reproductive options. It is also important to encourage prior to testing that the patient inform other family members of results as it may affect them as well. This may be a family stressor and counseling needs to be available [7].

Key Teaching Points

- Ask all reproductive-age women their pregnancy desires in order to reduce or eliminate risk and to gather information, including genetic screening, needed for a healthy pregnancy.

- Carrier screening and counseling ideally should be performed before pregnancy, and genetic screening should be offered to any woman considering pregnancy.
- Acceptable screening strategies can be based either on history-assessed risk or by offering expanded carrier/pan-ethnic screening with appropriate pre- and post-test counseling.

- ACOG recommends offering genetic screening to those of Ashkenazi Jewish descent for Canavan disease, familial dysautonomia, Tay Sachs disease, spinal muscular atrophy, and cystic fibrosis (the last two are recommended for everyone considering pregnancy). However, there are some who recommend a more complete list.

References

1. US Preventive Services Task Force. Folic acid supplementation: a evidence review. www.uspreventiveservicestaskforce.org/Home/GetFile/1/4292/folic-acid-evidencereview/pdf

2. Shipara SK, Dolan S. Genetic risks to the mother and the infant: assessment, counseling and management. *Matern Child Health J* 2006;**10**: S143–S146.

3. Centers for Disease Control and Prevention. Recommendations to improve preconception health and health care. A report of the CDC/ATSDR preconception care work group and the select panel on preconception care. *MMWR* 2006;**55**:1–23.

4. Grody WW, Thompson BH, Gregg AR et al. ACMG position statement on prenatal/preconception expanded carrier screening. *Genet Med* June 2013;**15**(6):482–483.

5. www.hhs.gov/hipaa/for-professionals/special-topics/genetic-information/index.html

6. American College of Obstetricians and Gynecologists. Carrier screening for genetic conditions. Committee opinion No. 691. *Obstet Gynecol* 2017;**129**(3): e41–e55.

7. American College of Obstetricians and Gynecologists. Counseling about genetic testing and communication of genetic test results. Committee opinion No. 693. *Obstet Gynecol* 2017;**129** (4):771–772.

A 40-Year-Old Woman with Chronic Hypertension on Atenolol Planning Pregnancy

L. David Moore

History of Present Illness

A 40-year-old, gravida 2, para 1, woman with hypertension presents for preconception counseling. She has been your patient for years, and you provided care for her during her previous pregnancies. She reports that although she is happy with her marriage, career, and child, she is curious about what her chances of having a healthy pregnancy are at her age. She would like to have another child, but wants to make an informed decision and maximize her health before attempting conception.

Her only current medical condition is hypertension, which was diagnosed last year and is treated by her internal medicine physician. She had a vaginal delivery at 38 weeks gestation 6 years ago that was complicated by preeclampsia. She also had one spontaneous abortion two years ago. She has not had any surgeries. Her medications include a multivitamin and atenolol 25 mg daily. For the past 18 months, she has used the levonorgestrel IUD for contraception. She reports no drug allergies. She is married and a nonsmoker.

Physical Examination

General appearance   Well-developed, well-nourished woman with no acute distress

Vital Signs

Temperature	37°C
Pulse	88 beats/min
Blood pressure	138/88 mmHg
Respiratory rate	20 breaths/min
Oxygen saturation	100 percent on room air
Height	65 inches
Weight	177 lb
BMI	29.5 kg/m^2
Physical Exam	deferred since counseling will be the focus of this visit.

How Would You Manage This Patient?

This patient has two medical issues that warrant attention during a preconception counseling visit: chronic hypertension and advanced maternal age (AMA). The patient was counseled that chronic hypertension is a risk factor for many obstetric complications, including superimposed preeclampsia, fetal growth restriction, and placental abruption. Infertility and early pregnancy loss are common for women with AMA, with 40 percent of clinically recognized pregnancies ending in a first-trimester loss at age 40. The patient was also counseled that fetal chromosomal abnormalities, including trisomies 13, 18, and 21 (Down syndrome), are more common as women age. At age 40, the likelihood of delivering an infant with any chromosome abnormality is 1:62. Both screening and invasive diagnostic tests for fetal chromosomal abnormalities

are available starting at ten weeks gestation. The cell-free DNA screening test yields a 93 percent positive predictive value for Down syndrome in patients who are 40 years old, without risk to the developing pregnancy. Initially, she hoped to have her IUD removed at the end of this visit, but instead decided to leave with her IUD in place and discuss these issues with her husband. She was informed that should they decide to attempt conception, atenolol should be discontinued, as some research linked this medication to fetal growth restriction. Labetalol (100 mg twice daily) would be instead prescribed during the preconception time period, as her chronic hypertension is well controlled on a similar medication.

Chronic Hypertension

Chronic hypertension is categorized as primary (essential) or secondary. Primary hypertension accounts for the overwhelming majority of cases and has no singular, identifiable cause, whereas secondary hypertension is caused by an underlying medical condition (such as renal disease). Once the diagnosis of chronic hypertension is established, the clinician should be aware if the patient has secondary hypertension or target-organ damage. These two factors are paramount in deciding which patients must continue antihypertensive therapy throughout pregnancy. Table 61.1 reviews target-organ damage and what tests are needed to assess for these conditions [1, 2].

During pregnancy, maternal blood pressure normally decreases, reaching a nadir in the late second trimester. This decrease is due to reduced systemic vascular resistance and occurs even with the expansion of maternal blood volume and increased cardiac output. Blood pressure then increases and may reach or surpass pre-pregnancy levels in the third trimester. This can lead to diagnostic difficulties if a patient with chronic hypertension presents for initial evaluation during the second trimester, since her chronic hypertension may be masked by normal pregnancy physiology. Blood pressure will rise as the gestation continues, and she may then be erroneously diagnosed with gestational hypertension or preeclampsia rather than superimposed preeclampsia. While chronic hypertension is a risk factor for placental abruption and fetal growth restriction, these conditions are more strongly associated with superimposed preeclampsia [1].

Preconception assessment for patients with chronic hypertension should include studies for platelet count, creatinine, liver enzymes, and a quantitative measure of proteinuria to use as a baseline to compare in case superimposed preeclampsia develops in the upcoming pregnancy. Physicians may also include an HbA1c level at this time to diagnose diabetes [1, 3]. With pregnancy, all chronic hypertensive patients should have an early glucose screening for diabetes. If this

Table 61.1 Target-organ damage and initial laboratory assessment of hypertension

Target organ	Assessment strategy
Heart	
Left ventricular hypertrophy	Baseline EKG
Angina or prior myocardial infarction	Echocardiogram indicated if warranted by other symptoms/findings
Prior coronary revascularization	Obtain echocardiogram for women with long-standing chronic hypertension (≥4 yrs)
Heart failure	
Brain	
Stroke or TIA	History and neurological examination
Chronic kidney disease	Baseline urine analysis
Peripheral artery disease	History and physical examination
Retinopathy	History and funduscopic examination
Other baseline tests to obtain with initial diagnosis of hypertension	Glucose, hematocrit, potassium, creatinine/GFR, calcium, HDL, LDL, and triglycerides

Source: Roberts J, August P, Bakris G et al. Hypertension in Pregnancy. Chronic Hypertension in Pregnancy and Superimposed Preeclampsia. Washington, DC: American College of Obstetricians and Gynecologists; 2013. pp. 51–69. American Medical Association. The Seventh Report of the Joint National Committee on Prevention, Detection, Evaluation, and Treatment of High Blood Pressure: the JNC 7 Report. JAMA. 2003;289(19):2560–2572.

Table 61.2 Common causes of secondary hypertension

Condition	Associated findings
Chronic kidney disease	Anemia, decreased GFR
Renovascular disease	Abdominal bruit, elevated plasma renin activity
Primary aldosteronism	Hypokalemia, elevated aldosterone to plasma renin activity ratio
Hypothyroidism	Decreased TSH
Hyperparathyroidism	Elevated serum calcium
Pheochromocytoma	Elevated plasma free metanephrines, palpitations headache, perspiration
Sleep apnea	Snoring, witnessed apnea, daytime somnolence
Chronic steroid therapy or Cushing syndrome	Cushingoid facies, central obesity, proximal muscle weakness, ecchymoses
Coarctation of the aorta	Delayed or diminished femoral pulses
Drug-induced or drug-related	Oral contraceptives, NSAIDs, decongestants, amphetamines, etc.

Source: Roberts J, August P, Bakris G et al. *Hypertension in Pregnancy.* Chronic Hypertension in Pregnancy and Superimposed Preeclampsia. Washington, DC: American College of Obstetricians and Gynecologists; 2013. pp. 51–69. American Medical Association. The Seventh Report of the Joint National Committee on Prevention, Detection, Evaluation, and Treatment of High Blood Pressure: the JNC 7 Report. *JAMA.* 2003;289(19):2560–2572. Rakel (ed.). Textbook of Family Medicine, Ninth Edition. Philadelphia: Elsevier; 2016.

early test is negative, then the standard glucose screening done at 24–28 weeks should still be administered. Additionally, all patients should take 81 mg of aspirin daily initiated between 12 and 28 weeks of gestation for the prevention of preeclampsia [4].

Only 10 percent of hypertensive patients have secondary hypertension. Patients with resistant hypertension, hypokalemia, palpitations, or no family history of hypertension, or <35 years of age may have secondary hypertension, and a thorough history and physical exam will help determine which tests are necessary. A workup for secondary hypertension should be included in preconception counseling if it was not previously addressed. Medical conditions that are common causes of secondary hypertension and their corresponding medical findings are listed in Table 61.2 [1, 2, 5]. The information included here is not extensive; other disease processes may cause secondary hypertension and there is a lack of consensus regarding diagnostic tests for many of these conditions. Referral to a physician experienced in diagnosing and treating hypertension is reasonable [1].

Chronic hypertension patients are then divided into low-risk and high-risk groups. The low-risk group consists of patients with uncomplicated, essential hypertension. The blood pressure goal for this group is <160 mmHg systolic and <105 mmHg diastolic. If patients in this group used antihypertensive medications prior to pregnancy, they may be discontinued in the first trimester. If blood pressure approaches the threshold for treatment, medications are restarted. Fetal growth restriction is common with hypertension and ultrasound examinations to monitor fetal growth are indicated. After the anatomic survey ultrasound is done at 18–22 weeks, fetal growth ultrasounds should start at 28–32 weeks and continue every 4 weeks. Antenatal fetal surveillance with non-stress tests or biophysical profiles should begin at 32–34 weeks, especially for patients who require antihypertensive medication. Delivery for patients in this group with no other complications should occur after 38 weeks gestation [1, 3].

The high-risk group of chronic hypertensive patients includes patients with target-organ damage, secondary hypertension, or uncontrolled hypertension. The blood pressure goal for this group is <140 mmHg systolic and <90 mmHg diastolic to avoid progression of disease. Concern for fetal growth restriction is heightened and serial growth ultrasounds should begin at 28 weeks and continue every 3–4 weeks. Additionally, antepartum fetal surveillance testing should start at 28 weeks and continue weekly or twice weekly. Delivery should occur at 37 weeks gestation [1, 3].

First-line antihypertensive medications in pregnancy include labetalol, nifedipine, and methyldopa. Labetalol, a nonselective β-blocker with vascular α-receptor blocking ability, is a first-line agent, but should be avoided in patients with asthma and congestive heart failure. The calcium channel blocker nifedipine is safe to use in pregnancy. Methyldopa, a centrally acting α-2 adrenergic agonist, has been used for decades and has many studies to attest its safety for mother and child. However, it may be less effective in preventing progression to severe hypertension in pregnancy and is rarely used outside of pregnancy [1, 3].

Some hypertensive medications should be avoided during pregnancy. In human studies, atenolol use in the first and second trimester has been associated with reduced fetal weight, making it an FDA category D medication. Patients desiring pregnancy should not take atenolol preconceptionally, and instead use labetalol or nifedipine. Angiotensin-converting enzyme (ACE) inhibitors and Angiotensin II receptor blockers (ARBs) are FDA category D medications as well and should be avoided if possible in women of reproductive age. These medications have been associated with fetal renal failure, oligohydramnios, and pulmonary hypoplasia when used in the second and third trimesters. Use in the first trimester may also increase the risk of congenital cardiac and central nervous system malformations [1].

Advanced Maternal Age

AMA is defined as pregnancy at 35 years of age or more. This population of patients deserves special attention in preconception counseling as increasing age is an individual risk factor for many antepartum comorbidities. Fundamental in patients desiring pregnancy after age 35 is counseling on decreased female fertility. Fecundity begins to decline at 32 years of age and declines more sharply after 37. Oocyte atresia is a continual process for every female starting at 20 weeks gestation in utero through menopause. The decrease in fecundity is primarily due to a decline in egg number and quality. Patients who are 35 years or older should have evaluation and treatment for infertility after attempting pregnancy for 6 months or earlier (if indicated), rather than 1 year. At age 40, patients may opt for immediate evaluation and treatment [6].

Rates of miscarriage also increase with age. At age 35, 20 percent of clinically recognized pregnancies will end in a first trimester loss compared to a 9–17 percent rate in women aged 20–30. This rate doubles to 40 percent at age 40. Chromosomal abnormalities are found in almost half of all early pregnancy losses [7]. Aneuploidy, the inheritance of either one extra or one fewer chromosome, is commonly caused by nondisjunction during meiosis. This occurs more commonly as women age and contributes to the increased risk of miscarriage [8].

While most aneuploidy patterns are incompatible with life, some fetuses will continue to develop and become viable. Fetuses with aneuploidy are likely to have congenital birth defects and functional abnormalities. Trisomy, the inheritance of an extra chromosome, accounts for almost half of all chromosomal abnormalities. This includes the most common autosomal trisomy, Down syndrome (Trisomy 21). At age 35 the likelihood of having an infant with Down syndrome is 1:353. It is 1:85 at age 40 [8].

Prenatal assessment for aneuploidy should be offered to all patients, regardless of age. However, with AMA patients, clinicians should be aware of the characteristics of the tests available. Some patients may choose an invasive diagnostic test such as chorionic villi sampling or amniocentesis over a screening test. Screening tests for aneuploidy include serum biochemical marker screening with or without ultrasound and cell-free fetal DNA. Among the choices for non-invasive screening tests, cell-free DNA may be a better choice given the low false-positive rate and better positive predictive value for women who will be 35 years or older at delivery. Some patients will choose to defer all prenatal testing [9].

Pregnancies in women over 35 are at risk for other comorbidities such as gestational diabetes, hypertensive disorders, and cesarean delivery. Though the overall absolute risk is low, the relative risk of perinatal mortality is increased for patients with AMA. In general, the physiological changes (elevated cardiac output, increased blood volume, and increased insulin resistance) that occur during pregnancy are tolerated well by younger women but may be overwhelming for older gravidas. These complications should be reviewed with patients who are considering delaying pregnancy until after 35 years of age, a growing trend [10].

Key Teaching Points

- During pregnancy, maternal blood pressure normally decreases, reaching a nadir in the late second trimester. Blood pressure then increases and may reach or surpass pre-pregnancy levels in the third trimester.
- Preconception assessment for patients with chronic hypertension should include studies for platelet count, creatinine, liver enzymes, and a quantitative measure of proteinuria to use as a baseline to compare in case superimposed preeclampsia develops in the upcoming pregnancy.
- Labetalol and nifedipine are first-line medications for chronic hypertension in pregnancy. ACE inhibitors, ARBs, and atenolol should not be prescribed to women of childbearing age, if possible.
- Fecundity begins to decline at 32 years of age and declines more sharply after 37. Rates of miscarriage also increase with age. At age 35, 20 percent of clinically recognized pregnancies will end in a first-trimester loss compared with

a 9–17 percent rate in women aged 20–30. This rate doubles to 40 percent at age 40.

- Patients who plan to deliver at age 35 or greater should be aware of the options for prenatal genetic diagnosis. Prenatal assessment for aneuploidy should be offered to all patients, regardless of age. However, with AMA patients, clinicians should be aware of the characteristics of the tests available.

- Pregnancies in women over 35 are at risk for other comorbidities such as gestational diabetes, hypertensive disorders, and cesarean delivery.

References

1. Roberts J, August P, Bakris G et al. *Hypertension in Pregnancy*. Chronic Hypertension in Pregnancy and Superimposed Preeclampsia. Washington, DC: American College of Obstetricians and Gynecologists; 2013. pp. 51–69.

2. American Medical Association. The seventh report of the Joint National Committee on Prevention, Detection, Evaluation, and Treatment of High Blood Pressure: the JNC 7 report. *JAMA* 2003;289(19):2560–2572.

3. Ankumah N, Sibai B. Chronic Hypertension in Pregnancy. *Clin Obstet Gynecol* 2017;60(1):206–214.

4. Practice Advisory on Low-Dose Aspirin and Prevention of Preeclampsia: Updated Recommendations – ACOG [Internet]. Acog.org. 2016 [cited November 6, 2016]. Available from: www.acog.org/about-acog/news-room/practice-advisories/practice-advisory-low-dose-aspirin-and-prevention-of-preeclampsia-updated-recommendations

5. Rakel (ed.). *Textbook of Family Medicine*, Ninth Edition. Philadelphia: Elsevier; 2016.

6. American College of Obstetricians and Gynecologists. Committee opinion No. 589. Female age-related fertility decline. *Obstet Gynecol* 2014;123 (3):719–721.

7. American College of Obstetricians and Gynecologists. Early pregnancy loss. Practice bulletin No. 150. *Obstet Gynecol* 2015;125(5):1258–1267.

8. American College of Obstetricians and Gynecologists. Screening for fetal aneuploidy. Practice bulletin No. 163. *Obstet Gynecol* 2016;127(5): e123–e137.

9. Dashe J. Aneuploidy screening in pregnancy. *Obstet Gynecol* 2016;128 (1):181–194.

10. Sauer M. Reproduction at an advanced maternal age and maternal health. *Fertil Steril* 2015;103(5):1136–1143.

A 30-Year-Old Woman with a History of Diabetes Controlled on Oral Agents Planning Pregnancy
(Counseling and Evaluation)

Saul D. Rivas

History of Present Illness

A 30-year-old, gravida 2, para 2, presents to clinic because she is interested in becoming pregnant. She has a three-year history of type 2 diabetes mellitus (T2DM) and has been treated with metformin 1,000 milligrams twice daily. She had good control of her glucose levels at her last checkup one year ago, but since then has not been performing self-monitoring. She has no other medical conditions, including known hypertension or cardiovascular disease. She does not exercise regularly, and although she has received nutritional counseling in the past, she does not adhere to healthy eating habits. Her only other medication is a daily combined oral contraceptive pill (COC) for contraception, and while on COCs she has been having regular periods every 28 days that are light and last 5 days. She denies any known drug allergies. She has had two previous vaginal deliveries, both complicated by gestational diabetes (GDM) but without complications during pregnancy or at delivery. She had no difficulty with fertility, and conceived within six months with each of her previous pregnancies once she discontinued her birth control pills. She is married and denies tobacco, alcohol, or drug use. She has a family history of type 2 diabetes mellitus and hypertension.

Physical Examination

General appearance	Well-developed, obese woman in no distress
Vital Signs	
Temperature	37.0°C
Pulse	80 beats/min
Blood pressure	125/85 mmHg
Respiratory rate	12 breaths/min
Oxygen saturation	100 percent on room air
Height	64 inches
Weight	175 pounds
BMI	30 kg/m^2
Abdomen	soft, non-distended, non-tender
Skin	mild acanthosis nigricans on the neck and axillae
Laboratory studies:	
HgbA1c	7.0 percent (53 mmol/mol)
Cr	0.6

How Would You Manage This Patient?

This patient has T2DM and her glycated hemoglobin (HgbA1c) of 7.0 percent shows she has not been optimally controlled on oral medication. Her weight, family history, and previous history of GDM are significant risk factors for her diagnosis. However, the only modifiable risk factor was her weight. She was, therefore, referred to a nutritionist for dietary counseling and started on an exercise regimen with the goal of reducing her weight. She received counseling on the importance of these interventions in achieving and maintaining a healthy pregnancy. Laboratory assessment of renal and thyroid function was performed using a complete metabolic panel and a thyroid-stimulating hormone measurement, respectively. Given that it had been a year since her last HgbA1c measurement, this was repeated and found to be higher at 8 percent. She was given education and supplies for daily glucose self-monitoring. She was also transitioned from metformin to an insulin regimen with a goal of decreasing her HgbA1c to less than 6.5 percent. She was referred to an ophthalmologist for a funduscopic exam. She was also started on a daily prenatal vitamin with 0.4 milligrams folic acid. After six months with the changes to her medication, diet, and physical activity level, her HgbA1c was 6 percent and she stopped her COC to attempt pregnancy.

Managing a Patient with Diabetes Who Is Planning Pregnancy

Pre-gestational Diabetes Counseling and Evaluation

Pre-gestational diabetes mellitus (PGDM), mainly T2DM, affects approximately 1 percent of pregnancies [5]. T2DM is characterized by a state of hyperglycemia due to insulin resistance. In contrast, T1DM is characterized by a deficiency in insulin due to destruction of the islet beta-cells in the pancreas. The prevalence of T2DM is thought to be increasing in part due to the increasing prevalence of obesity in worldwide populations. With the increase in the number of women with PGDM, it is also becoming more common to encounter patients on oral hypoglycemic medications in the preconception period or early in pregnancy. The metabolic issues associated with insulin resistance in T2DM can contribute to infertility due to ovulatory dysfunction, making glucose control important in the preconception period. Women with T2DM are at high risk for developing hypertension and preeclampsia among other complications.

Preconception counseling in women with PGDM has been demonstrated to minimize risks to the mother and the fetus through improved glycemic control [5]. Therefore, patients with PGDM should have a thorough evaluation when considering pregnancy. Evaluation should include a comprehensive history with the aim of optimizing glucose control as well as identifying and managing any comorbidities. Patients with T1DM have a higher risk of other autoimmune conditions such as hypothyroidism. Patients with T2DM have a higher risk of hypertension and hyperlipidemia. There are several well-documented risks that diabetic mothers face when pregnant. Type 1 DM is associated with more severe complications such as nephropathy, retinopathy, neuropathy, and ketoacidosis [1]. This is related to the typical earlier age of onset of T1DM, which makes it more likely that by the time a woman reaches her reproductive years, the disease process is in a more severe stage.

During pregnancy, complications from diabetes can affect both the embryo/fetus and/or the mother. Diabetic mothers have higher rates of first trimester miscarriage, congenital malformations, intrauterine fetal growth restriction, macrosomia, birth trauma, stillbirth, and iatrogenic preterm delivery [1]. In the neonate, the risk for complications such as hypoglycemia, polycythemia, hyperbilirubinemia, hypocalcemia, and morbidity/mortality from congenital malformations or severe prematurity is higher [1].

The likelihood of pregnancy complications due to PGDM is closely linked to blood glucose control both before and during pregnancy. The importance of glucose control in the preconception period has been demonstrated to improve perinatal outcomes and decrease the frequency of fetal anomalies. Patients who have normal or near normal HgbA1c values have similar baseline rates of fetal anomalies compared to nondiabetic patients. In contrast, women who have HgbA1c values of 10 percent or greater have a 20–25 percent rate of fetal anomalies [5]. The current recommendations for glycemic control in the preconception period is to achieve HgbA1c values <6.5 percent (48 mmol/mol). Women should be encouraged to perform self-monitoring of blood glucose levels fasting, 1 or 2 hours after the start of each meal, and at bedtime once they achieve pregnancy [3]. Fasting target glucose values should be ≤95 mg/dL (5.3 mmol/L) and ≤140 mg/dL and ≤120 mg/dL for 1 and 2 hour postprandial, respectively [3]. Currently, there are no recommendations for self-monitoring of glucose levels in the preconception period, unless they are on insulin therapy and already perform testing for this reason.

Counseling regarding exercise and nutrition is important for women with PGDM who are planning pregnancy. Obese and overweight women should receive nutritional counseling aimed at weight reduction. A focus on a balanced diet made up of lean meats, nonfat dairy products, vegetables and fruits, and whole grains is recommended. Caloric intake in pregnancy should be reduced by one-third of prepregnancy caloric intake while maintaining a minimum intake of 1,600–1,800 kcal/d [3]. A multivitamin with folic acid supplementation should be started at least a month prior to the patient attempting conception. Current recommendations are for 400 µg of folic acid daily for normal risk patients or 4 mg for patients who have had a previous pregnancy affected by a neural tube defect or take certain antiepileptic medications.

Women with PGDM who already exercise regularly should be encouraged to continue and those who do not should be encouraged to start an exercise program. The current recommendation is for pregnant patients to perform at least 150 minutes per week of moderate-intensity aerobic exercise (e.g., brisk walking) spread throughout the week as long as there are no contraindications [4]. Prior to conception, women should be encouraged and provided education on tobacco, alcohol, and illicit drugs cessation.

PGDM patients are often on oral hypoglycemic medications – typically metformin or glyburide. Although small studies suggest that the use of these medications in pregnancy is probably effective and safe, current recommendations are to use these medications with caution and on an individualized basis in pregnancy [5]. The use of insulin has been studied extensively in pregnancy and has been found to be safe and effective at the time of conception as well as during the pregnancy. In the preconception period, patients on oral hypoglycemics should be switched to insulin therapy to provide continuity into pregnancy to achieve glucose control while minimizing hypoglycemic events [1]. This is usually accomplished by administering a basal dose of long-acting insulin in combination with short-acting, bolus insulin before meals.

PGDM patients often also have other comorbidities such as hypertension, hyperlipidemia, or hypothyroidism. Therefore, it is important to review the other medications they are taking and modify them to minimize teratogenic effects, and providers should perform medication reconciliation with appropriate changes to medications that are safe in pregnancy [2]. Common hypertensive medications such as ACE inhibitors and angiotensin receptor blockers should be replaced with beta-blockers or calcium channel blockers such as labetalol or nifedipine prior to attempting conception. Statins should be discontinued in women with hyperlipidemia who are planning pregnancy due to the risk of contributing to congenital malformations.

Discontinuation of exposures such as tobacco, alcohol, and drug use should be encouraged. Measurement of height and weight with nutrition and exercise counseling should also be included. Laboratory testing to include screening for renal disease and establish baseline glucose levels should also take place. A discussion on the importance of these changes to the well-being of the patient and her future baby will build rapport and help facilitate a healthier pregnancy.

Key Points

- Preconception counseling in women with PGDM has been demonstrated to minimize risks to the mother and the fetus through improved glycemic control.
- In the preconception period, glucose control should be targeted to a HgbA1c of less than 6.5 percent.
- Obese and overweight women should receive nutritional counseling aimed at weight reduction.
- A multivitamin with folic acid supplementation should be started at least a month prior to the patient attempting conception. Current recommendations are for 400 µg of folic acid daily for normal risk patients.
- Patients should be encouraged to continue or start an exercise program. The current recommendation is for pregnant patients to perform at least 150 minutes per week of moderate intensity aerobic exercise (e.g., brisk walking) spread throughout the week.

- Patients on oral hypoglycemic medications – typically metformin or glyburide – should be switched to insulin therapy to provide continuity into pregnancy to achieve glucose control while minimizing hypoglycemic events prior to conception.
- A review of the patient's medications should be performed with the goal of transitioning to medications that are safe in pregnancy. ACE inhibitors and angiotensin receptor blockers should be replaced with beta-blockers or calcium channel blockers such as labetalol or nifedipine prior to attempting conception.
- Statins should be discontinued in women with hyperlipidemia who are planning pregnancy due to the risk of contributing to congenital malformations.
- Referral to an ophthalmologist should be made.

References

1. Pridjian G. Pregestional diabetes. *Obstet Gynecol Clin N Am* 2010;37:143–158.

2. American Diabetes Association. Management of diabetes in pregnancy. Sec. 13. In Standards of Medical Care in Diabetes. *Diabetes Care* 2017;40: S114–S119.

3. Blumer I, Hadar E, Hadden DR et al. Diabetes and pregnancy: an endocrine society clinical practice guideline. *J Clin Endocrinol Metab* 2013;98:4227–4249.

4. American College of Obstetricians and Gynecologists. Physical activity and exercise during pregnancy and the postpartum period. Committee opinion no. 650. *Obstet Gynecol* 2015;126: e135–e142.

5. American College of Obstetricians and Gynecologists. Pregestational diabetes mellitus. Practice Bulletin No. 60. *Obstet Gynecol* 2005;105:675–685.

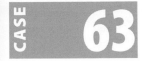

A 14-Year-Old Adolescent with a Large Labia

Roshanak Zinn

History of Present Illness

A 14-year-old female presents to your office complaining of a one-year history of vaginal discomfort and irritation. She reports her labia have been enlarging to the point where she now has discomfort wearing swimsuits or certain clothes. She feels a rubbing sensation when she walks, and sometimes her labia stick to her underwear. She usually removes all hair from her vulva by shaving. She does not have any rash, redness, or vaginal discharge. Her mother has seen the area and thinks it does not look normal.

Privately, the patient tells you that she has never been sexually active.

She denies any history of medical problems or any surgical history. She reports her menarche was at age 12 years, and her periods are regular. She is in eighth grade and is active in volleyball.

Physical Examination

General appearance	Well-developed adolescent in no distress
Respiratory	nonlabored respirations
Abdomen	soft, non-tender, non-distended
Breast	Tanner V, symmetric, no lumps
Pelvic	Normal external genital anatomy without rashes or lesions
	Tanner IV pubic hair
	Normal intact annular hymen
	No vaginal discharge or erythema
	Mildly asymmetric labia minora, right greater than left
	On stretch, the right labium measures 5 cm from midline and the left labium measures 4 cm from midline
	Wet prep: negative for clue cells, hyphae, or motile trichomonads

How Would You Manage the Patient?

This patient has mild labial hypertrophy, which is a normal variation and is not pathologic. In addition, she has no evidence of yeast vaginitis or other condition that may cause vulvovaginal discomfort.

The initial management involved reassuring the patient and her mother of the wide variety of normal vulvar anatomy. She was directed to resources online and in print to view images of normal vulvar anatomic variations. For her discomfort and vulvar irritation, she was advised to make some behavioral modifications, such as wearing looser clothing and supportive underwear. In addition, she was advised to avoid irritants in her personal hygiene regimen, such as harsh or scented soaps, scented pads or panty liners, detergents, and certain hair removal methods that can cause vulvar irritation. She was also advised to use a topical, over-the-counter barrier ointment such as petroleum jelly or zinc oxide to reduce chaffing.

At her follow-up visit, her symptoms of irritation had resolved, and she had no additional concerns.

Labial Hypertrophy in Adolescents

Increasing numbers of girls and women are seeking care due to concerns about genital appearance. Possible reasons for the increased attention to this area include increased access to images of genital anatomy online, trends in removal of pubic hair with resultant increased awareness of variation in genital anatomy, and awareness of the availability of labial cosmetic surgery [1, 2].

Usual patient concerns include pain or chronic irritation of the vulva, discomfort wearing certain clothing, concern that there is a "bulge" appearance that can be seen through clothing, embarrassment when changing clothes in front of peers, or self-consciousness with sexual activity. Parents may bring children to be seen for this condition when the adolescent's anatomy appears different from her parent's expectation of normal.

Labial hypertrophy is a poorly defined and subjective condition. When measured on stretch from the midline, labial size is known to vary greatly, from approximately 1 to 5 cm [3]. There is no consensus on what labial size constitutes hypertrophy or "abnormal" labia; however, most studies on labiaplasty have defined their own minimum measurements that diagnose labial hypertrophy, with variation between 3 cm and 5 cm [4].

In adolescents with symptoms of external vaginal irritation, the differential diagnosis includes vulvovaginitis due to yeast, bacterial vaginosis, or trichomoniasis, as well as vulvar dermatoses such as lichen sclerosus. In patients who complain solely of anatomic concerns or "extra skin" in the vulvar area, the differential includes anatomic abnormalities such as clitoromegaly, overgrowth of mucosal tissues such as hymenal tags or hymenal septa, and vulvar cysts such as Bartholin's gland cysts.

The initial workup for vulvar irritation in the setting of concern for labial hypertrophy should include a thorough history, with specific attention to symptoms of irritation, itching, and effect of symptoms on daily activities. Physical examination should include a thorough external genital exam with careful attention to all vulvar and vaginal anatomy and the relationship between vulvar structures. An evaluation for yeast, bacterial vaginosis, and trichomoniasis should be performed with a wet prep in patients who have symptoms of discharge or irritation.

Once the diagnosis has been confirmed and underlying infectious or dermatologic conditions have been ruled out,

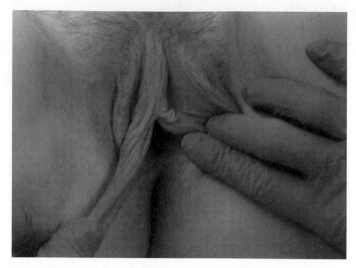

Figure 63.1 An adolescent patient with severe right labial hypertrophy (over 10 cm on stretch) that caused significant quality of life issues (preventing her from wearing jeans or riding a bike) despite conservative measures, including use of topical emollients.

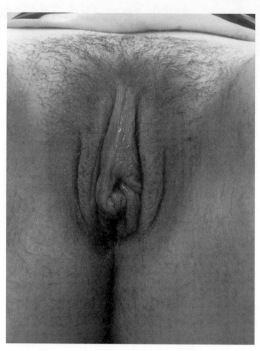

Figure 63.2 The immediate postoperative appearance of the patient in Figure 63.1 after linear resection. Note the entire labia minora was not removed but was resected to be similar to the left side.

the management of patients presenting with labial hypertrophy should be tailored to the presenting complaint. Patients who present with symptoms of discomfort can be counseled to wear clothing that is less form-fitting, wear supportive undergarments, make adaptations during exercise to increase comfort, improve personal hygiene to decrease irritation, or use topical emollients if there is chronic external irritation. The current trends of pubic hair removal and resultant exposure and irritation of labia can be discussed, and patients who shave or otherwise remove their pubic hair should be discouraged from continuing this practice.

If the primary concern is about labial appearance, the first step should be patient reassurance about a wide variety of normal vulvar appearances. Patients can be referred to a number of resources such as websites that have a variety of photographs of normal vulvar anatomy for comparison [11, 12]. Patients can also be reassured that increases in labial size during the pubertal years are common. Informative handouts and displays can help patients view variations in labial anatomy [5–7]. If there is concern for excessive preoccupation with a minor physical abnormality, the patient should be screened for body dysmorphic disorder using a standardized questionnaire or referred to a mental health professional [8, 13].

Labial Surgery in Adolescents

In recent years, increasing awareness about labiaplasty in the general population has led to an increase in requests for this procedure. In adolescent patients, surgery is performed only in extreme cases, as in the patient depicted in Figure 63.1, and should be performed by a practitioner with experience in labial surgery. Labial surgery exclusively for cosmetic purposes should not be performed in an adolescent population [1, 9].

There are multiple labial reduction techniques described in the literature. Two common variations are of linear resection (either straight or curvilinear) along the edge of the labia minora and wedge resection or de-epithelialization. The linear resection techniques will result in a linear scar along the exposed edge of

the labia minora. Wedge resection techniques have the benefit of preserving the natural edge of the labia minora [9, 10] but may have a higher rate of complications. Figure 63.2 demonstrates the immediate postoperative appearance of a patient who underwent a linear resection of the right labia minora.

Typical surgical risks include scarring, dyspareunia, altered sensation during sexual intercourse, dissatisfaction with appearance, and regrowth of labia minora, especially if the procedure is performed at a young age. Typical complications would include bleeding, wound breakdown, and infection. There are studies reporting an overall low rate of complications and high patient satisfaction; however, these studies are often retrospective surveys of complications and satisfaction rates and lack long-term follow-up data [9].

Key Teaching Points

- There is a wide variation in normal external genital anatomy.
- Labial hypertrophy is poorly defined but typically considered when the labia minor measure greater than 5 cm on stretch.
- In adolescents, the first approach to concerns about labial hypertrophy should be reassurance about anatomic variations and conservative measures aimed at symptom management.
- Body dysmorphic disorder should be considered in individuals presenting with concerns about genital appearance and be screened for using available screening questionnaires.
- Labial surgery in adolescents is reserved for extreme, medically indicated cases and should not be performed for cosmetic purposes alone.

References

1. Committee on Adolescent Health Care. Committee Opinion No. 686: Breast and Labial Surgery in Adolescents. *Obstet Gynecol* 2017 January;129(1): e17–e19.

2. Bercaw-Pratt JL, Santos XM, Sanchez J et al. The incidence, attitudes and practices of the removal of pubic hair as a body modification. *J Pediatr Adolesc Gynecol* 2012 February;25(1):12–14.

3. Lloyd J, Crouch NS, Minto CL et al. Female genital appearance: "normality" unfolds. *BJOG Int J Obstet Gynaecol* 2005;112:643–646.

4. Clerico C, Lari A, Mojallal A, et al. Anatomy and aesthetics of the labia minora: the ideal vulva? *Aesthetic Plast Surg* 2017 March 10. doi: 10.1007/s00266-017–0831-1. Epub ahead of print.

5. NASPAG Handouts for Patients. Labial Hypertrophy. http://c.ymcdn.com/sites/www.naspag.org/resource/resmgr/Patient/Labial_Hypertrophy_Patient_H.pdf, accessed 4/2017.

6. www.nickkarras.com/petals-book.html

7. www.greatwallofvagina.co.uk/home

8. Brohede S, Wingren G, Wijma B et al. Validation of the body dysmorphic disorder questionnaire in a community sample of Swedish women. *Psychiatry Res* 2013 December 15;210(2): 647–652.

9. Runacres SA, Wood PL. Cosmetic labiaplasty in an adolescent population. *J Pediatr Adolesc Gynecol* 2016 June;29 (3):218–222.

10. Reddy J, Laufer MR. Hypertrophic labia minora. *J Pediatr Adolesc Gynecol* 2010 February;23(1):3–6.

11. www.greatwallofvagina.co.uk/home

12. www.labialibrary.org.au/

13. http://bddfoundation.org/helping-you/questionnaires/

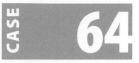

A 16-Year-Old Adolescent with Acne, Hirsutism, and Irregular Menses

Eduardo Lara-Torre

History of Present Illness

A 16-year-old old nulligravid female presents to your office for acne, excessive hair growth, and irregular menses. She reports menarche at age 13, with initial regular bleeding every 28 days that would last for 5 days. For the last 12 months, her menses have become irregular, with intervals between 28 and 90 days. Her menses have also become heavier and last 7–9 days. Her last menstrual period was six weeks ago. She denies any recent or prior sexual activity.

Over the past year, she reports an increase in hair growth on her face, lower back, and around her umbilicus, and she has to shave her legs more often. She denies deepening of the voice, but has noticed her acne is worsening. She currently has facial and upper back acne that is not responding to oral antibiotics or over-the-counter topical therapy. She reports a weight gain of 15 pounds in the past year, although she denies significant changes in her diet or activity level.

Her family history is significant for hypertension on her father's side and diet-controlled diabetes in her mother. She denies any other significant cardiovascular disease or history of deep vein thrombosis.

Physical Examination

General appearance	Well-appearing, no acute distress, overweight

Vital Signs

Temperature	98.5°F (36.9°C)
Blood pressure	110/65 mmHg
Pulse	64 beats/minute
Respiration	20 breaths/minute
Weight	185 pounds
Height	5 ft 3 in
BMI	32.8 kg/m²
Cardiovascular	Regular rate and rhythm without murmurs, rubs, or gallops
Lungs	Clear to auscultation bilaterally, no wheezing
Abdomen	Soft, non-tender, non-distended. Bowel sounds are present
Pelvic	Deferred
Skin	Moderate inflammatory acne lesions in different stages of healing on the face, neck, upper back, and upper chest, with signs of scarring around the mandible. Acanthosis nigricans of the back of the neck and the folds of the arms. Increased amount of hair in the upper lip and chin, as well as the sideburns. Shaved hair follicles around the areola bilaterally, suprapubic and upper abdomen, as well as on her lower back. Both arms and legs are shaved.

Laboratory Studies

Urine pregnancy test	Negative
FSH	4.8 mIU/mL (4.7–21.5 mIU/mL)
Testosterone	78 ng/dL (< 55 ng/dL)
17-hydroxy progesterone	80 ng/dL (<200 ng/dL)
DHEAS	250 mcg/dL (37–307 mcg/dL)
TSH	1.55 uIU/mL (0.51–4.94 uIU/mL)
Prolactin	19 ng/mL (2.8–29.2 ng/mL)

Imaging

A transabdominal pelvic ultrasound was performed showing a 7 cm uterus with normal ovarian size and appearance. Three to four sub-centimeter ovarian cysts were seen bilaterally. There was no free fluid in the pelvis.

How Would You Manage This Patient?

This patient underwent laboratory and imaging examinations to rule out specific medical conditions that could cause irregular menses and androgen excess. Given the lack of specific findings and the mild elevation of testosterone, the diagnosis of polycystic ovarian syndrome (PCOS) can be presumed. Although she has acanthosis nigricans, suspicious for hyperinsulinemia, insulin level testing was not performed, as it would not significantly change initial management. She was, however, tested for metabolic syndrome, including screening for diabetes with a two-hour glucose tolerance test and lipid profile screening, which were both negative.

The patient was prescribed combined oral contraceptive pills to regulate her menses and decrease the circulating free testosterone that causes her acne and hirsutism. She was advised on nonmedical interventions for hair removal, including depilation (above the skin) and epilation (beneath the skin) methods to help remove the already present hair. In addition to the hormonal management, the patient was counseled regarding the importance of healthy lifestyle, including calorie intake restriction and modification, as well as increase in physical activity. A referral to a dietician and the physical therapy group at the local gym was made.

At her six-month follow-up, she reports regular, light menses without cramping. She is following a low carbohydrate diet and walking an extra 30 minutes a few times a week, and she has lost 5 pounds. She reports her acne is much improved, as it is now only on her face and responds to topical therapy. She has not seen an increase in hair growth, and after undergoing frequent waxing, she has seen a better cosmetic result on her facial and abdominal hair.

Polycystic Ovarian Syndrome in Adolescents

Polycystic ovarian syndrome (PCOS) affects 6–15 percent of reproductive-age women and is responsible for more than 70 percent of cases of hyperandrogenism [1, 2]. Although its origin is not clear, evidence suggests PCOS is caused by an interaction of inherited traits, environmental factors, alterations in steroids and metabolism, and adaptations of excess energy supply [3, 4]. Although the criteria in adults have been well established to include polycystic ovarian morphology (PCOM), anovulation, and hyperandrogenism [5], the diagnosis of the condition in adolescents is controversial. The findings associated in adults are common normal findings in adolescents and are not necessarily diagnostic of PCOS. In order to establish better guidelines in the diagnosis and management of patients with suspected PCOS, multiple medical societies and its representatives created consensus guidelines in an attempt to unify specialists caring for these patients [6].

The evaluation of patients with suspected PCOS should include a complete personal and family history as well as appropriate laboratory testing to rule out other conditions, including nonclassical adrenal hyperplasia (see Box 64.1). Androgen excess in adolescents generally presents with hirsutism, moderate inflammatory acne, and menstrual irregularities. Mild facial hirsutism and acne are normally present in adolescents in their postpubertal stage and are not considered clinical evidence of hyperandrogenism. On the other hand, moderate or severe acne and hirsutism require laboratory evaluation before initiating therapy. Available assays to evaluate androgen levels have not been consistently reliable to measure levels in children and women. Each available measuring system has established normative levels, and abnormal values would depend on the assay utilized. Measurement of total and/or free testosterone seems the most widely available test for androgen assessment and can be used to determine hyperandrogenism in adolescents. Elevated androgens, without clinical findings, should not be considered hyperandrogenism in adolescents [6].

Irregular menses are most often the result of anovulatory cycles, which are common within the first two years after menarche and are not necessarily caused by PCOS or androgen excess. Patients who have persistent cycle lengths of less than 20 days or greater than 45 days after the first two years postmenarche warrant an evaluation. Similarly, patients with recurrent cycles greater than 90 days apart, or who started menses after age 15 (or 2–3 years after thelarche), should be assessed for PCOS. Patients presenting with oligomenorrhea or amenorrhea may benefit from follicle-stimulating hormone (FSH) testing to evaluate for premature ovarian insufficiency.

Unlike adults, the presence of multiple follicles in the ovary is not considered a diagnostic criterion for PCOS and can be a normal finding in adolescents. Data regarding ovarian morphology come from ultrasounds performed via the transvaginal approach, which is not commonly performed in non-sexually active adolescents. Obesity in these patients makes the transabdominal images not reliable, and could provide inaccurate information. For these reasons, ultrasound is not

Box 64.1 Laboratory testing in the evaluation of patients with suspected polycystic ovarian syndrome

FSH+

HCG

Testosterone (free and/or total)

17-OHP*

SHBG

DHEAS

Androstenedione

TSH

Prolactin

Fasting and 2-hour 75 g oral glucose tolerance test

Fasting lipid profile

FSH: follicle-stimulating hormone; LH: luteinizing hormone; HCG: human chorionic gonadotropin; 17-OHP: 17-hydroxyprogesterone; SHBG: steroid hormone binding globulin, DHEAS: dehydroepiandrosterone sulfate; TSH: thyroid-stimulating hormone.

+ Performed in the setting of oligomenorrhea and amenorrhea
* Performed in the morning

included as diagnostic criteria in this population during the evaluation for PCOS.

Patients suspected of having PCOS may also have clinical (acanthosis nigricans) and laboratory evidence of hyperinsulinemia. This condition is common in adolescents and should not play a role in the diagnosis of PCOS; however, detection of impaired glucose tolerance may be an opportunity to address the long-term effects of the condition, including diabetes and metabolic syndrome. This will allow initiating evaluations for these comorbidities, and placing interventions to improve the metabolic disturbances, including lifestyle modifications with diet and exercise. To address these concerns, screening for glucose intolerance and lipid abnormalities is indicated. A fasting and two-hour 75 g load glucose tolerance test and a fasting lipid profile will allow for early identification and management of the comorbidities.

Management of menstrual irregularity and the symptoms related to androgen excess is generally the main concern for these patients [8, 9]. Cyclic administration of combined estrogen-progesterone oral contraceptive pills (COC) is considered the first-line management for most adolescents [10]. By suppressing ovarian function, androgen production decreases. In addition, circulating estrogen increases the production of steroid hormone binding globulin (SHBG), thus decreasing free testosterone and its end organ effects. The cyclic shedding of the endometrium prevents the long-term effects of chronic anovulation, including endometrial hyperplasia and cancer, and provides reliable scheduled menses. Those with contraindications to estrogen may use progesterone-only products, but the reduction in circulating androgen is less.

Although COC has a significant impact in new hair growth and future outbreaks of acne, hair that is already present may still require mechanical and chemical treatment. For refractory cases, other medications, such as spironolactone, may be utilized as an adjuvant to further decrease hirsutism. Adjuvant use of chemical and mechanical hair removal methods is also recommended.

Along with hormonal management, lifestyle modifications, including weight loss, are beneficial to manage PCOS and the long-term effects of the condition. Menstrual irregularities respond well to weight loss through diet and exercise, and should also be utilized as first-line treatment, particularly in patients with obesity. A reduction of as little as 6.5 percent of total body weight has been shown to return menstrual regularity [11]. The use of insulin sensitizing agents, such as metformin, has been used in adolescents to manage the metabolic disturbance present in adolescents, and is best reserved for those with concomitant glucose impairment [8]. Contraceptive needs for the adolescent should also play a role in the treatment selection, as many of these patients may wrongly perceive they are unable to conceive given their anovulatory cycles.

Key Teaching Points

1. There is significant overlap between the normal changes associated with puberty and the findings associated with PCOS, making its diagnosis difficult in adolescents.
2. PCOS is a diagnosis of exclusion, and the proper evaluation for the other conditions presenting in a similar fashion should be performed.
3. When selecting management options, addressing both the immediate needs (menstrual regulation and decrease in acne and hair growth) as well as the potential long-term effects of the adolescent (metabolic syndrome, infertility) are warranted.
4. The use of combined oral contraceptive pills is considered first-line therapy for the treatment of adolescents with PCOS.
5. Lifestyle modifications (diet and exercise) should also be included in the initial approach to PCOS.
6. Obesity, hyperinsulinemia, and insulin resistance are not part of the diagnostic criteria for adolescents with suspected PCOS, but they should be screened for and addressed in the context of long-term disease prevention.

References

1. Fauser BC, Tarlatzis RW, Rebar RS et al. Consensus on women's health aspects of polycystic ovary syndrome (PCOS): the Amsterdam ESHRE/ASRM-sponsored 3rd PCOS consensus workshop group. *Fertil Steril* 2012;97:28–38.e25.

2. Carmina E, Rosato F, Janni A, Rizzo M, Longo RA. Extensive clinical experience: relative prevalence of different androgen excess disorders in 950 women referred because of clinical hyperandrogenism. *J Clin Endocrinol Metab* 2006;91:2–6.

3. Rosenfield RL. Identifying children at risk of polycystic ovary syndrome. *J Clin Endocrinol Metab* 2007;92:787–796.

4. Franks S. Polycystic ovary syndrome in adolescents. *Int J Obes (Lond)* 2008;32:1035–1041.

5. Johnson T, Kaplan L, Ouyang P, Rizza R. National Institutes of Health Evidence-Based Methodology Workshop on Polycystic Ovary Syndrome (PCOS). *NIH EbMW Report. Bethesda, National Institutes of Health* 2012;1:1–14.

6. Witchel SF, Oberfield S, Rosenfield RL et al. The diagnosis of polycystic ovary syndrome during adolescence. *Horm Res Paediatr* 2015;83:376–389.

7. American College of Obstetricians and Gynecologists. Polycystic ovary syndrome. ACOG practice bulletin no. 194. *Obstet Gynecol* 2018; 131:e157–71.

8. Javed A, Chelvakumar G, Bonny AE. Polycystic ovary syndrome in adolescents: a review of past year evidence. *Curr Opin Obstet Gynecol* 2016;28:373–380.

9. Rosenfield RL. The diagnosis of polycystic ovary syndrome in adolescents. *Pediatrics* 2015;136:1154–1165.

10. Legro RS, Arslanian SA, Ehrmann DA et al. Diagnosis and treatment of polycystic ovary syndrome: An endocrine society clinical practice guideline. *J Clin Endocrinol Metab* 2013;98: 4565–4592.

11. Ornstein RM, Copperman NM, Jacobson MS. Effect of weight loss on menstrual function in adolescents with polycystic ovary syndrome. *J Pediatr Adolesc Gynecol* 2011;24:161–165.

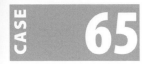

65 An Eight-Year-Old Girl with Persistent Vulvar Itching

Laura A. Parks

History of Present Illness

An eight-year-old girl presents with her mother with complaints of persistent vulvar itching. The girl has been seen by her pediatrician several times for this complaint without improvement of her symptoms. The girl states that she just cannot stop scratching because her vulva is so intensely itchy. Her mother reports that the patient has been scratching and rubbing her vulva more frequently over the last few months, and the discomfort seems to be worse at night. The mother and daughter deny any odor or discharge on the girl's underwear. The girl has been treated empirically for yeast infections twice and for bacterial infection once, but her mother states that the pediatrician was unable to find a source of the itching and that all the swabs and cultures have been negative. None of the treatments have helped, and the mother thought that the cream to treat a yeast infection made the girl's vulva burn and feel more painful.

The girl has had no medical problems. Prior surgery includes tonsillectomy at age five years. She has no known allergies and does not take any medications other than a daily vitamin. She was delivered vaginally at full term and has met all her developmental and physical milestones. She is doing well in third grade. She lives at home with her mother, father, and younger brother, and there is no concern for sexual abuse.

Physical Examination

General appearance	Well-appearing, well-nourished child

Vital Signs

Temperature	37.0°C
Pulse	85 beats/min
Respiratory rate	22 breaths/min
BP	90/64 mmHg
Weight	64 pounds
Height	49 inches
BMI	18.7 kg/m²
Abdomen	Soft, non-tender, non-distended
Breasts	Tanner 1

Gynecologic Exam

External genitalia	Prepubertal, Tanner Stage 1. Hypopigmentation from clitoral hood to perineum and spreading around perianal region with sharp borders. Tissue appears paper thin (see Figure 65.1).
Labia	Normal appearing in size and shape. Mild ecchymosis and superficial erosions noted on lower aspect of labia minora/majora.
Urethral meatus	Normal size and location, no lesions, no prolapse.
Urethra	No masses, no tenderness.

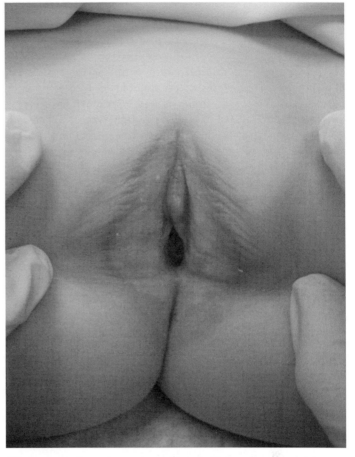

Figure 65.1 Lichen sclerosus in prepubertal girl. Courtesy of Diane Merritt

Bladder	No masses, no tenderness.
Vagina	Visualized, no abnormal discharge. Hymen appreciated with normal prepubertal appearance, appropriate hygiene.
Anus/perineum	Thin, hypopigmented skin.

Laboratory Studies (from Outside Pediatrician)

Vaginal bacterial culture	Normal flora
Fungal culture	Negative

How Would You Manage This Patient?

The patient has lichen sclerosus (LS), the diagnosis of which is based on clinical symptoms and physical examination. When LS is diagnosed in a child, the physician must first describe the disease to the patient and her parent and explain how to treat it. The goal is to preserve normal anatomy and help minimize pruritic symptoms. Vulvar biopsy is not indicated at this time and should only be done if LS is refractory to treatment or the diagnosis is in doubt.

This patient was treated with a high-potency corticosteroid ointment, clobetasol 0.05 percent, applied in a thin layer to the affected area twice daily. In addition to this pharmacological treatment, good vulvar care was recommended, including minimizing the use of any harsh soaps, body wash, harsh detergents, and/or dryer sheets. Further, oral diphenhydramine (25 mg every 6 hours) was recommended to relieve her pruritus symptoms. She was instructed to follow-up four weeks later, at which time her symptoms and clinical exam findings were resolved. The topical corticosteroids were tapered to a lower-potency steroid for two weeks, followed by 1 percent hydrocortisone ointment, to use daily. The patient was instructed to follow up every 6–12 months for intermittent monitoring of disease and to call if symptoms returned. This patient continued to have an excellent response to the steroid ointment taper and remained symptom-free six months later.

Childhood Lichen Sclerosus

LS is a benign inflammatory dermatologic skin condition primarily affecting the anogenital region in children. It is chronic, progressive, and characterized by marked inflammation, epithelial thinning, and skin changes. Although genital LS primarily occurs in postmenopausal women, about 10–15 percent of cases are in prepubertal children [1]. This bimodal age distribution appears to correlate with hypoestrogenic physiologic states. The etiology of LS is unclear, but it is accepted as an autoimmune disorder. LS has been associated with other autoimmune diseases such as alopecia, vitiligo, type 1 diabetes, and autoimmune thyroiditis [2].

Children with LS typically present with symptoms of intense pruritus, vulvar irritation or pain, dysuria, bleeding from excoriations from scratching, and painful bowel movements. The itching and irritation can be so intense that the patients cannot stop scratching. The irritation and discomfort also tend to be worse at night. Oftentimes, these patients are misdiagnosed as having other conditions with similar symptoms, such as urinary tract infections, pinworms, and/or yeast infections.

The diagnosis of LS in the pediatric population is based on history and physical exam. The differential diagnosis for LS includes lichen planus, vitiligo, psoriasis, eczema, and contact dermatitis. Classic vulvar LS appears as hypopigmented (white or pink) plaques with distinct borders. The tissue can become paper thin and is sometimes described as being similar to parchment paper or cigarette paper. The affected region most frequently surrounds the labia majora and minora but can also extend past the perineum and surround the anus. This pattern is typically referred to as a key-hole or figure-of-eight pattern. Figure 65.1 demonstrates the typical appearance of LS in a pediatric patient.

Scratching or rubbing may induce vulvar purpura with ecchymoses or fissures. If left untreated, scarring can occur, resulting in labial fusion, buried clitoris, and narrowing of the vaginal introitus [3]. The vagina is not affected by LS.

In children, biopsy should be conducted only if the condition is not improved with treatment or if the diagnosis is unclear [4]. Of note, LS is sometimes mistakenly diagnosed as sexual abuse, as they can share similar physical exam findings. As these two diagnoses can coincide, it is important to take a thorough history, and if there are any concerns for abuse, the child should be evaluated by a health-care provider trained in child abuse evaluation and management.

Treatment goals for LS are primarily medical and include suppression of symptoms and resolution of the signs of the disease, including atrophy, hyperkeratosis, fissuring, and ecchymosis. The most commonly used medication for treatment of LS is a topical super-potency corticosteroid ointment, such as clobetasol propionate 0.05 percent or betamethasone valerate 0.1 percent [5]. Few studies have evaluated the efficacy of topical steroids for LS in the pediatric population; however, a 2011 Cochrane Review by Chi et al. included a small number of pediatric patients [6]. Although the authors were unable to make specific recommendations for children, the evidence indicated that topical steroids were more effective than placebo, and clinical experience and subsequent studies appear to confirm that topical corticosteroids should be considered first-line therapy in these patients. To improve absorption and decrease risk of contact dermatitis, ointments rather than creams are recommended for the application of these steroids. The ointment should be applied sparingly to the affected area twice daily.

After a month of use, the patients typically become asymptomatic, as occurred in the above patient, and can begin to taper off the clobetasol ointment. This can be done in several ways, and there is no clear consensus on the optimal regimen. Some advocate decreasing to daily application of the clobetasol ointment for two weeks, then twice a week for two weeks. The patient is then instructed to either use a once weekly maintenance dose or to resume treatment with any flares. Other alternatives to a clobetasol taper include switching to a mid-potency steroid for two weeks, followed by a daily maintenance dose of hydrocortisone 1 percent ointment, with methylprednisolone aceponate 0.1 percent ointment used on the weekends [7]. It is thought by some experts that continued low- or mid-potency topical corticosteroid steroid use should be continued until puberty to prevent recurrence, progression, and scarring.

Topical calcineurin inhibitor therapy with tacrolimus or pimecrolimus has been reported as a successful adjunctive treatment for LS, particularly for maintenance therapy; however, it has not been shown to be effective as initial therapy. In addition, an FDA black box warning indicated a possible relationship between its long-term use and skin cancer and lymphoma.

Surgical management is not indicated for first-line treatment of LS. However, surgery may be an option for patients with long-standing untreated or refractory disease who have developed significant scarring that causes pain, urinary tract retention, or dyspareunia. As this is a rare procedure to treat the end-stage tissue damage of LS, it is best to refer to a specialist with experience in treating this complication. It is advised that the underlying LS be well-controlled prior to moving forward with surgical management, and the patient should be educated on the need to continue topical steroid ointment therapy after surgery to prevent recurrence of disease.

LS is a chronic dermatologic condition of the vulva that can recur even after appropriate treatment. The rates of recurrence for LS in children have been reported to range from almost half to nearly 80 percent after treatment [8]. Even during symptom-free periods of time, changes in the appearance of the vulva can be noted. In adults, there is a small increased risk of developing squamous cell carcinoma with LS. It is unknown if there is a similar risk for young girls diagnosed with LS [9]. Close follow-up is therefore recommended for patients with vulvar LS. In children with LS, long-term follow-up with a gynecologist is recommended every 6–12 months to monitor for symptoms and evaluate for recurrence.

Key Teaching Points

1. LS can be diagnosed in the pediatric population based on symptoms and appearance on physical exam, with vulvar biopsy reserved only for those cases refractory to treatment or atypical appearing lesions.

2. Initial therapy for LS should begin with a high-potency topical steroid ointment, such as clobetasol 0.05 percent, and continued until symptoms are resolved. Steroids may then be tapered, and maintenance therapy with a low-potency topical steroid may be considered to prevent recurrence.

3. Surgical management is rarely indicated and should only be performed in patients with severe architectural changes that result in significant pain or recurrent infection.

4. Follow-up for children with LS should occur every 6–12 months with a gynecologist to monitor symptoms and evaluate for recurrence.

References

1. Powell J. Wonjnarowska F. Childhood vulvar lichen sclerosus: an increasingly common problem. *J Am Acad Dermatol* 2001;44:803.

2. Lagerstedt M Karvinen K. Joki-Errila M. Childhood lichen sclerosus, a challenge for clinicians. *Pediatr Dermatol* 2013;30:444.

3. Bercaw-Pratt JL, Boardman LA, Simms-Cendan JS, North American Society for Pediatric and Adolescent Gynecology: Clinical recommendation: pediatric lichen sclerosus. *J Pediatr Adolesc Gynecol* 2014 April;27:111–116.

4. Dendrinos ML, Quint EH. Lichen sclerosus in children and adolescents. *Curr Opin Obstet Gynecol* 2013 October;25:370–374.

5. Casey GA, Cooper SM, Powell JJ. Treatment of vulvar lichen sclerosus with topical corticosteroids in children: a study of 72 children. *Clin Exp Dermatol* 2015;40:289.

6. Chi CC, Kirtschig G, Baldo M et al. Topical interventions for genital lichen sclerosus. *Cochrane Database Syst Rev* 2001; (12) CD008240.

7. Dinh H, Purcell SM, Chung C, Zaenglein AL. Pediatric lichen sclerosus: a review of the literature and management recommendations. *J Clin Aesthet Dermatol* 2016;9(9):49–54.

8. Smith, SD, Fischer, G. Childhood onset of vulvar lichen sclerosus does not resolve at puberty: a prospective case series. *Pediatr Dermatol* 2009;26:725.

9. Tong LX, Sun GS, Teng JM. Pediatric lichen sclerosus: A review of the epidemiology and treatment options. *Pediatr Dermatol* 2015 September–October;32(5):593–599. doi: 10.1111/pde.12615. Epub May 4, 2015.

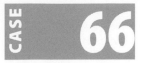

A Four-Year-Old Girl with Recurrent Vulvar Discharge and Itching

Sarah H. Milton

History of Present Illness

A four-year-old girl is referred from her pediatrician for evaluation of vaginal discharge. The discharge has been occurring on and off for several months. She also complains of itching and occasional burning pain associated with the discharge. She denies vaginal bleeding, abdominal pain, dysuria, or any other associated symptoms, and she has no recent history of upper respiratory infection. She is accompanied by her mother who confirms this history and adds that the discharge has a foul odor. The patient has been treated with oral fluconazole as well as oral metronidazole, but there has been no improvement in her symptoms.

She lives at home with her younger brother, mother, and father. The mother and patient both deny any abuse history or concerns for victimization. She attends preschool during the day. She is healthy and takes no medications.

Physical Examination

General appearance   Well-appearing child, alert and oriented, not in acute distress

Vital Signs

Temperature	37.0°C
Pulse	102 beats per minute
Blood pressure	90/65 mmHg
Respiratory rate	22 breaths/minute
Oxygen saturation	100 percent on room air
Height	32 inches
Weight	42 lb
BMI	20 kg/m^2
Abdomen	Soft, non-tender, non-distended, no masses, no rebound or guarding
Breasts	Tanner Stage 1
Genitourinary	Tanner Stage 1 pubic hair. Scant white discharge and mild erythema on bilateral labia and surrounding vaginal introitus. Normal hymen and distal vagina without discharge. No blood or foreign body noted. Vaginal mucosa thin and atrophic appearing consistent with prepubertal status.

Laboratory Studies

Saline microscopy	Normal
Culture	Mixed urogenital flora

How Would You Manage This Patient?

This patient has nonspecific vulvovaginitis. Her history is not suggestive of sexual abuse, and neither her history nor examination showed any evidence of a retained foreign body in the vagina. Culture of the discharge is negative for a specific bacterial pathogen. Given the suspected diagnosis of nonspecific vulvovaginitis, the patient and her mother were carefully educated on hygiene measures including front-to-back wiping, good handwashing, and daily soaks in a clean warm bath followed by a topical barrier ointment nightly. These measures resulted in improvement of her discharge and itching within 48 hours, and at a two-month follow-up visit, she was symptom free.

Nonspecific Vulvovaginitis in Children

Vaginal discharge is one of the most common reasons that prepubertal girls seek gynecologic care. While newborns and neonates may have some physiologic leukorrhea due to maternal estrogen, vaginal discharge in childhood is pathologic. The interval between the neonatal period and puberty is characterized by a hypoestrogenic state with resultant changes in the vaginal mucosa and bacterial flora of the vagina. These changes predispose girls in this age group to colonization of the vagina with oropharyngeal or gastrointestinal bacteria that can proliferate and cause discharge. This colonization is further hastened by poor hygiene practices in young children, including improper toileting, wiping, and handwashing practices.

The differential diagnosis of a child with vaginal discharge includes infection with a specific pathogen, abuse with resultant infection, or vulvar dermatoses, including lichen sclerosus. Importantly, vulvovaginal candidiasis and bacterial vaginosis do not commonly occur in prepubertal girls, and treatment for these conditions should not be undertaken in this age group. The differential diagnosis of a child with vaginal discharge also includes a retained vaginal foreign body, and this must be reasonably excluded in a child with persistent discharge [1, 2]. A foreign body, if trapped in the vagina, can cause irritation of the vaginal walls and lead to malodorous vaginal discharge and/or vaginal bleeding. Rarely, tumors of the vagina in prepubertal children can lead to vaginal discharge with associated bleeding and must be considered in the differential diagnosis, particularly in refractory cases [1, 2].

Vulvovaginitis in children is characterized by vulvar and/or vaginal irritation and inflammation that is often accompanied by vaginal discharge. The vulva may be primarily affected or it may be secondarily affected as a result of the discharge from the inflamed vagina. In addition to discharge, symptoms of vulvovaginitis include vulvar puritis, irritation, pain, and/or burning. Some girls may have associated light vaginal bleeding or vulvar erythema [2]. These symptoms warrant a careful history from the patient and her caregivers. History should be obtained regarding the duration, onset, and presence of any symptoms associated with the discharge. Symptoms that have been waxing and waning for several months are more consistent with a nonspecific vulvovaginitis, whereas severe, acute symptoms are more common with specific bacterial pathogens.

Further, the clinician should clarify any risk for foreign body insertion into the vagina from the patient and caregiver. Given the ease with which the prepubertal vagina can become colonized with oropharyngeal or gastrointestinal bacteria, a history should also clarify the girls' toileting habits, including wiping direction, and any recent gastrointestinal or upper respiratory infection in the patient. Lastly, both the patient and the caregiver should be interviewed independently to assess for any concerns regarding victimization or sexual abuse.

A full physical examination should be performed. Careful attention should be devoted to assignment of pubertal stage to the patient, as the differential diagnosis of vaginal discharge differs after puberty. Genitourinary examination in the prepubertal patient can be challenging to the inexperienced provider. Depending on the child's level of comfort, several positions can be used to visualize the external genitalia and the lower vagina.

1. Frog-Leg Position: child lays supine on the exam table with soles of feet aligned, knees flexed, and hips abducted.
2. Lithotomy Position: child sits on a parent's lap in traditional lithotomy position, the parent provides support to the posterior thighs.
3. Knee-Chest Position: child lies prone, brings knees up to chest with knees slightly apart.

Regardless of the position, visualization of the lower vagina and the hymen commonly require labial traction. Labial traction is performed by gently grasping the labia majora bilaterally and exerting gentle outward traction [1]. Vaginal discharge is more commonly visualized cephalad to the hymen in prepubertal girls. Discharge that is located on the vulva and external genitalia is more consistent with smegma, which is normal sebaceous material commonly visualized in labial folds in prepubertal girls. In addition to visualization of discharge, the vulva should also be carefully examined for the presence of rashes, hypopigmentation, or erythema. A culture for aerobic and anaerobic organisms should be obtained if true vaginal discharge is visualized. Care should be taken to avoid palpation/manipulation of the hymen when obtaining culture of the discharge, as the hymen is particularly sensitive in prepubertal girls. This often requires two providers, one to provide labial traction and a second to obtain the culture cephalad to the hymen while avoiding/minimizing manipulation of the hymen. Care should be taken that young girls consent to these examinations and are comfortable with the physician–patient relationship and their own autonomy.

In patients who are intolerant of an external pelvic examination or are unwilling to cooperate, examination may be deferred until a follow-up visit, particularly in girls who present with chronic vulvovaginitis. In more acute cases, or when vaginal bleeding is present, conscious sedation or examination under anesthesia may be warranted. In patients with a history concerning for sexual abuse or in those with refractory or recurrent discharge, screening for sexually transmitted infections is indicated.

In prepubertal children, vaginal culture does not commonly reveal a specific organism as the causative agent for vulvovaginitis, hence the term "nonspecific." In cases where a specific organism is identified, it is often an oropharyngeal or gastrointestinal pathogen. The most common bacteria isolated in cases of pediatric vulvovaginitis in children are Group A Beta hemolytic *Streptococci*, *Haemophilus influenzae*, *Staphylococcus aureus*, coagulase negative *Staphylococci*, *Enterococcus* spp, *Escherichia coli*, Virdan *Streptococci* [3]. Poor hygiene practices and wiping methods in children account for translation of fecal material to vulva and vagina and result in over-proliferation of gastrointestinal bacteria leading to discharge [4]. This pathogenesis has been validated by studies that show fecal bacteria were more commonly isolated in girls under the age of six with vaginal discharge, the age in which toileting habits can be more inconsistent [5]. Similarly, poor handwashing and genital touching can lead to transmission or oropharyngeal bacteria to the external genitalia.

The diagnosis of nonspecific vulvovaginitis in children is made based on history and examination and is a diagnosis of exclusion. The management of nonspecific vulvovaginitis is centered on patient education and behavior modification. Particular attention is focused on toileting and education regarding appropriate front-to-back wiping technique. Good handwashing should also be emphasized given the known association between vaginal discharge and the presence of gastrointestinal and oropharyngeal bacteria on vaginal culture in girls with vulvovaginitis. Daily baths with emphasis on soaking in clean bath water can help alleviate symptoms. Avoidance of tight-fitting clothing has also been recommended [1, 2]. Topical emollients, such as clear petroleum jelly, can be used on the irritated vulvar skin nightly to decrease symptoms and to deter scratching and further translocation of bacteria [2].

In cases where the vaginal culture reveals a specific organism, a course of appropriately targeted antibiotics should be administered, with concurrent attention to aforementioned behavioral changes to prevent recurrence. If acute symptoms do not improve within 48 hours of initial conservative management, initiation of an antihistamine or hydroxyzine to break the itch/scratch cycle may be considered. Further, in refractory cases, empiric treatment with antibiotics targeting the commonly isolated vaginal pathogens can be undertaken, even in the setting of a negative culture.

In cases where a vaginal foreign body is visualized, it should be carefully removed. Removal can generally be facilitated in the office setting by using vaginal lavage. This is performed using a flexible urinary catheter attached to a 50 cc syringe filled with warm, sterile water or saline. The catheter is gently passed above the hymen, and the vagina is irrigated to flush out the foreign body. If in-office removal and/or lavage is unsuccessful or is poorly tolerated by the patient, an examination under anesthesia and vaginoscopy are indicated [1].

Vaginoscopy is performed in the ambulatory operating room setting under anesthesia. A cystoscope or hysteroscope is placed into the vagina, and sterile fluid is infused into the vagina while the vaginal introitus is occluded. This allows for visualization of the upper vagina and cervix in prepubertal girls and is favored over speculum examination in this age group as it facilitates improved visualization and avoids unnecessary trauma. Vaginoscopy should also be considered in prepubertal girls with recurrent unexplained vaginal discharge and in girls with vaginal bleeding in whom precocious puberty has been excluded. In the absence of precocious puberty, vaginal bleeding in a prepubertal girl is most commonly attributed to a vaginal foreign body; however, trauma or a vaginal tumor, including but not limited to sarcoma botryoides, must be considered and excluded [1].

Key Teaching Points

- Vaginal discharge is a common problem in prepubertal girls; however, an inciting infecting organism is rarely identified.

- Nonspecific vulvovaginitis is diagnosed based on history and physical examination, and the mainstay of treatment is education on behavior modification, improved hygiene, and topical bland emollients.
- Yeast vaginitis and bacterial vaginosis generally do not occur in prepubertal girls; therefore, treatment for these is not indicated.
- Persistent vaginal discharge despite appropriate conservative measures warrants additional investigation with vaginal cultures and possibly vaginoscopy.
- If discharge is associated with vaginal bleeding, a more extensive workup is indicated and concern for foreign body is heightened. Precocious puberty should be reasonably excluded, and vaginoscopy should be considered to further evaluate bleeding.

References

1. Sanfilippo J, Lara-Torre E, Edmonds K, Templeman C. *Clinical Pediatric and Adolescent Gynecology*. New York, NY: Informa Health Care;2009.
2. Zuckerman A, Romano M. Clinical recommendation: vulvovaginitis. *J Pediatr Adolesc Gynecol* 2016;29:673–679.
3. Stricker T, Navratil F, Sennhauser FH. Vulvovaginitis in prepubertal girls. *Arch Dis Child* 2003;88:324–326.
4. Cemek F, Odabas D, Senel U, Kocaman AT. Personal hygiene and vulvovaginitis in prepubertal children. *J Pediatr Adolesc Gynecol* 2016 June;29 (3) 223–227.
5. Randelovic G, Mladenovic V, Ristic L et al. Microbiological apsects of vulvovaginitis in prepubertal girls. *J Formos Med Assoc* 2012;111:392–396.

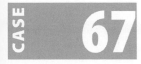

A 15-Year-Old with Painful Vulvar Ulcers

Sarah A. Shaffer

History of Present Illness

A 15-year-old nulligravid female presents to your clinic with her mother for one-day history of painful genital ulcers. She denies a history of genital, oral, or other skin lesions. She is not sexually active, and she denies any history of prior intercourse or sexually transmitted infections. She has a subdermal contraceptive implant for the treatment of dysmenorrhea. She is currently symptomatic with an upper respiratory infection and had a negative rapid antigen test for group A *Streptococcus* two days ago. She reports a sore throat, rhinorrhea, nonproductive cough, and low-grade fever. She denies nausea, emesis, dysuria, change in bowel movement, or abnormal uterine bleeding. Her vulvovaginal pain is reported as a 7 out of 10 on the pain scale and increases to a 9 when she urinates. The patient's past medical and surgical histories are negative. She has no known drug allergies, and her only medication is the etonogestrel implant.

Physical Examination

General appearance	Well-nourished and well-groomed, alert and oriented, cooperative but in mild distress and moderate discomfort

Vital Signs

Temperature	37.7°C
Pulse	94 beats/min
Blood pressure	131/75 mmHg
Respiratory rate	14 breaths/min
BMI	19.39 kg/m^2
HEENT	Normo-cephalic, injected conjunctiva bilaterally, erythematous nasal mucosa, swollen tonsils bilaterally, erythematous larynx
Respiratory	Normal effort, occasional dry cough, clear to auscultation bilaterally without wheeze
Abdomen	Soft, non-distended, non-tender; two 10–15-mm, mobile, non-tender inguinal lymph nodes on the right
Skin	No rash, lesions, or scars; no pigmentation changes

Pelvic

External genitalia	Normal anatomic structures; inner right labia minora with a painful, shallow ulcer, 12 mm in largest diameter, with well-demarcated, erythematous border, and no eschar; left posterior fourchette with a painful, shallow ulcer, 17 mm in largest diameter, with moist, white-gray, partially sloughed eschar
Perineum	Without lesion or pigmentation change
Vagina/cervix/ uterus/adnexa	No speculum exam or bimanual performed due to patient discomfort, subjectively increased amount of non-malodorous yellow-white vaginal discharge

Laboratory Studies

WBCs	11.9 k/mm^3
Hgb	13.2 g/dL
Hct	39 percent
Platelet count	203 k/mm^3
Urine pregnancy test	declined

How Would You Manage This Patient?

This immunocompetent adolescent female presents with an acute onset of ulcerative genital lesions in the setting of what appears to be a viral upper respiratory infection. She was interviewed away from her mother and again reported no history of sexual activity or abuse. Given her denial of sexual activity and recent viral illness, an outbreak of noninfectious acute genital ulcers (AGU), also referred to as Lipschutz ulcers, was suspected. Herpes simplex virus (HSV) polymerase chain reaction (PCR) testing was performed on the lesion, and she was started empirically on a course of oral acyclovir. In addition, she was offered testing for other STIs but declined.

Supportive therapy for her symptoms was initiated, including twice daily sitz baths, topical lidocaine, and oral naproxen sodium. In addition, she was offered topical zinc oxide to use as a protective barrier until the ulcers healed. Two days later, the HSV PCR returned as negative; therefore, she was advised to discontinue the acyclovir. The patient was scheduled to follow up in one week, at which time her pain and ulcers were significantly improved. At four weeks, she was asymptomatic and the ulcers were completely resolved.

Evaluation and Management of Lipschutz Ulcer

Since the initial case series published by Lipschutz in 1913, understanding of the AGU described has progressed very little. Aphthae or aphthosis of the vulva and/or vagina are other terms for Lipschutz ulcers; AGU will be used here [1]. The sparse literature on this topic describes young, often premenarchal and/or virginal women with genital ulcers [2]. A concomitant illness is frequently identified, and reports of AGU have been associated with Epstein Barr virus (EBV)/infectious mononucleosis [1], cytomegalovirus (CMV), influenza A/B, salmonellosis/paratyphoid fever, and mumps. The etiology and/or causative agent of AGU is unknown despite literature describing associated conditions. In addition, the incidence

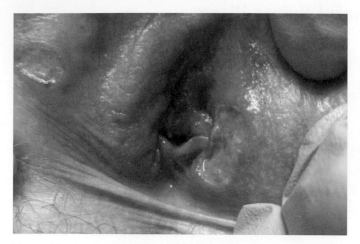

Figure 67.1 Acute genital ulcer, Lipschutz ulcer, with a clean base.

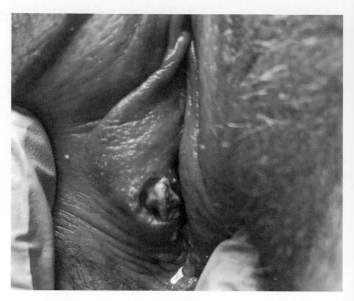

Figure 67.2 Acute genital ulcer, Lipschutz ulcer, with a moist eschar of sloughed tissue.

and prevalence of AGU is unknown as patients may not divulge their symptoms or present for care due to fear, shame, and embarrassment.

Young women with AGU typically present with acute onset of a single or few painful vulvar and/or vaginal ulcers ranging in size from less than 1 cm to 4–5 cm at largest diameter. The lesions are generally shallow with a sharply demarcated border. There may be a "clean base" with little necrotic burden, (Figure 67.1) or there may be an overlying moist eschar of sloughed tissue (Figure 67.2); however, the lesions are not friable. Cases with an increased amount of vaginal discharge should trigger suspicion for concomitant vaginal lesions, which are less common. Edema and erythema of the external genitalia may be significant, and there may be associated, localized cellulitis. The most common locations of AGU are the medial labia minora and the posterior fourchette. Ulcers in these areas are frequently exposed to urine; therefore, patients should be queried about their ability to urinate as well as any pain with urination. Mirror-image or "kissing" ulcers may be identified on the labia or in the lower vagina.

Systemic symptoms usually include fever, malaise, fatigue, and headache. In one report, all prior symptoms were present in 75 percent or more of study subjects, and 50 percent or more additionally reported gastrointestinal or respiratory symptoms [3]. Some patients have simultaneous oral aphthae, while others will present a history of oral and/or genital ulcers.

A sexual history (including sexual abuse) should be obtained along with inquiry into prior and/or similar episodes. Physical examination should include evaluation for other skin and mucosal ulcers (e.g., oral), including an external pelvic examination. For younger patients, a supine frog-leg or knee-chest position can facilitate visualization of the necessary structures while minimizing need for instrumentation and manipulation of painful tissue. A speculum examination is not routinely performed if external ulcers can be seen and sampled. Photo documentation is extremely useful and should be discussed prior to the examination. Lymphadenopathy may be noted and, while it should be documented, is most often a nonspecific finding.

The differential diagnosis of AGU must include STIs, including HSV, syphilis, lymphogranuloma venereum, chancroid, and granuloma inguinale. The likelihood of these depends on the patient's sexual history and the disease prevalence in the region. Non-penetrative sexual and nonsexual transmission of HSV can occur. One must also consider ulcerative vulvar dermatoses like erosive lichen planus, lichen sclerosus, and lichen simplex chronicus. Immune blistering disorders of the skin are usually diagnosed in an older population of patients; younger patients with bullous pemphigoid, linear IgA disease, mucous membrane pemphigoid/cicatricial pemphigoid, bullous systemic lupus erythematosus, and benign familial pemphigus (Hailey-Hailey disease) have been described. The possibility of a fixed drug eruption should also be considered, along with systemic diseases like inflammatory bowel diseases, particularly Crohn's disease, Behcet's disease (multiorgan inflammatory disorder), and leukemia [4].

Transient systemic illnesses due to common viruses like CMV and EBV are thought to act as precipitating factors for AGU. Although the ulcers may be caused by a direct cytotoxic effect to the vulvar epithelium, there is more evidence to suggest these ulcers are the result of local inflammation and microthrombi that cause tissue necrosis as a localized manifestation of a systemic illness [1], possibly in people with unidentified predisposing factors.

Available reports describe an expansive array of tests to consider the broad differential, but the vast majority of tests are negative or, at most, nonspecific [2]. Table 67.1 summarizes the diagnostic testing for acute genital ulcers as described in the literature. A "full work-up" for every patient would be expensive and is generally not helpful for the classic presentation of an otherwise healthy, young, not-yet sexually active female in whom the absolute need for various STI testing is debatable.

Although there is no standard work-up, collection of a sample from the ulcer for HSV PCR or viral culture is routinely

Table 67.1 Acute genital ulcer – diagnostic testing described in the literature. The majority of these tests do *not* contribute to the diagnosis and they rarely alter the required treatment

Reference	Common STIs	Uncommon STIs	EBV & CMV	Routine lab work	Culture	Nutrient levels	Biopsy
Vieira-Baptista, et al. 2016	Yes	No	Yes; convalescent testing if initial indeterminate	Per patient presentation & history	No	No	No
Huppert 2010	HSV; other per demographics/ not with first episode	Per demographics/ not with first episode	EBV serology; CMV optional	CBC minimum (evaluation of systemic disease)	Not with first episode	Not with first episode	Not with first episode
Farhi, et al. 2009	Yes	Per patient presentation & history	EBV serology; other not routine	Yes, also kidney function	Not routine	Not routine	Per patient presentation & history
Moreira Gomes, et al. 2007	Unclear	Unclear	Unclear	Per patient presentation & history	Yes	No	Yes
Huppert, et al. 2006	No; HSV = exclusion criteria	No	Yes; also convalescent testing (minimum 14 days later)	Yes (per funding = not all subjects)	Yes; also Gram stain	No	Yes

Common STIs = herpes simplex virus (HSV), syphilis, human immunodeficiency virus
Uncommon STIs = lymphogranuloma venerum, granuloma inguinale, chancroid
EBV & CMV – IgM and IgG for both; convalescent testing only if noted
Routine lab work = CBC, electrolytes, liver function
Cultures = viral, bacterial, fungal
Nutrient levels = iron, folate, vitamin B12, vitamin D
Biopsy = punch biopsy (3–4 mm) at border of lesion

recommended. In circumstances where discomfort or other factors limit direct sampling of a lesion, or the age of the lesion may limit the reliability of the result, HSV serology should be performed. Judicious screening for common STIs should be considered if the patient is sexually active or if HSV testing is positive. This includes HIV, as HSV is a common co-infection.

In the "classic" patient, serology for EBV and/or CMV, bacterial culture and biopsy of the lesion will rarely alter the diagnosis or the treatment plan; therefore, these tests are not routinely advised. While common viral illnesses have been implicated in AGU, testing for them is rarely timely, and results are often negative or indeterminate. Most studies report collection of routine lab work including a complete blood count, electrolyte panels, and liver or kidney function testing. While this might assist in identifying a previously undiagnosed systemic condition, such a finding would be rare, and these tests are unlikely to alter the plan of care [1, 3, 4]. Physical evidence or medical history suggestive of systemic disease warrants evaluation by a specialist. Only in unusual situations, including prolonged healing of AGU or recurrence of AGU in a short time frame, should other testing be considered such as biopsy of the ulcer or a broader panel of blood work.

It is reasonable to initiate empiric treatment for HSV with oral antivirals per published protocols while awaiting the results of HSV testing, as was done in the above patient [5]. If testing for HSV is negative, the course of antiviral therapy should be discontinued. If cellulitis or superinfection (bacterial or fungal) is suspected, appropriate therapy should be initiated with antibiotics and/or antifungals.

The main goal of treatment is pain relief until the ulcer heals spontaneously. The average duration of healing is 14–21 days [1–3]; however, some ulcers heal more slowly. Topical analgesics (e.g., lidocaine or xylocaine gel) may be sufficient for pain relief when used with vulvar comfort measures discussed below. Compounded lidocaine 2 percent, epinephrine 1:1000, and tetracaine 2 percent (LET) in a petroleum or gel base has been described [2, 3]. LET can be applied in a thin layer to the ulcer(s) several times daily. Prescription strength doses of acetaminophen and ibuprofen or naproxen sodium, administered on a schedule, are also recommended if topical analgesics are insufficient. Oral narcotics should be employed sparingly (no more than 5–7 days total duration) and only if other analgesics provide inadequate pain relief.

The use of topical corticosteroid ointments is described in recent literature, but there are no existing studies to demonstrate benefit in duration of analgesic use, time to healing, or other parameters [2]. No studies have evaluated the use of intralesional corticosteroid injections for treatment of AGU.

Likewise, while amlexanox paste (topical anti-inflammatory/ immunomodulator used for oral aphthae) is suggested in several sources [2], it has never been studied for AGU.

Vulvar care and comfort measures must be counseled in detail. Sitz baths are soothing and soften adherent tissue, allowing exudative crust to slough. Voiding at the end of bathing or using a spray bottle to dilute urine with water can decrease pain with urination. Likewise, rinse bottles can be used after voiding or defecation to minimize wiping near inflamed tissue. Skin protectants in the form of petroleum or zinc oxide can be used as a barrier against friction from clothing and common chemical irritants while also retaining moisture in the vulvar epithelium. Patients should also be advised to avoid wearing underwear and/or tight-fitting clothing to diminish friction, heat, and pressure.

In sexually active patients, repeat STI testing should be recommended three to six months after initial testing. Patients should also be counseled on the increased risk of HIV transmission in the presence of STI-related genital ulcers [5, 6].

Follow-up is suggested weekly or every 14 days until the ulcer is re-epithelialized and pain has resolved [2]. Healing of AGU generally occurs without scarring. Recurrence has not been well documented in the literature; however, one series of 20 patients reported a 35 percent rate of recurrence [3]. It is not known whether recurrences are milder or if they are suggestive of a different disease etiology or future course.

Key Teaching Points

- Classic AGU, or Lipschutz ulcers, present as painful, acute ulcer(s) in young women, often in the setting of another viral illness and prior to the onset of sexual activity.
- Lipshutz ulcers are not caused by a sexually transmitted infection; however, HSV should be ruled out during the initial evaluation, and empiric treatment with acyclovir is reasonable until HSV has been excluded.
- Treatment of AGU consists of pain relief and vulvar comfort measures.
- Acute genital ulcers heal spontaneously, do not routinely recur, and generally do not lead to any long-term sequelae.

References

1. Farhi D, Wendling J, Molinari E et al. Non-sexually related acute genital ulcers in 13 pubertal girls: a clinical and microbiological study. *Arch Dermatol* 2009;145(1):38–45.

2. Huppert JS. Lipschutz ulcers: evaluation and management of acute genital ulcers in women. *Dermatol Ther* 2010;23 (5):533–540.

3. Huppert JS, Gerber MA, Deitch HR et al. Vulvar ulcers in young females: a manifestation of aphthosis. *J Pediatr Adolesc Gynecol* 2006;19 (3):195–204.

4. Vieira-Baptista P, Lima-Silva J, Beires J, Martinez-de-Oliveira J. Lipschutz ulcers: should we rethink this? An analysis of 33 cases. *Eur J Obstet Gynecol Reprod Biol* 2016;198:149–152.

5. Prevention CfDCa. Sexually Transmitted Diseases Treatment Guidelines. MMWR. 2010;59(RR-12):18–26.

6. Gomes CM, Giraldo PC, Gomes Fde A et al. Genital ulcers in women: clinical, microbiologic and histopathologic characteristics. *Braz J Infect Dis* 2007;11 (2):254–260.

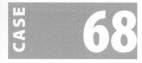

A 15-Year-Old Adolescent Who Is Unable to Use a Tampon

Celeste Ojeda Hemingway

History of Present Illness

A 15-year-old adolescent female presents to the office indicating she has difficulty using tampons. She is accompanied by her mother to the appointment. The patient reports that she started her first period at age 11, and after having initially irregular periods, she has had regular monthly periods for the last few years. Her last menstrual period was ten days ago. The patient's periods typically last 5–6 days, and she uses 4–5 pads per day on her heaviest day. She reports some cramping at the beginning of her cycle, which is relieved by over-the-counter medications, and she feels the amount of bleeding is manageable. Two months ago, the patient attempted to use tampons for the first time. She initially tried tampons with a cardboard applicator, and after finding it uncomfortable, her mom purchased tampons with plastic applicators. She attempted placement with the new tampons, but was again unsuccessful. She was finally able to place a light-days tampon with a plastic applicator but experienced extreme discomfort with what she describes as a "very difficult" removal. The patient's medical history is notable only for seasonal allergies and surgeries for ear tubes as a child. She does not take any prescription medications and has no known allergies to medications.

The patient was interviewed with her mother out of the room. She denies ever being sexually active or having plans to become sexually active in the near future. She does not smoke and denies alcohol use. She feels safe at home and denies depression. She confides that she really wants to be able to use tampons more easily so she can swim and exercise without bulky pads. The patient consents to a pelvic examination and requests her mom be present.

Physical Examination

General appearance	Well-appearing, appropriately developed young woman in no distress

Vital Signs

Temperature	37.6°C
Pulse	92 beats/min
Blood Pressure	104/66 mmHg
Height	63 inches
Weight	122 lb
BMI	21.6 kg/m^2
Cardiovascular	Regular rate and rhythm
Pulmonary	Symmetric breath sounds, clear to auscultation bilaterally
Abdomen	Soft, non-distended, non-tender without guarding or rebound
Breasts	Tanner stage IV
Skin	Mild acne, no lesions or rashes

External genitalia	Tanner stage III, normal-appearing labia majora and minora, initially difficult to visualize a vaginal opening; with gentle traction and moistened q-tip probe, bilateral orifices identified lateral to the midline which admit q-tip and allow visualization of a central vertical septum at the level of the hymen (Figure 68.1)

Laboratory Studies

Urine analysis	Negative for nitrites, leukocyte esterase, blood, and leukocytes
Imaging	None requested.

How Would You Manage This Patient?

The patient is an appropriately menstruating adolescent with a septate hymen. The septate hymen with its bilateral small openings allows egress of monthly menses, and given her menstrual pattern, there is no immediate suspicion for other

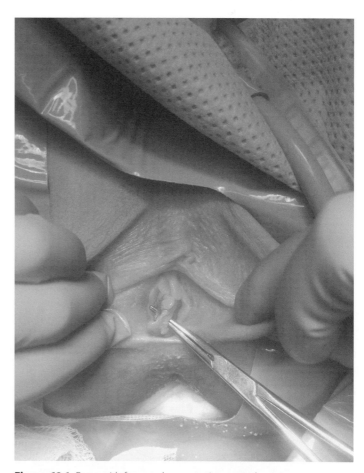

Figure 68.1 Exam with forceps demonstrating vertical septum.
Image reprinted with permission from Paula J Adams Hillard MD, Stanford University School of Medicine, published by Medscape Drugs and Diseases (http://emedicine.medscape.com/), 2017, available at: http://emedicine.medscape.com/article/269050-overview

abnormalities. She is an active young woman with an interest in using tampons during menses. The patient and her mother were counseled on her diagnosis of a septate hymen with the assistance of visual aids. They were reassured that given the patient's history, additional abnormalities of the genital tract are unlikely. The patient's treatment options were reviewed along with the benefits and risks of each. The patient was offered expectant management or surgical excision of the hymenal septum. After discussion, both the patient and her mother were in agreement to undergo surgical excision. The patient subsequently underwent outpatient surgical excision of a hymenal septum under anesthesia, and the pelvic examination under anesthesia that followed excision revealed an otherwise unremarkable vagina, cervix, and uterus. The patient was seen postoperatively with a normal-appearing vaginal opening and was encouraged to use tampons when she was ready.

Septate Hymen

Hymenal abnormalities are relatively uncommon, affecting approximately 2 percent of females. Non-obstructing variants of hymenal abnormalities include cribiform hymen, microperforate hymen, and septate hymen (Figure 68.2). The estimated incidence of septate hymen among children and adolescents ranges from 0.7 to 2.7 percent in descriptive studies. Vertical hymenal septa are the most common configuration followed by diagonal, then horizontal septa [1]. Because an imperforate hymen will block egress of menses, the diagnosis of imperforate hymen is typically made in early adolescence due to amenorrhea with accompanying cyclic pelvic pain. In contrast, non-obstructing hymenal abnormalities typically allow for normal menstrual flow. Therefore, these abnormalities are often identified much later in adolescence or even in adulthood. While non-obstructing variants of hymenal abnormalities are sometimes identified in the prepubertal period, they more commonly present with complaints of difficult tampon insertion, painful tampon removal, difficulty achieving vaginal penetration with intercourse, or painful intercourse.

The hymenal structure develops embryonically from invagination of the urogenital sinus, an endodermal layer, which will ultimately form the lower portion of the vagina. A non-obstructing hymenal abnormality, such as a septate hymen, is most likely the result of incomplete canalization of the hymenal tissue in-utero or incomplete vacuolization of the sinovaginal bulbs [2]. While a concomitant upper genital tract abnormality such as a vaginal septum or müllerian abnormality is not common, evaluation for further abnormalities can be undertaken as clinically indicated. For example, a patient with a non-obstructing hymenal abnormality and concomitant amenorrhea would require additional evaluation for the etiology of her amenorrhea. In addition, an obstructive müllerian anomaly should be considered in a patient with persistent or worsening dysmenorrhea despite appropriate treatment.

A hymenal abnormality is typically diagnosed in the office setting with a thorough examination of the external genitalia. In an adolescent or adult patient, this can usually be achieved with examination in the dorsal lithotomy position with the patient's feet in stirrups. The examiner places his or her thumbs on the inferior aspects of the labia majora and applies gentle downward and outward traction to visualize the hymenal structure. If needed, the hymen can be probed with a moistened q-tip or smaller probe to confirm patency. For pediatric patients, examination of the hymenal structure can be achieved with frog-leg positioning (lying on mom's abdomen if appropriate) or knee-chest position again with the assistance of gentle traction as described above, a small probe, cough, Valsalva, or a small amount of irrigation [3].

Microperforate, cribiform, or septate hymen can be managed expectantly if the patient or family desires. This is especially appropriate in the prepubertal period. Surgical management should generally be deferred until puberty when the patient's own endogenous estrogen production is sufficient to prevent postoperative adhesion of the vaginal epithelium. It is possible, particularly with a septate hymen, that the future insertion of tampons, removal of tampons, or vaginal intercourse will sever the septum and eliminate the need for

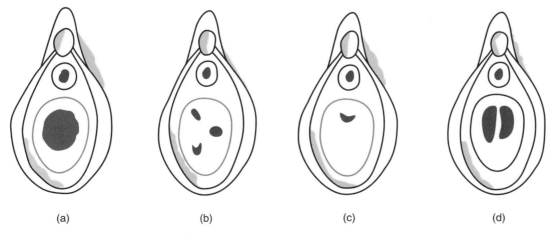

(a)   (b)   (c)   (d)

Figure 68.2 Non-obstructing hymenal abnormalities. A. Normal-appearing hymen, B. Cribiform hymen, C. Microperforate hymen, and D. Septate hymen.

surgery. However, this could prove to be both painful and anxiety-provoking for the patient. With consistent tampon use or vaginal intercourse, it is also possible that the septum may become attenuated, and one side of the hymenal opening is able to comfortably accommodate tampon usage and intercourse. It is appropriate to offer surgical intervention at the patient and family's discretion, especially after menarche.

The literature also offers serial dilation as a nonsurgical treatment option for non-obstructing hymenal abnormalities. The use of a series of lubricated dilators to gradually open the orifice of the microperforate hymen has been described [4], and by extension, these could be similarly used to dilate one of the lateral orifices created by a septate hymen. This would require a more mature, motivated patient. If dilators were to successfully create an accommodating vaginal opening, removal of the attenuated septum may still be required if it interfered with comfortable intercourse or tampon use.

Office-based excision of septate hymen is described in the literature and is an appropriate option for some patients. Under local anesthesia, the hymenal septum is excised with scissors or scalpel and absorbable suture employed for hemostasis. With younger patients, however, it is more common to perform surgical excision of a hymenal septum under sedation in an outpatient surgical setting. With the patient in dorsal lithotomy position in stirrups, the hymenal septum is isolated by passing narrow (Vanderbilt/tonsil or similar) forceps

behind the septum. If needed, a red rubber catheter can be placed intraoperatively to clearly identify and avoid the urethra. The septum is excised with transection of the septum superiorly and inferiorly using needle point cautery [5]. Sutures are only placed if required for hemostasis. If appropriate, after excision of the hymenal septum, a vaginal exam with a single digit or small speculum can be performed to evaluate the upper vaginal tract. A short course of topical estrogen to prevent postoperative adhesion may be used in the rare prepubertal patient undergoing excision of a septate hymen. However, as mentioned previously, it is preferable to perform excision after puberty.

Key Teaching Points

- Non-obstructing hymenal abnormalities such as a septate hymen may present with difficulty inserting or removing tampons, difficulty with vaginal penetration during intercourse, or without symptoms as an incidental finding.
- Surgical management of a microperforate, cribiform, or septate hymen identified after menarche may be undertaken immediately or deferred based on patient preference.
- While upper vaginal or müllerian abnormalities are unlikely to be diagnosed in patients with a septate hymen, evaluation should be undertaken as clinically appropriate.

References

1. Berkowitz CD, Elvik SL, McCann J et al. Septate hymen: variations and pitfalls in diagnosis. *Adolesc Pediatr Gynecol* 1991;4:194–197.
2. Shulman LP, Elias S. Developmental abnormalities of the female reproductive tract: pathogenesis and nosology. *Adolesc Pediatr Gynecol* 1988;1:230–238.
3. Emans SJ. Office evaluation of the child and adolescent. In: Emans SJ, Laufer MR, editors. *Emans, Laufer, Goldstein's Pediatric and Adolescent Gynecology*, 6th Edition. Philadelphia: Lippincott Williams & Wilkins; 2012. pp. 1–20.
4. Segal TR, Fried WB, Krim EY, Parikh D, Rosenfeld DL. Treatment of microperforate hymen with serial dilation: a novel approach. *J Pediatr Adolesc Gynecol* 2014; 28(2): e21–e22.
5. Gebhart JP, Breech LL, Hurst BS, Rock JA. Congenital vaginal abnormalities. In: Baggish MS, Karram MM, editors. *Atlas of Pelvic Anatomy and Gynecologic Surgery*, 4th Edition. Philadelphia: Elsevier; 2016. pp. 779–798.

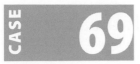

A Six-Year-Old Girl with Breast Development (Precocious Puberty)

Shelly Holmstrom

History of Present Illness

A six-year-old girl presents to your office with concerns about significant breast development over the last six months. Her mother notes that the patient is the tallest girl in her class and estimates that her daughter has grown about 3 inches in the last year. She reports no headaches, visual changes, abdominal pain, or any other associated symptoms.

Her past medical and surgical histories are negative. She has no known drug allergies and does not take any medications. The patient lives with her mother and younger sister, and she started first grade this year. Her family history is significant for diabetes mellitus in both maternal grandparents; there is no history of thyroid disease or early puberty.

Physical Examination

General appearance	Well-developed, well-nourished girl in no acute distress

Vital Signs

Temperature	37°C
Pulse	90 beats/min
Blood pressure	105/60 mm Hg
Respiratory rate	14 breaths/min
Oxygen saturation	100 percent on room air
Height	45 inches
Weight	52 lb
BMI	18.1 kg/m^2 (94th percentile)
Neck	Full range of motion, no thyromegaly, no acanthosis nigricans
Cardiac	Regular rate and rhythm, no murmurs
Lungs	Clear to auscultation bilaterally
Breasts	Tanner stage 2, symmetric, no masses, nodes, or discharge.
Abdomen	soft, non-tender, non-distended, no guarding, no rebound
External genitalia	Tanner stage 2, normal female external genitalia with estrogenized labia. Patient would not allow an internal exam.
Recto-vaginal	declined by patient

Laboratory Studies

LH 11.0 mIU/mL

Reference Range (mIU/mL):	Infants <3.0; Prepubertal <7; Follicular 1.1–11.1; Mid-cycle 17.5–72.9; Luteal 0.4–15.1

FSH 7.8 mIU/mL

Reference Range (mIU/mL):	Infant female<5.0; Prepubertal female <11.0; Adult 0.4–15.1

Estradiol 2.2 ng/dL	Tanner Staging//Reference Range (ng/dL)

Tanner 1// 0.5–2.0
Tanner 2// 1.0–2.4
Tanner 3// 0.7–6.0
Tanner 4// 2.1–8.5
Tanner 5// 3.4–17
TSH 2.4 µU/mL Reference Range (µU/mL):   0.5–5.0

Imaging

Bone age	9 years of age (>2 standard deviations above the mean for her age)
Pelvic ultrasound	Uterus measures 3.5 cm × 1.2 cm × 1.0 cm. Right ovary cubic volume is 3.4 cm^2 and left ovary cubic volume is 2.5 cm^2.

How Would You Manage This Patient?

This patient has central precocious puberty, as evidenced by sequential maturation of breast and pubic hair, her puberty range blood tests, and her increased bone age that is greater than two standard deviations above the mean for her age of 6 years. A magnetic resonance imaging (MRI) of the brain was ordered to evaluate for a central nervous system (CNS) lesion and was negative.

Since she presented at 6 years of age, this patient was treated with GnRH agonist therapy to halt further pubertal development. **Leuprolide** depot was given intramuscularly (IM) every 28 days at a dose of 7.5 mg (calculated by using approximately 0.3 mg/kg/dose). The patient and her family were warned of possibility of vaginal bleeding with the transient stimulation of the pituitary–ovarian axis with the first dose. She did well, with no further progression of secondary sexual characteristics until her therapy was stopped at age 11 years.

Precocious Puberty Evaluation

Precocious puberty is defined as the onset of secondary sexual development before age 8 years in girls and age 9 years in boys. These age limits are set at 2–2.5 standard deviations below the mean age of onset of puberty. In most populations, the onset of pubertal development is 10.5 years in girls and 11.5 years in boys with a standard deviation of ~1 year [1]. This chapter will focus on the evaluation and management of precocious puberty in girls.

Pubertal development in triggered when the hypothalamic–pituitary–ovarian (HPO) axis is activated in girls. The hypothalamus begins to increase the pulsatile secretion of gonadotropin-releasing hormone (GnRH), which stimulates the production of follicle-stimulating hormone (FSH) and luteinizing hormone (LH) by the pituitary gland. FSH promotes the development of follicles in the ovary and LH stimulates ovarian estradiol production by the ovary. Moreover, estradiol is the hormone responsible for progressive breast development, growth spurt, and rapid bone age advancement. Pubic and axillary hair development is independent of the

Table 69.1 Classification of precocious puberty

	Central precocious puberty	Peripheral precocity	Benign or nonprogressive variants
Alternative nomenclature	Gonadotropin-dependent precocious puberty True precocious puberty	Gonadotropin-independent precocious puberty Peripheral precocious puberty	Isolated breast development Isolated pubic and/or axillary hair
Cause	Early maturation of hypothalamic–pituitary–ovarian axis	Endogenous or exogenous source of excess hormones	Early activation of the hypothalamic–pituitary–adrenal axis
Pathology	80%–90% of cases are idiopathic; most others due to CNS lesions (see Table 69.2)	Excess secretion of estrogens and androgens from the ovary, adrenal glands, or tumor; exogenous sources of sex hormones (see Table 69.2)	Can be a normal variant of pubertal development

activation of the HPO axis and is related to the increase in secretion of weak adrenal androgens, primarily dehydroepiandrosterone-sulfate (DHEA-S).

Several studies have highlighted the racial/ethnic and body mass index (BMI) differences in the timing of pubertal development [2, 3, 4, 5]. Biro and colleagues [4] showed that in a sample of 7- to 8-year-old girls, 23 percent black, 15 percent Hispanic, and 10 percent white girls had breast development. Moreover, the Rosenfield study demonstrated overweight girls have earlier development of breast and pubic hair and a slightly earlier menarche as compared to normal weight girls [5].

A thorough evaluation is suggested for girls younger than 8 years of age presenting with secondary sexual development. Initially, central versus peripheral precocity or benign nonprogressive variants, as classified in Table 69.1, should be determined to further guide the evaluation. The potential etiologies of central versus peripheral precocity are listed in Box 69.1. Central precocious puberty (CPP) development follows the normal sequence of events (breast development, peak height velocity, menarche) but at an earlier age. Girls with peripheral precocity, however, are more likely to deviate from the normal sequence and pace of pubertal development.

A medical history should focus on when the initial pubertal changes were seen and the sequence of development. Timing of pubertal development of parents and siblings should be obtained as well. Additional questions should assess for linear growth rate, headaches, changes in vision, seizures, abdominal pain, and prior CNS disease or trauma. Exogenous exposure to sex steroids or compounds with sex-steroid-like properties should also be explored as a possibility.

Physical examination should document height, weight, and height velocity to date on a standard growth chart. Moreover, visual fields should be assessed, as an abnormality may be suggestive of a CNS mass. A careful skin examination should be conducted to look for café-au-lait spots that can be associated with neurofibromatosis or McCune–Albright syndrome.

Secondary sexual development should be assessed using the sexual maturity rating or Tanner staging. This staging system

Box 69.1 Etiology of precocious puberty

Central Precocious Puberty

1. Idiopathic
2. CNS lesions

    a. Space-occupying lesions

    - Congenital defects
    - Hydrocephalus
    - Suprasellar/arachnoid cysts
    - Hamartoma (gonadotropin-releasing hormone secreting)
    - Septo-optic dysplasia

    b. Tumors

    - Optic glioma
    - Ganglioneuroma
    - Ependymoma
    - Craniopharyngioma
    - Dysgerminoma

    c. Infection/inflammation

    - Postencephalitis
    - Brain abscess
    - Post-meningitis
    - Granulomas

    d. Injury

    - Post-head trauma
    - Postirradiation

    e. Syndromes

    - Tuberous sclerosis
    - Neurofibromatosis (often with optic glioma)

    f. Prolonged exposure to sex steroids

    - Late/incompletely treated adrenal hyperplasia
    - Postexposure to androgens/estrogens (tumors)

Box 69.1 (cont.)

Peripheral Precocity

1. Exposure to topical or ingested androgens or estrogens
2. Severe primary hypothyroidism
3. Ovarian tumors
    a. Granulosa/theca cell
    b. Germ cell
    c. Sertoli/Leydig
    d. Gonadoblastoma
4. Ovarian cysts
    a. Idiopathic
    b. McCune–Albright
5. Adrenal tumors

rates breast and pubic hair development in girls. The breast assessment should include direct palpation of the breast tissue to differentiate true breast development from adipose tissue as well as evaluation of the nipple-areolar complex.

Radiographic assessment of bone age should be performed to assist the development of a differential diagnosis in girls with development of secondary sexual characteristics confirmed by physical examination. A significant advance in bone age, defined as two standard deviations beyond chronological age, is more likely in girls with CPP or peripheral precocity as opposed to benign pubertal variant.

Initial laboratory evaluation in girls with secondary sexual development includes basal LH, FSH, and estradiol levels. These laboratory results can assist with differentiating CPP from peripheral precocity (see algorithm in Figure 69.1).

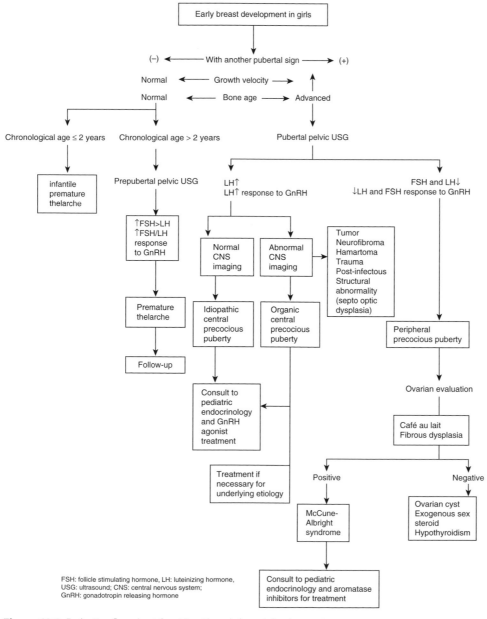

Figure 69.1 Evaluation flow sheet for girls with early breast development.
Berberoglu, M. Precocious puberty and normal variant puberty: Definition, etiology, diagnosis and current management. *J Clin Res Pediatr Endocrinol*. 2009 June; 1(4):164–174. Published online December 8, 2010.

Table 69.2 Clinical characteristics of forms of early pubertal development

	CPP	Peripheral precocity	Benign or nonprogressive precocious puberty
Physical examination: Advancement through pubertal stages (Tanner stage)	Progression to next pubertal stage in 3 to 6 months	Progression	No progression in Tanner staging during 3 to 6 months of observation
Growth velocity	Accelerated	Accelerated	Normal for bone age
Bone age	Advanced	Advanced	Normal to mildly advanced
Serum estradiol concentration	Prepubertal (<16 pg/mL) to increased	Increased in ovarian causes or exogenous estrogen exposure	Prepubertal (<16 pg/mL)
Basal (unstimulated) serum LH concentration¶	Pubertal (>2–3 mIU/mL)	Suppressed or prepubertal (<2 mIU/mL)	Prepubertal (<2 mIU/mL)
GnRH (or GnRHa) stimulation test	LH peak elevated (in the pubertal range) Higher stimulated LH to FSH ratio	No change from baseline or LH peak in the prepubertal range	LH peak in the prepubertal range Lower stimulated LH to FSH ratio

CPP: central precocious puberty (also known as gonadotropin-dependent precocious puberty); LH: luteinizing hormone; GnRH: gonadotropin-releasing hormone; GnRHa: gonadotropin-releasing hormone agonist; FSH: follicle-stimulating hormone.

Basal LH is the best test to evaluate for activation of the hypothalamic–pituitary–ovarian axis. LH concentrations in the prepubertal range are consistent with peripheral precocity or a benign variant, such as premature thelarche. LH levels above 2–3 mIU/mL are highly sensitive and specific to CPP. Serum levels of FSH are less useful in discriminating between CPP and benign pubertal variants. FSH levels are typically higher in children with CPP when compared with benign pubertal variants; however, considerable overlap exists between these two groups of girls. Patients with peripheral precocity have FSH levels that are in the prepubertal range. Very high levels of estradiol in the setting of low (suppressed) LH and FSH are consistent with a peripheral source, such as an ovarian tumor or cyst.

A GnRH stimulation test helps differentiate between CPP and benign pubertal variant. Once baseline LH, FSH, and estradiol levels are measured, girls are given the GnRH agonist leuprolide acetate at the dose of 20 mcg/kg. An LH level is then measured 60 minutes after the GnRH agonists. LH levels above 3.3–5 mIU/mL are suggestive of CPP.

Measurement of serum adrenal steroids is useful in girls with isolated precocious pubarche to differentiate between peripheral precocity and benign premature adrenarche. Concentration of DHEA-S >135 mcg/dL or testosterone >35 ng/dL warrants further evaluation for causes of peripheral precocity, such as nonclassical congenital adrenal hyperplasia or virilizing adrenal tumor.

Brain MRI is recommended for girls with suspected CPP because of higher rates of CNS abnormalities [6]. Pelvic ultrasound may be useful to differentiate between CPP and benign pubertal variants and will evaluate for an ovarian tumor or cyst in girls with progressive peripheral precocity. Girls with CPP have greater uterine and ovarian volumes as compared to girls with isolated premature thelarche.

A summary of the evaluation appears in Table 69.2. Once the diagnosis is made, the patient should be referred to a pediatric endocrinologist or other provider with experience treating precocious puberty.

Key Teaching Points

- Precocious puberty is defined in girls as the onset of secondary sexual development before age 8 years
- Precocious puberty can be classified as one of three types: CPP, peripheral precocity, and benign or nonprogressive pubertal variants
- A thorough history, physical examination (including Tanner staging), and a radiographic bone age are the initial steps in evaluation
- Additional laboratory testing and radiologic imaging that should be performed to further assist in determining the diagnosis include
  - Serum basal LH, FSH, and estradiol levels
  - GnRH stimulation test
  - Pelvic ultrasonography
  - Serum adrenal steroid levels (if isolated precocious pubarche)
  - Brain MRI (if CPP)

References

1. Kaplowitz P, Bloch C, The SECTION ON ENDOCRINOLOGY. Evaluation and referral of children with signs of early puberty. *Pediatrics* 2016;137(1): e20153732.

2. Herman-Giddens ME, Slora EJ, Wasserman RC et al. Secondary sexual characteristics and menses in young girls seen in office practice: a study from the Pediatric Research in Office Settings network. *Pediatrics* 1997;99(4):505–512.

3. Wu T, Mendola P, Buck GM. Ethnic differences in the presence of secondary sex characteristics and menarche among US girls: the Third National Health and Nutrition Examination Survey, 1988–1994. *Pediatrics* 2002;110(4):752–757.

4. Biro FM, Galvez MP, Greenspan LC et al. Pubertal assessment method and baseline characteristics in a mixed longitudinal study of girls. *Pediatrics* 2010;126(3).

5. Rosenfield RL, Lipton RB, Drum ML. Thelarche, pubarche, and menarche attainment in children with normal and elevated body mass index. *Pediatrics* 2009;123(1):84–88.

6. Berberoglu, M. Precocious puberty and normal variant puberty: definition, etiology, diagnosis and current management. *J Clin Res Pediatr Endocrinol* 2009 June; 1 (4):164–174. Published online December 8, 2010.

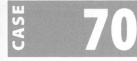

A 13-Year-Old Adolescent with Primary Amenorrhea and Cyclic Abdominal Pain (Imperforate Hymen)

James Casey

History of Present Illness

A 13-year-old female presents to the clinic with cyclic abdominal pain for the past four months. She describes the pain as dull, in her lower abdomen, and crampy. It is associated with low back pain, dysuria, and occasional dyschezia. The pain lasts approximately 7–10 days and resolves on its own. It has been recurring monthly and worsening with each episode. She has used ibuprofen without success.

She reports thelarche and pubarche at age 11 years, with normal pubertal progression, but she has not yet started menstruating. She has a history of mild, intermittent asthma and had an appendectomy at eight years of age. Her medical history is otherwise unremarkable, and she has no known allergies to medications. During discussion with her parents out of the room, the patient states she is not sexually active and has not previously attempted intercourse.

Physical Examination

General appearance   Well developed, well nourished

Vital Signs

Temperature	37.1°C
Pulse	92 beats/min
Blood pressure	96/60 mmHg
Respiratory rate	12 breaths/min
Oxygen saturation	100 percent on room air
Height	60 inches
Weight	120 lb
BMI	23.4 kg/m^2
Chest	Tanner stage IV breast development
Abdomen	Thin, soft, non-tender, mildly distended, no guarding, no rebound
External genitalia	Pubertal hair present. Normal appearing labia minor and majora. Urethra is normal in appearance.
Vagina	A discreet hymenal ring is not identified; there is a smooth, distensible mass with a bluish-tint bulging from the introitus.
Cervix	Unable to be visualized
Uterus	Unable to be visualized
Adnexa	Limited exam by vaginal mass/bulge.

Laboratory Studies

Urine pregnancy test	negative

Imaging

Pelvic ultrasound shows 6 cm uterus with endometrial fluid collection measuring 1.0 cm and significant hematocolpos extending to the perineum, normal appearing ovaries.

How Would You Manage This Patient?

This patient has a classic presentation of an imperforate hymen. She presents with cyclic abdominal pain at the time of expected menarche with a bluish-tint vaginal bulge seen on physical exam, and ultrasound imaging showing hematometra and hematocolpos and otherwise normal female pelvic organs. Physical exam shows expected pubertal changes in all other aspects (thelarche, pubarche) without acute concern for endocrinologic origin for her primary amenorrhea.

The patient and her parents were counseled on the need for surgical correction with hymenectomy, and informed consent was obtained from both the patient and her parents. She was posted urgently for examination under anesthesia and hymenectomy in the operating room under general anesthesia. The procedure was performed by incising and draining the hematocolpos, excising the imperforate hymen in an annular fashion, and suture ligation of the incised base circumferentially with interrupted, resorbable suture. She was discharged to home the same day, with resolution of her abdominal pain, and she recovered without incident. At her follow-up visit, she reported regular menses without dysmenorrhea.

Imperforate Hymen

An imperforate hymen is the most common obstructive vaginal anomaly and affects up to 1 in 2,000 females. It results from incomplete degeneration of the central portion of the hymen during fetal development. There is no significant genetic component described with imperforate hymen, though rare familial association has been described. Incomplete regression of the hymen can lead to a spectrum of hymenal abnormalities in addition to an imperforate hymen, which include a focal hymenal septum, a microperforate hymen, or a cribriform hymen. These abnormalities, however, do not cause menstrual obstruction and therefore do not cause cyclic pelvic pain or amenorrhea. Instead, they typically present as inability to use a tampon or have vaginal intercourse.

The hallmark presentation of imperforate hymen is cyclic lower abdominal and pelvic pain that begins at the time of expected menarche, which is generally 1–2 years after thelarche. This pain worsens over time in the face of primary amenorrhea. Other common symptoms are the result of menstrual retention within the vagina, cervix, and uterus and include back pain, dyschezia, and occasionally dysuria. The inability to place a tampon may be reported, though complete obstruction is associated with functional primary amenorrhea by patient history, negating the need for tampon use. If sexually active, the patient may offer an inability to complete vaginal intercourse.

221

While less common than imperforate hymen, additional diagnoses on the differential include a transverse vaginal septum, distal vaginal atresia/agenesis, cervical agenesis, complete labial agglutination due to irritation or trauma, or a large obstructive vaginal mass. Vaginal atresia occurs when a segment of the vaginal canal is embryologically obliterated with an atretic vaginal segment >1 cm in length [1].

Physical exam of the external genitalia reveals a classic blue-tinted bulge at the vaginal introitus. While this is the most common presentation, evaluation may also include a less prominent vaginal bulge. A thorough examination is required in all cases. Visual inspection will confirm a distensible membrane obscuring the vagina. In patients with a history consistent with an obstructive anomaly but no bluish bulge visible at the introitus, further imaging is warranted, generally with MRI, to clearly define the anatomy before surgical correction is attempted. Although a transverse vaginal septum and distal vaginal atresia are also managed surgically, the correction is more technically challenging and requires postoperative vaginal dilation to maintain vaginal patency. In these cases, it is often preferable to use hormonal menstrual suppression until the patient is mature enough to comply with postoperative care and to refer to a provider with experience in these procedures.

Prior to menarche, patients are generally asymptomatic, as the imperforate hymen does not impact daily function or activity. Occasionally, an imperforate hymen may be identified in newborn females on a focused pediatric newborn screening; however, it is not generally externally visible. The presence of a vaginal bulge in newborn females with imperforate hymen may present due to estrogen-dependent mucous buildup within the vagina [2]. If there is associated significant swelling of the vaginal membrane or concern for compression of the urethra, an incision and drainage may be performed with removal of excess hymenal tissue [3]. Surgical excision is discussed in detail below.

The primary treatment of an imperforate hymen involves surgical correction, which should preferably be performed in the newborn or post-pubertal period [4]. If the diagnosis is incidentally made in childhood, surgery should be delayed until puberty. Since most patients present with symptomatic menstrual obstruction, the procedure is generally performed urgently in order to relieve the patient's pain, as it was in the above patient. Regardless of the timing of the procedure, it is generally completed under anesthesia, with the goal of restoration of a patent vagina and relief of the obstruction, with removal of collected menses or other material within the vagina.

When the diagnosis is made incidentally in the newborn period, surgical correction may be performed at that time or delayed until adolescence. Rarely, newborns with imperforate hymen will be symptomatic, with findings that may include urinary retention or ureteral obstruction. In these cases, immediate surgical correction is indicated and can often be performed using needle-tip electrocautery with only local anesthesia with topical emla cream.

Several approaches to incising the imperforate hymen have been utilized, including vertical, elliptical, cruciate, stellate, and circumferential sharp excisions. Prior to incision, a thorough exam under anesthesia is performed, identifying the urethra and opening of the Bartholin's and Skene's glands, and confirming the diagnosis by the presence of a bulge at the introitus. An initial incision is made in the center of the bulge with a scalpel or electrocautery to allow for release of the hematocolpos, which is often brown and thick in consistency, and irrigation of the vagina. If a cruciate incision is used for hymenal excision, it should be performed as an "X" rather than a "+" to avoid both inadvertent incision toward the urethra at 12 o'clock and toward the lateral pudendal arteries at 3 and 9 o'clock [5]. The imperforate hymen is opened and excised to restore a normal vaginal opening. Trans-illumination and digital palpation will help demarcate the borders of the thin hymenal band from the surrounding vaginal wall during excision. The base of the hymenal ring is then sutured with resorbable suture, such as vicryl or monocryl, to reapproximate the mucosal edges at the hymenal ring. This is performed with interrupted sutures, as a running suture has greater risk for hymenal stricture or scar tissue formation. An overly aggressive and lateral dissection risks the inadvertent occlusion of the Bartholin's or Skene's glands during suture ligation.

A small central incision followed by sequential dilation with a Foley catheter or dilators has also been described; however, this approach may require weeks of active treatment, insufficient dilation, and is not the standard of care. Several approaches with a single vertical incision or an elliptical incision have also been described for culturally dependent preservation of "virginity." It is important to incorporate an understanding and appreciation of cultural goals; however, patients and their families should be informed that hymenectomy is recommended as the safest and most beneficial approach to treating imperforate hymen, with excellent long-term outcomes. Nonetheless, the patient's wishes should ultimately be respected.

Postoperative care involves pelvic rest, routine Sitz baths, and avoidance of tight-fitting clothing or manipulation of the area until healing is complete. Topical estrogen cream is occasionally used nightly for two weeks postoperatively to aid with healing; however, this is not needed in post-pubertal patients. While data are limited, topical estrogen cream should be considered in patients with concern for systemic medical issues that impede healing.

Key Teaching Points

- Imperforate hymen should be suspected in a young reproductive age adolescent female with cyclic abdominal pain and primary amenorrhea.
- The differential diagnosis of cyclic pelvic pain in patients with primary amenorrhea also includes more significant obstructive anomalies; therefore, the absence of the classic bluish bulge at the introitus should prompt further evaluation prior to surgical correction.
- Surgical correction should occur during times of existing estrogenized vaginal tissue (newborn and post-pubertal).
- Expectant management with counseling for later surgery should be provided if an imperforate hymen is discovered incidentally in childhood.
- Primary treatment involves surgical excision of the imperforate hymen in the operating room, with good long-term results.

References

1. Vallerie AM, Breech LL. Update in Müllerian anomalies: diagnosis, management, and outcomes. *Curr Opin Obstet Gynecol* 2010;22:381–387.

2. Atencio FP, Yabes-Almirante C. Abnormalities in Development. Atlas of Pediatric and Adolescent Gynecology. JP Medical Ltd. 2012;32–49.

3. Creighton SM. Common congenital anomalies of the female genital tract. *Reviews in Gynaecological Practice* 2005;5:221–226.

4. Laufer MR, Barbieri RL, Falk, SJ. Diagnosis and management of congenital anomalies of the vagina. *UpToDate®* 2015; Literature current through April, 2017.

5. Wheeless CR, Roenneburg ML. *Atlas of Pelvic Surgery*. Lippincott Williams & Wilkins. 1997.

6. Lardenoije C, Aardenburg R, Mertens H. Imperforate hymen: a cause of abdominal pain in female adolescents. *BMJ Case Rep* 2009.

7. Sucato GS, Murray PJ. Pediatric and Adolescent Gynecology. *Atlas of Pediatric Physical Diagnosis*. Saunders, an imprint of Elsevier Inc. 2012; 693–730.

8. Dietrich JE, Millar DM, Quint EH. Obstructive reproductive tract anomalies. *J Pediatr Adolesc Gynecol* December 2014;27 (6):396–402.

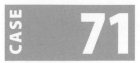

A 17-Year-Old Adolescent with Secondary Amenorrhea

Courtney Rhoades

History of Present Illness

A 17-year-old female, gravida 0, presents to your office with her mother. She states her mother is making her come to the gynecologist because she has not had a period in the last six months. The patient denies concern about her amenorrhea. She denies any prior or recent sexual activity. Menarche was at age 14, with subsequent monthly menses, lasting three days and without cramping. Her periods stopped when she started running with the track team in high school. Her grades are good, but lately she has been getting behind in her school work. Her mother is concerned because she feels her daughter is preoccupied with exercise. She states her daughter comes home from track practice and continues to work out rather than doing homework. She also has been reclusive and not interacting with the family. The patient states she is enjoying getting into shape and is exercising so that she can improve her track times. Her friends have made comments about how great she looks, so she doesn't understand why her mother can't be happy for her. She denies vomiting after eating and states she is just "cutting back" on her caloric intake. Her mother is concerned that she does not seem to be eating at all and mentions her daughter weighed 120 lb at the pediatrician's office at her last visit less than a year ago.

Her past medical history is significant for mild asthma, for which she uses an albuterol rescue inhaler. Her surgical history is positive only for an appendectomy at the age of 12. She has no drug allergies. She denies using any over-the-counter medications. Her mother's height is 65 inches, and she has a history of anxiety and depression. Her father is 70 inches and has hypertension.

Physical Examination

| General appearance | Slender build with a flat affect, appears tired |

Vital Signs

Temperature	37.0°C
Pulse	55
BP	110/60
Respiratory Rate	16
Height	65 inches
Weight	99 lb
BMI	16.5 kg/m^2 (less than 1 percentile for age)
Skin	Generally appears dry, finger nails well cared for without discoloration
HEENT	Good dentition, no chips or discoloration, thyroid without nodularity or enlargement
Cardiac	slow rate, normal rhythm without murmur
Breast	Tanner stage 3
Abdomen	Thin soft non-tender, no guarding or rebound
External genitalia	No lesions, Tanner stage 4
Vagina	No lesions, hymen intact
Cervix	Without lesions, nulliparous
Uterus	Normal size and mobile on bimanual exam
Adnexa	No masses and non-tender

Laboratory Studies

Urine pregnancy test	Negative
Hg	10 g/dl
Chemistry panel	Normal
TSH and prolactin	Normal
FSH	.2 IU/L
Estradiol	20 pg/ml

How Would You Manage This Patient?

This patient has secondary amenorrhea with a low follicle-stimulating hormone and estradiol, consistent with hypogonadotropic hypogonadism. She has lost a substantial amount of weight in a short time frame and has a BMI below the first percentile. Given her clinical history of amenorrhea, her severe caloric restriction and excessive exercise, and her physical and laboratory findings, this patient has anorexia nervosa (AN) as the underlying cause of her hypothalamic amenorrhea.

The patient was given the SCOFF questionnaire and scored a 2, which is a positive test, supporting the diagnosis of an eating disorder. The patient was counseled on the need to decrease her exercise and increase her nutritional intake. She was informed of the severe impact that weight restriction can have on her body with long-lasting consequences. These include cardiac arrhythmias that can lead to death, electrolyte imbalances, poor bone deposition and risk for osteoporosis, shortened stature, infertility, and difficulty with carrying a baby to term. She does not have electrolyte issues or thyroid changes, and she is cooperative and has great family support, so inpatient treatment is not indicated.

She was given a referral to a multidisciplinary eating disorder center near her home, and her family was encouraged to be active participants in her care. She was started on calcium, vitamin D, iron, and vitamin C supplementation to help with her anemia and mitigate any damage to her bone density. She was advised that although this will be an issue that will need to stay on top of for the rest of her life, she will likely resume menses once she improves her nutritional state and is back to greater than 90 percent of her ideal body weight.

Amenorrhea due to Anorexia Nervosa

AN is characterized by loss of significant body weight through restriction of energy intake. This is accompanied by a fear of weight gain, even though the patient is below normal weight, and a disturbance in how she perceives her body shape.

Box 71.1 The SCOFF screening tool for eating disorders

The SCOFF questions

Do you make yourself **S**ick when you feel overly full?

Do you worry that you lost **C**ontrol over how much you eat?

Have you recently lost more than **O**ne stone (14 lb) in a three-month period?

Do you believe yourself to be **F**at when others say you are too thin?

Would you say **F**ood dominates your life?

*Each yes =1 point; a score of 2 indicates likely diagnosis of anorexia nervosa or bulimia with 94.7%–100% sensitivity and 87.5% specificity.

Morgan JF, Reid F, Lacey JH. The SCOFF questionnaire: assessment of a new screening tool for eating disorders [Internet]. BMJ. British Medical Journal Publishing Group; 1999

Severity is defined by the DSM-5. A BMI of greater than 17 kg/m^2 is mild, 16–16.99 kg/m^2 is moderate, and less than 15.99 kg/m^2 is severe. The DSM-5 further subtypes the disorder into restrictive type and binging and/or purging type [1].

The prevalence of AN among women is about 4 percent [2], and it affects all racial and socioeconomic groups. While it does occur in men, 90 percent of patients arc women. For women, it can happen during any stage of life, but 40 percent of all cases of AN occur between 15 and 19 years, and 90 percent of eating disorders will present before the age of 25 [3].

Menstrual dysfunction is reported in 90 percent of patients with AN [4], and patients with AN will often not present due to weight loss or struggles with food but instead complain of symptoms from hypogonadotropic hypogonadism. Excessive weight loss, exercise, and anxiety can cause a reduction in gonadotropin-releasing hormone pulsatility and gonadotropin production. These changes result in a hypogonadal state of low luteinizing hormone, follicular-stimulating hormone, and estrogen levels and in symptoms of anovulation and amenorrhea, as seen in this patient [3]. The fecundability of women with AN is less than half that of healthy women, and women presenting to infertility clinics have a much higher incidence of eating disorders than the general population [5]. Once pregnant, women with eating disorders tend to improve; however, women with active disease are more likely to have preterm deliveries, small for gestation babies, microcephaly, and birth defects [3].

Low body weight reduces bone density as well. The annual decline of bone density, as long as the patient is underweight, is between −2.6 percent and −2.4 percent for the spine and hip, increasing the risk for fracture sevenfold after six or more years with AN. In addition, starvation can cause cardiac changes such as bradycardia, hypotension, electrolyte-induced arrhythmias, and orthostatic hypotension. Cold intolerance, hair loss, dry skin, and acrocyanosis are also common. Patients may also present with complaints of bloating, constipation, and generalized abdominal pain.

Making the diagnosis is key. Patients suspected of an eating disorder should have an assessment of orthostatic vitals, serum electrolytes, EKG, and mental check for suicidal intent and be given the SCOFF questionnaire (Box 71.1), which is both sensitive and specific for an eating disorder [6].

Patients with AN benefit most from a multidisciplinary approach, which should include specialists in nutrition, psychiatry, and social work who have experience treating patients with AN. The environment at home, work, or school is a main influencer on eating issues, so it is important to address any social issues in treatment. Family-based treatment is the most effective for children and adolescents, and improving nutrition is the goal regardless of age [8].

Women with AN are generally best treated in the outpatient setting. Criteria for inpatient admission are based on medical indications of instability, including a heart rate of less than 50, cardiac arrthymias, and/or hypothermia. In addition, when a patient fails to respond to outpatient treatment, is hemodynamically unstable, or has electrolyte abnormalities, inpatient treatment should be considered. Patients with eating disorders are often also dealing with psychological issues such as depression. Since suicide is a leading cause of death for eating disorder patients, inpatient treatment is recommended in AN patients with possible suicidal ideation [8].

While the gynecologist may look at the return of regular menses as the objective, it is important to not use hormonal treatment to treat amenorrhea. Instead, one should allow time for the patient's nutritional status to improve and thus allow for the return of normal menses. While estrogen deficiency contributes to the net bone reabsorption, studies of women with eating disorders placed on oral estrogen or oral contraception did not demonstrate recovery of their bone loss. Women who take oral contraceptives or other hormonal remedies to resume menses may get a false sense of well-being and thereby have a reduced incentive to continue treatment. They should be encouraged to achieve normal ideal body weight [4]. If contraception is desired, long-term reversible methods are recommended due to the high risk of unintended pregnancy in adolescents and possible adverse bone mineral density effects of low-dose estrogen contraceptive pills and depot medroxyprogesterone acetate [8].

Half of teens with AN have low bone density. This is due to slow bone formation, in contrast to the low bone density of menopause, which is from a decrease in bone formation and an increase in degradation. Bisphosphonates and other bone density treatments are not recommended in premenopausal patients who have not completed their childbearing due to long half-lives and potential deposition of the medication in the bone itself. Treatment, therefore, is concentrated on weight-bearing exercise, dietary supplementation, and improved nutrition. The recommended supplementation of calcium of 1,300–1,500 mg/day and Vitamin D 400 IU/day has been made by the Society of Adolescent Medicine for AN patients [3].

The longer the time to treatment and weight recovery, the poorer the prognosis; however, when diagnosed early, 80 percent of patients with AN recover [8]. When the duration of illness is shorter and the environment is positive, the patients are less likely to relapse. AN also has the highest rate of death among eating disorders, and 20 percent of those deaths are from suicide [9]. To decrease this risk, patients will need both psychological support and medical follow up for the five to six years that recovery can take [3]. Therefore, gynecologists can have a profound effect on this disease if they identify it early and encourage proper treatment.

Key Teaching Points

1. Providers should screen for eating disorders in female patients, especially in ages 14–19 years.
2. Menstrual irregularities, particularly secondary amenorrhea, can be caused by eating disorders such as AN.
3. Menstrual dysfunction is reported in 90 percent of patients with AN, who often present to gynecologists with symptoms related to hypogonadotropic hypogonadism, and not because of weight loss or struggles with food.
4. Treatment for AN is centered on improving nutrition and restoring ideal body weight. A family-centered, multidisciplinary treatment approach is optimal for AN, with involvement of nutrition, psychiatry, and social work.
5. Oral contraceptives or other hormonal treatments have not been shown to improve bone density in women with AN and should not be prescribed. The goal should be to improve body weight and restore spontaneous menses.
6. In patients with eating disorders who desire contraception, implants or intrauterine devices should be encouraged as first line.

References

1. American Psychiatric Association. Diagnostic and statistical manual of mental disorders (DSM-5). 5th ed. Arlington, VA.: American Psychiatric Publishing; 2013.

2. Smink F, van Hoeken D, Hoek H. Epidemiology of eating disorders: incidence, prevalence and mortality rates. *Curr Psychiatry Rep* 2012;14(4):406–414.

3. Andersen A, Ryan G. Eating disorders in the obstetric and gynecologic patient population. *Obstet Gynecol* 2009;114 (6):1353–1367.

4. Boisseau C. Identification and management of eating disorders in gynecology: menstrual health as an underutilized screening tool. *Am J Obstet Gynecol* 2016;215 (5):572–578.

5. Linna M, Raevuori A, Haukka J et al. Pregnancy, obstetric, and perinatal health outcomes in eating disorders. *Am J Obstet Gynecol* 2014;211(4):392. e1–392.e8.

6. Morgan JF, Reid F, Lacey JH. The SCOFF questionnaire: assessment of a new screening tool for eating disorders. *BMJ* 1999;319:1467–1468.

7. Witkop C, Warren M. Understanding the spectrum of the female athlete triad. *Obstet Gynecol.* 2010;116(6):1444–1448.

8. Sieke E, Rome E. Eating disorders in children and adolescents: what does the gynecologist need to know? *Curr Opin Obstet Gynecol* 2016;28(5):381–392.

9. Arcelus J. Mortality rates in patients with anorexia nervosa and other eating disorders. *Arch Gen Psychiatry* 2011;68 (7):724.

A 53-Year-Old Woman with a 3 cm Dermoid Cyst Noted as an Incidental Finding on CT

Jacob Lauer

Case Description

A 53-year-old postmenopausal woman is referred to you for evaluation and management of a 3 cm ovarian mass. She had previously presented to the emergency department with hematuria and flank pain where she underwent a CT scan of the abdomen and pelvis to evaluate for nephrolithiasis. A small stone was visualized as well as a 3 cm cyst of the right ovary, suspected to be a mature cystic teratoma (dermoid cyst). She was managed expectantly and passed the stone without intervention.

Her obstetric history is significant for two uncomplicated vaginal deliveries. She has been menopausal for approximately two years. Prior to menopause she describes normal menses at regular intervals and has had minimal menopausal symptoms.

Her past medical history is complicated by hypothyroidism for which she takes levothyroxine. She has no past surgical history. She is married and sexually active with her husband and denies pain with intercourse. Normal age-related screening studies are up-to-date and normal as documented in the record.

Review of symptoms is negative for vaginal bleeding, change in bowel habits, pain with intercourse, or abdominal pain or bloating.

Physical Examination

General appearance Well-developed, well-nourished female in no apparent distress.

Vital Sign

Temperature	98.6°F
Pulse	80 beats/min
Respiratory rate	16 breaths/min
Blood pressure	112/68 mm Hg
Height	5'6"
Weight	154 lb

BMI 24.9 kg/m^2

Abdomen	Soft non-tender, no palpable mass, normal bowel sounds
Vulva/Vagina	Normal external genitalia with minimal atrophy, vaginal mucosa pale. No significant discharge
Cervix	Normal appearing
Adnexa	Non-tender and non-palpable bilaterally

How Would You Evaluate and Manage This Patient?

Based on the patient's normal history and physical exam, an ultrasound was obtained which showed a small complex ovarian mass containing elements consistent with a small mature cystic teratoma. The mass was unilocular with no internal vascularity on doppler (see Figure 72.1). CA-125 was obtained and noted to be 30 pg/ml, which is in the normal range. Based on the CT imaging, sonographic imaging, a normal CA-125, and the lack of associated symptoms, the patient was counseled for surveillance with a repeat ultrasound in three months.

Mature Cystic Teratoma in a Postmenopausal Female

Mature cystic teratomas are a common and benign germ cell tumor of the ovary. They are the most common type of germ cell tumor to arise from the ovary and although they are most common in premenopausal women, they are seen in postmenopausal women as well. The majority of patients are asymptomatic at the time of diagnosis and thus they are a common incidental finding on CT or ultrasound imaging studies.

These tumors arise from primordial germ cells of the ovarian tissue. They typically contain a combination of well-differentiated ectodermal, endodermal, and mesodermal tissue. Though diagnosis can only be made with certainty based on histologic review, the unique composition of these tumors leads to a characteristic appearance on ultrasound (Figures 72.1 and 72.2). This allows for a highly accurate imaging-based diagnosis with specificity reported to be 98 percent [1]. The most common ultrasound finding is an echogenic tubercle projecting into the cyst lumen. This is often referred to as a "Rokitansky nodule." A hemorrhagic cyst or an endometrioma may also be considered in the sonographic differential. In cases where a confident diagnosis cannot be made with ultrasound, other imaging modalities can be considered. CT and MRI are highly sensitive in detecting fat, and thus

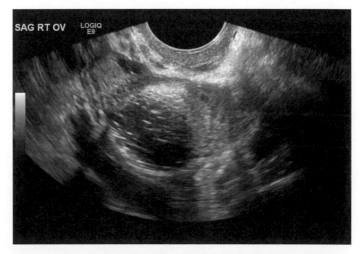

Figure 72.1 Transvaginal ultrasound demonstrating a small 3 cm mature cystic teratoma of the right ovary.

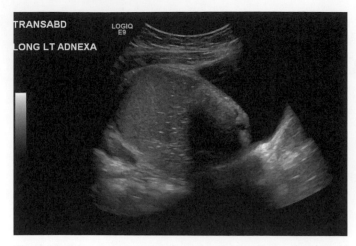

Figure 72.2 Transabdominal ultrasound demonstrating a large 11 cm mature cystic teratoma of the left ovary.

diagnosis of a mature cystic teratoma with these modalities is generally straightforward [2, 3]. Ultrasound is used most often in surveillance of these tumors. If the initial diagnosis is made by CT or MRI, obtaining a baseline ultrasound can allow for more straightforward comparison with future imaging.

Complications from mature cystic teratomas are rare, though they can become quite large and lead to ovarian torsion and pain. Cyst rupture has been reported to occur and although rare, can lead to a chemical peritonitis either through an acute or chronic process [4]. Malignant transformation is rare but can occur and is most likely a squamous cell carcinoma arising from the ectoderm.

In a postmenopausal woman with a newly diagnosed ovarian cyst, a serum CA-125 aids in the assessment for a possible malignancy. This tumor marker is of most use in identifying women with a non-mucinous epithelial ovarian cancer. The sensitivity of CA-125 for predicting malignancy has been reported to be 35–91 percent and the specificity 67–90 percent. The wide variation in these values is due to the inclusion of both postmenopausal and premenopausal women in the studies. Because of the higher incidence of ovarian cancer in postmenopausal women, CA-125 is a more useful marker in this population [5, 6]. Case reports describing malignant transformation of a mature teratoma into a squamous cell carcinoma do describe elevations in carcinoembryonic antigen, but there are no studies to validate use of this tumor marker in the routine workup of a mature cystic teratoma [7]. For a postmenopausal patient with imaging consistent with a mature cystic teratoma and a normal CA-125, the clinician

can be reasonably certain of the diagnosis and proceed with appropriate management. Based on current evidence, use of additional serum laboratory studies is of limited value.

The primary treatment of symptomatic or large mature cystic teratomas of the ovary is surgical excision. This can be accomplished either laparoscopically or through an open technique, though the majority of cases are amenable to a laparoscopic approach. Laparoscopy is associated with improved surgical outcomes, including less blood loss and a shorter hospital stay. The cyst is more likely to be ruptured with laparoscopy than with an open procedure and caution should be taken in these circumstances to thoroughly irrigate the abdomen and pelvis, but cases of chemical peritonitis in the event of cyst rupture are exceedingly rare [8]. For premenopausal women, cystectomy is typically preferred. In postmenopausal patients or patients who have completed childbearing, oophorectomy can be considered.

Conservative management of suspected mature cystic teratomas of the ovary is evidence based [9]. Appropriate candidates are patients who are asymptomatic, have small cysts, and have no imaging or laboratory findings to suggest a possible malignancy. There is no widely agreed-upon criteria for determining which size of cysts should be conservatively managed. Some guidelines suggest cysts less than 10 cm can be managed without surgery while other studies use criteria of 6 cm or less [1, 10]. As cyst size increases, patients are more likely to be symptomatic and will also assume more risk of complication such as ovarian torsion. If conservative management is chosen, serial imaging should be used to assess for stability. The ideal interval of repeat imaging is not known. One prospective study utilized ultrasound at three months after initial diagnosis and then every six months for the first two years. Ultrasound was continued annually if the cyst remained stable [10]. Some experts advocate for discontinuing imaging after 24 months for stable lesions in patients who remain asymptomatic [11].

Teaching Points

1. Ultrasound is the preferred imaging modality for suspected mature cystic teratomas due to its low cost and lack of radiation exposure. CT and MRI also have high diagnostic accuracy.

2. Asymptomatic, small mature cystic teratomas may be managed conservatively.

3. For symptomatic or large mature cystic teratomas, surgical excision via laparoscopic cystectomy or oophorectomy is the preferred route.

References

1. Practice Bulletin No. 174: Evaluation and management of adnexal masses. *ObstetGynecol* 2016 November;128(5): e210–e26. PubMed PMID: 27776072. Epub 2016/ 10/25.eng.

2. Outwater EK, Siegelman ES, Hunt JL. Ovarian teratomas: tumor types and imaging characteristics. *RadioGraphics*

2001;21(2):475–490. PubMed PMID: 11259710.

3. Guerriero S, Mallarini G, Ajossa S et al. Transvaginal ultrasound and computed tomography combined with clinical parameters and CA-125 determinations in the differential diagnosis of persistent ovarian cysts in premenopausal women.

Ultrasound in Obstetrics & Gynecology: The Official Journal of the International Society of Ultrasound in Obstetrics and Gynecology 1997 May;9(5):339–343. PubMed PMID: 9201878. Epub 1997/ 05/01.eng.

4. Koshiba H. Severe chemical peritonitis caused by spontaneous rupture of an

ovarian mature cystic teratoma: a case report. *J Reprod Med* 2007 October;52 (10):965–967. PubMed PMID: 17977177. Epub 2007/ 11/06.eng.

5. Pepin K, del Carmen M, Brown A, Dizon DS. CA 125 and epithelial ovarian cancer: role in screening, diagnosis, and surveillance. *Am J Hematol Oncol* 2014;10(6):22–29.

6. Grzybowski W, Beta J, Fritz A et al. [Predictive value of CA 125 in detection of ovarian cancer in pre- and postmenopausal patients]. *Ginekologia Polska* 2010 July;81(7):511–515. PubMed PMID: 20825052. Epub 2010/09/10. Wartosc predykcyjna stezenia CA 125 w diagnostyce raka jajmnika u kobiet przed i po menopauzie. pol.

7. Takagi H, Ichigo S, Murase T, Ikeda T, Imai A. Early diagnosis of malignant-transformed ovarian mature cystic teratoma: fat-suppressed MRI findings. *J Gynecol Oncol* 2012 April;23 (2):125–128. PubMed PMID: 22523630. Pubmed Central PMCID: PMC3325347. Epub 2012/ 04/24.eng.

8. Briones-Landa CH, Ayala-Yanez R, Leroy-Lopez L et al. [Comparison of laparoscopic vs. laparotomy treatment in ovarian teratomas]. *Ginecol Obstet Mex* 2010 October;78 (10):527–532. PubMed PMID: 21966769. Epub 2011/10/05. Comparacion del tratamiento laparoscopico vs laparotomia en teratomas ovaricos. spa.

9. Hoo WL, Yazbek J, Holland T et al. Expectant management of ultrasonically diagnosed ovarian dermoid cysts: is it possible to predict outcome? *Ultrasound Obstet Gynecol* 2010;36(2):235–240.

10. Alcazar JL, Castillo G, Jurado M, Garcia GL. Is expectant management of sonographically benign adnexal cysts an option in selected asymptomatic premenopausal women? *HumReprod (Oxford, England)* 2005 November;20 (11):3231–3234. PubMed PMID: 16024535. Epub 2005/ 07/19.eng.

11. Suh-Burgmann E, Kinney W. Potential harms outweigh benefits of indefinite monitoring of stable adnexal masses. *Am J Obstet Gynecol* 2015 12//;213(6):816. e1–816.e4.

A 60-Year-Old Woman with a 4 cm Simple Ovarian Cyst

Tara Harris

History of Present Illness

A 60-year-old woman, gravida 2, para 2, is referred from her primary care physician (PCP) for an ovarian cyst found on imaging. The patient was initially seen by her PCP for left-sided abdominal pain. CT scan of the abdomen and pelvis obtained at initial evaluation revealed evidence of diverticulosis and a 4 cm simple-appearing right ovarian cyst. She presents for consultation due to concern for the ovarian cyst. Her pain has since completely resolved with dietary changes. She denies feeling pelvic fullness, early satiety, or bloating.

Her past medical history is significant for chronic hypertension, which is well controlled with metoprolol. She takes no other medications. Her prior surgical history includes a postpartum bilateral tubal ligation. Menstrual history includes menarche at age 13, regular cyclic menses, and menopause at age 53. Her most recent cervical cancer screening is current and showed normal cytology with negative high-risk HPV cotesting. She has no family history of ovarian, breast, or colon cancer.

Physical Examination

General appearance	Well-developed, overweight female in no acute distress

Vital Signs

Temperature	37.0°C
Pulse	65 beats/min
Blood pressure	132/81 mm Hg
Respiratory rate	18 breaths/min
Oxygen saturation	98% on room air
BMI	25.6 kg/m^2
Neck	No masses or lymphadenopathy
Axillae	No masses or lymphadenopathy
Chest	Clear to auscultation bilaterally
Abdomen	Soft, non-tender, non-distended, normal active bowel sounds, no palpable masses, no hepatosplenomegaly, no fluid wave
External genitalia	Unremarkable, no lymphadenopathy
Vulva/vagina	No lesions, scant discharge and loss of ruggae and pale appearing
Cervix	No lesions or cervical motion tenderness
Uterus	Six-week size, mobile, non-tender, no masses
Adnexa	Right ovary approximately 4 cm by 3 cm in size, mobile and non-tender. Left ovary not palpable.

How Would You Manage This Patient?

The source of the patient's previous left-sided abdominal pain has been identified as diverticulosis and managed successfully by her primary care physician. As the patient is asymptomatic and the ovarian cyst is small and simple-appearing on CT, management should be guided by risk of malignancy. Further evaluation of the adnexal mass would include serum testing and a transvaginal ultrasound. The ovarian cyst was characterized on ultrasound as a simple, unilocular 4 cm right ovarian cyst. The left ovary was noted as a normal postmenopausal ovary, and no free fluid was noted in the pelvis (Figure 73.1). Her CA 125 level was reported as 12 U/mL. As these findings were consistent with a benign cyst, the recommendation was made to repeat the ultrasound imaging in three months. At follow-up ultrasound imaging, the cyst was noted to be slightly smaller at 3 cm but otherwise unchanged. The patient remained asymptomatic. Continued expectant management was recommended. Follow-up imaging revealed resolution of the cyst.

Adnexal Masses in the Postmenopausal Patient

Approximately 15–20 percent of women will develop ovarian masses [1]. Most ovarian masses are benign, but the risk of malignancy increases sharply with age. There is a 3.5-fold increase of ovarian cancer in postmenopausal women compared with premenopausal women [2]. A strong family history of breast and/or ovarian cancer is also an important risk factor, especially if the history is suggestive of *BRCA1* or *BRCA2* mutations. The lifetime risk for ovarian cancer is estimated to be 1.3 percent in the general population, but increases to 39 percent for women with *BRCA1* mutations and up to 17 percent for women with *BRCA2* mutations [3]. Risk factors for malignancy also include early menarche, late menopause, endometriosis, nulliparity, and/or primary infertility.

Although postmenopausal patients with adnexal masses have a much higher risk of malignancy than premenopausal patients, the most common adnexal mass in a postmenopausal patient is a benign serous cystadenoma. Unilocular ovarian cysts, such as the one in this case, occur in approximately 5–14 percent of postmenopausal women and are almost universally benign [1].

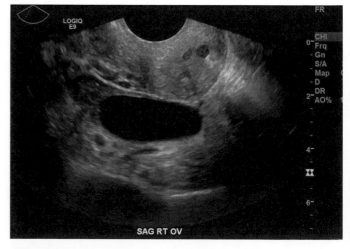

Figure 73.1 Ultrasound of 4 cm simple ovarian cyst.

A comprehensive history and physical examination is critical in the evaluation of a patient with an adnexal mass, including detailed gynecologic and family history as well as an in-depth review of systems. Ovarian cancer may be asymptomatic, but symptoms such as early satiety, urinary frequency or urgency, pelvic pain, generalized abdominal pain, or bloating may be present, particularly in later stages. For patients with adnexal masses, exams should include not only a thorough abdominal and pelvic exam but also palpation of lymph nodes and chest auscultation. A recto-vaginal exam may be necessary depending on the patient's history, the characteristics of the mass, and other exam findings. Signs such as a fluid wave may be indicative of ascites, and any firm, nodular, or fixed mass warrants further investigation.

Transvaginal ultrasound is the preferred imaging modality for the initial evaluation of adnexal masses [4]. Though ultrasound has a low positive predictive value for malignancy, it can identify features of an adnexal mass which may be concerning for malignancy (Box 73.1). Several algorithms that use various clinical and ultrasound features to create risk-scoring systems have attempted to predict the probability of malignancy. Most of these systems accurately discern benign masses from malignancies; however, the results of a 2014 meta-analysis found that the International Ovarian Tumor Analysis (IOTA) Logistic Regression model 2 (with a risk cutoff of 10 percent) and the IOTA Simple Rules model both demonstrate high sensitivity and specificity and thus may be considered [5]. Though transvaginal ultrasound is the recommended imaging modality for the evaluation of adnexal masses, CT is more suitable for assessing the presence of other signs of possible malignancy (e.g., pelvic and/or periaortic lymph node enlargement, ascites, peritoneal or omental implants, hepatic masses) or for other potential sources of metastatic disease.

Serum marker testing may also be beneficial in evaluating the likelihood of malignancy. Cancer antigen 125 (CA 125) is a monoclonal antibody associated with epithelial ovarian cancers, and to date it is the most studied ovarian tumor marker. Unfortunately, its use as a marker for ovarian malignancy has limitations due to its poor sensitivity and specificity. CA 125 can be expressed by nonmalignant tissues and in patients with conditions such as pregnancy, pelvic inflammatory disease, endometriosis, systemic lupus erythematosus, adenomyosis, inflammatory bowel disease, and uterine fibroids. CA 125 is elevated in 50–80 percent of patients with epithelial ovarian

cancer depending on disease stage [4], but is often normal in patients with other types of ovarian malignancies (i.e., germ cell, mucinous, or stromal cancers). Despite these limitations, CA 125 can be useful in the evaluation of adnexal masses, particularly for postmenopausal patients. Consultation with a gynecologic oncologist is appropriate for patients with a postmenopausal adnexal mass and a CA 125 level greater than 35 U/mL [4]. The American College of Obstetricians and Gynecologists previously recommended that premenopausal patients with an adnexal mass and CA 125 level greater than 200 U/mL be referred to a gynecologic oncologist; however, its most recent statement acknowledges that there is not an evidence-based cutoff and that the entire clinical picture should be considered when determining the need for referral [4].

Additional tumor marker testing may be indicated if there is suspicion of a non-epithelial ovarian malignancy. Serum biomarker panel testing may also be valuable in the workup of patients with adnexal masses. Panel testing is not recommended during the initial evaluation of patients with adnexal masses but can be used to identify patients who would benefit from consultation with a gynecologic oncologist. Serum biomarker panels such as the multivariate index assay have improved sensitivity and negative predictive value over CA 125 or clinical impression alone for the diagnosis of ovarian malignancy [4]. The Risk of Ovarian Malignancy Algorithm is more sensitive and specific in the detection of ovarian malignancy when compared to CA 125 alone [4]. Although the studies evaluating serum biomarker panel tests have been promising, their clinical utility is still in question.

After evaluation of a patient with an adnexal mass, the clinician must decide if the patient is a candidate for observation or if concerns for malignancy necessitate surgical intervention. In asymptomatic patients with benign-appearing cysts and with no suspicious laboratory findings, observation is generally recommended. Most of these masses are benign and many will resolve or regress spontaneously, even in women aged 50 and older [1, 6, 7]. Although estimates on the rates of resolution of these cysts vary, 69.4 percent of ovarian tumors measuring less than 10 cm spontaneously resolved in one study of 3,259 women aged 50 and older with unilocular cystic ovarian tumors [6]. Therefore, observation in these cases is reasonable; however, there currently are no accepted standards regarding the timing and duration of repeat imaging. In one study of 1,363 women aged 50 and older undergoing ultrasound observation of a complex adnexal mass, all but one of the masses later determined to be malignant demonstrated growth by seven months [7]. Although there is currently no clinical standard, some experts recommend limiting the observation of stable masses without solid components to one year [8].

For symptomatic patients and those with findings concerning for cancer, surgical management is indicated. If there is high clinical suspicion for malignancy, surgical intervention is best performed by a gynecologic oncologist with appropriate staging and debulking procedures. If the mass is believed to be benign, minimally invasive procedures are generally preferred; however, care should be taken to avoid intraoperative cyst rupture and spillage with subsequent iatrogenic upstaging of

---

Box 73.1 Ultrasound findings concerning for malignancy

- High-color Doppler flow
- Size greater than 10 cm
- Solid or mixed components
- Mural nodularity
- Presence of septations
- Septations greater than 3 mm in thickness
- Papillary excrescences
- Free fluid in pelvis

an undiagnosed malignancy. Concern exists for spillage with minimally invasive procedures; however, studies have found that the rates of spillage between patients undergoing laparoscopy versus laparotomy for clinically benign masses were equivalent [4]. Moreover, there were statistically significant improvements in pain control, length of hospital stay, and recuperation time with patients undergoing laparoscopic procedures [4]. Therefore, a minimally invasive approach is favored when appropriate.

Key Teaching Points

- Most ovarian masses are benign, even in postmenopausal patients.

- There are specific ultrasound findings that are more concerning for malignancy.
- CA 125 levels have limitations, but may be useful in the evaluation of adnexal masses, especially for postmenopausal patients.
- Many ovarian masses will spontaneously resolve and can be expectantly managed.
- There is currently no clinical standard for the expectant management of adnexal masses; however, some have suggested limiting the observation of stable masses without solid components to one year.
- If there is a high clinical suspicion of malignancy, surgical intervention is best performed by a gynecologic oncologist.

References

1. van Nagell Jr. JR, Miller RW. Evaluation and management of ultrasonographically detected ovarian tumors in asymptomatic women. *Obstet Gynecol* 2016;127:848–858.

2. Kinkel K, Lu Y, Mehdizade A, Pelte M-F, Hricak H. Indeterminate ovarian mass at US: incremental value of second imaging test for characterization – meta-analysis and Bayesian analysis. *Radiology* 2005;236:85–94.

3. The National Cancer Institute. BRCA1 and BRCA2: Cancer risk and genetic testing fact sheet. 2015. www.cancer.gov /about-cancer/causes-prevention/ genetics/brca-fact-sheet. (Accessed April 4, 2017.)

4. American College of Obstetricians and Gynecologists. Evaluation and management of adnexal masses. Practice Bulletin No. 174. *Obstet Gynecol* 2016;128:1193–1195.

5. Kaijser J, Sayasneh A, Van Hoorde K et al. Presurgical diagnosis of adnexal tumors using mathematical models and scoring systems: a systematic review and meta-analysis. *Hum Reprod Update* 2014;20:449–462.

6. Modesitt SC, Pavlik EJ, Ueland FR et al. Risk of malignancy in unilocular ovarian cystic tumors less than 10 cm in diameter. *Obstet Gynecol* 2003;102:594–599.

7. Suh-Burgmann E, Hung YY, Kinney W. Outcomes from ultrasound follow-up of small complex adnexal masses in women over 50. *Am J Obstet Gynecol* 2014;211:623.e1–623.e7.

8. Suh-Burgmann E, Kinney W. Potential harms outweigh benefits of indefinite monitoring of stable adnexal masses. *Am J Obstet Gynecol* 2015;213:816.e1–816.e4.

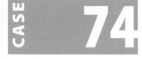
A 25-Year-Old Woman with a 2 cm Simple Asymptomatic Cyst Noted Incidentally on Ultrasound

Sarah A. Wagner

History of Present Illness

A 25-year-old nulligravid woman presents to the office for consultation due to an ovarian cyst. She reports menstrual cycles every 28 days, but started having intermenstrual bleeding three months ago. She describes the bleeding as light, mid-cycle, and lasting for two days. She sought the advice of her primary care physician, who ordered a pelvic ultrasound. The ultrasound identified a 2 cm simple ovarian cyst; therefore, she was referred for further management.

The patient is not taking hormonal contraceptives, as she is trying to conceive. She has no significant medical or surgical history. She has no family history of breast, ovarian, uterine, or colon cancer. She denies a history of sexually transmitted infections or pelvic inflammatory disease. She also denies a previous history of ovarian cysts, fibroids, or abnormal pap tests. Her periods are usually monthly, lasting five days with minimal discomfort. The patient's last menstrual period was three weeks ago and was normal. Her pelvic ultrasound was performed ten days before her visit.

Physical Examination

Vital Signs

Blood pressure	126/72
Heart rate	75
Temperature	98.6°F
Height 67 inches	
Weight	145 lb

General appearance	Well-appearing woman who appears to be her stated age, in no apparent distress
Neck	Supple, no masses, thyroid palpable and normal size, no lymphadenopathy
Lungs	Clear to auscultation bilaterally
Heart	Regular rate and rhythm, without murmurs, rubs, or gallops
Abdomen	Soft, non-tender, non-distended, without rebound or guarding
Vulva	Normal external female genitalia, no lesions. No groin lymphadenopathy
Vagina	Well rugated, no lesions, scant physiologic discharge
Cervix	Normal-appearing, no lesions, no cervical motion tenderness
Uterus	Small, anteverted, non-tender, mobile
Adnexae	Ovaries palpated bilaterally, non-tender, no masses identified

Labs

Gonorrhea and chlamydia	Negative
Cervical cytology	Negative one year ago
Pelvic ultrasound	The uterus measures 7.5 × 4.5 × 5 cm. The myometrium appears homogenous. The endometrial stripe measures 8 mm and is tri-laminar. The right ovary measures 2.4 × 3.2 × 2.1 cm and has normal vascular flow. The left ovary measures 4.5 × 3.6 × 4.1 cm and has a 2 × 2.2 × 2.1 cm simple-appearing cyst within. The ovary has normal vascular flow. There is scant free fluid present in the cul de sac.

How Would You Manage This Patient?

This patient has a small, simple ovarian cyst that was incidentally identified and is asymptomatic. She has no evidence of cervicitis, and her cervical cancer screening is up-to-date and negative. Given her negative workup, with a normal-appearing uterus on ultrasound, the mid-cycle bleeding is most likely due to the physiologic drop in estradiol related to ovulation. Considering her menstrual pattern, the ultrasound was performed just prior to ovulation. Based on the timing and appearance on ultrasound, her ovarian cyst is most likely a follicular cyst.

In women with physiologic, asymptomatic ovarian changes, the most appropriate management is patient education and reassurance. This patient was counseled on the menstrual cycle and the expected appearance of the ovary in different phases of the cycle. She was reassured that her ovaries appear to be functioning properly and that no further imaging was necessary. In addition, because she is trying to conceive, she was educated about timed intercourse, given routine preconception counseling, and advised to begin taking prenatal vitamins.

Simple Ovarian Cysts in Premenopausal Women

When evaluating a patient with an ovarian cyst, special care should be taken to elicit a thorough gynecologic and family history. A review of systems, with particular focus on pain, bloating, early satiety, bowel symptoms, and pressure symptoms, can help to qualify the urgency of evaluation and workup, as well as assist in narrowing the differential diagnosis. A comprehensive physical exam including a thorough pelvic exam should be performed. The identification of lymphadenopathy, a fluid wave, or a firm or fixed adnexal mass should trigger a prompt evaluation for malignancy.

Pelvic ultrasound is the preferred modality to evaluate an incidentally found adnexal mass. Experienced sonographers should be able to qualify adnexal masses to help guide management. When possible, it is ideal to perform ultrasounds in reproductive-age women between day 5 and day 10 of the menstrual cycle in order to reduce the possibility of identifying a normal developing follicle [1]. If the imaging shows thin walls and the absence of complex findings, these cysts are almost always benign. An ultrasound that demonstrates a cyst with thick vascular septations, excrescences, solid components, or low-resistance Doppler flow is concerning for malignancy [2].

Benign pelvic masses can arise from gynecologic and non-gynecologic causes. From the gynecologic origins, masses can develop from the ovary, fallopian tube, and uterus. The ovary can produce many different varieties of benign cystic masses, including functional cysts, endometriomas, mature teratomas, and cystadenomas; however, the differential diagnosis of adnexal cysts would also include hydrosalpinges and paratubal cysts. It is estimated that about 7 percent of women worldwide will have an ovarian cyst at some time in their lives [3].

Most ovarian cysts in premenopausal women are incidentally discovered, are benign, and will resolve without intervention within six months. Ovarian cysts are typically divided into two categories: functional cysts and neoplastic cysts. A majority of ovarian cysts are functional, with follicular cysts and corpus luteal cysts being most common. Follicular cysts occur when a developing follicle does not rupture and continues to grow. They are typically unilocular and have a thin, smooth wall. Most are asymptomatic unless they rupture or undergo torsion. Corpus luteal cysts, which occur after a developing follicle ruptures in ovulation, can appear simple or complex on ultrasound. Internal echoes and thick walls can be present. Though they can grow to be quite large (up to 8 cm), corpus luteal cysts almost always resolve without intervention.

Cystadenomas are neoplastic cysts that can have serous or mucinous cells lining them, and these cells determine the contents of the cyst. The appearance on ultrasound varies, as they can be simple or have complex features with multilocular characteristics. Serous cystadenomas are more common than mucinous, and are more frequently bilateral. Differentiating serous from mucinous cystadenomas on imaging can be challenging; however, mucinous cystadenomas can grow to be very large and are more commonly multiloculated. Symptoms of benign neoplastic ovarian cysts may include pain and bloating, but these generally only present when a cyst grows quickly, becomes very large, or undergoes torsion. Cystadenomas are more likely to be persistent than functional cysts.

The management of the simple ovarian cyst depends on its size and whether or not the cyst is growing or is symptomatic. Simple cysts that are 3 cm or less generally represent follicular or other physiologic cysts, which are a normal finding and do not require follow-up or intervention. Similarly, cysts that are 5 cm or less do not require any additional treatment unless they are symptomatic. Annual pelvic examination is recommended, and repeat ultrasonography can be considered if any new symptoms or findings develop.

Simple cysts that are greater than 5 cm but less than 10 cm can be conservatively managed and monitored with serial ultrasonography, as the risk of malignancy in these cases is extraordinarily low. It is reasonable to initially perform repeat imaging in 6–12 weeks, with subsequent management dependent on whether the cyst resolves or persists. In cases where repeat ultrasonography documents resolution, no further follow-up is warranted. When repeat ultrasonography demonstrates persistence, serial ultrasounds should be performed every 6 to 12 months to ensure that the cyst is not enlarging or developing characteristics that may be concerning for malignancy. In cases where the cyst is larger than 10 cm, it is generally recommended to treat the patient surgically with cystectomy or oophorectomy. Nonetheless, simple cysts of this size have been noted to spontaneously resolve when managed with serial ultrasonography [4]. In cases in which an adnexal mass is going to be conservatively managed with observation, it is critical to educate the patient on signs and symptoms of adnexal torsion. The threshold for surgery should always be lowered when the cyst is associated with pain or other symptoms concerning for torsion.

Key Points

- Pelvic ultrasound is the preferred modality to evaluate an adnexal mass, performed between day 5 and day 10 of the menstrual cycle.
- Findings that indicate benign pathology include a unilocular cyst with thin walls.
- Most ovarian cysts in premenopausal women are benign and will resolve without intervention within six months.
- Simple cysts that are 3 cm or less are a normal finding and do not require follow-up or intervention.
- Simple cysts up to 10 cm can be conservatively managed and monitored with ultrasound.
- Indications for surgical management include >10 cm in diameter, complex findings on pelvic ultrasonography, and pelvic pain.

References

1. Timor-Tritsch IE. Adnexal masses. In: Timor-Tritch IE, Goldstein SR, eds. *Ultrasound in Gynecology*. Philadelphia. Churchill Livingstone. 2007;100.

2. Barroihet L, Vitonis A, Shipp T, Muto M, Benacerraf B. Sonographic predictors of ovarian malignancy. *J Clin Ultrasound* 2013 June;41 (5):269–274.

3. Farghaly SA. Current diagnosis and management of ovarian cysts. *Clin Exp Obstet Gynecol* 2014;41(6):609–612.

4. American College of Obstetricians and Gynecologists. Evaluation and management of adnexal masses. Practice bulletin no. 174. *Obstet Gynecol* 2016;128 (5):1193–1195.

5. Alcazar JL, Castillo G, Jurado M et al. Is expectant management of sonographically benign adnexal cysts and option in selected asymptomatic premenopausal women? *Hum Reprod* 2005;20(11):3231.

6. Glanc P, Benacerraf B, Bourne T et al. First international consensus report on adnexal masses: management recommendations. *J Ultrasound Med* 2017 May;36(5):849–863. doi: 10.1002/jum.14197. Epub 2017 Mar 7.

A 25-Year-Old Woman with Endometriosis and a 4 cm Endometrioma

Mostafa A. Borahay

History of Present Illness

A 25-year-old, gravida 0, para 0, female presents to the office with gradually worsening painful menses and lower abdominal pain, predominantly on the right side. She describes her pain as aching in nature and worse during menstrual periods and sexual intercourse. She rates the pain as 7/10 at its worst. She states the pain used to be relieved by ibuprofen, but that is no longer the case. She denies frequency, burning, or other urinary complaints. She has normal bowel movements. She denies fever, chills, or fatigue.

The patient gives history of endometriosis diagnosed a few years ago during a diagnostic laparoscopy for pelvic pain, with temporary postoperative improvement reported after excision of the endometriosis implants. She does not have history of other medical problems or surgeries. She drinks alcohol socially, but denies smoking or illicit drug use. She has no known drug allergies. She has been married for the last three years and is not using condoms or any other form of contraceptives. Although they are not actively trying, she and her husband are open to the possibility of pregnancy.

Physical Examination

General appearance	Well developed, well nourished, alert and oriented, in no acute distress

Vital Signs

Temperature	37.1°C
Pulse	86 beats/min
Blood pressure	113/72 mmHg
Respiratory rate	16 breaths/min
Oxygen saturation	100% on room air
Height	66 inches
Weight	128 lb
BMI	20.7 kg/m^2
Abdomen	Thin, soft, non-distended, no guarding, mild tenderness in right lower quadrant on deep palpation, no rebound
External genitalia	Unremarkable
Vagina	Unremarkable
Cervix	Nulliparous, closed, no active bleeding or discharge
Uterus	Anteverted, limited mobility, normal size, mild tenderness on bimanual examination
Adnexa	Fullness and tenderness in the right adnexa

Laboratory Studies

WBCs	7,800/μL
Hb	11.9 g/dL
Hct	36.2%

Imaging	Transvaginal pelvic ultrasound shows a normal uterus with endometrial thickness 6 mm and no myometrial abnormalities. There is a 3.6 cm right ovarian cyst with homogenous low-level internal echoes. Left ovary appears normal with no free fluid (Figure 75.1).

How Would You Manage This Patient?

The patient has a history of endometriosis with symptoms, signs, and imaging findings consistent with a right ovarian endometrioma. The combination of classic symptoms of endometriosis (dysmenorrhea, pelvic pain, dyspareunia, and infertility) and an ovarian cyst with homogenous low-level internal echoes is highly suggestive of an endometrioma. Differential diagnosis also includes hemorrhage into a functional cyst or a benign tumor. Cancer is unlikely in this case given her age and the benign appearance of the mass on ultrasound. The ultrasound was repeated six weeks later, and the cyst was unchanged.

The patient was thoroughly counseled on the risks and benefits of different management options. She opted for surgical management, and an uncomplicated laparoscopic right ovarian cystectomy was performed. Histopathologic examination confirmed the diagnosis of endometrioma. The patient's pain improved postoperatively, and she was started on oral contraceptives to decrease the risk of recurrence. She continued to do well over a one-year follow-up.

Ovarian Endometrioma

Endometriosis is a chronic gynecologic condition where endometrial glands and stroma grow outside the uterine cavity.

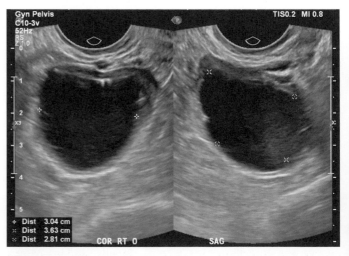

Figure 75.1 Ultrasound image of an endometrioma showing the typical homogenous low-level internal echoes.

It affects 6–10 percent of reproductive-age women, 38 percent of infertile women, and 71–87 percent of women with chronic pelvic pain. Ovarian endometriomas are cystic invaginations of ovarian surface containing blood and endometrial tissue inside. They are considered to form as a result of chronic bleeding in ovarian endometriotic lesions. The incidence of ovarian endometriomas is unclear. They induce fibrosis and are usually firmly attached to ovarian tissues and surrounding structures. Endometriomas are usually associated with pain and infertility, although some are asymptomatic [1]. They can be felt on pelvic exam as a tender mass or "fullness" at the vaginal fornix.

Pelvic ultrasound is usually the initial imaging modality of choice in the evaluation of adnexal masses. An ovarian endometrioma appears as a cyst with homogenous low-level internal echoes suggestive of old blood (Figure 75.1). Transvaginal ultrasound has a high diagnostic accuracy for ovarian endometriomas [1]. In addition, ultrasound can potentially identify associated endometriotic lesions, such as deep infiltrating endometriosis of the rectum or rectovaginal septum. Magnetic resonance imaging can be useful in equivocal cases [1].

Differential diagnosis of an endometrioma includes hemorrhage into a functional cyst, a benign tumor, or ovarian cancer. A repeat ultrasound in 6–12 weeks is generally recommended, as resolution would suggest the diagnosis of a functional cyst. Although CA 125 can be a helpful tool in the evaluation of an adnexal mass in postmenopausal patients, it has significant limitations in premenopausal patients [2]. CA 125 can be elevated in endometriosis and may reach levels as high as 1,000 units/mL or more with an endometrioma [2]. It can also be elevated in other noncancerous conditions such as fibroids, pelvic inflammatory disease, cirrhosis, peritoneal disease, or even pregnancy. Previously, the American College of Obstetricians and Gynecologists (ACOG) used 200 units/mL as a cutoff to refer premenopausal patients to gynecologic oncologists. However, there is no evidence to support a certain threshold, and ACOG currently recommends integrating CA 125 levels into the clinical picture [2]. Thus, it appears that CA 125 has limited role in the diagnosis of endometriosis or endometriomas.

Several considerations should be discussed when counseling patients about endometrioma treatment. First, there is a small but real risk of being or becoming malignant (clear-cell, endometrioid, or serous). The risk of malignant transformation of ovarian endometriosis is estimated to be 0.6–0.8 percent. In addition to the risk of malignant transformation of endometriosis, there is also the risk of misdiagnosing ovarian cancer as an endometrioma. Second, they can undergo rupture and torsion. Third, ovarian endometriomas can gradually destroy ovarian tissue and cause low ovarian reserve and infertility. Fourth, surgically resecting endometriomas is almost invariably associated with removal of ovarian tissues and may further lower ovarian reserve and contribute to infertility. Finally, endometrioma recurrence is common, and studies showed 11–30.4 percent recurrence at two years and up to 50 percent at five years after laparoscopic cystectomy [3, 4].

The treatment of endometriomas should be individualized according to patient characteristics, including presence of pain, infertility, plans for in vitro fertilization (IVF)/intracytoplasmic sperm injection (ICSI), and suspicion of malignancy. Treatment options include expectant management, endometrioma excision (ovarian cystectomy), and oophorectomy with/without hysterectomy. In most cases, endometriomas are surgically removed to alleviate symptoms, improve spontaneous pregnancy, and exclude malignancy.

Some cases of ovarian endometriomas can be managed expectantly, especially in asymptomatic women with small cysts (generally considered 3 cm or less in diameter) displaying typical ultrasound findings and prior diagnosis of endometriosis by laparoscopy. The frequency and duration of ultrasound follow-up of these cases are uncertain [2]. These cases usually receive the medical and hormonal treatments typically used for endometriosis such as oral contraceptive pills or progestins.

Surgery may be indicated in symptomatic cases, large or growing endometriomas, or when malignancy is suspected [2]. When surgery is planned, there is clear evidence that minimally invasive approaches (laparoscopic and robotic-assisted) have advantages over laparotomy, including less blood loss and pain, lower risk of postoperative adhesions, and faster recovery. Referral to surgeons with extensive experience in minimally invasive gynecologic surgery can be beneficial in complex cases. Certain cases with ultrasound findings suspicious for malignancy may benefit from collaboration with a gynecologic oncologist and availability of intraoperative frozen section.

Complete cyst excision of the endometrioma with ovarian cystectomy is associated with better improvement in pain, lower recurrence, and better spontaneous pregnancy rates compared with cyst aspiration (fenestration) with ablation/coagulation of cyst wall [5]. During surgery, every effort should be made to preserve normal ovarian tissue and minimize the use of tissue coagulation, which may reduce ovarian function and ovarian reserve. This is particularly important in younger patients and those attempting pregnancy.

There is no evidence that surgical removal of endometriomas before planned IVF/ICSI improves the pregnancy rate [6]. This, in addition to the potential negative effects of endometrioma removal on ovarian reserve and the costs and risks associated with surgery, made many experts recommend proceeding directly to IVF/ICSI and skipping endometrioma excision in these patients [7]. The decision for surgery before IVF/ICSI in women with endometriomas should be individualized, taking into account factors as pain, improving access for oocyte retrieval, and removal of an associated hydrosalpinx.

There is evidence that postoperative long-term ovarian suppression (at least 24 months) reduces symptoms and endometrioma recurrence. This includes oral contraceptives (whether cyclic or continuous), progestins (oral or parenteral), and GnRH agonists. Levonorgestrel intrauterine system has also been shown to decease dysmenorrhea after endometriosis surgery. Therefore, it is recommended to use one of these modalities postoperatively in those not attempting pregnancy [1, 8]. There is no evidence that preoperative ovarian suppression affects outcomes [1].

Finally, certain patients who do not desire future fertility and have severe intractable symptoms and/or recurrent disease after multiple prior conservative surgeries may be candidates for definitive surgical treatment. If the uterus was removed and ovaries conserved, the risk of recurrence of symptoms and repeat surgery after about 58 months was 62 percent and 31 percent, respectively. However, if the uterus and both ovaries were removed, the risk of recurrence of symptoms and repeat surgery was only 10 percent and 4 percent, respectively. The risk of recurrence of endometriosis after hysterectomy and bilateral adnexectomy is estimated to be up to 15 percent. Postoperative estrogen therapy in these cases is not contraindicated, as there is no evidence that it increases the risks of endometriosis recurrence. During definitive surgery, every effort should be made to remove all visible disease, especially when present on bowel, as small and large bowels are the most common sites of recurrence. Due to independent growth in a hypoestrogenic state, medical treatment is usually less effective for recurrent disease after definitive surgical treatment and repeat surgery is usually indicated. Patients should be counseled about the low but possible risk of endometriosis symptom recurrence after hysterectomy with bilateral adnexectomy [1].

Key Teaching Points

- An ovarian endometrioma should be suspected when imaging shows an ovarian cyst with homogenous low-level internal echoes, particularly with dysmenorrhea, pelvic pain, dyspareunia, infertility, and/or previous diagnosis of endometriosis by laparoscopy.
- Expectant management is reasonable, especially in patients who are asymptomatic and/or have small endometriomas without concern for malignancy.
- Surgical resection of an ovarian endometrioma is usually indicated to alleviate pain and rule out malignancy.
- Complete surgical removal of an endometrioma is preferred over simple drainage and coagulation of cyst wall.
- During surgery, every effort should be made to preserve normal ovarian tissue.
- Postoperative ovarian suppression, using combined oral contraceptives, systemic progestins, a levonorgestrel IUD, or a GnRH agonist, is recommended to reduce endometrioma recurrence in patients not currently desiring pregnancy.

References

1. American College of Obstetricians and Gynecologists. Management of endometriosis. Practice bulletin no. 114. *Obstet Gynecol* 2010;116(1):223–236.

2. American College of Obstetricians and Gynecologists. Evaluation and management of adnexal masses. Practice bulletin no. 174. *Obstet Gynecol* 2016;128 (5): e210–e26.

3. Maul LV, Morrision JE, Schollmeyer T, Alkatout I, Mettler L. Surgical therapy of ovarian endometrioma: recurrence and pregnancy rates. *JSLS* 2014;18(3).

4. Guo SW. Recurrence of endometriosis and its control. *Hum Reprod Update* 2009;15(4):441–461.

5. Dan H, Limin F. Laparoscopic ovarian cystectomy versus fenestration/coagulation or laser vaporization for the treatment of endometriomas: a meta-analysis of randomized controlled trials. *Gynecol Obstet Invest* 2013;76 (2):75–82.

6. Benschop L, Farquhar C, van der Poel N, Heineman MJ. Interventions for women with endometrioma prior to assisted reproductive technology. *Cochrane Database Syst Rev* 2010(11): CD008571.

7. Garcia-Velasco JA, Somigliana E. Management of endometriomas in women requiring IVF: to touch or not to touch. *Hum Reprod* 2009;24 (3):496–501.

8. Koga K, Takamura M, Fujii T, Osuga Y. Prevention of the recurrence of symptom and lesions after conservative surgery for endometriosis. *Fertil Steril* 2015;104 (4):793–801.

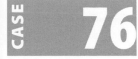

A 25-Year-Old Woman with Abrupt Onset of Pelvic Pain, Nausea and Vomiting, and Adnexal Masses (Torsion)

Todd R. Jenkins

History of Present Illness

A 25-year-old nulligravid woman with a last menstrual period three weeks ago presents to the office reporting acute onset of right lower quadrant pain for the last four hours. She describes the pain as constant, sharp, stabbing, and radiating into her right flank. She rates the pain an 8 out of 10 and notes associated nausea and vomiting since the onset of the pain. She denies any bowel or bladder dysfunction. She is currently not sexually active and denies any history of sexually transmitted infections or recent exposures. She is not using any contraception. She denies any significant past medical or surgical history and has no known drug allergies.

Physical Examination

General appearance	Well-developed, well-nourished female in moderate distress.

Vital Signs

Temp:	98.2°F
Pulse	110 beats/min
Respiratory rate	24 respirations/min
Blood pressure	126/80 mmHg
Oxygen saturation	98% on room air
Chest	Clear to auscultation bilaterally. Equal respirations bilaterally
CV	Tachycardia with regular rhythm. No murmurs or arrhythmias noted.
Abdomen	Tense, diffuse tenderness to mild palpation; no distension noted; voluntary guarding noted. Tenderness with palpation improved with Valsalva maneuver. No rebound appreciated. No masses appreciated.
Pelvic	Normal external female genitalia. Vagina with physiologic discharge, cervix with mild ectropion, but no significant discharge. Mild–moderate cervical motion tenderness noted. Anteverted, anteflexed uterus without abnormalities. Left adnexa without mass or tenderness. Right adnexa with significant tenderness and questionable mass; however, exam limited by guarding. Rectovaginal exam confirms pelvic fullness.
Extremities	No calf tenderness or edema
Neurologic	Alert and oriented × 3; anxious mood

Laboratory

WBCs	9,500/µL with 72% neutrophils
Platelet count	251,000/µL
Hb	12.2 g/dL
Electrolytes, liver function tests, and lipase	Within normal limits
Urinalysis	Moderate ketones and trace protein
Urine pregnancy test	Negative

Imaging

Pelvic ultrasound	Anteverted, anteflexed uterus measuring 8.2 × 5.3 × 4.8 cm with a symmetric endometrial thickness of 12 mm. The left ovary measures 3.3 × 3.1 × 2.9 cm and is without abnormalities. The right ovary is enlarged and measures 8.6 × 6.9 × 7.5 cm. It contains solid and cystic components. The cyst has a heterogeneous echotexture and contains numerous hyperechoic areas. Peripheral edema is noted within the ovary. Doppler flow is present in both ovaries. No free fluid is noted. Findings are concerning for a mature teratoma. Clinical correlation is recommended.

How Would You Manage This Patient?

This patient presents with acute right-sided pelvic pain with associated nausea and vomiting. Once pregnancy has been ruled out, the differential diagnosis of a patient with acute pelvic pain includes many gynecologic and nongynecologic conditions such as appendicitis, kidney stones, ruptured physiologic cysts, gastroenteritis, colitis, necrosis of a leiomyoma, and pelvic inflammatory disease [1]. However, in this patient with acute pain, nausea and vomiting, and a complex adnexal mass with no evidence of infection, ovarian torsion should be the primary diagnostic concern.

This patient was posted urgently for diagnostic laparoscopy, which was both diagnostic and therapeutic. Intraoperative findings confirmed right ovarian torsion. De-torsion of the adnexal mass and ovarian cystectomy were performed, and the patient was discharged later that day with resolution of her symptoms. She was doing well at her postoperative visit, and the pathologic evaluation of the ovarian cyst confirmed a mature cystic teratoma.

Ovarian Torsion

Ovarian torsion is "caused by the twisting of an ovary on its pedicle with subsequent lymphatic and venous stasis, leading to ischemia, potential necrosis, and loss of function" [2]. The true incidence of ovarian torsion is not known, as only cases that are correctly diagnosed and treated surgically can be evaluated. It has been estimated, however, that up to 3 percent of female patients with acute abdominal pain will have ovarian torsion [3, 4].

Ovarian torsion can occur across the age spectrum from in-utero to postmenopausal women, but it is most commonly diagnosed in women of reproductive age [4]. Risk factors for ovarian torsion include a history of ovarian torsion, polycystic ovarian syndrome, previous tubal ligation, ovarian hyperstimulation syndrome, and pregnancy, in which up to 20 percent of cases of torsion occur [3, 5]. In up to 60 percent of cases of ovarian torsion, the ovary is enlarged secondary to a benign ovarian cyst, such as a mature teratoma, hemorrhagic cyst, or a serous cystadenoma. It is important to recognize that torsion can occur in normal-sized ovaries as well, particularly in younger women. Some studies have suggested that torsion is more common in patients with ovarian masses > 5 cm. The risk of torsion in patients with an endometrioma or malignancy is low, however, secondary to associated adhesive disease or the fixed nature of these masses [3, 6]. Torsion occurs more commonly on the right side as a result of the mobile cecum and ileum as compared to the left side, where the relatively fixed sigmoid colon is in close proximity to the left ovary [2, 3, 4, and 6].

While the presentation can be quite varied, most patients with ovarian torsion present with the acute onset of abdominal pain (90–100%), nausea (70%), vomiting (45%), flank pain (20%), and fever (20%) [3]. Patients are usually normothermic, and those in severe pain may demonstrate slight tachycardia and an elevated blood pressure. Abdominal and pelvic exam may demonstrate a palpable mass; however, due to voluntary guarding and other patient factors, a mass may not be palpable. To date, a laboratory test that definitively confirms the diagnosis of ovarian torsion has not been identified.

The most commonly used imaging study to aid in the diagnosis of adnexal torsion is a pelvic ultrasound, with or without Doppler analysis [3]. Ultrasonography often demonstrates an ovarian mass, unilateral ovarian enlargement, peripheral cystic structures on the ovary, and a small-to-moderate amount of free fluid in the pelvis (see Figure 76.1). Some authors have described the "whirlpool sign," created by the twisted vascular pedicle, and a "follicular ring sign," defined as perifollicular hyperechoic prominent margins, as suggestive of ovarian torsion [6, 7]. The "follicular ring sign" is thought to be the result of significant hemorrhage and edema that occur around the follicles. In most situations, however, both of these signs disappear as arterial flow is compromised, so they may not reliably be present.

During the process of ovarian torsion, venous and lymphatic outflow is disrupted first. This disruption in the drainage system of the ovary leads to ovarian swelling, resulting in a heterogeneous and edematous appearance on ultrasound. Arterial flow is initially spared since the muscular arterial wall resists compression. Over time, however, the artery is eventually compressed, leading to an absence of Doppler flow. Arterial occlusion is a late occurrence; therefore, the presence of vascular flow does not exclude torsion, particularly if the clinical presentation is suspicious. Studies have

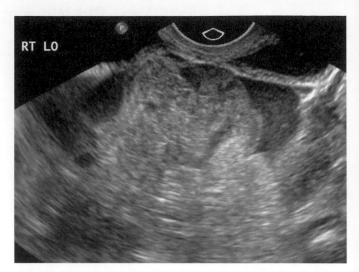

Figure 76.1 Ultrasound image of a torsed right ovary demonstrating an ovarian mass and peripheral cystic structures on the ovary.

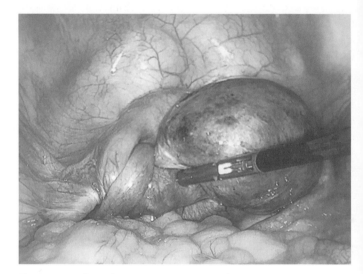

Figure 76.2 Classic laparoscopic appearance of ovarian torsion.

demonstrated normal Doppler flow in up to 61 percent of torsion cases [6].

Many patients who originally present to the emergency department with abdominal pain undergo CT imaging as the first diagnostic imaging technique. On CT, ovarian torsion can present with "multiple peripheral follicles in an asymmetrically enlarged ovary, decreased adnexal enhancement on the side of torsion following administration of IV contrast, a twisted vascular pedicle, pelvic free fluid, inflammatory fat stranding adjacent to the ovary, and/or uterine deviation towards the side of the torsion" [6]. As with other imaging modalities, the absence of these findings on CT imaging does not exclude ovarian torsion.

Ovarian torsion is a surgical emergency, and treatment with a laparoscopic approach is generally recommended [3]. The decision to operate should be made based on clinical suspicion. This should incorporate history, physical exam, and imaging and should not be solely based on Doppler findings [8]. Even with compelling clinical findings for ovarian torsion, the diagnosis of ovarian torsion is confirmed in only 10–44 percent of cases [3].

Laparoscopy is recommended as the best diagnostic and therapeutic approach for the management of ovarian torsion [1, 3]. Figure 76.1 demonstrates the classic appearance of ovarian torsion. Conservative surgery with de-torsion of the mass is recommended, even in the presence of a bluish-black, dusky ovary. The ovary may not return to a normal appearance during the initial laparoscopy; however, postoperative studies have demonstrated normal follicular development, normal Doppler flow, and normal appearance at six weeks postoperatively in 90 percent of patients [1, 3]. In the minority of patients who do not regain ovarian function, a second laparoscopic procedure may be indicated. De-torsion was previously not recommended due to theoretical concerns regarding the spread of vascular emboli at the time the ovarian pedicle is untwisted. This dogma has subsequently been proven false, as pulmonary embolism in cases of adnexal torsion are exceedingly rare [1]. As with all decisions regarding management of the ovaries at surgery, factors such as age, future fertility, menopausal status, and the particular ovarian disease identified should affect management.

There is no consensus regarding the need for cystectomy or oophoropexy at the time of laparoscopy for ovarian torsion. Most authors recommend cystectomy if possible; however, this is often challenging secondary to tissue edema and the resultant loss of surgical planes. Patients in whom a cystectomy is not performed should be counseled that recurrent torsion and/or a second laparoscopy may be necessary. Torsion recurrence rates have been reported to vary between 10.7 percent and 19.2 percent [4]. Those patients who experience ovarian torsion with a normal ovary appear to be at increased risk of recurrent ovarian torsion. A retrospective study by Pansky et al. revealed a recurrence rate of 60 percent in patients with a normal ovary at the initial torsion event compared to 8 percent in those with torsion in the presence of ovarian pathology [9]. As a result of this high rate of ovarian torsion recurrence, some authors recommend oophoropexy in women with torsion of normal adnexa in an attempt to limit ovarian mobility and prevent recurrent adnexal torsion [4]. At this time, however, neither the efficacy nor the best technique for oophoropexy has been demonstrated [3].

Key Points

- Ovarian torsion has been estimated to occur in 3 percent of female patients presenting for care with acute abdominal pain.
- Risk factors include a history of ovarian torsion, polycystic ovarian syndrome, previous tubal ligation, ovarian hyperstimulation syndrome, and pregnancy.
- The most common presenting symptoms of ovarian torsion are abdominal pain (90–100%) and nausea (70%) with or without vomiting (45%).
- In up to 60 percent of ovarian torsion cases, the ovary is enlarged secondary to a benign ovarian cyst, such as a mature teratoma, hemorrhagic cyst, or a serous cyst adenoma.
- Since arterial occlusion is a late occurrence, the presence of vascular flow does not exclude ovarian torsion.
- Ovarian torsion is a surgical emergency. Laparoscopy with de-torsion of the mass is the treatment of choice. There is no consensus regarding the need for cystectomy or oophoropexy.

References

1. Spinelli C, Piscioneri J, Strambi S. Adnexal torsion in adolescents: update and review of the literature. *Curr Opin Obstet Gynecol* 2016;27:320–325.

2. Ashwal E, Hiersch L, Krissi H et al. Characteristics and management of ovarian torsion in premenarchal compared to postmenarchal patients. *Obstet Gynecol* 2015;126:514–520.

3. Sasaki KJ, Miller CE. Adnexal torsion: review of the literature. *J Min Invasive Gynecol* 2014;21:196–202.

4. Melcer Y, Sarig-Meth T, Maymon R et al. Similar but different: A comparison of adnexal torsion in pediatric, adolescent, and pregnant and reproductive-age women. *J Women's Health* 2016;25 (4):391–396.

5. Boswell K, Silverberg KM. Recurrence of ovarian torsion in a multiple pregnancy: conservative management via transabdominal ultrasound-guided ovarian cyst aspiration. *Fertil Steril* 2010;94:1910e1–1910e3.

6. Lourenco AP, Swenson D, Tubbs RJ, Lazarus E. Ovarian and tubal torsion: imaging findings on US, CT, and MRI. *Emerg Radiol* 2014;21:179–187.

7. Sibal M. Follicular ring sign: a simple sonographic sign for early diagnosis of ovarian torsion. *J Ultrasound Med* 2012;31:1803–1809.

8. Ginath S, Shalev A, Keidar R et al. Differences between adnexal torsion in pregnant and nonpregnant women. *J Min Invasive Gynecol* 2012;19:708–714.

9. Pansky M, Smorgick N, Herman A, Schneider D, Halperin R. Torsion of normal adnexa in postmenarchal women and risk of recurrence. *Obstet Gynecol* 2007;109:355–359.

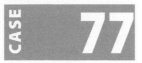

A 30-Year-Old Woman with Fever, Abdominal Pain, Vaginal Discharge, and Adnexal Mass (Tubo-Ovarian Abscess)

Joseph E. Peterson

History of Present Illness

A 30-year-old, gravida 1, para 0, female presents for an unscheduled office visit. She reports a two-week history of progressively worsening abdominal pain. She describes a predominately dull, cramping ache with occasional sharp spikes in intensity, particularly with movement and sex. The pain initially localized to the right side but recently spread throughout her lower abdomen and pelvis. She has taken ibuprofen and acetaminophen with some relief. Although the pain is "tolerable" and she has continued working, she feels it has progressed and is now worried she may have "some STD like before." She denies any exacerbation or alleviation with defecation or urination though she does feel like she is urinating more frequently. Her appetite is normal; she denies any change in bowel habits. She has a new sexual partner of two months, but vaginal penetration has become too painful for intercourse, especially with deep penetration. Her partner also noted a vaginal discharge with foul odor, further precipitating abstention. She reports that she has felt fevers and chills that awaken her at night.

Her family history is noncontributory and she reports no significant medical or surgical history.

Her sexual history includes first coitus at 12 years of age, 25 lifetime partners, and a history of being treated twice for unknown vaginal infections. Her last menstrual period was approximately one week prior to the onset of pain. She notes her cycles are usually 27–30 days. She reports some recent spotting. She uses birth control pills for contraception.

She denies tobacco or ethanol and reports infrequent marijuana use. Her current medications include only the above-noted ibuprofen and acetaminophen and oral contraceptives. Her only allergy is reported to be nausea with penicillin.

Physical Examination

Vital Signs

Temperature	99.9°F
Pulse	87
Blood pressure	98/67
Respiratory rate	18
Oxygen saturation	99% on room air
Height	60 inches
Weight	105 lb
BMI	20.5 kg/m²
General	Well-developed, well-nourished female. Alert and oriented. No acute distress but appears somewhat uncomfortable when walking and sitting on the exam table
Abdomen	Thin, soft, tender throughout, right greater than left, non-distended, voluntary guarding, mild focal rebound tenderness in right lower quadrant
External genitalia	Normal external female genitalia
Vagina	Normal, estrogenized epithelium with rugae
Cervix	Nulliparous-appearing, with foul-smelling, green, muco-purulent discharge present at the cervical os

Bimanual

Uterus	Anteverted, mobile, normal size and contour, cervical motion tenderness present that lateralizes to the right
Adnexa	Palpable enlarged right adnexa with report of acutely increased tenderness on palpation

Laboratory Studies

Urine pregnancy test	Negative
Saline wet prep	Negative for trichomonads or yeast. Multiple clue cells and clusters of WBCs
KOH wet prep	Positive amine odor. No budding yeast
GC/CT PCR	Pending
HIV	Pending
Serology	
WBC	16,200/μL
Hgb	13.1 g/dL
Hct	38.9%
CRP	8 mg/dL
ESR	50 mm/hr
Imaging	Transvaginal ultrasound shows normal-sized uterus and trilaminar endometrium of normal thickness. Left ovary 2.8 cm in largest dimension. Right adnexa with complex-appearing mass, 5×7 cm with hypoechoic, multi-loculated areas, obscuring normal ovarian and tubal appearance. Hyperemia of tubal complex noted on doppler imaging. Cul de sac with 0.5 cm of fluid.

How Would You Manage This Patient?

This patient has pelvic inflammatory disease (PID) with an apparent tubo-ovarian abscess (TOA) on imaging. Her clinical presentation, particularly in light of her sexual history, makes PID a likely diagnosis even without supportive laboratory or imaging results. The criteria for diagnosis of PID include non-specific signs and symptoms that can be supported with laboratory and imaging studies when available (Table 77.1). Testing for sexually transmitted infections (STIs) at the time of physical exam should be performed. Even without laboratory evidence, empiric treatment should be initiated as soon as PID is suspected.

After imaging confirmation of a tubo-ovarian complex, the patient was counseled on the risks to future fertility and possible incomplete treatment and resolution of the TOA requiring prompt, adequate surgical or procedural treatment. Even though clinically afebrile, due to the presence of a TOA, parenteral antibiotic treatment was recommended. Since there is minimal cross-sensitivity with second- and third-generation cephalosporins [1] and the patient's allergy to penicillin was reported as mild, first-line cefoxitin and doxycycline were utilized.

As the patient did not appear septic and the abscess was not ruptured, nor did she have a clearly accessible fluid collection, drainage was not undertaken as an initial step in her treatment.

She remained afebrile and her symptoms were noted to be improving the day after initiating treatment. Parenteral antibiotics were then continued for 36 additional hours. On hospital day 2, GC/CT PCR returned as positive for both gonorrhea and chlamydia. The patient was discharged home with oral doxycycline and metronidazole on hospital day 3 to complete a 14-day course of therapy. She was seen in the office two weeks later with resolution of symptoms. Ultrasound follow-up showed an adnexal complex still present, but with decreasing size and vascular flow.

She was advised to have her sexual partner(s) tested and treated for gonorrhea and chlamydia before resumption of any sexual activity. As required by state law, her infection was reported to the local health department by the testing laboratory.

Tubo-ovarian Abscess

PID incidence and prevalence are declining, estimated at less than 5 percent as of 2015 [2]. Mortality from TOAs is nearly nonexistent compared to the mid-twentieth century [3].

However, the severity of the sequelae of PID and associated TOAs (ectopic pregnancy, hydrosalpinx and associated tubal factor infertility, chronic pelvic pain, sepsis, and death) warrant a low diagnostic threshold for empiric treatment. When compared to laparoscopy, clinical diagnosis has a positive predictive value of 65–90 percent [1].

Though this patient's case was relatively straightforward, PID and even TOA may present an unclear picture to the clinician. The signs, symptoms, and diagnostic criteria of PID, even with the development of TOA, are nonspecific (see Box 77.1), sharing significant overlap with symptoms and signs of other intra-abdominal pathologies. Similarly, the presentation of a patient with TOA at times may be no more severe or different than one with mild PID. She may present with no fever, no severe pain, or even a normal white blood cell count. Alternatively, TOAs may present primarily with acute peritonitis when ruptured or with overt sepsis.

However, if the suspicion of TOA is heightened in a patient with a clinical diagnosis of PID secondary to palpation of an adnexal mass with tenderness on exam, a pelvic ultrasound should be obtained. Once TOA is confirmed, inpatient treatment with parenteral antibiotics is indicated. This recommendation contrasts with traditional recommendations for initial *outpatient* management of a patient with PID who otherwise presents with mild symptoms, lacking a high fever or severe abdominal pain. Early parenteral treatment, for premenopausal, unruptured, nonseptic patients with TOA less than 9 cm in size, will likely be effective without invasive drainage or surgery in two out of three cases [4].

Due to the polymicrobial nature of PID and TOAs, broad-spectrum antibiotic coverage should be used [1]. PID/TOA may effectively be treated by many regimens, as noted by the CDC and confirmed in a Cochrane review of the literature [5], of which the parenteral regimens should be used specifically when TOA is confirmed (see Box 77.1). Likely antecedent or concurrent infection with *Neisseria gonorrhoeae* and *Chlamydia trachomatis* requires antibiotic coverage for these organisms as well. Additional coverage of anaerobic bacteria with a specific medication such as metronidazole has not been shown to be necessary if the regimen administered includes

Table 77.1 Criteria for diagnosis of pelvic inflammatory disease

Minimum criteria (at least one must be present)	Additional criteria increasing suspicion	Additional criteria increasing specificity or establishing diagnosis
Cervical motion tenderness Adnexal tenderness	Oral temperature >38.3° C (>101° F)	Endometrial biopsy showing endometritis
Uterine tenderness	Large amount of WBCs on saline wet prep Mucopurulent cervical discharge or friability Elevated ESR Elevated CRP Documented infection with gonorrhea or chlamydia	Ultrasound or MRI showing thickened, fluid-filled tubes, tubo-ovarian complex, hyperemia on Doppler studies, +/− free fluid Laparoscopic or open surgical findings consistent with PID

Adapted from the Centers for Disease Control and Prevention 2015 STD Treatment Guidelines

> **Box 77.1** Treatment regimens for tubo-ovarian abscess
>
> **Recommended parenteral regimen**
>
> Cefotetan 2 g IV q12 *and*
>
> Doxycyline 100 mg IV/PO q12
>
> OR
>
> Cefoxitin 2 g IV q6 *and*
>
> Doxycycline 100 mg IV/PO q12
>
> OR
>
> Clindamycin 900 mg IV q8 *and*
>
> Gentamicin 2 mg/kg then 1.5 mg/kg q8 IV/IM
>
> **Alternate parenteral regimen**
>
> Ampicillin/Sulbactam 3 g IV q6 *and*
>
> Doxycycline 100 mg IV/PO q12
>
> Adapted from the Centers for Disease Control and Prevention 2015 STD Treatment Guidelines

anaerobic coverage. However, following appropriate parenteral treatment for TOAs, oral clindamycin or metronidazole should be administered in addition to doxycycline to complete 14 days of therapy, as the combination provides better anaerobic coverage than doxycycline monotherapy.

Once parenteral treatment is initiated, the patient's symptoms and clinical signs should be monitored for improvement. However, if improvement is not noted within 24–48 hours after initiation of parenteral treatment, drainage or surgical management of the tubo-ovarian complex may be necessary. Imaging-guided percutaneous drainage of a discrete fluid collection may be possible in consultation with interventional radiological specialists. Conservative management in this manner is successfully managed in the majority of cases [6]. Alternately, if interventional radiology is not available, or no discrete fluid collection is present (the abscess is multiloculated), and surgical intervention is required, laparoscopic surgery may be undertaken to drain or to remove the abscess and adnexal structures. Open abdominal surgery may be required if the necessary surgical expertise for the laparoscopic approach is unavailable. Surgical intervention should be isolated to removing the affected organs such as the affected adnexa versus total hysterectomy and oophorectomy. Conservative management is preferred when surgically treating TOAs. The inflammatory changes, edema, and distortion of tissue planes may result in more morbidity than with benign hysterectomy. Conservative surgical management also lessens the impact on hormonal function and future fertility. However, if the patient no longer desires fertility and has

advanced infection, a hysterectomy with bilateral salpingo-oophorectomy may be preferred.

Non-barrier contraceptive methods are more often associated with PID and TOA. Intrauterine device (IUD) use, when compared to combined hormonal contraception, does not *further* increase the risk for PID/TOA though this hypothetical risk was previously espoused. Studies have shown that this specific risk is only increased over baseline within the first three weeks after IUD insertion [7].

When counseling regarding resumption of intercourse, the patient should be counseled that her partner may be an asymptomatic vector for STIs and should therefore be tested and/or treated prior to resumption of any sexual activity with the patient regardless of her testing status.

Gonorrhea and chlamydia are found with vaginal testing in approximately half of the PID cases. TOAs are more likely to harbor group A and B *Strep, E. Coli, Klebsiella, Proteus, Haemophilus, Bacteroides, Prevotella, Peptococcus,* and *Peptostreptococcus.* The absence of gonorrhea and chlamydia on cervical testing, however, does not preclude the diagnosis of either PID or TOA resulting from an ascending genital tract infection with either or both organisms. A preceding lower genital tract infection with gonorrhea or chlamydia also puts the patient at risk for ascending infection with normal vaginal flora [1, 8].

Since PID and TOAs are more common in younger women, the finding of either in a postmenopausal patient should warrant surgical evaluation and treatment due to the increased risk of additional pathologies in the differential diagnosis such as fibroids, diverticulitis, and the concurrent risk of genitourinary or gastrointestinal tract cancers [2, 9].

Key Teaching Points

- Though unruptured TOAs rarely are associated with death, TOA can become a life-threatening situation via rupture and sepsis. Prompt treatment with parenteral antibiotics and access to surgical drainage is essential.
- Similar to the broad-spectrum antibiotic coverage for PID, a similar strategy should be utilized for TOA (see Box 77.1) as etiologies include both STI and ascending polymicrobial infections.
- Unlike PID treatment, treatment for TOA should *begin* in the inpatient setting with parenteral antibiotics and progress to surgical management if no improvement is seen within 24–72 hours.
- Surgical management, when indicated, should be conservative and need not result in hysterectomy with oophorectomy except in the postmenopausal patient where a TOA may represent a more worrisome etiology and pathology.

References

1. Centers for Disease Control and Prevention 2015 STD Treatment Guidelines: Pelvic Inflammatory Disease. Accessible at www.cdc.gov/std/tg2015/pid.htm.

2. Centers for Disease Control and Prevention STD Surveillance 2015. Accessible at www.cdc.gov/std/stats15/std-surveillance-2015-print.pdf.

3. Collins CG, Frank GN, Cerha HT. Ruptured tuboovarian abscess. *Am J Obstet Gynecol* 1956;72:820–829.

4. Lareau SM, Beigi RH. Pelvic inflammatory disease and tubo-ovarian

abscess. *Infect Dis Clin North Am* 2008;22:693–708.

5. Savaris RF, Fuhrich DG, Duarte RV, Franik S, Ross J. Antibiotic therapy for pelvic inflammatory disease. *Cochrane Database Syst Rev* 2017, Issue 4. Art. No.: CD010285. DOI: 10.1002/14651858. CD010285.pub2

6. Gjelland K, Ekerhovd E, Granberg S. Transvaginal ultrasound-guided aspiration for treatment of tubo-ovarian abscess: A study of 302 cases. *Am J Obstet Gynecol* 2005; 193: 1323–30.

7. Grimes DA. Intrauterine device and upper-genital-tract infection. *Lancet* 2000;356:1013–1019.

8. Sweet RL. Treatment of Acute Pelvic Inflammatory Disease. *Infect Dis Obstet Gynecol* Vol. 2011, Article ID 561909, 13 pages, 2011. doi:10.1155/2011/561909

9. Protopas AG et al. Tubo-ovarian abscesses in postmenopausal women: gynecological malignancy until proven otherwise? *Eur J Obstet Gynecol Reprod Biol* 2004;114:203–209.

Further Reading

Ness RB et al. Effectiveness of inpatient and outpatient treatment strategies for women with pelvic inflammatory disease: results from the Pelvic Inflammatory Disease Evaluation and Clinical Health (PEACH) randomized trial. *Am J Obstet Gynecol* 2002;186:929–937

Ross, J. Pelvic Inflammatory Disease. *Am Fam Physician*. 2014 November 15;90(10): 725–726.

Grandson, M. Pelvic inflammatory disease. *Am Fam Physician*. 2012, April 15;85(8):791–796.

A 45-Year-Old Woman with Pelvic Pain One Year after TLH/BSO for Endometriosis (Ovarian Remnant)

Todd R. Griffin

History of Present Illness

A 45-year-old female, gravida 2, para 2, presents to the office with an eight-month history of persistent pelvic pain. The pain has been worsening over the last few months; it was initially cyclic but is now constant with exacerbations. She is also complaining of dyspareunia and at times dysuria. The patient underwent a total laparoscopic hysterectomy/bilateral salpingoophorectomy (TLH/BSO) for endometriosis one year prior to this presentation. At the time of surgery, she had dense adhesions from four prior laparoscopies for endometriosis. Prior to her surgery she had been using oral contraceptives without symptomatic improvement. She currently denies any fever, chills, nausea, vomiting, change in bowel habits, or loss of appetite. She describes the pain as constant and rates it at 7 out of 10 – increasing to 9 out of 10 when it worsens. She uses ibuprofen as needed for the pain but it no longer helps.

Her surgical history is significant for four prior laparoscopies and an appendectomy. She has no significant past medical history. She has been married for 14 years and has 2 children ages 12 and 9. She has no known drug allergies. Her current medications include oral estrogen, a multivitamin, and ibuprofen.

Physical Examination

General appearance	Well-developed, well-nourished woman who is in mild discomfort but alert and oriented

Vital Signs

Temperature	37.0°C
Pulse	82 beats/min
Blood pressure	112/72 mmHg
Respiratory rate	16 breaths/min
Height	66 inches
Weight	145 lb
BMI	23.4 kg/m^2
Abdomen	Thin, soft, tender in lower abdomen, non-distended, no guarding, no rebound tenderness
External genitalia	Unremarkable
Vagina/Cuff	Well-healed vaginal cuff, no obvious lesions visualized
Cervix/Uterus	Absent
Adnexa	Discomfort on palpation of bilateral adnexal regions, left ≫ right.

Laboratory Studies

WBCs	8,800/μl
Hb	12.1 g/dl
Hct	37.1%
Bun/Cr	11.0/0.9
Urinalysis and urine culture	Both negative
FSH	7 mIU/ml
Imaging	Transvaginal ultrasound reveals an absent uterus and cervix; a small amount of free fluid in the pelvis, the right pelvis is unremarkable, the left pelvis shows a 2.3 complex solid and cystic lesion.

How Would You Evaluate and Manage This Patient?

This patient likely has ovarian remnant syndrome. Her persistent pelvic pain that worsens cyclically after a TLH/BSO for endometriosis in combination with ultrasound imaging makes ovarian remnant syndrome a likely diagnosis. Her normal follicle-stimulating hormone (FSH) may be secondary to her estrogen therapy. The oral estrogen was discontinued and the FSH rechecked after ten days. The FSH was unchanged, indicating retained functional ovarian tissue. The patient underwent operative laparoscopy with resection of the cystic mass. Intraoperative evaluation and pathologic evaluations confirmed the diagnosis of ovarian remnant syndrome. After the surgery, the patient's pain resolved.

Ovarian Remnant Syndrome

Ovarian remnant syndrome (ORS) was first formally described by Shemwell and Weed in 1970 [1]. They noted that incomplete removal of all ovarian tissue at the time of bilateral salpingoophorectomy (BSO) may result in pelvic cystic masses and chronic pain syndromes. ORS is a gynecologic condition defined as the presence of a pelvic mass with residual functional ovarian tissue after a previous oophorectomy, often in combination with a hysterectomy [2]. ORS should not be confused with residual ovarian syndrome or supernumerary ovary syndrome, where an ovary is intentionally left in place after gynecologic surgery and causes pain or where extra ovaries develop embryologically (rare syndrome), respectively.

The incidence of ORS is unknown and has been difficult to determine as most publications are case reports or case series. Definitive diagnosis is obtained from surgical removal and histologic confirmation of remnant ovarian tissue (presence of corpus luteum, dystrophic ovarian lesions, and hemorrhagic and follicular cysts) [2]. Inadvertent and incomplete removal of the ovarian tissue at the time of the primary surgery leads to ORS. There are a number of predisposing factors to the development of ORS, including dense pelvic adhesions from prior surgeries, pelvic inflammatory disease, inflammatory bowel diseases, and most importantly endometriosis. Endometriosis increases the risk of embedded functional ovarian tissue on adjacent tissue or structures. This poses a challenge for the operating surgeon who must diligently dissect the ovary off any adjacent structures such as the pelvic side wall or ureter. Failure to ligate the ovarian vessels well away from the ovary increases the chance of retaining a viable piece of ovary behind. To minimize this risk, surgeons should abide by three operative principles: opening the retroperitoneal space widely to allow for complete resection of the ovary, avoiding blunt dissection of ovarian adhesions, and resecting dense fibrotic ovarian adhesions involving adjacent peritoneum or viscera [1].

Patients with ORS most often present within the first five years after oophorectomy with a chronic pain syndrome but less frequently may present with an asymptomatic pelvic mass. In the largest published series of ORS patients (183) reported by the Mayo Clinic, the presenting symptoms include chronic pelvic pain (84%), dyspareunia (26%), cyclic pelvic pain (9%), dysuria (7%), and tenesmus (6%) [3]. The increased volume of remnant ovarian tissue in premenopausal women can lead to compression of adjacent structures, such as the peritoneum, bowel, and ureter, leading to pain. Additionally, pain can develop through the continued production of hormones and stimulation of ectopic endometriotic implants by the ovarian remnant. ORS is more commonly noted in young premenopausal women who undergo surgery. The absence of menopausal symptoms after BSO in these patients should raise the suspicion for ORS.

The diagnosis of ORS can often be difficult, but the use of laboratory and hormonal analysis, specifically estradiol and FSH levels, can be helpful. Often premenopausal patients who have undergone BSO are placed on estrogen therapy. In order to assess for ovarian remnant syndrome, estrogen therapy should be discontinued for at least ten days prior to hormonal testing to avoid any misinterpretation. In two separate published series (183 and 30 patients), approximately 59–71 percent of patients had premenopausal levels of estradiol and FSH. It is important to note that FSH levels (< 35–40 IU/dl) can confirm the diagnosis of ORS in patients with prior BSO; however, postmenopausal levels of estradiol and FSH do not completely exclude the diagnosis of ORS [2]. Ovarian tissue has been pathologically confirmed in surgical specimens in patients with postmenopausal hormone levels. Provocation of the remnant ovarian tissue through the use of clomiphene can be utilized in patients where the diagnosis is still uncertain. In two small studies, imaging was able to identify cystic structures after the administration of 50 mg of clomiphene citrate twice daily for ten days in 67–75 percent of patients. Once again, lack of a response to clomiphene does not rule out ORS. Anovulatory patients may not respond to clomiphene stimulation; similarly, not all ovarian remnant tissue will respond [1]. Additionally, provocation can be helpful at the time of surgery to aid in identification of the remnant tissue. Hormonal and provocation studies are clearly useful in the diagnosis of ORS.

Imaging is critical in the diagnosis of ovarian remnant syndrome. In the series of patients described by the Mayo Clinic (186 patients), a pelvic mass was found in 93 percent of the patients on ultrasound, 92 percent of those who had a computed tomography, and 78 percent of those who had magnetic resonance imaging. This led the authors to conclude that pelvic imaging, in any form, was recommended for first-line evaluation [3]. The combination of imaging, hormonal studies, and provocation studies is very helpful in the diagnosis of ORS. MRI images of ovarian remnants can be seen in Figures 78.1 and 78.2.

With a presumptive diagnosis of ORS, there are a number of different treatment options that have been reported. These include medical therapies, radiotherapies, and surgical therapies. Medical therapies include medications that are aimed at suppressing ovarian function. These include the use of continuous oral contraceptives, danazol, gonadotropin-releasing hormone analogues (GnRH-a), and the use of progesterone. The use of these agents has had mixed results. In the series of 186 patients from the Mayo Clinic, 50 percent of patients had some improvement with medications but ultimately all patients continued to have significant symptoms requiring further treatment. Medical therapies may be helpful in patients where surgery is contraindicated or in cases of endometriosis-associated ureteral obstruction [4]. Radiotherapy has been utilized in an attempt to castrate the residual tissue. A number of series with mixed and conflicting results have led experts to discourage the use of radiation therapy for ORS due to the potential deleterious effects of pelvic radiation. The one area where it might be useful is in a patient with significant comorbidities that would preclude a surgical approach [2]. In addition, for both medical and radiation therapy, the lack of pathologic diagnosis could lead to the misdiagnosis of a potential borderline or malignant process.

Surgical removal remains the gold standard for both diagnosis and treatment of symptoms, simultaneously excluding a potential malignancy [2]. Surgical management can be complex and requires extensive surgical dissection, including ureterolysis and enterolysis. One retrospective study published in 2012 compared open laparotomy versus laparoscopy versus robotic approach to surgical excision for ORS. They demonstrated that the rates of pain improvement were 93 percent, 94 percent, and 72 percent for the laparotomy, laparoscopy, and robotic approaches, respectively. The authors demonstrated that the laparoscopic and robotic approaches had reduced blood loss, lower postoperative complications, and shorter length of stay when compared to open approaches [5]. ORS is often commonly associated with deep endometriosis; preoperative imaging with pelvic MRI can help to identify these areas. Due to the complexity of the surgery, preoperative planning is imperative and may require involvement of other surgical services, including colorectal and urology. The surgical approach traditionally requires identification of the ovarian vessels with high re-ligation of the vessel above the aortic bifurcation. The ureter should be mobilized laterally to allow for complete peritonectomy of the ovarian remnant tissue. A more conservative surgical approach has been endorsed by others in that similar relief of pain symptoms

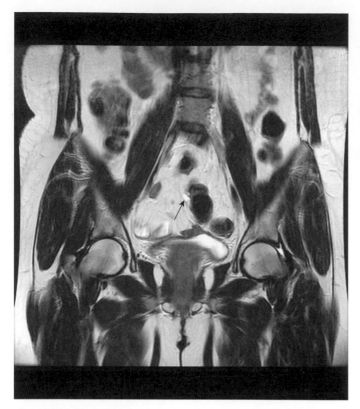

Figure 78.1 Pelvic MRI – T2 coronal view (arrow points to ovarian remnant).

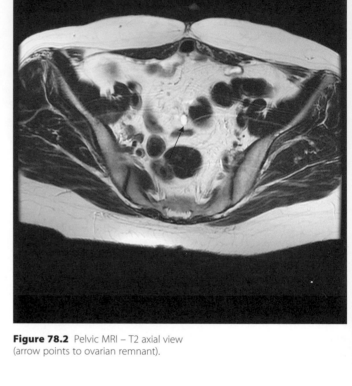

Figure 78.2 Pelvic MRI – T2 axial view (arrow points to ovarian remnant).

(97% versus 89%) can be achieved with a lower risk of complications [2]. In either approach, the surgical planning should be thorough and the surgeon should be skilled in pelvic surgery to ensure the best surgical outcome.

Ovarian remnant syndrome can be debilitating for a patient and continues to remain a diagnostic and therapeutic challenge for experienced clinicians. It should always be in the differential diagnosis of women who have chronic pain after bilateral oophorectomy, especially if intraoperatively there were dense pelvic adhesions or in cases performed for endometriosis. Ideally, prevention remains key to this disease. Proper surgical technique at the initial surgery is critical to decrease retained ovarian tissue and thus the development of ovarian remnant syndrome.

Key Points

- ORS is an important differential diagnosis in patients with pelvic pain or a pelvic mass after bilateral oophorectomy in which the initial surgery was complicated by dense adhesion or endometriosis.
- Laboratory studies (FSH and estradiol), hormonal provocation studies, and imaging studies (pelvic ultrasound, computed tomography, and/or magnetic resonance imaging) are key tools to aid in the diagnosis of ovarian remnant syndrome.
- ORS is best treated surgically by clinicians experienced in pelvic surgery through excision of the remaining and surrounding tissue. Medical therapy may be helpful in patients where surgery is not an option.

References

1. Magtibay PM, Magrina J. Ovarian remnant syndrome. *Clin Obstet Gynecol* 2006 September;49(3):526–534.

2. Kho R, Abrao M. Ovarian remnant syndrome: etiology, diagnosis, treatment and impact of endometriosis. *Curr Opin Obstet Gynecol* 2012 August;24 (4):210–214

3. Magtibay PM, Nyholm JL, Hernandez JL, Podratz KC. Ovarian remnant syndrome. *Am J Obstet Gynecol* 2005 December;193(6):2062–2066.

4. Vilos GA, Marks-Adams JL, Vilos AG et al. Medical treatment of ureteral obstruction associated with ovarian remnants and/or endometriosis: report of three cases and review of the literature. *J Minim Invasive Gynecol* 2015 March–April;22 (3):462–468.

5. Zapardiel I, Zanagnolo V, Kho RM, Magrina JF, Magtibay PM. Ovarian remnant syndrome: comparison of laparotomy, laparoscopy and robotic surgery. *Acta Obstet Gynecol Gynecol Scand* 2012 August;91 (8):965–969.

A 21-Year-Old Woman at Five Weeks EGA with Left Lower Quadrant Pain

Lisa M. Keder

History of Present Illness

A 21-year-old female, gravida 1, para 0, presents to the office with left lower quadrant pain. Her last menstrual period was approximately five weeks ago. She denies any light-headedness, fever, urinary problems, or gastrointestinal symptoms. She describes the pain as crampy, intermittent, and mild in intensity. Her past medical history is significant for a prior history of chlamydia. Surgical history is significant for an appendectomy. She is sexually active with one partner with whom she has been in a six-month relationship. They have been using condoms inconsistently. Her urine pregnancy test is positive. She is planning to return to an out-of-state college in two weeks.

Physical Examination

General appearance	Tearful adult woman, who appears comfortable sitting upright

Vital Signs

Temperature	37.1°C
Pulse	72 beats/min
Blood Pressure	110/72 mmHg
Respiratory rate	16 breaths/min
Height	62 inches
Weight	120 lb
BMI	21 kg/m^2
Abdomen	Normal bowel sounds, thin, soft, non-distended, no guarding or rebound, mildly tender on deep palpation of the left lower quadrant
External genitalia	Normal
Vagina	Normal rugae, normal discharge
Cervix	Ectropion present, no bleeding noted, no cervical motion tenderness
Uterus	Retroverted, non-tender, mobile, normal in size
Adnexa	No palpable masses, left slightly tender to palpation

Laboratory Studies

Urine pregnancy test Positive

Imaging

Transvaginal ultrasound shows a normal-sized uterus with endometrial thickness of 8 mm, a 2.5 cm simple cyst in the left ovary, and a normal right ovary. There is no free fluid in the cul de sac.

How Would You Manage This Patient?

The clinical scenario of a positive pregnancy test with ultrasound that shows no pregnancy is called a pregnancy of unknown location (PUL). PUL is often an interim diagnosis. With further follow-up, PUL may be diagnosed as an intrauterine pregnancy (IUP), spontaneous abortion, or ectopic pregnancy. However, on occasion, a location will never be identified. Since the patient is clinically stable without an acute abdomen, further evaluation can occur in the outpatient setting. Blood work, including a quantitative β-hCG, CBC, and blood type, was ordered. The patient was instructed to call if she had a change in symptoms: specifically increasing pain, bleeding, or light-headedness.

Initial laboratory studies returned that afternoon included a hemoglobin of 12.2 g/dl, WBC of 11,100 /μl, and a β-hCG of 600 mIU/ml, and blood type O positive. The patient was instructed to return for a repeat β-hCG in 48 hours. At that time, the level had risen to 800 mIU/ml, a rise of 33 percent. The patient reports continued crampy pain and spotting since her last visit. On exam, her abdominal exam is unchanged, she has scant bleeding from the cervical os, and no cervical motion tenderness or adnexal masses are present. Ultrasound reveals a small amount of fluid in the uterine cavity, but is otherwise unchanged from the prior scan. The patient is consented for manual vacuum aspiration in the office due to a PUL with inappropriately rising β-hCG. Direct examination of the uterine contents does not show chorionic villi. The β-hCG is repeated 24 hours after the surgery and has fallen to 200, and the pathology examination does not show chorionic villi. Because of the significant drop in HCG, this clinical scenario likely represents a completed abortion, or a resolving persistent PUL and serial HCG was not required. On follow-up two weeks later in the outpatient office, the patient has a negative urine pregnancy test. A levonorgestrel intrauterine device is placed and the patient is instructed to use a backup method or abstinence for seven days.

Pregnancy of Unknown Location

PUL describes a situation in which a pregnancy test is positive, but there is no evidence of either an intrauterine or an extrauterine pregnancy on transvaginal ultrasound. Additionally, the patient has not had prior imaging during this pregnancy showing an IUP nor symptoms suggesting a completed abortion. Women with this diagnosis often present to medical facilities because they are symptomatic due to pain or light bleeding. On occasion, they simply have a positive pregnancy test and imaging that does not identify a pregnancy. Since a PUL, especially in a symptomatic woman, may lead to a diagnosis of ectopic pregnancy, it is important that the patient be closely followed. Moreover, the correct diagnosis has implications for future pregnancy prognosis and management. However, it is not always possible to come to a firm diagnosis as some patients may have had early spontaneous abortions or may have

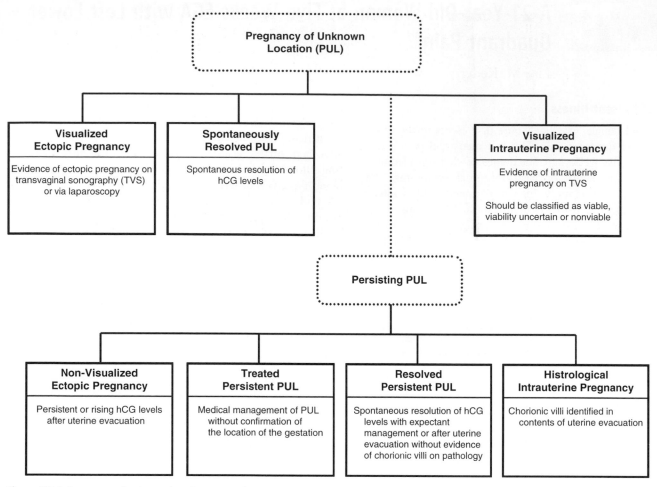

Figure 79.1 Pregnancy of unknown location nomenclature.
Reprinted from Fertility and Sterility, Vol 95 Issue 3, Barnhart et al., Pregnancy of unknown location: a consensus statement of nomenclature, definitions, and outcome. pp 857–866, Copyright 2011, with permission from Elsevier.

spontaneously resolving ectopic pregnancies and the location cannot be confirmed (Figure 79.1) [1].

In the diagnosis of PUL, appropriate evaluation will be directed by a careful history including the date of last menses, duration of normal menstrual cycle, date of first positive pregnancy test, and characterization of pain and bleeding. Examination should include the amount of bleeding, with inspection of the cervix for dilation and tissue presence. Bimanual exam should be performed to for cervical motion tenderness, adnexal masses, or tenderness. Basic laboratory tests include a quantitative β-hCG, CBC, and blood type. Ultrasound exam is best performed transvaginally, which is more sensitive than transabdominal scanning in the identification of early pregnancy. Ultrasound evaluation of a symptomatic patient in pregnancy requires careful examination not only of the uterus but also of the adnexa.

Both the absolute value of a quantitative β-hCG and its relative rise over time are useful in assessing a PUL. The discriminatory level of β-hCG is the value at or above which an ultrasound should be diagnostic of an IUP. In most cases, an IUP is detected on ultrasound when the β-hCG level is 2,000 or higher [2]. This assumes a singleton IUP. In multiple gestations, the β-hCG could be higher at any particular point in

gestation. The discriminatory value depends upon the skill of the ultrasonographer, the equipment, and the patient herself. Thus, it is a relative concept [3]. Uterine position or malformation, the presence of fibroids, and patient obesity can all affect the quality of imaging. One center's experience described a patient with β-hCG of 2317 with no IUP visualized, who went on to develop a normal, singleton pregnancy. The authors then modeled the association of β-hCG and visualization of the gestational sac. They found that the probability of detecting a sac would be 99 percent at a level of 3,510, suggesting that the discriminatory value in their institution may be higher, and the concept should be used cautiously [4]. An accurate assessment of gestational age based on last menstrual period is a better predictor of ultrasound landmarks than is a single measurement of β-hCG, since the level has a wide range of normal values at any point in pregnancy.

With a value at or above the discriminatory β-hCG, ultrasound interpretation is based on the predictable sequence of anticipated developmental events [5]. A gestational sac is first seen at approximately five weeks gestational age and is described by the mean sac diameter (the average of sagittal, transverse, and anteroposterior diameters of the sac). Subsequently, the yolk sac, a circular structure about 3–5 mm

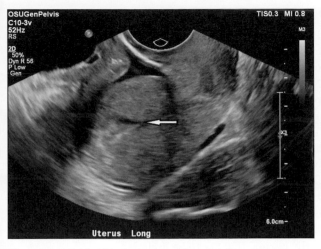
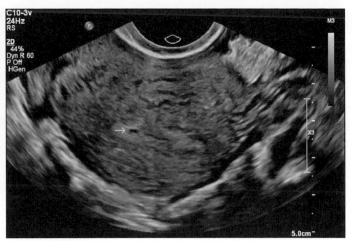

Figure 79.2 Fluid within the uterine cavity mimicking a gestational sac.

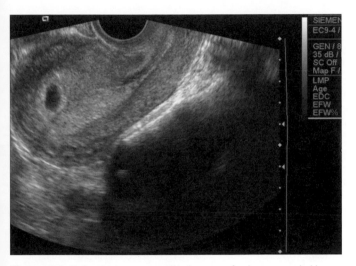

Figure 79.3 Early pregnancy, gestational sac near fundus surrounded by endometrium.

in diameter, becomes visible at approximately 5.5 weeks gestation [6]. Definitive diagnosis of an IUP is dependent upon the presence of a gestational sac in the upper uterus. Skilled ultrasonographers may identify an early gestational sac by the fact that an ovoid lucency is present, implanted eccentric from the midline endometrial echo, and surrounded by a decidual reaction that is brighter than the endometrium itself. However, an intrauterine fluid collection can be mistaken for a gestational sac. Fluid will be in the midline and not have a decidual halo. Additionally, a "beak sign" may be present. This is a visible tapering of the fluid at its distal end in the endometrial cavity as seen in the sagittal plane (Figures 79.2 and 79.3).

In a compliant, stable patient with a nondiagnostic ultrasound and level below the discriminatory value, follow-up β-hCG testing is useful. The β-hCG is repeated in 48 hours. Initial work by Kadar suggested that a minimum rise of 66 percent occurs over a 48-hour period for a normal pregnancy. [7] A subsequent study found that 99 percent of viable pregnancies would have a rise of 53 percent or more when the

starting level was less than 5,000.[8] Recent research examining a more diverse patient population found that the rate of rise varies dependent upon the initial value and patient's race and age, as well as presence of bleeding. This study found that a minimal (first percentile rise at 48 hours) of 49 percent is expected when the initial value is less than 1,500, 40 percent when initial values are 1,500–3,000, and of 33 percent for values over 3,000 [9]. If such a rise does not occur, the pregnancy is abnormal, but the location is still indeterminate. Repeat transvaginal ultrasound should be considered, especially if there is any change in symptoms. In the absence of adnexal findings suggestive of an ectopic pregnancy and with an abnormally rising β-hCG potential management strategies include continued observation, uterine evacuation, or treatment with methotrexate. Uterine evacuation by manual vacuum aspiration or suction dilation and curettage can be both diagnostic and therapeutic. Direct visualization of the uterine aspirate by floating the tissue in saline may identify villi and thus resolve the question of pregnancy location. However, microscopic fresh tissue inspection or permanent pathology exam is sometimes necessary. If the health-care provider fails to identify villi and the suspicion for ectopic pregnancy is low, the β-hCG should be repeated the day following surgery. A decline of greater than 30 percent is highly suggestive that a failed IUP has been removed [10]. However, since ectopic pregnancies may have spontaneously falling β-hCGs, the clinician may want to continue to follow the level until resolution, dependent upon the clinical presentation and baseline suspicion for ectopic pregnancy. Failure of the level to drop after surgical evacuation of the uterus suggests ectopic pregnancy. This may then be managed medically or surgically and would fall into the category of a treated PUL. If uterine evacuation is not performed, in the setting of an abnormally rising β-hCG, the patient should be followed with serial lab studies or treated with methotrexate. In either of these approaches, ectopic pregnancy has not been ruled out and careful follow-up is essential. Methotrexate should only be given if the clinician is certain that a normal early IUP is not in the differential diagnosis. In a patient with a β-hCG that was initially below the discriminatory value, spontaneously falls, and eventually drops to zero, a resolving PUL is the diagnosis. The implantation site of the pregnancy has never been determined. The patient must be aware that an ectopic pregnancy was still within the differential diagnosis and close follow-up is warranted in subsequent pregnancy.

Decisions regarding management of PULs should be made in conjunction with the patient's desires regarding the pregnancy and guided by the preexisting likelihood of ectopic pregnancy, the likelihood that the patient will be compliant with follow-up, and her access to emergent medical care. If the patient does not have an ongoing pregnancy, preconceptual care or contraception should be addressed at the time of diagnosis and in follow-up.

Key Teaching Points

- PUL is often an interim diagnosis, which on further evaluation will lead to determination of viable or failed IUP or ectopic gestation.
- Normal rise in β-hCG is dependent upon the starting value, but should be at least 49 percent for initial values less than 1,500.
- The β-hCG discriminatory level is a relative concept affected by multiple technical considerations, but is a helpful adjunct in interpreting ultrasound findings.
- Uterine evacuation can help differentiate failed IUP from ectopic pregnancy.
- Methotrexate may be used for treatment only when an early, normal IUP has to be excluded.

Reference

1. Barnhart K, van Mello NM, Bourne T et al. Pregnancy of unknown location: a consensus statement of nomenclature, definitions, and outcome. *Fertil and Steril* 2011;95: 857–866.

2. van Mello NM, Mol F, Ankum, WM et al. Ectopic pregnancy: how the diagnostic and therapeutic management has changed. *Fertil Steril* 2012;98:1066–1073.

3. Condous G, Kirk E, Van Huffel S et al. Diagnostic accuracy of varying discriminatory zones for the prediction of ectopic pregnancy in women with pregnancy of unknown location. *Ultrasound Obstet Gynecol* 2005;26: 770–775.

4. Connolly AM, Ryan DH, Stuebe AM, Wolfe HM. Reevaluation of discriminatory and threshold levels for serum b-hCG in early pregnancy. *Obstet Gynecol* 2013;121:65–70.

5. Bree RL, Edwards M, Bohm-Velez M et al. Transvaginal sonography in the evaluation of normal early pregnancy: correlation with hCG level. *Am J Roentgenol* 1989;153:75–79.

6. Goldstein I, Zimmer EA, Tamir A et al. Evaluation of normal gestational sac growth: appearance of embryonic heartbeat and embryo body movements using transvaginal technique. *Obstet Gynecol* 1991;77:885–888.

7. Kadar N, Caldwell BV, Romero R. A method of screening for ectopic pregnancy and its indications. *Obstet Gynecol* 1981;58:162–166.

8. Barnhart K. Early pregnancy failure: beware the pitfalls of modern management. *Fert Steril* 2012;98: 1061–1065.

9. Barnhart K, Guo W, Cary M et al. Differences in serum human chorionic gonadotropin rise in early pregnancy by race and value at presentation. *Obstet Gynecol* 2016;128:504–511.

10. Shaunik A, Kulp J, Appleby DH et al. Utility of dilation and curettage in the diagnosis of pregnancy of unknown location. *Am J Obstet Gynecol* 2011;204:130. e1–130.e6.

A 30-Year-Old Woman with Postpartum Flatal and Fecal Incontinence

K. Lauren Barnes and Lori R. Berkowitz

History of Present Illness

A 30-year-old female, gravida 1, para 1, presents to your clinic for a six-week postpartum visit following a vaginal delivery. After asking how she is doing, she awkwardly admits to having issues with unintentional loss of gas.

She passes flatus without intending to on a frequent basis, and experienced an episode of accidental bowel leakage that stained her underwear when she had loose stools. She denies loss of urine, pelvic pain, or constipation, but does have urgency prior to defecating, which causes her to rush to the bathroom. She very rarely has diarrhea. These issues are making her anxious to go out in public and cause significant embarrassment. She had a third-degree perineal laceration during the birth of her child.

She is otherwise healthy and has had no surgeries. She takes no medications. She has no allergies. She does not smoke, drink alcohol, or use other substances or drugs.

Physical Examination

General appearance	Well-developed, well-nourished woman, appearing anxious

Vital Signs

Pulse	74 beats/min
Blood pressure	122/64 mmHg
Respiratory rate	12 breaths/min
Height	63 inches
Weight	140 lb
BMI	24.8 kg/m^2
Abdomen	Soft, non-tender, non-distended. No rebound or guarding
External genitalia	Normal-appearing labia majora and minora bilaterally. Well-healed perineal laceration with no discharge or erythema
Vagina	Pink, rugated with no bleeding or discharge.
Cervix	Normal-appearing parous cervix, closed with no active bleeding or discharge
Rectal examination	Mildly decreased external sphincter tone, no stool in rectal vault. Perianal reflexes with positive anal wink.
Labs/Imaging	None

How Would You Manage This Patient?

The patient has postpartum flatal incontinence and had fecal incontinence with diarrhea after a vaginal delivery that was complicated by external anal sphincter injury from a third-degree perineal laceration. Initial recommendations included dietary changes targeted at minimizing episodes of urgency and diarrhea, which were contributing to her symptoms. The patient kept a food diary that identified dietary irritants, ate small, frequent meals, started stool-bulking agents, and treated her rare diarrhea with Loperamide. She was also referred to pelvic floor physical therapy. She returned to clinic two months later noting no further episodes of fecal incontinence and rare flatal incontinence.

Postpartum Flatal and Fecal Incontinence

Anal incontinence is the term encompassing both flatal and fecal incontinence. Flatal incontinence is the involuntary loss of gas, and affects approximately one in four women in the postpartum period. Fecal incontinence often presents with loss of liquid stool and occurs in about one in ten women postpartum [1]. Though extremely common, anal incontinence is more of a taboo subject than urinary incontinence, and patients rarely bring up this issue to providers without being directly asked. The problem frequently is undiagnosed and can be profoundly distressing to a patient. If symptoms persist, it can negatively impact quality of life, social activities, and emotional health, and cause difficulty in sexual relationships that can last for years [1]. Fecal incontinence has greater impact than flatal incontinence alone [2].

The etiology of anal incontinence is complex, as continence is achieved by multiple methods. The increased burden of pregnancy on the pelvic floor can cause anal incontinence, with many women complaining of involuntary loss of gas and stool prior to delivery. Up to one-third of women describe flatal or fecal loss during the last four weeks of pregnancy [1]. This prenatal anal incontinence, which is thought to be caused by nerve damage, is highly predictive of postpartum incontinence. No interventions have been successful for prevention. Labor and delivery events are important, with a number of identifiable risk factors for later anal incontinence (Box 80.1). Vaginal delivery with disruption of pelvic floor support and damage to the external anal sphincter is a major cause of flatal and fecal incontinence (Figure 80.1). Obstetric anal sphincter injuries (OASIS) with vaginal delivery are a risk factor for anal incontinence, with the highest rates of anal incontinence occurring in woman with OASIS, although not all women with OASIS experience such symptoms [4]. Twenty-seven percent of primiparous women have anal sphincter defects on endoanal ultrasound, but only 29 percent of these patients are symptomatic [5]. Because of damage to the pelvic floor prior to delivery, cesarean does not completely protect against anal incontinence. Seven percent of women continue to experience fecal incontinence at six months after cesarean delivery, with 4.5 percent of women persistently having accidental bowel leakage 3–5 years after delivery [1, 6]. Changes in transit

Box 80.1 Risk factors for anal Incontinence

OASIS (Obstetric Anal Sphincter InjurieS)

Forceps delivery

Midline episiotomy

Long duration of pushing

Maternal age >35 at delivery

Persistent occiput posterior position at delivery

Birth weight >4 kg or 8 lb 13 oz

Bols EM, Hendriks EJ, Berghmans BC et al. A systematic review of etiological factors for postpartum fecal incontinence. Acta Obstet Gynecol Scand. 2010 March;89(3):302–14. doi: 10.3109/00016340903576004.

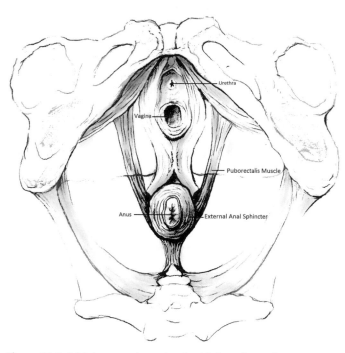

Figure 80.1 Pelvic bones and muscles of pelvic floor. Anatomic structures are indicated.
(Illustration by Joseph Werkmeister)

of stool through the terminal rectum and anus due to diarrhea or constipation can exacerbate the dysfunction from the structural damage and lead to loss of gas or stool. A 2010 Cochrane review does not support elective cesarean delivery to prevent anal incontinence [7].

The diagnosis is usually made based on history and physical examination. Laboratory studies are not typically helpful and imaging rarely adds to the diagnosis or initial management. History should determine if the incontinence is fecal or flatal and should determine inciting causes. The term "accidental bowel leakage" is recommended as it tends to be more acceptable to patients and may increase the number of women who

admit to the problem. Loss of solid versus liquid stool is helpful in estimating the degree of pelvic floor dysfunction, as loss of solid stool indicates more damage to the mechanisms of continence. Timing of symptoms, urgency, constipation, diarrhea, inciting medications, and underlying gastrointestinal conditions should be elicited. If the patient reports a history of chronic diarrhea, screening for underlying inflammatory bowel disease, irritable bowel syndrome, Celiac disease, lactose intolerance, and infectious causes may be indicated. Physical exam should target the pelvic floor. If the patient sustained a recent perineal laceration, the vaginal mucosa and perineal body should be inspected to ensure they are healing appropriately. The anal wink or anocutaneous reflex can be tested by stroking the skin surrounding the anus with a Q-tip, which should cause contraction of the external anal sphincter. Absence of this reflex indicates damage to the afferent or efferent nerves of S2-4 spinal arc. Rectal exam should be performed to determine the tone of the external anal sphincter, and presence of hemorrhoids or impacted stool. If examination is consistent with complete breakdown of the perianal body, rectal prolapse, or rectal exam concerning for malignancy, referral to a specialist is indicated.

Initial treatment for anal incontinence targets avoiding the identified inciting triggers for flatal and fecal loss. In women with fecal urgency as primary symptoms, small meals and stool bulking with powder-based supplementation can lead to symptomatic improvement. Methylcellulose 1–2 g in 8 oz of water daily or psyllium 1 capful (3.4 g in 8 oz of water) is a safe and effective option. The patient can maintain a food diary to identify and avoid triggers such as artificial sweeteners, lactose, fatty foods, gluten, spicy food, alcohol, or caffeine. This diary should also include episodes of both flatal and fecal loss, stool consistency, and symptoms of fecal urgency. Medications to slow colonic transit time, such as Loperamide 2 mg daily until stools are more formed, can be used sparingly when diarrhea is the trigger as long as there is low concern for underlying medical conditions that suggest referral to a specialist is warranted. We typically recommend using Loperamide 2 mg two to three times per week for at most 1–2 months and then slowly discontinue. Referral to pelvic floor physical therapy is beneficial for the entire pelvic floor and is recommended for initial therapy in women with low external anal sphincter tone and second-line therapy for those with a normal rectal tone. The goal of the therapy is to target both fast and slow twitch muscle fibers and contract the genital hiatus in order to stimulate pudendal nerve function. A Cochrane review suggests that some elements of biofeedback therapy and sphincter exercises may have a therapeutic effect, though data are limited [7]. Generally, symptoms will improve within 6–12 months with interventions. A long-term study with 12-year follow-up demonstrated lower rates of fecal incontinence one year after delivery with pelvic floor physical therapy. However, 43 percent of women who reported fecal incontinence three months postpartum still had symptoms 12 years after delivery and the benefit of physical therapy was not seen at that time [8]. Improvement and long-term continence are unpredictable.

This patient had vast improvement in her symptoms with conservative first-line management. If anal incontinence persists or worsens despite initial interventions, she could be referred to a specialist in Female Pelvic Medicine and Reconstructive Surgery or a colorectal specialist for further evaluation and management. Diagnostic studies can include anoscopy, defecography, anorectal manometry, pelvic and endoanal ultrasound, or colonoscopy, depending on the constellation of symptoms. Anal plugs, vaginal inserts, and scheduled bowel retraining have also been used for persistent anal incontinence, but adherence to these methods is poor overall or not well described in the literature. For persistent or severe anal incontinence, anal sphincteroplasty, injectable bulking agents, surgical placement of slings around the rectum, or sacral nerve stimulation can be used. Surgical outcomes are not well described, but generally lack long-term success [7]. Biofeedback and pelvic floor exercises as well as sacral nerve root implants demonstrate improvement in short-term symptoms, but long-term data are lacking as well [9].

If symptoms of anal incontinence are persistent at the time of the next pregnancy, many women and providers consider cesarean delivery, as the symptoms can worsen with subsequent vaginal deliveries. If anal sphincter injury occurred during the first pregnancy, the risk of repeat anal sphincter injury and long-term anal incontinence increases [6, 10]. Many women with persistent, severe incontinence opt for elective cesarean delivery in hopes to prevent long-term symptoms [6]. Currently, no recommendation regarding the route of delivery for women with history of incontinence after first delivery or continued symptoms has been universally accepted, so there should be a discussion and shared decision making between the patient and the provider.

Key Teaching Points

- Using the term "accidental bowel leakage" may be more acceptable for patients and encourage more honest discussion of symptoms.
- Flatal and fecal incontinence are extremely common after both vaginal and cesarean deliveries and typically improve over time.
- Initial office management should include a comprehensive examination, but no imaging studies.
- First-line medical management includes fiber supplementation for stool bulking, identifying dietary triggers, and pelvic floor physical therapy.
- Cesarean is not recommended for primary avoidance of anal incontinence, but can be considered for subsequent deliveries for patients with severe, persistent symptoms.

References

1. Borello-France D, Burgio KL, Richter HE et al; Pelvic floor disorders network. Fecal and urinary incontinence in primiparous women. *Obstet Gynecol* 2006 October;108 (4):863–872.

2. Lo J, Osterweil P, Li H et al. Quality of life in women with postpartum anal incontinence. *Obstet Gynecol* 2010 April;115(4):809–814. doi: 10.1097/ AOG.0b013e3181d4160d.

3. Bols EM, Hendriks EJ, Berghmans BC et al. A systematic review of etiological factors for postpartum fecal incontinence. *Acta Obstet Gynecol Scand* 2010 March;89(3):302–314. doi: 10.3109/ 00016340903576004.

4. Jangö H, Langhoff-Roos J, Rosthøj S, Sakse A. Mode of delivery after obstetric anal sphincter injury and the risk of long-term anal incontinence. *Am J Obstet Gynecol* 2016 June;214(6):733. e1–733.e13. doi: 10.1016/j. ajog.2015.12.030. Epub 2015 Dec 22.

5. Oberwalder M, Connor J, Wexner SD, Meta-analysis to determine the incidence of obstetric anal sphincter damage. *Br J Surg* 2003;90 (11):1333–1337.

6. Ng K, Cheung RY, Lee LL, Chung TK, Chan SS. An observational follow-up study on pelvic floor disorders to 3–5 years after delivery. *Int Urogynecol J* 2017 February;14:1–7.

7. Norton C, Cody JD. Biofeedback and/ or sphincter exercises for the treatment of faecal incontinence in adults. *Cochrane Database Syst Rev* 2012 July ;11(7):CD002111. doi: 10.1002/14651858.CD002111.pub3.

8. Glazener CMA, MacArthur C, Hagen S et al. Twelve-year follow-up of conservative management of postnatal urinary and faecal incontinence and prolapse outcomes: randomised controlled trial. *BJOG* 2014;121:112–120.

9. Brown SR, Wadhawan H, Nelson RL. Surgery for faecal incontinence in adults. *Cochrane Database Syst Rev* 2013 July;2(7):CD001757. doi:10.1002/14651858.CD001757. pub4.

10. Nelson RL, Furner SE, Westercamp M, Farquhar C. Cesarean delivery for the prevention of anal incontinence. *Cochrane Database Syst Rev* 2010 February;17 (2):CD006756. doi: 10.1002/ 14651858.CD006756.pub2.

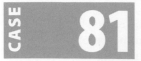
A 46-Year-Old Woman with Leakage of Urine

Cynthie K. Wautlet

History of Present Illness

A 46-year-old female, gravida 3, para 3, presents with complaint of leaking urine. The leakage began four years ago and has been increasing in frequency. She leaks 2–3 times daily, triggered by lifting, laughing, and sneezing. She changes protective undergarments 2–3 times per day. She is upset by these symptoms, concerned about malodor, and bothered by leakage at work and home. She reports no dysuria, continuous leakage, nocturia, slow stream, straining, or post-void leakage. She denies recurrent urinary tract infections or pelvic surgery. She does not experience involuntary passage of flatus or stool.

Her history is significant for three term vaginal births. Menses are regular. She is sexually active with one male partner, without sexual concerns, and has an IUD for birth control. She reports no diabetes, neurological disorders, or vascular disease. She is a nonsmoker and takes no prescription medications.

Physical Examination

General appearance	Alert, comfortable

Vital Signs

Pulse	82 beats/min
Blood pressure	130/78 mmHg
BMI	31 kg/m^2
Abdomen	Non-tender, non-distended, no palpable mass
External genitalia	Normal, no atrophy
Urethra	No diverticulum or mass
Vagina	Anterior vaginal wall prolapse with straining, leading edge 2 cm above the hymen (POP-Q Stage I)
Cervix	Normal
Uterus	Small, anteverted
Supine cough stress test	Leak of urine and urethral mobility observed simultaneous with cough
Voided volume	270 mL
Post-void residual urine volume (PVR)	40 mL

Laboratory Studies

Urinalysis	Negative
Urine culture	No growth

How Would You Manage This Patient?

This patient has uncomplicated stress urinary incontinence (SUI). She is having the classic symptom, involuntary leakage of urine from the urethra simultaneous with effort and sneezing. Positive cough stress test, negative urinalysis, normal post-void residual, absence of pelvic organ prolapse beyond the hymen, and absence of other bladder storage and voiding symptoms confirm the diagnosis. Urodynamic testing is not necessary before initiating treatment. Therapy should be directed at alleviating bothersome symptoms and improving quality of life. The patient is a candidate for conservative therapies with behavioral and lifestyle modification, pelvic floor muscle exercises with or without pelvic floor physical therapy, and an incontinence pessary. With appropriate counseling, she may opt for primary surgical management.

The patient was counseled thoroughly about the likelihood of symptom control with various treatments and the risks and benefits of each, including surgery. She wished to reduce incontinence episodes but preferred to avoid surgery. The patient was instructed to reduce caffeine intake, avoid constipation, perform pelvic floor muscle (Kegel) exercises, and keep a voiding diary to determine if leakage was more likely to occur at higher bladder volumes. She was advised of the benefits of moderate weight loss to reduce incontinence episodes for obese women and agreed to increase physical activity and manage her diet. She was provided written information about pessaries and surgical management. She returned in eight weeks for follow-up. She reported improvement in her symptoms to the point that they were tolerable and not interfering with her daily activities. She was counseled that her symptoms may worsen with age and additional treatment could be initiated as necessary. Her symptoms will be reviewed at her periodic well-woman visits.

Stress Urinary Incontinence

SUI occurs when urine involuntarily leaks from the urethra simultaneous with effort, physical exertion, sneezing, or coughing. Overall, incontinence affects 44–57 percent of adult women in the United States, up to 75 percent of US female nursing home residents, and millions of women worldwide [1, 2]. Prevalence increases with older age, higher body mass index, increasing parity, postmenopausal status, and medical conditions such as neurologic disease or poorly controlled diabetes. This patient was at risk for SUI given her age and obesity. Urgency and mixed (coexisting stress and urgency) incontinence are also common. The differential diagnosis also includes extra-urethral incontinence from fistulas or ectopic ureter, functional incontinence due to cognitive or mobility impairment, incontinence from chronic urinary retention ("overflow"), postural, coital, and occult (revealed after reduction of prolapse). Establishing the correct diagnosis is important since prognosis and treatment options vary considerably.

This patient sought care due to distress at work and home. Urinary incontinence often has a negative impact on quality of life and can be debilitating. Many women avoid seeking care due to stigma and other barriers, so providers should screen for incontinence at periodic well-woman visits [1]. Questionnaires to assess distress and symptom severity can be administered at the first visit and serially to define goals and monitor response to therapy. Several validated tools are available, including the Urogenital Distress Inventory and Incontinence Impact Questionnaire (IIQ) [1, 3].

History should include duration of symptoms, frequency, precipitating factors, protective pad use, and fluid intake. Leakage occurring only with increased intra-abdominal pressure is consistent with SUI. However, leakage immediately preceded or accompanied by a strong urge to void is concerning for urge incontinence and leakage without provocation is concerning for fistula. Bladder storage (urgency, incomplete bladder emptying, and continuous leakage) and voiding symptoms (hesitancy, slow stream, intermittency, straining, spraying, need to re-void, postmicturition leakage, position-dependent micturition, and dysuria) should be assessed to determine whether SUI is complicated [3, 4]. Complicated SUI is also diagnosed when history of any of the following is identified: previous incontinence surgery, complex urethral surgery, radical pelvic surgery, prior pelvic radiation therapy, recurrent UTIs, poorly controlled diabetes, neurological disease, or dementia. This patient had no such history and no additional storage or voiding symptoms, consistent with uncomplicated SUI.

Physical examination should be performed to characterize any abdominal or pelvic masses, urethral abnormalities (such as mass or diverticulum), vulvovaginal atrophy, or fistula. The International Federation of Gynecology and Obstetrics (FIGO) recommends that pelvic organ prolapse be assessed using either the POP-Q or, in practice settings where complexity of POP-Q is prohibitive, the simplified version S-POP [5, 2]. In addition, a minimum of four additional assessments should be performed [1, 3, 2]:

(1) Cough stress test

(2) Assessment of urethral mobility

(3) Urinalysis or dipstick

(4) Measurement of post-void residual urine volume (PVR)

When feasible, many clinicians instruct patients to arrive with a comfortably full bladder to facilitate evaluation. Cough stress test and urethral mobility evaluation are first performed during supine pelvic examination. While the urethral meatus is visualized, the patient is instructed to relax, then cough. Urinary leakage and excessive downward urethral displacement simultaneous with cough are consistent with SUI. When the cough stress test is negative, it should be repeated with the patient standing and with a full bladder. To be valid, there must be adequate urine volume at the time of the test. Bladder volume can be evaluated with a bladder scanner to ensure at least 300 mL of urine is present or the bladder can be backfilled under sterile conditions to a minimum of 300 mL before the test is repeated. The cotton swab test is traditionally used to evaluate for urethral hypermobility. A lubricated cotton swab is inserted through the urethra to the bladder neck and displacement >30 degrees from horizontal with Valsalva is considered hypermobile. Measurement of POP-Q point Aa, while important in the evaluation of prolapse, is not recommended by FIGO as a test for urethral hypermobility [2]. Urine dipstick or urinalysis should be performed to rule out infection

and significant hematuria. PVR should be assessed either with a bladder scanner or sterile catheter immediately after voiding. Though controversy exists, FIGO and ACOG agree that PVR <150 mL is normal. Complicated SUI is diagnosed when office evaluation reveals pelvic organ prolapse beyond the hymen, genitourinary fistula, urethral diverticulum, absence of urethral mobility, or PVR>150 mL.

For uncomplicated SUI, as was diagnosed in this case, urodynamic testing is not indicated prior to management [3, 2]. In cases where the diagnosis remains unclear after thorough office examination or SUI is complicated, for example by advanced prolapse beyond the hymen, prior incontinence surgery, or pelvic radiation therapy [1, 3], urodynamic testing or specialist referral (where available) is advised.

A simple bladder diary recorded by the patient for 1–3 days should be recommended after the initial office visit and provides information about frequency of leakage episodes, related fluid intake, and precipitating factors. This information assists in confirming the diagnosis, initiating lifestyle modifications, and monitoring response to treatment. A free online version is available for download (see www.niddk.nih.gov/health-infor mation/health-topics/urologic-disease/daily-bladder-diary/Do cuments/diary_508.pdf).

Currently, there is no effective pharmacologic therapy for SUI. All patients are candidates for conservative management with lifestyle modifications, pelvic floor (Kegel) exercises, and behavioral therapy. Obese women have a fourfold higher risk for SUI compared with normal weight women. Obese women assigned to an intensive weight-loss program reduced the frequency of incontinence episodes by 70 percent or more compared with controls [6], so weight loss should be advised when indicated. Observational studies demonstrate that caffeine intake, constipation, and carbonated beverage consumption are each independently associated with incontinence episodes, so reducing or eliminating these triggers may be of benefit [1]. Women with excessive (>2 L) daily fluid intake, leakage at higher bladder volumes, or nocturia identified on the bladder diary can be advised to limit fluid intake to 2 L daily, time voids (see bladder training below), or decrease fluid intake before bedtime. Pelvic floor muscle (Kegel) exercises are commonly recommended with or without pelvic floor physical therapy or biofeedback to strengthen voluntary muscles of the pelvic floor. An online video series is available to teach techniques: www.nrsg101.com/kegel-exercise.html. Instructions are also available through the National Association for Continence: www.nafc.org/kegel. Regardless of regimen, pelvic floor muscle training alone or in combination with other therapies is effective for reducing incontinence episodes, improving quality of life, and restoring continence with 50 percent satisfaction at one year [1]. Behavioral therapy with bladder training employs a fixed voiding schedule with progressively increasing time between voids. A 2004 Cochrane review [7] concluded that bladder training may be considered first-line therapy for stress, urge, and mixed incontinence with a 50 percent reduction in mean incontinence episodes. Instructions for patients and providers are available through the National Association for Continence: www.nafc.org/blad

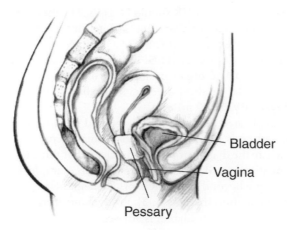

Figure 81.1 Woman's pelvis with vagina, bladder, and pessary.
National Institute of Diabetes and Digestive and Kidney Diseases, National Institutes of Health

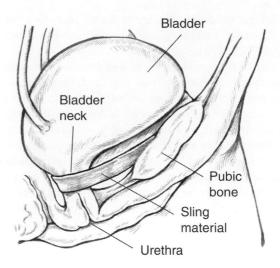

Figure 81.2 Side view of female bladder supported by a sling to prevent urinary incontinence. The sling is wrapped around the urethra, and the ends are attached to the pubic bone. Labels point to the bladder, bladder neck, pubic bone, sling material, and urethra.
National Institute of Diabetes and Digestive and Kidney Diseases, National Institutes of Health

der-retraining. Response to conservative management can be evaluated longitudinally using a voiding diary or validated tools such as the Patient Global Impression of Improvement and Patient Global Impression of Severity measures [8]. This patient preferred conservative treatment and, at least over the short term, was satisfied with her improvement. Close follow-up is important since incontinence symptoms may vary over time, with approximately 50 percent of women in conservative management crossing over to surgery within one year [1].

Patients with SUI with or without prolapse can be offered a pessary trial [1], which this patient initially declined. Patients who fail conservative therapy, desire future fertility, and wish to avoid or delay surgery are good candidates. Incontinence pessaries support the proximal urethra and bladder neck to increase urethral resistance (Figure 81.1) and often contain a knob for anterior positioning under the urethra, though many shapes and sizes exist. Pessaries should be fitted by a trained clinician. Undue pressure from a large pessary creates risk for vaginal erosion or urinary obstruction, while a pessary that is too small will be ineffective.

Surgery can be considered first-line treatment for patients who have completed thorough office evaluation, have uncomplicated SUI, decline conservative management or pessary, are medically cleared for surgery, and are appropriately counseled about the risks, benefits, and outcomes of surgical management. A 2009 Cochrane review of surgeries for uncomplicated SUI concluded that pubovaginal slings (Figure 81.2), Burch colposuspension, and mid-urethral slings were equally effective [9]. Synthetic mid-urethral slings are also highly effective

[10] and are currently the most commonly performed incontinence procedures given reduced operative time and shorter recovery. Long-term effectiveness and safety of the transobturator (TOT) and retropubic (TVT) mid-urethral approaches are similar [11].

Key Teaching Points

- The classic symptom of SUI is involuntary urine leakage from the urethra simultaneous with physical exertion or effort, coughing, or sneezing.
- In addition to history and physical examination, minimum initial office evaluation for women with incontinence includes urinalysis or dipstick, cough stress test, assessment of urethral mobility, and measurement of PVR.
- If the initial supine cough stress test is negative, the test should be repeated with the patient standing and with a full bladder.
- For women with uncomplicated SUI, urodynamic testing is not indicated prior to therapy. In cases where the diagnosis is unclear or SUI is complicated, urodynamic testing or specialist referral is recommended.
- Management options include lifestyle modifications, pelvic floor (Kegel) exercises, behavioral therapy, and incontinence pessaries. Appropriately counseled patients may opt for primary surgical management.

References

1. The American College of Obstetricians and Gynecologists. Urinary incontinence in women. Practice bulletin no. 155. *Obstet Gynecol* 2015;126: e66–e81.

2. Medina CA, Costantini E, Petri E et al. Evaluation and surgery for stress urinary incontinence: a FIGO working group report. *Neurourol Urodyn* 2017;36:518–528.

3. The American College of Obstetricians and Gynecologists. Evaluation of uncomplicated stress urinary incontinence in women before surgical treatment. Committee opinion no. 603. *Obstet Gynecol* 2014;123: 1403–1407.

4. Haylen BT, de Ridder D, Freeman RM et al. An international urogynecological association (IUGA)/International continence society (ICS) joint report on

the terminology for female pelvic floor dysfunction. *Int Urogynecol J* 2010;21:5–26.

5. Manonai J, Mouritsen L, Palma P et al. The inter-system association between the simplified pelvic organ prolapse quantification system (S-POP) and the standard pelvic organ prolapse quantification system (POPQ) in describing pelvic organ prolapse. *Int Urogynecol J* 2011;22(3):347–352.

6. Subak LL, Wing R, West DS et al. Weight loss to treat urinary incontinence in overweight and obese women. *N Engl J Med* 2009;360(5):481.

7. Wallace SA, Roe B, Williams K et al. Bladder training for urinary incontinence in adults. *Cochrane Database Syst Rev* 2004,Issue 1. Art. No.: CD001308. DOI: 10.1002/14651858. CD001308.pub2.

8. Yalcin I, Bump RC. Validation of two global impression questionnaires for incontinence. *Am J Obstet Gynecol* 2003 July;189(1):98–101.

9. Ogah J, Cody JD, Rogerson L. Minimally invasive synthetic suburethral sling operations for stress urinary incontinence in women. *Cochrane Database Syst Rev* 2009;7:CD006375.

10. Ford AA, Rogerson L, Cody JD, Ogah J. Mid-urethral sling operations for stress urinary incontinence in women. *Cochrane Database Syst Rev* 2015,Issue 7. Art. No.:CD006375. DOI: 10.1002/14651858.CD006375. pub3.

11. Leone Roberti Maggiore U, Finazzi Agrò E, Soligo M et al. Long-term outcomes of TOT and TVT procedures for the treatment of female stress urinary incontinence: a systematic review and meta-analysis. *Int Urogynecol J* 2017.DOI:10.1007/ s00192-017–3275-x.

A 48-Year-Old Woman with Microscopic Hematuria and Negative Urine Culture

Kimberly S. Gecsi

History of Present Illness

A 48-year-old woman, gravida 3 para 3, presents to the office for an annual exam. She states that two months ago she had a urinary tract infection that was diagnosed by her primary care physician. Her physician told her she had "some blood in her urine." She reports that she gets urinary tract infections frequently, about three times per year. She would like a test today to ensure that the blood has resolved. She denies dysuria, flank pain, abdominal pain, gross hematuria, or vaginal bleeding. Her last menstrual period was two weeks ago.

Her past medical history is significant for hypothyroidism. Her past surgical history is negative. She reports no history of STDs or abnormal pap tests. She had three full-term vaginal deliveries followed by a tubal ligation. She is an avid runner, completing her first half marathon last month, and denies tobacco use, alcohol, or drugs. She is sexually active with her husband and lives with him and her three children. She works as a lawyer.

Physical Examination

General appearance	Well-developed, well-nourished in no distress

Vital Signs

BP	110/70 mmHg
Weight	130 lb
Height	65 inches
BMI	21 kg/m^2
Abdomen	Soft, non-tender, non-distended, no costo-vertebral angle tenderness
External genitalia	Normal vulva and urethra
Vagina/cervix	Normal, no blood
Uterus	Anteverted, small, mobile, non-tender
Adnexa	Non-tender, no masses

Laboratory Studies

Urinalysis (dipstick):

Leukocytes	Negative
Nitrite	Negative
Urobilinogen	Negative
Protein	Negative
pH	6.5
Blood	1+ (small)
Specific gravity	1.005
Ketones	Negative
Bilirubin	Negative
Glucose	Negative
Urine culture (from two months prior)	No growth

How Would You Manage This Patient?

The patient has evidence of blood on a urine dipstick test. She does not report symptoms of a urinary tract infection currently, and had a negative culture from her visit with her PCP two months prior. She does not report any symptoms that suggest a urinary stone as a cause of the hematuria. While infection and stones are common causes of transient hematuria, in patients without evidence of those diagnoses, depending on the amount of blood, it may be important to investigate for other causes.

Evidence of blood on a urine dipstick necessitates evaluation with a formal urinalysis and microscopy. In a nonsmoking woman under age 50, further workup is only recommended if the microscopic evaluation reveals >25 RBCs per high-power field (hpf) [1].

The patient's urinalysis and microscopic evaluation are as follows:

Urinalysis

Color	Yellow
Appearance	Clear
Specific gravity	1.020
pH	7.0
Protein	Negative
Glucose	Negative
Blood	Moderate (2+)
Ketones	Negative
Bilirubin	Negative
Urobilinogen	<2.0 mg/dL
Nitrite	Negative
Leukocyte Esterase	Negative

Microscopic Evaluation

WBCs	1/hpf
RBCs	40/hpf
Epithelial cells	<1/hpf
Casts	Negative

Given the presence of 40 RBCs/hpf, she was informed of the finding of microscopic hematuria. She had no evidence of glomerular disease on her urinalysis and a repeat urine culture was also negative. She was scheduled for imaging with a computerized tomography (CT) urogram and referred to urology for cystoscopy. No definitive cause of her microscopic hematuria was identified. A repeat urinalysis is planned in one year.

Microscopic Hematuria with a Negative Urine Culture

Unexplained hematuria is fairly common. Some studies have demonstrated asymptomatic microscopic hematuria in up to 40 percent of patients [2]. In patients under the age of 35, hematuria is usually transient and of no consequence. In nonsmoking women under 50, the risk of urinary tract malignancy is very low [1].

Microscopic hematuria is defined as the presence of three or more RBCs per hpf from a spun specimen in the absence of a color change to the urine. It is frequently identified incidentally when a urinalysis is ordered for another reason. While microscopic evaluation is the gold standard, urine dipsticks can reliably detect microscopic hematuria of 1–2 RBCs/HPF. Several contaminants can cause false positive urine dipsticks for hemoglobin including semen, agents used to clean the perineum, and myoglobinuria. Contamination with menstrual blood can also cause false positives on both dipstick and microscopic evaluation. If menstrual contamination is suspected, the test can be repeated after menses or after inserting a tampon prior to specimen collection. Because of the increased incidence of benign causes of hematuria in young women, and the low risk of urinary tract cancers, different cutoff values are used for prompting further evaluation. In nonsmoking women under age 50, a cutoff of >25 RBCs/HPF was recommended for determining the need for further evaluation. Women older than 50 and men with ≥3 RBCs/HPF should also be evaluated.

The most common causes of microscopic hematuria include infections and stones. Vigorous exercise or recent trauma can also cause transient hematuria. History can help determine if any of these are potential causes. A history of fever or dysuria should raise suspicion of infection and unilateral flank pain should raise concerns for a stone. A urine culture should be sent to test for infection and a urinalysis should be repeated approximately six weeks after completion of antibiotic therapy to confirm resolution of the hematuria [3]. Patients with possible stones should undergo imaging with noncontrast CT or ultrasound. In asymptomatic patients with recent trauma or frequent exercise, a urine dipstick can be repeated after a period of no exercise.

The first step in evaluation of microscopic hematuria is to send the urine for urinalysis and microscopy. This will help determine if the bleeding is from a glomerular or nonglomerular cause. Signs of glomerular bleeding include the presence of red cell casts and abnormal red cell morphology. The presence of proteinuria exceeding 500 mg/day also suggests a glomerular cause of hematuria. The timing of the proteinuria is important. If proteinuria was present prior to the onset of hematuria, a cause other than glomerular disease may be present and a full evaluation may be warranted. If glomerular bleeding is suspected, a referral to a nephrologist is recommended. Causes of glomerular bleeding are typically from immune-mediated injury to the glomeruli. Diseases such as IgA nephropathy, basement membrane nephropathy, post-infectious glomerulonephritis, and hereditary nephritis (Alport syndrome) are common causes of glomerular hematuria [4]. A renal biopsy can determine the cause, but may not be necessary in patients without evidence of progressive disease. Proteinuria, increased serum creatinine, or a rise in blood pressure would be concerning for a progressive disease. A renal biopsy is also not indicated in patients without evidence of glomerular disease.

Patients with non-glomerular hematuria should undergo evaluation for potential malignancy. Prior to this evaluation, a urine culture should be performed to rule out infection.

Patients with transient or persistent hematuria and an elevated risk of malignancy should be referred for urologic evaluation. Risk factors for malignancy, as determined by the American Urological Association (AUA), are listed in Box 82.1[5]. In one study, 1.9 percent of women with microscopic hematuria between the ages of 50 and 59 had malignancy identified, and this increased to 4.5 percent in women aged 60–69 [6].

Imaging is recommended to evaluate for lesions in the kidney, collecting system, ureters, bladder, or urethra. Multidetector computerized tomography urography (CTU) is the recommended imaging modality. Conventional CT, ultrasound, intravenous pyelography (IVP), and magnetic resonance imaging can also be used in patients who are not candidates for CTU, such as patients who are pregnant or patients with an elevated creatinine. Multidetector CTU is preferred because it combines the benefits of CT scanning with IVP imaging and provides global imaging of the urinary tract. The radiation dose is high, about double the dose of an IVP, but lower dose protocols are being developed [7]. Cystoscopy is also recommended in addition to radiologic imaging to fully evaluate the bladder and urethra for potential causes of bleeding and to rule out malignancy in these areas. Cystoscopy has very low morbidity and the AUA guidelines recommend cystoscopy in patients at elevated risk for malignancy with an otherwise negative workup [5].

A cause for hematuria is often not identified. Recommendations for follow-up after a negative workup are based upon expert opinion and should include annual urinalysis [8]. After two negative evaluations screening can be discontinued. If the hematuria persists for 3–5 years, a repeat urologic workup is warranted. In a study of 421 patients with unexplained microscopic hematuria and a negative initial workup, about 5 percent had an identifiable cause of the hematuria within 3 years [9]. In patients with glomerular disease, protein

---

Box 82.1 Risk factors for malignancy in patients with asymptomatic hematuria

Male gender

Age (> 35 years)

Past or current smoking

Occupational or other exposure to chemicals or dyes (benzenes or aromatic amines)

Analgesic abuse

History of gross hematuria

History of urologic disorder or disease

History of irritative voiding symptoms

History of pelvic irradiation

History of chronic urinary tract infection

History of exposure to known carcinogenic agents or chemotherapy such as alkylating agents

History of chronic indwelling foreign body

excretion, serum creatinine, and blood pressure should be monitored for signs of progressive disease.

Screening for hematuria is not recommended. The United States Preventive Services Task Force does not recommend screening because there is insufficient evidence to balance the benefits and harms in asymptomatic adults [10]. Previously, it had recommended against screening (level D recommendation) because the prevalence of undetected, asymptomatic, early disease is relatively low, there is little evidence that hematuria is a sensitive test for localized disease, and there is little evidence that early treatment of local disease results in better prognosis.

Key Teaching Points

- Unexplained hematuria is fairly common, and in nonsmoking women under 50, the risk of urinary tract malignancy is very low.
- In the absence of other risk factors, women under 50 should only undergo further workup if microscopic analysis reveals >25 RBCs/hpf.
- Multidetector CTU and cystoscopy are the recommended imaging modalities to fully evaluate the urogenital tract.
- Screening for hematuria is not recommended.

References

1. Asymptomatic Microscopic Hematuria in Women. Committee on Gynecologic Practice and American Urologic Society. ACOG Committee Opinion, 703, June 2017.

2. Loo RK, Lieberman SF, Slezak JM et al. Stratifying risk of urinary tract malignant tumors in patients with asymptomatic microscopic hematuria. *Mayo Clin Proc* 2013;88:129–138.

3. Mariani AJ. The evaluation of adult hematuria: a clinical update. In: AUA update series 1998; volume XVII, lesson 24. Houston: AUA Office of Education, 1998:185–192.

4. McGregor DO, Lynn KL, Bailey RR et al. Clinical audit of the use of renal biopsy in the management of isolated microscopic hematuria. *Clin Nephrol* 1998;49:345–348.

5. Diagnosis, evaluation, and follow-up of asymptomatic microhematuria (AMH) in adults: American Urological Association (AUA) Guideline. www.auanet.org/guidelines/ asymptomatic-microhematuria- (2012-reviewed-and-validity- confirmed-2016)

6. Khadra MH, Pickard RS, Charlton M et al. A prospective analysis of 1,930 patients with hematuria to evaluate current diagnostic practice. *J Urol* 2000;163:524–527.

7. Eikefjord EN, Thorsen F, Rørvik J. Comparison of effective radiation doses in patients undergoing unenhanced MDCT and excretory urography for acute flank pain. *AJR Am J Roentgenol* 2007;188:934–939.

8. Murakami S, Igarashi T, Hara S, Shimazaki J. Strategies for asymptomatic microscopic hematuria: a prospective study of 1,034 patients. *J Urol* 1990;144:99–101.

9. Grossfeld G, Wolf JS, Litwin MS et al. Asymptomatic microscopic hematuria in adults: summary of the AUA best practice policy recommendations. *Am Fam Physician* 2001;63:1145–1154.

10. *Final Recommendation Statement: Bladder Cancer in Adults: Screening.* U.S. Preventive Services Task Force. April 2017. www.uspreventiveservices taskforce.org/Page/Document/Recom mendationStatementFinal/bladder-can cer-in-adults-screening

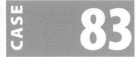

A 55-Year-Old Woman with Urinary Urgency and Negative Urinalysis and Culture

Julie Zemaitis DeCesare

History of Present Illness

A 55-year-old white female, gravida 0, presents to your office complaining of loss of urine. Upon questioning, she states that the symptoms started about five years ago, shortly after she completed menopause. Her symptoms are so severe that she has restricted activities that she previously enjoyed, including her walking club and gardening. She voids on average 15–20 times per day, including three episodes of nocturia night. She has episodic incontinence, and feels like her incontinence is worse when her bladder is full. Her symptoms are provoked by running water, and she feels like she cannot leave her home because she needs to be close to bathroom facilities.

She has no other medical problems. She has never had surgery. She takes no medications and has no allergies. She does not use tobacco products or drink alcohol, but she drinks six 8-ounce glasses of sweet tea per day.

Physical Examination

General appearance	Thin, white woman in no distress

Vital Signs

Temperature	37.0°C
Pulse	92 beats/min
Blood pressure	110/72 mmHg
Respiratory rate	16 breaths/min
Oxygen saturation	100 percent on room air
Height 60 inches	
Weight	100 lb
BMI	19.5 kg/m^2
External genitalia	Normal appearing with sparse pubic hair
Vagina	Mucosa with minimal rugae, grade 1 cystocele, no rectocele
Cervix	Normal appearing
Uterus	Minimal prolapse, smooth contour, freely mobile. Normal size
Adnexa	No masses appreciated,
Urethral q-tip angle	Minimal deflection
Cough stress test	Negative
Postvoid residual	25 cc

Lab Values

Normal urinalysis and negative urine culture

How Would You Manage This Patient?

This patient has overactive bladder as evidenced by her urgency symptoms and lack of prolapse on physical exam. As her urinary incontinence is impairing her quality of life, it requires evaluation and management. You recommend lifestyle modifications, including restricting intake of caffeinated beverages and overall restriction of fluid intake. You also recommend timed voids to avoid overdistention of her bladder. She is referred to a local physical therapist that specializes in pelvic floor dysfunction, and a regimen of pelvic floor training with biofeedback is initiated.

The patient returns after two months. Her symptoms are minimally improved, but she is unhappy with the amount of time required for her pelvic floor physical therapy sessions. You initiate Oxybutynin XL 5 mg per day. She returns in six weeks stating that she has had dry mouth and dry eyes, but her urinary incontinence symptoms are improved. She is happy that she does not need to spend time going to physical therapy, and her symptoms are controlled to the point where she is able to participate in many of her previous activities.

Overactive Bladder

Overactive bladder (OAB) impacts approximately 18 million women per year, and accounts for about 7 percent of all ambulatory visits made by women [1]. For many women, the problem can prevent normal activities and simple treatment can restore quality of life. Less than half of women with weekly incontinence voluntarily disclose their incontinence to their provider. Questions about incontinence should be included in the routine review of systems. The stigma and psychological impact of the condition are underestimated and significant.

Normal micturition occurs when the smooth detrusor muscle, which surrounds the bladder wall, contracts and triggers an automatic relaxation of the urethral sphincter muscles. This process is normally under voluntary control unless the bladder is extremely full. In cases of overactive bladder, the detrusor muscle contracts when the bladder is not full, often at random [2]. This makes the patient feel a sudden urge to void with resultant episodic incontinence. Most patients describe an overwhelming urge to void with difficulty getting to the bathroom in time to prevent leakage.

Initial evaluation of incontinence includes obtaining a complete history, having the patient complete a bladder diary, and performing a physical examination. The history should focus on symptom severity and the impact on the patient's quality of life. It is useful for the patient to complete a bladder diary prior to the office encounter. The patient should record in the bladder diary her oral intake, number of voiding episodes, and number of incontinence episodes. This information should be recorded for at least three to five days. Validated questionnaires can be used to help identify the type and severity of the incontinence. Examples include the Incontinence Quality of Life and the Incontinence Severity Index questionnaires.

The physical examination should assess pelvic support, urethral mobility, post-void residual, and provoked incontinence.

Pelvic exam (including a rectal exam) should include assessing the amount of prolapse. Pelvic floor muscle strength and tone should be assessed. A q-tip test assesses urethral mobility, a feature of stress incontinence. It is performed by placing a lidocaine gel coated q-tip within the urethra and measuring the deflection of the q-tip from baseline at rest to the angle of deflection when the patient is bearing down. A normal angle (deflection of less than 30 degrees) generally rules out urethral hypermobility as a cause for the incontinence. A cough stress test is performed by asking the patient to cough and observing if there is leakage of urine. A negative cough stress test makes stress incontinence less likely. A high post-void residual (PVR) indicates a neurological cause of bladder dysfunction. Generally, a PVR less than 150 cc is considered normal. PVR can be measured with bladder catheterization or ultrasound measurements. The measurement should be taken after the patient voids, starting with a full bladder. Bladder filling can be done spontaneously or by filling the bladder through a catheter.

Usual lab tests include a urinalysis and culture to diagnose cystitis as a cause of the incontinence. Microscopic hematuria should be further evaluated. Consensus supports referral to a urological specialist when more than 25–30 red blood cells per high power field are identified in women aged 35–50 who do not report a history of smoking [3]. Multichannel urodynamic studies should be reserved for complex cases in which an initial office diagnosis is unclear or in patients failing usual therapy.

Table 83.1 lists pharmacological and non-pharmacological treatment options. First-line treatment involves noninvasive lifestyle and behavior modification, including bladder retraining and dietary modifications. A large clinical trial that included women with all types of incontinence (overactive bladder, stress and mixed) demonstrated a 50 percent reduction in urinary symptoms in women undergoing behavior therapy compared to 15 percent reduction in controls [4]. Behavior therapy is noninvasive and well tolerated, and is a good first-line option. Obesity can be a major contributor, and if present, weight loss should be employed as an initial strategy. Fluid restriction to less than 2 liters per day can also improve incontinence, and should be encouraged. Avoiding oral intake several hours before bed is useful in women with episodes of nocturnal incontinence. A fluid intake diary can help the patient identify and eliminate triggers.

Reduction or avoidance of caffeinated beverages can improve symptoms, and data support that as little as one cup of coffee per day may exacerbate overactive bladder symptoms [5].

Pelvic floor physical therapy has been shown to subjectively improve symptoms of urinary leakage, and verbal or biofeedback has been shown to improve the results of the therapy. Physical therapy has virtually no side effects, but the treatment effects are variable and the improvement often disappears when the therapy is stopped [6]. Referral and collaboration with a provider with specialized training in pelvic floor physical therapy is important. It is reasonable to start with nonmedical therapy; however, pharmacologic therapy may be initiated first line in select patients.

Antimuscarinic medications, which inhibit parasympathetic M2 and M3 receptors, are first-line pharmacotherapy. It is reasonable to start with these agents in well-counseled patients who decline behavior and lifestyle modifications. These medications also increase the storage capacity of the bladder and reduce urgency symptoms. Common agents include oxybutynin, solifenacin, and tolterodine tartrate (Table 83.2). Newer-generation medications like solifenacin have a better side effect profile, but tend to be more expensive. Compliance is improved with sustained release forms of the medication. These medications have frequent side effects, including dry mouth, constipation, and somnolence. Less common side effects include nausea, dry eyes, and headache. These medications only provide a minimal decrease on the number of voiding episodes, which is commonly the most bothersome symptom [7]. A recent systematic review suggested that anti-muscarinic medications only reduced daily voids by two episodes, and had minimal impact on the patient's reported bladder symptoms [8]. Combining medication and behavioral-based treatments as first line to enhance symptom control has been proposed. Studies do not support that combining these two treatments gives better clinical results than anti-muscarinic therapy alone [9].

Additional treatments are available for patients failing first-line therapy, but are more invasive or expensive. Botulinum Toxin A injections have shown promise, but overtreatment can lead to urinary retention. Acupuncture has been effective in limited trials. Mirabegron is a relatively new pharmacological agent that works as a B3 receptor agonist and could be initiated after failing

Table 83.1 Treatment options for overactive bladder

Nonpharmacologic	Pharmacologic
Weight loss	Propantheline
Pelvic floor	Oxybutynin
Biofeedback	Tolterodine tartrate
Acupuncture	Mirabegron
Neuromodulation	Botulinum Toxin A

Table 83.2 Suggested first-line medications for overactive bladder

Drug	Dose
Tolterodine tartrate	2 mg twice daily
Tolterodine tartrate XL	4 mg daily
Oxybutynin	5 mg two to three times daily
Oxybutynin XL	5 mg daily
Solifenacin	5 mg daily

commonly prescribed first-line agents. Nerve modulators, including posterior tibial nerve stimulation and sacral neuromodulation, can be used when behavioral and pharmacologic therapy have failed.

Key Teaching Points

- OAB is often not voluntarily reported by patients. Screening questions should be included in the review of systems.

- Evaluation includes a complete history, a physical exam assessing pelvic support and urethral mobility, and a bladder diary with a symptom log. A validated incontinence tool is also useful.

- Treatment should be tailored to the patient. Symptomatic relief can be obtained with pelvic floor physical therapy, biofeedback, and dietary modifications.

- Pharmacological therapy can be beneficial, but most agents have significant side effects.

References

1. Olivera C, Meriwether K, El-Nashar S et al. Nonantimuscarinic treatment for overactive bladder: a systematic review. *Am J Obstet Gynecol* 2016 July;215(1):34–57.

2. Yamaguch O. Antimuscarinics and overactive bladder: other mechanism of action.

3. Committee Opinion No 703: Asymptomatic Microscopic Hematuria in Women.

4. Subak LL, Quesenberry CP, Posner SF, Cattolica E, Soghikian K. The effect of behavioral therapy on urinary incontinence: a randomized controlled trial. *Obstet Gynecol* 2002 July;100 (1):72–78.

5. Gleason JL, Richter HE, Redden DT et al. Caffeine and urinary incontinence in US women. *Int Urogynecol J* 2013 February;24 (2):295–302. doi: 10.1007/s00192-012-1829-5. Epub 2012 June 15.

6. Wallace SA, Roe B, Williams K, Palmer M. Bladder training for urinary incontinence in adults. *Cochrane Database Syst Rev* 2004,Issue 1. Art. No.: CD001308. DOI: 10.1002/14651858. CD001308.pub2.

7. American College of Obstetricians and Gynecologists. Urinary incontinence in women. Practice bulletin no. 155. *Obstet Gynecol* 2015;126: e66–e81.

8. Reynolds WS, McPheeters M, Blume J et al. Comparative effectiveness of anticholinergic therapy for overactive bladder in women: a systematic review and meta-analysis. *Obstet Gynecol* 2015;125:1423–1432.

9. Gormley EA, Lightner DJ, Burgio KL et al. Diagnosis and treatment of ovractive bladder (non-neurogenic) in adults: AUA/SUFU guideline. Linthicum (MD): American Urological Association Education and Research, Inc.; 2014 May. 57 p. www.guideline.gov /summaries/summary/48226 Accessed 5/8/17.

A 30-Year-Old Woman with Frequency, Urgency, Nocturia, and Pressure Relieved by Urination

(Painful Bladder Syndrome – Evaluation and Initial Management)

Jaclyn van Nes

History of Present Illness

A 30-year-old female, gravida 2, para 2, presents to the office for a problem visit. She complains of urinary frequency and urgency. She reports the symptoms have been present for several months, but feels they are getting worse. On further questioning, she says she also has pelvic pressure symptoms that are relieved when she empties her bladder. She says she gets up frequently at night to use the bathroom and has noticed pain with intercourse. She denies new sexual partners and denies fever or chills. She is frustrated because she has been treated recently for several urinary tract infections without resolution of her symptoms.

Her past medical history is significant for asthma and irritable bowel disease. Her surgical history includes removal of her tonsils as a child. She is married and has been with her husband for seven years. Her husband has had a vasectomy. The patient denies known drug allergies, takes a multivitamin, and uses an albuterol inhaler as needed.

Physical Examination

General appearance	Well-developed, well-nourished female in no acute distress. Alert and oriented.

Vital Signs

Temperature	37.0°C
Pulse	78 beats/min
Blood pressure	112/68 mmHg
Respiratory rate	16 breaths/min
Oxygen saturation	100 percent on room air
Height	64 inches
Weight	130 lb
BMI	22.3 kg/m^2
Abdomen	Soft, non-tender, no rebound or guarding
External genitalia	Normal, no lesions, normal urethra
Pelvic exam	Normal uterus, normal adnexa, mildly tender to palpation at anterior vagina

Laboratory Studies

Urinalysis	Negative

How Would You Manage This Patient?

The patient likely has painful bladder syndrome. This diagnosis is suggested by her history of urinary symptoms with negative workup for other etiologies and lack of resolution of symptoms despite treatment for urinary tract infection. Given her suggestive symptoms, the Pelvic Pain and Urgency/Frequency Patient Symptom Scale (PUF Questionnaire) was given. She had a score of 20, which correlates well with the presence of painful bladder syndrome. She was counseled on the diagnosis and given education and resources. Self-care and behavior modifications were initiated, including application of local heat or cold to the bladder area and an elimination diet. The patient was given instructions for bladder training and was referred to a physical therapist.

She returned for follow-up six weeks later and reported improvement in her symptoms and identification of dietary triggers. The patient removed the triggers from her diet, but admitted to compliance issues with the bladder training exercises. She felt her symptoms, while better, were not adequately improved. She was started on hydroxyzine at night for continued nighttime symptoms and pentosan polysulfate daily. Six months later, she reported occasional symptom flares but significant overall symptom improvement and improved quality of life.

Painful Bladder Syndrome

Painful bladder syndrome, also referred to as interstitial cystitis, is defined as "an unpleasant sensation (pain, pressure, discomfort) perceived to be related to the urinary bladder, associated with lower urinary tract symptoms of more than six weeks duration, in the absence of infection or other identifiable causes" [1]. Some patients will have a waxing and waning course and occasional spontaneous resolution of symptoms. Others will have a chronic course that requires long-term care. The pathophysiology of painful bladder syndrome is unknown. It is thought to be autoimmune in nature and related to increased permeability of the glycosaminoglycan layer of the bladder urothelium, which allows toxic elements to reach the bladder and cause irritation and dysuria [2]. The syndrome is often seen in patients with coexisting problems such as irritable bowel disease, fibromyalgia, inflammatory bowel disease, atopic allergies, and systemic lupus erythematosus [3, 2]. It mostly affects women in their thirties and forties with a female-to-male ratio of 5:1 [3]. The syndrome is important to recognize as it can be a debilitating illness for patients. The impact of the syndrome on patients' quality of life can be comparable to rheumatoid arthritis or end-stage renal disease [4]. Economic costs can be significant as well; mean annual health-care costs with painful bladder syndrome are 2 to 2.4 times greater than age-matched controls. The annual cost for painful bladder syndrome in the United States was estimated to be $750 million in 2,000 [2, 4]. The true financial impact is likely underestimated due to variations in diagnosis and difficulty measuring aspects such as missed work and productivity.

Painful bladder syndrome is a diagnosis of exclusion. Patients often present after several months or years of treatment for urinary tract or pelvic infections without symptom resolution. Treatable causes such as urinary tract infection, overactive bladder, urethral calculi, and endometriosis should be ruled out. The differential diagnosis also includes bladder carcinoma, sexually transmitted infections, mycobacterium tuberculosis infection, pelvic radiation, urethral diverticulum, and pelvic floor muscle dysfunction [2].

A thorough history and physical exam are important and will guide the clinician in obtaining a correct diagnosis. Patients often present with a history of treatment for multiple urinary tract infections and chronic dysuria. Although symptoms may vary, many patients describe pressure or pain symptoms near the bladder often worsened when the bladder is full and improved after bladder emptying. Patients may also describe urinary frequency and urgency. A detailed urinary symptom history should be obtained, including number of voids per day, urgency symptoms, and pain symptoms. A sexual history should also be reviewed, including complaints of dyspareunia. The physical exam includes an abdominal and pelvic exam. The external genitalia should be examined, a bimanual exam performed to rule out masses, and the pelvic floor support assessed. Many patients with painful bladder syndrome experience discomfort with palpation during the pelvic exam; however, the physical exam findings are variable.

Validated instruments such as the interstitial cystitis (IC) symptoms quantitation questionnaire [5] and the pelvic PUF questionnaire [6] have been developed to aid in the diagnosis and should be administered to patients with suggestive symptoms and physical findings. The questionnaires vary somewhat, but both focus on quantifying the bladder symptoms and how bothersome they are for the patient. While useful in assisting with the diagnosis, they are not required. These questionnaires are readily available and can be easily completed by the patient in the office. The potassium sensitivity test was developed as an additional diagnostic tool for painful bladder syndrome. It is not widely used due to discomfort and the potential to cause an exacerbation of patient symptoms.

A urinalysis should be completed on all patients. A urine culture should be performed if symptoms or the urinalysis suggest infection. Further laboratory testing should be guided by the history and physical exam and may include testing for sexually transmitted diseases, yeast or bacterial vaginal infections, and imaging, including pelvic ultrasound.

Once the diagnosis of painful bladder syndrome is likely, the patient should be counseled on the expected course of the syndrome and initial treatment options. Initial treatments are conservative and involve behavior modifications, including stress reduction. Examples of lifestyle changes that may improve symptoms are fluid restriction or hydration, dietary changes, and application of heat or cold to the bladder or perineum [4]. As the behavior modifications are low-risk, patients are instructed to trial each separately while monitoring for symptom improvement. The patient should be counseled to monitor for triggers and avoid vigorous activities or foods that are associated with worsening of symptoms. Acidic and spicy foods should be avoided, as should caffeinated and alcoholic beverages. Artificial sweeteners may trigger or worsen symptoms as well. Patients can be counseled to start with a strict elimination diet and add back foods and drinks while monitoring for symptom flares. A multidisciplinary approach may help provide maximum treatment benefits [4]. Psychological stress may contribute to poor treatment success and involvement of a mental health professional may be helpful. A physical therapist familiar with pelvic floor techniques and chronic pelvic pain can be helpful as well. Nonprescription analgesics such as nonsteroidal anti-inflammatory drugs (NSAIDs) and short-term use of the urinary analgesic phenazopyridine may also be utilized as first-line treatment agents. Because of limited supporting data for other treatments and the low risk and cost of these treatments, the American Urological Association recommends them as first line for all patients presenting with symptoms of painful bladder syndrome [4].

Further pharmacologic and surgical treatment options are available if a patient has failed initial empiric therapy. There are no specific recommendations for how much time is allowed for symptom improvement, and escalation to second-line treatments should be guided by the patient's symptoms and clinician's judgment. Pentosan polysulfate (Elmiron) 100 mg three times daily is FDA-approved for the relief of pain in patients with chronic IC. It is thought to work by replacement of the glycosaminoglycan layer of the bladder urothelium, although the exact mechanism of action is unknown. It is the most studied pharmacologic therapy for use with interstitial cystitis/painful bladder syndrome. Effectiveness studies demonstrated varying results, with 21–56 percent of patients showing clinically significant improvement with pentosan polysulfate versus 13–49 percent showing improvement with placebo. Given a low adverse event rate, pentosan polysulfate is considered an option for second-line treatment. Hydroxyzine 10–75 mg daily has been shown to have benefit alone and in combination with pentosan polysulfate, with clinical improvement rates ranging from 23 to 92 percent. Cimetidine 300–400 mg twice daily may also be considered, but large effectiveness data are lacking. Amitriptyline 25 mg titrated up to 100 mg daily has also shown benefit, but it can have significant side effects. Use of gabapentin and prednisone has also been described. The American Urological Association recommends against long-term use of steroids due to the risks of adverse events and small studies showing benefit; short-term therapy for flares could be considered [2, 4]. A key point in the management of painful bladder syndrome as discussed in the American Urological Association Guidelines is that a treatment plan will likely be multimodal and may incorporate first- and second-line agents simultaneously. The recommendations stress that care for painful bladder syndrome be individualized and that pain symptoms be adequately addressed to minimize effects on patients' quality of life [4]. This may involve multiple conservative and medical therapies at once. A helpful treatment algorithm is available on the American Urological Association website.

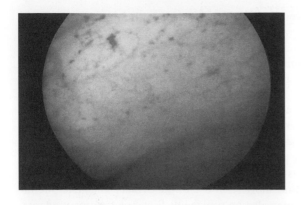

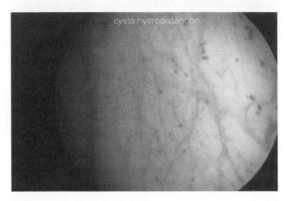

Figure 84.1 Glomerulations (petechial red areas) as seen on cystoscopy.

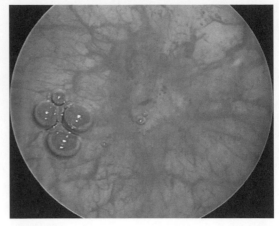

Figure 84.2 Hunner's ulcer (reddened lesion on the bladder) seen on cystoscopy.

Cystoscopy should be reserved for those patients who have failed other treatment modalities or whose diagnosis is unclear. Cystoscopy with hydrodistention of the bladder can be both diagnostic and therapeutic. Exact therapeutic benefits are unknown due to lack of randomized trials although patients have reported clinically significant relief of symptoms up to 56 percent at 2–3 months [2]. Due to the discomfort of the hydrodistention, it should be undertaken in the operating room with the patient under anesthesia. Cystoscopic evaluation may identify lesions characteristic to painful bladder syndrome such as glomerulations (Figure 84.1), hypervascularity, and Hunner's ulcers (Figure 84.2). Cystoscopy can also aid in ruling out other causes for the patient's symptoms. Fulgaration of Hunner's lesions should be performed at the time of cystoscopy and instillation of intravesical treatment solutions such as dimethyl sulfoxide (DMSO), steroids, heparin, and local anesthetics can be helpful [3]. Intravesical therapy can be performed in the operating room or in the physician's office, and may be taught to patients for home self-therapy

Key Teaching Points

- Painful bladder syndrome or IC is an important diagnosis to include in the differential of women who present with pelvic pain and dysuria.
- Painful bladder syndrome is a diagnosis of exclusion. Validated questionnaire instruments may help in the diagnosis.
- First-line treatments include behavioral modifications such as dietary changes, fluid intake adjustments, and application of heat or cold, as well as NSAIDs and urinary analgesics.
- Second-line therapy includes prescription medications, such as pentosan polysulfate, hydroxyzine, amitriptyline, and cimetidine.

References

1. Hanno P, Dmochowski R. Status of international consensus on interstitial cystitis/bladder pain syndrome/painful bladder syndrome: 2008 snapshot. *Neurourol Urodyn* 2009;28:274–286.

2. Deniseiko Sanses, T. Painful bladder syndrome/interstitial cystitis. *J Pelvic Med Surg* 2007;13:321–336.

3. Swift SE. Painful Conditions of the Lower Urinary Tract Including Painful Bladder Syndrome. In: Bent A, Cundiff G, Swift S. Ostergard's Urogynecology and Pelvic Floor Dysfunction. Philadelphia, PA: Lippincott Williams & Wilkins; 2008:106–118.

4. Hanno P, Burks D, Clemens Q et al. Diagnosis and treatment of interstitial cystitis/bladder pain syndrome. American Urological Association (AUA) Guideline. 2011. www.auanet.org/guidelines/interstitial-cystitis/bladder-pain-syndrome. Accessed 6/26/17.

5. O'Leary MP, Saint GR, Fowler FJ et al. The interstitial cystitis symptom index and problem index. *Urology* 1997;49 (5A Suppl):58–63.

6. Parson CL, Dell J, Stanford EG et al. Increased prevalence of interstitial cystitis: previously unrecognized urologic and gynecologic cases identified using a new symptom questionnaire and intravesical potassium sensitivity test. *Urology* 2002;60:573–578.

A 25-Year-Old Woman with Recurrent Urinary Tract Infections

Jonathan Emery

History of Present Illness

A 25-year-old woman, gravida 0, presents to her gynecologist's office with a three-day history of pain and burning with urination. She also notes mild urinary frequency for the past 24 hours. Her last menstrual period was ten days ago. She denies fever or blood in her urine and notes her vaginal discharge is of normal consistency. She is sexually active and has been monogamous with her male partner for the past 18 months and notes consistent condom use for contraception. She denies any prior history of sexually transmitted infections, though she admits to an abnormal pap test that was positive for human papilloma virus at age 21, which resolved on repeat testing. Her last intercourse prior to presentation was four days ago.

She has no prior surgeries and denies chronic medical issues except that she has had 3 urinary tract infections (UTIs) over the previous 12 months, most recently 6 weeks ago. Her initial UTI was diagnosed in an urgent care setting, and another was diagnosed with a positive urine culture for *E. coli* and subsequently treated by her primary care physician. She takes only ibuprofen as needed for headaches and denies medical allergies. She does not smoke nor use drugs.

Physical Examination

General appearance	Well-developed, well-nourished female who is in no acute distress.

Vital Signs

Temperature	36.7 C
Pulse	88 beats/min
Blood pressure	116/68 mmHg
Weight	125 lb
BMI	22.3 kg/m^2
Abdomen	Soft with normal bowel sounds. Nontender and non-distended, without guarding or rebound. No costovertebral angle tenderness
External genitalia	Normal genitalia without vesicles, ulcers, or condylomata
Vagina	Normal vaginal mucosa with minimal white, non-odorous discharge
Cervix	Nulliparous, closed, and without bleeding or erythema
Uterus	Small, mobile, and non-tender
Adnexa	No fullness or tenderness

Laboratory Studies

Urine pregnancy test	Negative
Urinalysis	Significant for large blood and positive for nitrites.
Wet mount	Negative for trichomonads; absent clue cells
Potassium hydroxide (KOH)	Negative for hyphae

How Would You Manage This Patient?

Based on this patient's history of irritative urinary symptoms and a urinalysis that is positive for blood and nitrites, she meets criteria for the office diagnosis of UTI. Further supporting the diagnosis is that she is not pregnant and is without evidence of vaginitis or acute infective vulvitis, both of which can also cause irritative voiding symptoms. Since the patient is afebrile and does not have systemic symptoms, she is a candidate for outpatient oral antibiotic therapy. She was treated with a 3-day course of trimethoprim/sulfamethoxazole, twice daily, and was instructed to continue to void immediately after intercourse. Since this is her fourth infection in 12 months, she meets criteria for recurrent UTIs. Therefore, she was also given a prescription for nitrofurantoin 100 mg to be taken after intercourse for the next six months as a method to effectively decrease recurrent infections.

Recurrent UTIs

Recurrent UTIs have been defined as having greater than two infections in six months or three or more infections in one year [1]. This patient meets criteria for recurrent UTI, as evidence is present that this is a new infection and not a relapsing infection, which would require further evaluation. The American Congress of Obstetricians and Gynecologists notes that a recurrent UTI with the same microbe after appropriate treatment is classified as a relapse. Alternatively, reinfection is a recurrent UTI caused by an organism identified in a previous culture with an intervening negative urine culture [2]. Recurrent UTI may also be caused by a newly identified (or different) isolated microorganism. The majority of UTI recurrences present as cystitis, as in this patient, and are a result of reinfection. These generally occur within the first three months after initial infection. The lifetime prevalence of UTI in women is estimated to be over 50 percent, with some estimates as high as 80 percent. Estimates for recurrent episodes of UTI range from 25 to 50 percent in the first 6–12 months after the initial episode [2].

Risk factors for recurrent UTI include frequent sexual intercourse (three or more acts of intercourse per week), use of spermicide, and/or new sexual partner. Also, a history of the first UTI prior to age 15 years increases one's risk for recurrent UTI. In addition, while the patient in this case is premenopausal, there is an increased incidence of recurrent UTIs in postmenopausal women, notably in those who are estrogen-deficient and/or have urinary retention. There are genetic and/or biologic factors that also play a role in the development of recurrent UTIs. Increased predisposition to colonization of the vagina with uropathogens has been documented in women with recurrent infections, and non-secretor and P1 phenotypes have been shown to be genetic determinants that increase risk.

It is well documented that colonization of the vagina by rectal flora, commonly with intercourse, is a critical event in

269

Table 85.1 Standard treatments for uncomplicated urethritis and cystitis

Antimicrobial	Dose	Duration
Trimethoprim-sulfamethoxazole	160 mg trimethoprim–800 mg sulfamethoxazole	Twice daily for 3 days
Nitrofurantoin	100 mg	Twice daily for 7 days
Fosfomycin	3 g single dose (powder)	One dose

the development of an initial UTI. It is felt that this pathogenic sequence is also involved in women who develop recurrent UTIs. Greater than two-thirds of all UTIs are caused by *Escherichia coli,* and women with an initial *E. coli* UTI are more likely to experience a second UTI within six months as compared with women whose initial UTI was caused by a different organism. Use of the spermicide nonoxonyl-9 or other factors that lead to a diminution of *Lactobacillus* species and subsequent decrease in hydrogen peroxide production has also been shown to increase risk for recurrent UTI [3].

Once a urinary tract infection is diagnosed, treatment should be initiated immediately. Universally recognized standard treatments for uncomplicated urethritis and cystitis include a three-day course of trimethoprim/sulfamethoxazole, a five-day course of nitrofurantoin, or a one-day treatment with fosfomycin (Table 85.1). Treatment regimens of three or fewer days in duration are correlated with improved patient compliance, decreased side effects, and reduced risk of evolution to pyelonephritis [1]. In patients who are suffering from recurrent UTIs, the vast majority of recurrences represent reinfections, especially when they occur more than two weeks after resolution of symptoms. Since most recurrent UTIs are uncomplicated and caused by the same pathogens as an initial UTI, antimicrobial therapy should continue to be one of the approved therapies. In patients with recurrent infections who have been treated solely based on self-reported symptomatology or urinalysis, a midstream, clean catch urine culture should be obtained while the patient is symptomatic in order to verify an infection is present and to identify the causative organism. A colony count of greater than 100,000 colony-forming units (CFU) is the traditional threshold for infection; however, decreasing the required colony count in symptomatic patients to 1,000 to 10,000 CFU will improve sensitivity without significantly reducing specificity [2]. The decision to establish a definitive CFU cut-off should be determined by the provider, taking into account the clinical presentation. After a positive culture, choosing appropriate antimicrobial therapy should be done with culture results in mind.

For patients who present with multiple, recurrent episodes of UTIs, working to establish a strategy to prevent or reduce recurrences should be the goal. Initial management should include behavior modifications or adjustments, such as avoiding use of spermicides, either alone or in conjunction with

a diaphragm or condoms (including spermicide-coated condoms), as well as encouraging postcoital voiding. Although theoretically helpful, the latter action has not been shown to reduce recurrent UTIs. Consumption of cranberry juice (or related cranberry products) has shown promise in some studies at decreasing symptomatic UTIs. However, a Cochrane review in 2012 stated that the evidence cannot support use of cranberry juice for the prevention of UTIs [4]. Probiotic therapy has also been identified as an option to reduce recurrent infections, but data are few. It appears as though oral probiotic therapy is not likely to be of greater benefit than placebo at preventing recurrent UTI. More recent evidence with vaginal probiotics (specifically with *Lactobacillus* tablets), however, has shown promise in decreasing recurrent UTI, but more data are needed to confirm this.

Approaches to prevention have looked at use of antimicrobial prophylaxis in two main formats: daily (or continuous) and postcoital. Both have been studied and shown to be exceedingly effective for the prevention of symptomatic recurrent UTIs by approximately 95 percent [1]. Daily therapy can be used for a period of 6 to 12 months (or longer) but carries a greater risk of side effects (vaginal candidiasis, gastrointestinal symptoms) and cost. Also, discontinuation of the antibiotics will usually cause patients to return to having continued recurrences [5]. Postcoital prophylaxis, on the other hand, has been shown to be equally effective, with less overall medication burden and cost as well as diminution of side effects. It should be noted that postcoital medication is likely most effective if used in the first 2 hours after intercourse. Long-term effects of both methods include small risks of antibiotic resistance and possible rare side effects from prolonged nitrofurantoin exposure such as pulmonary fibrosis. Trimethoprim 40 mg/sulfamethoxazole 200 mg or nitrofurantoin 50–100 mg are considered first-line prophylactic medications, but cephalosporins (cephalexin 125–250 mg or cefaclor 250 mg) or trimethoprim 100 mg alone have been used [1, 3].

A third option for management of recurrent infections is so-called patient-initiated (or self) treatment [6], as studies have shown that women are able to self-diagnose with greater than 85 percent accuracy [3]. This is effective in patients who typically have three or fewer recurrences per year, are motivated, and are able to clearly identify symptoms. These patients are given a three-day course of antibiotics and instructed to begin treatment upon development of symptoms. While this means that the patient may typically suffer more recurrences, the overall use of antibiotics is decreased compared with prophylactic regimens.

In this case, the patient was prescribed a three-day course of antibiotics and given a prescription for a limited term of postcoital prophylaxis. In addition, she was counseled to use condoms without spermicide and consider vaginal probiotics as a follow-up measure. In patients with uncomplicated recurrent cystitis, like the woman described above, further evaluation with imaging of the urinary tract is not indicated. Patients who fail to respond, or develop worsening clinical status while on appropriate therapy, have persistent hematuria after clearing their infection, or meet any of the criteria listed in Box 85.1,

Box 85.1 Selected factors that warrant further evaluation in patients with recurrent UTIs

Hematuria (macroscopic or microscopic) persisting after clearance of infection, noted by resolution of symptoms or a negative urine culture

History of urinary tract malignancy

History of urinary tract surgery or trauma, or diverticular disease

History or presence of calculi*

Multidrug-resistant organism

Persistent symptoms and bacteriuria despite two weeks of culture-directed therapy

Pneumaturia or fecaluria

Presence of anaerobic organisms (with the exception of facultative anaerobes [e.g., Escherichia coli, Staphylococcus species])

Repeat episodes of pyelonephritis or treatment-resistant pyelonephritis

Symptoms of urinary obstruction

Voiding dysfunction (e.g., elevated post-void residual volume, incontinence)

*Consider further workup if urine culture shows presence of struvite stone-producing (urea-splitting) organisms (e.g., *Proteus, Klebsiella, Pseudomonas*).

Adapted or reprinted with permission from Common Questions about Recurrent

Urinary Tract Infections in Women, April 1, 2016, Vol 93, No 7, American Family Physician Copyright © 2016

American Academy of Family Physicians. All Rights Reserved.

require further evaluation with imaging. Renal ultrasonography is generally a reasonable first step to evaluate for obstruction or abscess; however, intravenous pyelography or contrast enhanced CT or MRI may be indicated in some cases.

Key Teaching Points

- Estimates for recurrent UTI range from 27 to 44 percent in the first 6–12 months after an initial UTI.

- *E. coli* accounts for greater than two-thirds of all UTIs, with other enteric flora as possible causative agents.
- Standard, proven antimicrobial therapies include trimethoprim/sulfamethoxazole, nitrofurantoin, and fosfomycin.
- Prophylactic use of daily or episodic (postcoital) antibiotics can decrease recurrences as well as patient-initiated therapy, but recurrent infections typically return when treatment is discontinued.

References

1. Arnold JJ, Hehn LE, Klein DA. Common questions about recurrent urinary tract infections in women. *Am Fam Physician* 2016;93:560–569.

2. American College of Obstetricians and Gynecologists. Treatment of urinary tract infections in nonpregnant women. Practice bulletin No. 91. *Obstet Gynecol* 2008;111:785–794.

3. Gupta K, Stamm WE. Pathogenesis and management of recurrent urinary tract infections in women. *World J Urol* 1999;17:415–420.

4. Jepson RG, Williams G, Craig JC. Cranberries for preventing urinary tract infections. *Cochrane Database Syst Rev.* 2012;October 17:10.

5. Albert X, Huertas I, Pereiro II et al. Antibiotics for preventing recurrent urinary tracts infection in non-pregnant women. *Cochrane Database Syst Rev* 2004;(3): CD001209.

6. Gupta K, Hooton TM, Roberts PL et al. Patient-initiated treatment of uncomplicated recurrent urinary tract infections in young women. *An Intern Med* 2001; 135:9–16.

An 80-Year-Old Woman with Total Procidentia with Vaginal Irritation

Madhurima Krishna Keerthy

History of Present Illness

An 80-year-old woman, gravida 7, para 7, presents to the office complaining of vaginal irritation that has been present for six months. She has noticed worsening of the symptoms recently. She has also noticed a vaginal "swelling" that has been present for the last 4–5 years. She has not been evaluated for these symptoms before.

Her past medical history is significant for hypertension controlled with a diuretic and an ACE inhibitor. She has diabetes that is not well controlled. She had seven full-term vaginal deliveries. Her largest infant was 4,150 g. She admits to constipation and having to apply pressure with her fingers in her vagina to evacuate her bowels completely. She has difficulty urinating and has to exert to void. She has had several urinary tract infections in the past few years.

Physical Examination

Height	160 inches
Weight	210 lb
BMI	41 kg/m²
Temperature	36. 8°C
HR	87 bpm
BP	140/90 mmHg

Physical Exam
Abdomen	Soft, non-tender, non-distended, obese

Pelvic Exam
External genitalia	Atrophic. Bulbocavernosus and anal wink reflexes present symmetrically.
Transverse genital diameter	Approximately 5 cm. Cervix and uterus protruding 8 cm beyond the introitus (Figure 86.1). Exposed skin with erythema and small ulcerations at the most dependent site. Prolapse reducible.

After reduction, inspection was again performed, which revealed a normal urethra. A bivalved speculum exam was placed, which revealed atrophic vaginal walls. Cervix appeared grossly normal with no lesions. Patient was asked to cough while slowly withdrawing the speculum and the descent of the cervix was noted to occur past the hymen and the introitus.

Bimanual exam revealed no adnexal masses. Pelvic floor muscle function was noted to be poor. Rectovaginal exam showed no rectal prolapse and confirmed bimanual exam findings.

Exam repeated with patient standing: Maximum prolapse 8 cm from introitus.

POP-Q assessment (Figure 86.2): Aa +3, Ba +8, C+8, D +8, Ba +3, Bp +8, TVL 10, GH 4.5, PB 1.5.

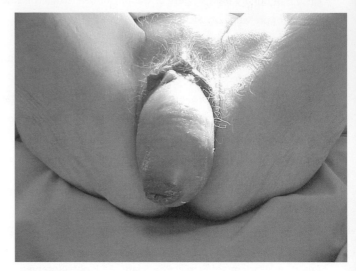

Figure 86.1 This image shows the extent of the prolapse. Cervix is noted at about 8 cm outside the introitus and there is erythema noted on the exposed area. (Image provided by Steven Cohen, MD)

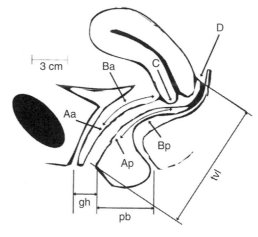

Figure 86.2 POP-Q measurement of a uterine procidentia. The difference between points Aa, Ba and Ap, Bp can be noted.
Figure from Bump RC, Mattiasson A, Bo K, Brubaker LP, DeLancey JO, Klorskov P, et al. The standardization of terminology of female pelvic organ prolapse and pelvic floor dysfunction *Am J Obstet Gynecol*, 1996;175:10–17, reprinted with permission from Elsevier

Cough stress test: negative for incontinence with prolapse reduced.

Postvoid residual volume by catheterization: 150 ml.

How Would You Manage This Patient?

This patient has Stage IV pelvic organ prolapse, also known as uterine procidentia. Due to coexisting voiding and defecatory dysfunction, expectant management is not ideal for this patient. After thorough discussion of options, the patient elected to proceed with pessary insertion. A 3-inch Gellhorn pessary was inserted and the patient was trained in removal and reinsertion. Vaginal estrogen was prescribed as adjunctive therapy. Urine culture was obtained as patient had voiding dysfunction with high residual volumes. Culture confirmed a urinary tract infection, which was treated. She was able to retain the pessary, which reduced the prolapse without causing incontinence. She was seen in follow-up in six weeks, at which time she remained comfortable. She had been counseled to remove and reinsert the pessary monthly, which she has done without problem. She had no vaginal discharge, odor, or bleeding. She was instructed to continue monthly pessary reinsertions and call if she expelled the pessary, had difficulty with insertion or removal, or developed vaginal discharge or bleeding. One-year follow-up was planned.

Uterine Procidentia

Pelvic organ prolapse is the descent of one or more aspects of the vagina and uterus: the anterior vaginal wall, posterior vaginal wall, the uterus (cervix), or the apex of the vagina (vaginal vault or cuff scar after hysterectomy) [1]. Procidentia is an extreme form where the uterus, cervix, and vagina prolapse through the introitus. The actual prevalence of procidentia is not known. According to the National Health and Nutrition Examination Survey, approximately 3 percent of women in the United States report symptoms of vaginal bulging [2]. However, in the studies that evaluated the severity of prolapse, very few cases with Stage III–IV prolapse, which encompasses uterine procidentia, were identified. Risk factors for procidentia are similar to other forms of pelvic organ prolapse, and include age, parity, vaginal birth, obesity, neurological disease, prior pelvic surgery, chronic constipation, and chronic cough. Modification of these risk factors will not improve procidentia, but may reduce the risk of failure if the patient chooses to undergo surgical management.

Common symptoms of procidentia include vaginal bulge, pressure, vaginal irritation, spotting, excessive discharge, and defecatory and sexual dysfunction. Patients often present with urinary complications such as recurrent infections, acute retention, incontinence, or pain or bleeding from bladder stones. Some patients may present with a history of stress urinary incontinence that improves or resolves with worsening of prolapse. Sudden onset pain can be a sign of incarcerated prolapse, which requires immediate evaluation and prompt reduction.

Evaluation

Evaluation of potential prolapse symptoms includes a thorough history, physical examination, and establishment of goals for treatment. History should assess the range of symptoms including pain, bleeding, irritation, urinary incontinence and retention, and defecatory problems. The impact of the prolapse on patient's quality of life can be assessed with structured tools like the Pelvic Floor Distress Inventory and the Pelvic Floor Impact Questionnaire, which can be used to monitor treatment and guide management decisions.

Physical examination should begin in the dorsal lithotomy position while the patient performs a Valsalva maneuver. If the patient states the full extent of prolapse is not appreciated, she should be asked to stand up and strain again. The extent of prolapse should be confirmed with the patient. Stress urinary incontinence should be evaluated using the cough stress test before and after reduction of prolapse. A neurological exam should include eliciting bulbocavernosus (by stroking laterally to the clitoris with cotton tip swab) and anal wink (by stroking the skin around the anus) reflexes to help diagnose coexisting neurological disorders. The prolapsed areas should be evaluated for ulcerations, keratinization, yeast vaginitis, and other signs of chronic exposure. A bimanual exam should be performed to assess for adnexal masses.

POP-Q should be assessed after reduction of the prolapse. POP-Q was developed to assess and document prolapse in individual compartments. Although its role has not been studied in nonsurgical patients, it can serve as a baseline measurement and be used to compare future measurements. This system has been noted to have interobserver reproducibility and is recommended by most international organizations, including the American Urogynecologic Society, the Society of Gynecologic Surgeons, and the International Continence Society. Stage IV of POP-Q represents uterine procidentia, where the most distal prolapse protrudes almost completely (at least, total vaginal length (TVL) = 2 cm). In this case, TVL was 10 cm and the most distal prolapse was noted to be 8 cm past the hymen (Figure 86.2). For a patient with procidentia, genital hiatus and TVL are the most important measurements.

Post-void residual should be calculated as many patients with procidentia have voiding difficulties. A basic urinalysis and culture are appropriate if patient has urinary symptoms. Evaluation for cervical and intrauterine malignancy should be performed in case of bleeding from the cervical os. Imaging is not recommended for routine evaluation. As chronic procidentia can cause obstruction to urinary outflow, renal sonogram or CT scan may be necessary to evaluate hydronephrosis, hydroureter, or bladder stones.

Management

Management options include observation, nonsurgical approaches, and surgery. The decision depends on the patient's goals, age, symptoms, medical comorbidities, complications of prolapse, and need for correction of concurrent incontinence.

Procidentia can be observed without treatment. These patients should be instructed to monitor the protruded areas for ulceration, skin changes, bleeding, and other changes and to seek medical attention if any of these things occur. Topical estrogen can be applied to the exposed areas. Twice-a-year follow-up is reasonable for patients with advanced prolapse as urinary and defecatory symptoms can worsen over time.

Pessaries are usually first-line management for advanced stage prolapse. They are ideal for management of women with uterine procidentia and vaginal vault prolapse, especially those who do not desire or have comorbidities that prohibit immediate surgery. Pessaries can also be used for patients with severe ulceration to allow healing prior to planned surgery. Management with a pessary was acceptable to 62 percent of patients with Stage III–IV prolapse [3]. Sexual activity and absence of concomitant stress urinary incontinence are associated with continued use. Age, parity, menopausal status, and prior prolapse surgery or hysterectomy is associated with discontinuation [4]. Observational studies have shown improvement in symptoms of prolapse and urinary and bowel symptoms with continued use [5].

About 75 percent of women were successfully fitted with a pessary after two office visits [6]. Pessary trial is often by trial and error. Vaginal introitus size and vaginal length can help determine the size of the pessary needed. The largest pessary that is comfortable should be inserted [7]. Pessaries can be broadly divided into two types: support (Ring, Lever, Gehrung) and space-filling (Gellhorn, Donut, Cube). A prospective observational study by Clemons et al. reported that most women with stage II and III prolapse (100 and 71 percent, respectively) were successfully fitted with ring pessaries and women with Stage IV prolapse with a Gellhorn pessary (space-filling pessary) (64 percent). The stage of the prolapse and the size of the vaginal introitus were used to guide pessary selection. If the vaginal introitus was 3–4 finger breadths and the stage was III–IV, Gellhorn pessaries were usually successful [6].

After a pessary is inserted in the office, the patient is asked to cough, ambulate, void, and strain on a toilet. This tests for expulsion and stress urinary incontinence. Once the pessary is noted to be a good fit, the patient is scheduled for 1–2 week follow-up. At this visit, patient is assessed for pain, pressure, vaginal bleeding, discharge, and difficulty in voiding or defecation. The pessary is removed, cleaned with water and soap, and a vaginal exam is performed for erosions. The patient is counseled to remove the pessary every 1–2 weeks for cleaning and asked to leave it out overnight. These patients are typically followed up in 1–2 months and then annually. If a patient cannot remove and reinsert the pessary for any reason, they should return every 3–6 months for cleaning at the physician's office. A UK-based physician survey showed that 23 percent changed their patient's pessaries every three to six months, 67 percent every six months, and 10 percent every 6–12 months [7].

Patients are instructed to identify and call if problems such as vaginal erosion or ulceration develop. Vaginal discharge occurs frequently from pH disturbance, inflammation, and atrophy. Vaginal estrogen or a pH-altering product can be used. If vaginal ulceration or erosion occurs, the pessary can be discontinued for 2–4 weeks and estrogen applied. Serious complications such as fistula formation are rare.

Vaginal estrogen alone is effective treatment of severe urogenital atrophy and has a role in treating vaginal keratinization and irritation due to chronic exposure [8]. However, there is limited evidence to support a role in treatment of procidentia [9].

Patients who need treatment and fail pessary may be candidates for surgery [10]. Surgery can be reconstructive or obliterative and is performed via several approaches, with or without graft materials. Le Fort's Colpocleisis is an obliterative procedure that can be performed in older women with comorbidities and those that do not plan to have vaginal intercourse in future.

Key Teaching Points

- Procidentia or Stage IV pelvic organ prolapse can present with vaginal bulge, irritation, and voiding or defecatory dysfunction, and can adversely impact quality of life.
- Nonsurgical management with vaginal estrogen and pessary should be offered as first-line management.
- Pessaries can be fit in 75 percent and are acceptable to 60 percent of patients with Stage III–IV prolapse.
- Space-filling pessaries are suitable for patients with advanced stage prolapse.
- Patients opting for expectant management should be followed to monitor for worsening voiding and defecatory dysfunction.

References

1. Haylen BT, de Ridder D, Freeman RM et al. An International Urogynecological Association (IUGA)/International Continence Society (ICS) joint report on the terminology for female pelvic floor dysfunction. International Urogynecological Association, International Continence Society. *Neurourol Urodyn* 2010;29:4–20.

2. Wu JM, Vaughan CP, Goode PS et al. Prevalence and trends of symptomatic pelvic floor disorders in U.S. women. *Obstet Gynecol* 2014;123:141–148.

3. Powers K, Lazarou G, Wang A et al. Pessary use in advanced pelvic organ prolapse. *Int Urogynecol J Pelvic Floor Dysfunct* 2006;17(2):160–164.

4. Brincat C, Kenton K, Fitzgerald MP, Brubaker L. Sexual activity predicts continued pessary use, *Am J Obstet Gynecol* July 2004;191(1).

5. Cundiff GW, Amundsen CL, Bent AE et al. The PESSRI study: symptom relief outcomes of a randomized crossover trial of the ring and Gellhorn pessaries. *Am J Obstet Gynecol* 2007;196:405.e1.

6. Clemons JL, Aguilar VC, Tillinghast TA et al. Risk factors associated with an unsuccessful pessary fitting trial in

women with pelvic organ prolapse. *Am J Obstet Gynecol* 2004;190:345.

7. Gorti M, Hudelist G, Simons A. Evaluation of vaginal pessary management: a UK-based survey. *J Obstet Gynaecol* 2009;29 (2):129–131.

8. Weber MA, Kleijn MH, Langendam M et al. Local oestrogen for pelvic floor disorders: a systematic review. *PLoS One* 2015;10:e0136265.

9. Ismail SI, Bain C, Hagen S. Oestrogens for treatment or prevention of pelvic organ prolapse in postmenopausal women. *Cochrane Database Syst Rev* 2010,Issue 9. Art. No.:CD007063. (Systematic review)

10. American College of Obstetricians and Gynecologists. Pelvic organ prolapse. Practice bulletin No. 176. *Obstet Gynecol* 2017;129: e56–e72.

A 60-Year-Old Woman Presenting with Difficulty with Defecation (Posterior Wall Defect)

Erica Nelson

History of Present Illness

A 60-year-old woman, gravida 2, para 2, presents with complaints of fullness in her vaginal area and difficulty emptying her bowels. The problem has progressively worsened over the past six months. She had two vaginal deliveries, the first with an episiotomy. She takes fiber daily to relieve constipation, which she has struggled with most her life. After defecation, she has a feeling of incomplete emptying and occasionally has smearing of her underwear. On very active days she notices rectal pressure, with a feeling of a soft mass in her vagina, which resolves at night. The exposed area feels dry and irritated. She denies bleeding, vaginal discharge, or vulvar symptoms. She denies urinary incontinence, urgency, or nocturia. She is hesitant to have intercourse because of the bulge and dryness.

Menopause was at age 51. She has no other medical problems or prior surgeries. She takes no medications other than the fiber.

Physical Examination

General appearance	Menopausal female in no acute distress

Vital Signs

Temperature	37.1°C
Pulse	80 beats/min
Blood pressure	110/68 mmHg
Height	64 inches
Weight	175 lb
BMI	30.0 kg/m^2
Abdomen	Soft, not distended, no palpable mass

Pelvic Exam

External genitalia	Normal appearing
Vagina and cervix	Normal without lesions.
Uterus	Normal size, mobile, non-tender
Adnexa	No masses and non-tender
Neurologic examination	Sensation intact. Bulbocavernosus and pudendal reflexes normal.

Pelvic Examination with Maximum Valsalva

Vagina	Anterior wall with minimal descent. Negative cough stress test. Cervix and vaginal apex descend less than 3 cm. Posterior wall descends as a smooth bulge to one centimeter beyond the introitus.
Rectal exam	Intact anal sphincter. Palpable defect in the distal rectovaginal septum.

How Would You Manage This Patient?

The patient has a distal rectocele or posterior vaginal wall defect. The rectocele was diagnosed on physical exam, where the posterior vagina was noted to be bulging and descending through the introitus. The defect was palpable on rectal exam. Her anterior vagina and cervix were well supported, indicating that she had an isolated rectocele. Her symptoms could all be attributed to the rectocele.

Management was guided by her symptoms, primarily her bulge symptoms and difficulty defecating. To improve her bowel habits, increased daily dietary fiber and water intake to at least 3 liters a day was recommended. If she got inadequate relief from this, she was asked to start an osmotic laxative such as MiraLax with the goal of daily bowel movements that do not require straining or splinting. She should have an urge to defecate and pass soft, intact stool without significant effort. The fiber and osmotic laxatives should be titrated by the patient to achieve the desired bowel movements while avoiding loose stools or diarrhea. She should be counseled to avoid straining with bowel movements and sitting on the toilet for prolonged periods of time.

The patient was instructed to perform Kegel exercise several times a day to see if this would relieve her symptoms. She was instructed she could discontinue if she did not observe improvement within several weeks. She was prescribed vaginal estrogen for her dryness and irritation symptoms.

She was counseled that the vaginal estrogen may help with dryness symptoms and water-based lubricants such as Astroglide or K-Y Jelly may further decrease friction and pain. She and her partner were encouraged to experiment with various positions which might decrease feelings of pressure and pain. She was reassured that sexual activity will not harm or worsen the rectocele and she could have sex without restriction.

She was brought back for follow-up in two months and reported improved bowel habits and decreased need for splinting. Her symptoms of dryness and discomfort with normal activities had improved. She still noted pressure in her vaginal area and the feeling of a bulge at the end of the day, but these symptoms are less bothersome. She and her husband are satisfied with their sexual relations. She feels her symptoms are adequately improved and no longer limit her activities. She was counseled to continue the interventions she was doing, and that other interventions such as pessaries and surgery were available if her symptoms worsen.

Posterior Wall Defects

Rectoceles are caused by defects of the rectovaginal septum, the layer of fascia between the vagina and the rectum. The septum extends from above the cervix to the perineal body. Defects result in herniation of the rectum into the vagina. Rectoceles are not usually isolated defects, but often are associated with an apical (cervix or vaginal cuff) or anterior (cystocele) prolapse [1].

The size and position of the defects vary and do not correlate with symptoms. Rectoceles are present in around 20–50 percent of parous women and up to 12 percent of nulligravid women [2, 3].

Most women with posterior wall defects are asymptomatic. Typical rectocele symptoms include pelvic or rectal pressure, vaginal fullness, fecal smearing, incontinence, and difficulty defecating, including constipation, incomplete emptying, or need for straining. Women typically become symptomatic when the leading edge protrudes beyond the hymeneal ring [1, 2, 4]. In extreme cases, patients may have to splint or place fingers in the vagina and push on the posterior wall to complete defecation. Since posterior wall defects are often accompanied by anterior and apical wall defect, women may also note urinary incontinence and sexual dysfunction, including pain, pressure, or avoidance of intercourse. Many patients, like this one, have isolated rectoceles with no other defects that need addressing.

Risk factors for rectoceles are primarily, but not exclusively, obstetrical. Obstetrical risk factors include operative vaginal deliveries, episiotomy, large perineal lacerations, and prolonged second stage of labor. The mechanisms of the childbirth leading to posterior wall defects include injury to the rectovaginal fascia and injury or stretching of the pudendal nerve. Non-obstetrical risk factors include obesity, chronic constipation or other defecation disorders, chronic cough, and repeated heavy lifting or straining. All these factors increase stretch and strain on the rectovaginal septum and pelvic floor leading to weakening and laxity of the tissue [1, 2]. This patient's only identified risk factors were her two vaginal births.

The diagnosis of rectocele is made on physical exam (Figure 87.1). Rectoceles are frequently found as incidental findings on routine examination of asymptomatic patients. Examination of the exposed prolapsed vagina may note atrophy, irritation, or ulcers. Vaginal examination is performed first without a speculum and descent of the posterior vagina noted with and without Valsalva. A Pelvic Organ Prolapse Quantification (POP-Q) examination should be performed to quantitate the extent of vaginal prolapse for all three compartments, which will help with monitoring over time. Rectal examination should be performed to assess the integrity of the rectal sphincter for weakness or injury. Pelvic muscle tone is assessed by asking the patient to contract her pelvic muscles and noting whether tone is absent, weak, or strong [2]. Additional diagnostic testing is not necessary unless the symptoms are complex, involve neurologic deficits, or the prolapse is large with significant sphincter or pelvic floor weakness. Defecography and manometry may assist in the evaluation of patients with complicated bowel habits, evaluation of anal sphincter integrity, and evaluation of large or recurrent posterior wall defects [5]. This patient needed no evaluation other than her physical examination. Her rare streaking was not suggestive of significant fecal incontinence, and no neurologic deficit was noted.

Management of the rectocele is aimed at relieving symptoms and improving quality of life. Initial management should focus on relieving specific symptoms with conservative measures. While there is a large evidence base for surgical management, there is little data to guide initial conservative management, and most interventions are empiric and low-risk, but not supported by data. Asymptomatic women should be reassured that no treatment is necessary, but they should avoid constipation and straining to decrease the risk of the rectocele worsening. Women with difficulty evacuating should have treatment for constipation with daily fiber or osmotic laxatives and adequate fluid intake [6] These measures should decrease the need for straining and prolonged sitting on the toilet. Local care is important for exposed vaginal mucosa, and topical estrogen may help with atrophy and dryness [2]. Sexual dysfunction may stem from embarrassment about the bulge or from dryness or irritation from the exposed tissue. Reassurance, estrogen, and supplemental lubrication may be adequate for many patients, as it was for this one [7]. For patients with weak pelvic floor muscles or who have failed behavioral modifications, pelvic floor biofeedback with physical therapy can improve the strength and tone of the pelvic floor thereby decreasing symptoms. Success rates near 70 percent after 8–12 weeks of treatment vary depending on patient commitment and experience of the therapist [8, 11].

Bulge symptoms may be improved with weight loss and minimizing heavy lifting. Some providers advocate a trial of Kegel's exercises. Pessaries can be useful for bulge symptoms.

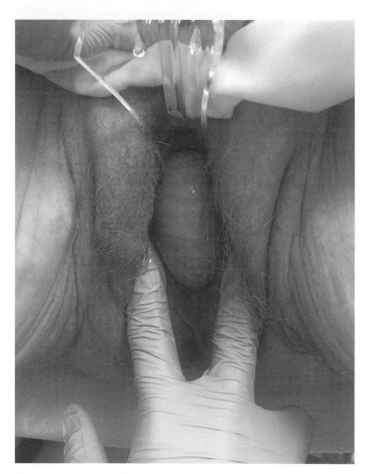

Figure 87.1 Rectocele. Posterior wall can be seen prolapsing through the introitus. This patient's prolapse is more extensive than the case patient. Image courtesy of Ashley Carroll, MD

Pessaries come in a variety of shapes and sizes including a ring, Gellhorn, donut, or balloon, and selection is motivated by ease of use and concomitant support defects. The ring pessary with support is the easiest to fit and for patients to manage and is adequate for many women. For women who cannot retain a ring pessary or where it does not adequately relieve the bulge, a bulkier pessary like a Gellhorn or balloon may be more effective. Pessaries can cause vaginal wall irritation or ulceration resulting in vaginal bleeding and extremely rarely, fistula. Topical estrogen may decrease irritation. The pessary should be removed, cleaned, and replaced regularly. Some patients can do this themselves and others will need this done by the provider. The pessary should be removed before sexual activity. Pessary removal and inspection of the vagina can be attempted as infrequently as every three months for geriatric patients with limited mobility [2].

Women should be reassessed 2–3 months after initiating conservative measures for assessment of improvement in their symptoms. When conservative management fails to adequately resolve symptoms, surgical treatments are available. Surgery can be transanal, transvaginal, or transabdominal depending on the training and preference of the surgeon. Surgical repairs involve levator muscle plication or site-specific repairs of the rectovaginal fascia. These repairs are performed with or without mesh or graft augmentation and a perineorrhaphy. Around 82–90 percent of women have success with their repair with decreased symptoms of defecation and vaginal pressure and improvement in quality of life. Complications of surgery include pain, dyspareunia with sexual dysfunction, constipation, incontinence, and recurrence of the defect [9, 10]. Nonsurgical treatments should be maximized before performing surgical repair, both to increase success and overall well-being and to avoid complications [11].

Key Teaching Points

- Rectoceles are common in parous women and management should be symptom focused. Asymptomatic rectoceles do not require treatment.
- Dietary modifications including increased fiber and water intake and use of osmotic laxatives may improve constipation and defecation symptoms.
- Localized vaginal estrogen applied daily for several weeks and then weekly can improve symptoms of dryness and discomfort from the prolapse.
- Women should be reassured that presence of a rectocele should not limit sexual activity and encouraged to use lubricants as needed. Water-based lubricants may alleviate discomfort.
- Surgical repair should be offered to women with inadequate symptom relief from nonsurgical treatments.

References

1. DeLancey JOL: Structural anatomy of the posterior pelvic floor compartment as it relates to rectocele. *Am J Obstet Gynecol* 1999;180:815–821.

2. American College of Obstetricians and Gynecologists. Pelvic organ prolapse. Practice bulletin No. 176. *Obstet Gynecol* 2017;129: e56–e72.

3. Dietz HP, Clarke B. Prevalence of rectocele in young nulliparous women. *Aust N Z J Obstet Gynaecol* 2005;45:391–394.

4. Swift SE, Tate SB, Nicholas J. Correlation of symptoms with degree of pelvic organ support in a general population of women: what is pelvic organ prolapse? *Am J Obstet Gynecol* 2003;189:372–377.

5. Brown Heidi, Grimes Cara. Current trends in management of defecatory dysfunction, posterior compartment prolapse, and fecal incontinence. *Curr Obstet Gynecol Rep* 2016 June;5 (2):165–171.

6. Bharucha AE, Dorn SD, Lembo A, Pressman A. American gastroenterological association medical position statement on constipation. *Gastroenterology* 2013;144:211–217.

7. Cundiff GW, Fenner D. Evaluation and treatment of women with rectocele: focus on associated defecatory and sexual dysfunction. *Obstet Gynecol* 2004;104:1403–1407.

8. Heit M, Rosenquist C, Culligan P et al. Predicting treatment choice for patients with pelvic organ prolapse. *Obstet Gynecol* 2003;101:1279–1283.

9. Olsen AL, Smith VJ, Bergstrom JO, Colling JC, Clark AL. Epidemiology of surgically managed pelvic organ prolapse and urinary incontinence. *Obstet Gynecol* 1997;89:501–506.

10. Houman J, Weinberger JM, Eilber KS. Native tissue repairs for pelvic organ prolapse. *Curr Urol Rep* 2017;18(1):6.

11. Hicks CW, Weinstein M, Wakamatsu M et al. In patients with rectoceles and obstructed defecation syndrome, surgery should be the option of last resort. *Surgery* 2014 April;155 (4):659–667.

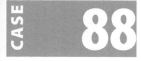

CASE 88

A 25-Year-Old Woman with Recurrent STDs (Human Trafficking)

Fay Chelmow and David Chelmow

History of Present Illness

A 25-year-old female, gravida 4 EAB 4 (elective abortion), presents to clinic complaining of vaginal discharge present for one week. She has had visits every several months over the last two years to multiple providers with diagnoses of gonorrhea, chlamydia, trichomonas, and genital warts. She reports being sexually active, and does not provide specific answers to questions about risk factors or living arrangements. She insists she is in a hurry and requests treatment so she can "get back to work." She answers "no" to all questions on the clinic's standard intimate partner violence screen on the intake form, and again replies "no" when asked by the provider. She smokes one pack per day. She denies substance use. She received depo medroxyprogesterone acetate 150 mg 8 weeks ago at her last visit to the clinic and takes no other medications.

Physical Examination

General appearance Well-appearing thin woman in no apparent distress. No visible bruising or signs of physical trauma.

Vital Signs

Temperature	37.0°C
Pulse	80 beats/min
Blood pressure	90/60 mmHg
BMI	24.2 kg/m^2
Abdomen	She has a tattoo in her left lower quadrant that says "Daddy." Soft, non-tender, non-distended, no guarding, rebound
External genitalia	Unremarkable
Vagina	Foul grey-white discharge
Cervix	Nulliparous, no mucopurulent cervicitis, no cervical motion tenderness
Uterus	Normal size, mobile, non-tender
Adnexa	Normal size, non-tender

Laboratory Studies

Urine pregnancy test	Negative
Wet mount	Motile trichomonads
KOH prep	No clue cells or hyphae.
Gonorrhea and chlamydia nucleic acid amplification tests (NAAT)	Obtained and returned negative the next day.

How Would You Manage This Patient?

The patient has trichomonas, which you treat with metronidazole. You counsel her regarding need for partner treatment and

sexually transmitted infection prevention. You are deeply concerned about the pattern of multiple abortions and recurrent sexually transmitted infections and her reticence to discuss her risks. Concerns include engaging in high-risk sexual behaviors, intimate partner violence, prostitution, and human sex trafficking. While the patient has not responded to any of your questions in a way that confirms the diagnosis, you are aware that traffickers often use tattoos to brand their victims, and decide to probe further. Using principles of trauma informed care, you aim to raise awareness, build trust, and facilitate the patient seeking help when ready.

You observe for behavioral cues and ask questions like those suggested by the University of Kansas Human Trafficking Medical Assessment Tool (Box 88.1). The patient listens to the questions, but makes no clear responses. You conclude by briefly expressing your concerns that she is at significant risk, and you are worried that she may be the victim of intimate partner violence or human trafficking. You give her your standard discharge paperwork, as well as two "shoe-sized," easy-to-hide cards, one with contact information for the local domestic violence shelter, and the other for the National Human Trafficking Resource Center hotline. You leave the exam room before she does. She leaves the discharge paperwork, but takes the shoe cards.

Human Sex Trafficking

Human sex trafficking, also known as commercial sexual exploitation (CSE), is defined by the Trafficking Victims Protection Act of 2000 as compelling a person to perform a commercial sex act through force, fraud, coercion, or where the person induced to perform the act is less than 18 years of age. A person under the age of 18 engaged in any commercial sex act is considered a victim regardless of whether force, fraud, or coercion is present. CSE is an egregious violation of human rights where victims are treated as commodities, and repeatedly bought, sold, and serially raped by an untold number of buyers who are usually unknown to the victim. Traffickers use ongoing humiliation to destroy a victim's self-esteem and anything that gives them reason to leave. The skillful use of force, fraud, and coercion by the trafficker can make a victim feel bonded to their trafficker and "personally responsible" for "choosing" to be prostituted [1].

The majority of CSE victims in this country are US citizens and almost half are under the age of 18 [2]. Children and teens are at increased risk of becoming victims because of their inability to fully comprehend the sophisticated and manipulative practices used by traffickers to target, recruit, and control. CSE occurs when victims are compelled or entrapped into the

Box 88.1 Questions to ask if human trafficking is suspected

- Is anyone forcing you to do something you don't want to do?
- Have you ever been forced to have sex to pay off a debt or for any other reason?
- Is anyone stopping you from coming and going as you wish?
- Does anyone hold your documents of identification for you?
- Has anyone lied to you about the type of work you would be doing?
- Is anyone threatening you or forcing you to stay at your job or at your home?
- Were you ever threatened with deportation or jail if you tried to leave your situation?

Questions derived from:

Center for the Human Rights of Children, Building Child Welfare Response to Child Trafficking. (Chicago: Loyola University Chicago, 2011). Available at www.luc.edu/media/lucedu/chrc/pdfs/BCWRHandbook2011.pdf

Connecticut Department of Children and Families, Practice Guide for Intake and Investigative Response to Human Trafficking of Children. (Hartford, CT: Connecticut Department of Children and Families, 2014). Available at www.ct.gov/dcf/lib/dcf/human trafficking/pdf/human_trafficking_pg_-_copy.pdf

Covenant House, Homelessness, Survival Sex and Human Trafficking: As Experienced by the Youth of Covenant House New York (New York: Covenant House, 2013). Available at https://d28whvbyjonrpc.cloudfront.net/s3fs-public/attachments/Covenant-House-trafficking-study.pdf

Mount Sinai Emergency Medical Department, Human Trafficking Information and Resources for Emergency Healthcare Providers (New York: Mount Sinai Hospital, 2005). Available at www.humantraffickinged.com/index.html

Ohio Human Trafficking Task Force, Human Trafficking Screening Tool (Columbus, OH: Ohio Department of Mental Health and Addiction Services, 2013). Available at http://mha.ohio.gov/Portals/0/assets/Initiatives/HumanTrafficking/2013-human-traffricking-screening-tool.pdf.

Polaris Project, Medical Assessment Tool. (Washington, DC: Polaris Project, National Human Trafficking Resource Center, 2010). Available at www.safvic.org/content/uploads/safvic/documents/Resources%20-%20HT/Medical%20Assessment%20Tool%20-%20HT.pdf

Vera Institute of Justice, Screening for Human Trafficking (New York: Vera Institute of Justice, 2014). Available at www.vera.org/sites/default/files/resources/downloads/human-trafficking-identification-tool-and-user-guidelines.pdf

Via Christi Health, Human Trafficking Assessment for Clinicians. (Wichita, KS: Via Christi Health, 2015). Available at www.viachristi.org/sites/default/files/pdf/about_us/2015–0625%20Human%20trafficking%20assessment_web.pdf

L.M. Williams and M.E. Frederick, Pathways into and out of commercial sexual victimization of children: Understanding and responding to sexually exploited teens (Lowell, MA: University of Massachusetts – Lowell, 2009). Available at http://traffickingresourcecenter.org/sites/default/files/Williams%20Pathways%20Final%20Report%202006-MU-FX-0060%2010–31-09 L.pdf

Wisconsin Statewide Human Trafficking Committee, Wisconsin Human Trafficking Protocol and Resource Manual (Madison, WI: Wisconsin Office of Justice Assistance, Violence Against Women Program, 2012). Available at www.endabusewi.org/sites/default/files/resources/Wisconsin%20Human%20Trafficking%20Protocol%20and%20Resource%20Manual.pdf

U.S. Department of Health and Human Services, The Campaign to Rescue and Restore Victims of Human Trafficking: HHS Human Trafficking Order Form (Washington, DC: U.S. Department of Health and Human Services, 2015). Available at http://archive.acf.hhs.gov/trafficking/about/form.htm

sex industry by traffickers who use physical and psychological violence, including an array of deceptive tactics, to exploit vulnerability. A CSE victim has no life predictability, agency, safety, or control, and cannot leave their trafficker without fear of violent retribution. CSE victims may be engaged in street and internet-based prostitution and pornography, as well as in "legitimate" businesses like escort services, massage parlors, and stripping. CSE victims can be involved in sex tourism, phone sex, and mail order bride industries. Despite being engaged in the sex trade, victims are *not* prostitutes, but are victims and survivors of CSE, entitled to protections under the law. Prostitution and CSE are different and the terms should not be used interchangeably.

Many gynecologists have seen CSE victims in their office and are not aware of this. Clinicians need to have a high index of suspicion because human trafficking is clandestine by nature. Studies estimate that anywhere from 28 to 88 percent of trafficked persons access medical services at some point during their exploitation, but are frequently not recognized [3,4]. Victims have limited access to preventative care and management of chronic conditions because entering a health-care system presents a high risk to the trafficker about exposing their crimes. Given these circumstances, it is likely that trafficking victims typically enter hospitals and clinics only when injuries and ailments are life threatening or debilitating enough to affect the victim's ability to make money. Health-care providers are one of the few groups of professionals who interact with victims while they are still under the control of their abuser, so the clinic visit may be the only chance a victim may have to be assisted in recognizing their exploitation, consider exit strategies, and reclaim their basic human right to freedom, health, and safety. CSE has a tendency to intersect with related crimes and can coexist with domestic violence, dating violence, survival sex, truancy, homelessness, running away, drug addiction, or any type of call to the police.

Health Consequences of CSE

Common physical and reproductive health manifestations are listed in Boxes 88.2 and 88.3. Mental health consequences include Stockholm syndrome, affective disorders, complex post-traumatic stress disorder, dissociative disorders, sleep disorders, psychosomatic syndromes, low self-esteem, substance use disorders, and suicide [5]. Victims can experience adverse health outcomes from torture tactics such as starvation, strangulation, forced drug use, dehydration, isolation, beatings, rape, and gang rape. Reactions to the trauma from human trafficking are wide ranging and can be severe and long lasting. The Substance Abuse and Mental Health Services Administration provides an extensive table (Exhibit 1.3–1) listing these consequences [6].

Box 88.2 Possible physical manifestations of human sex trafficking

- Deliberate injuries including cuts, bite marks, and bruises
- Traumatic injuries:
  - Bone fractures
  - Internal traumatic injuries including stab or gunshot wounds
  - Concussions and other traumatic brain injury
  - Facial and dental injuries
- Chronic pain
- Respiratory and gastrointestinal disorders from chronic stress
- Bladder damage, injury, or infection
- Unexplained scars and burns
- Drug-related health issues (e.g., asthma and Hepatitis C)
- Tattoos

Modified from Macias-Konstantopoulos [5] with permission.

Box 88.3 Reproductive health problems among human-trafficking victims

- Vaginal, perineal, and rectal injuries
- Menstrual pain and irregularities
- Vaginal discharge and infection from using items inserted into the vagina to block menstruation
- Spontaneous abortion
- Sexually transmitted infections
- Poor access to barrier protection and contraception
- Forced sterilization or use of contraceptive devices
- Lack of prenatal care
- Forced pregnancy and childbirth
- Unplanned and high-risk pregnancies
- Unsafe and forced abortions

Modified from Macias-Konstantopoulos [5] with permission.

Approach to the Human Sex Trafficking Victim: Trauma Informed Care

The victim's extensive history of trauma interferes with their ability to communicate and interpret and understand the world around them. They are reticent to disclose their victimization due to lack of perception of victim status, trauma bonding, fear, shame, distrust of authority figures, and language and cultural barriers. Trauma informed care assumes that the victim of CSE has been exposed to chronic and severe physical and psychological violence and that their behavioral responses are consequences of traumatic experiences. This care approach makes trauma the central problem or core event of the assessment, diagnosis, and treatment. Trauma informed care is grounded in an understanding and responsiveness to the impact of trauma and draws upon the victim's existing strengths and resources [6].

Building trust and showing empathy is key, as many victims are unwilling to reveal their victimhood, and some do not understand that they are victims. Clinicians may be the only persons who ever tell the victim that they have worth and the possibility of a better life. To mitigate the possibility of retraumatization, questions should start peripherally and clinicians should ask as an "information gatherer" instead of as an "interrogator." The focus of the conversation should be "What happened to you?" as opposed to "What's wrong with you?" [6]. The provider needs to be careful not to express surprise or disbelief when the victim shares their experiences, which may be far from the provider's personal experience or colored by somatization or psychiatric issues. Trauma informed care helps the clinician avoid "patient-blaming," which can be damaging to the victim's self-worth and recovery process. Box 88.4 lists sample messages that build trust and minimize blame.

Identifying the Human Trafficking Victim

The gynecologist is in a unique position to identify human trafficking since the most common reason a CSE victim will seek health care includes testing for sexually transmitted

> **Box 88.4** Messages for communicating with victims that counter victim blame and build trust
>
> - I believe you.
> - We are here to help you.
> - Our first priority is your safety.
> - Under the Trafficking Victims Protection Act of 2000, victims of trafficking can apply for special visas or could receive other forms of immigration relief.
> - We will give you the medical care that you need.
> - We can find you a safe place to stay.
> - You have a right to live without being abused.
> - You deserve the chance to become self-sufficient and independent.
> - We can help get you what you need.
> - We can help to protect your family.
> - You can trust me.
> - We want to make sure what happened to you doesn't happen to anyone else.
> - You have rights.
> - You are entitled to assistance. We can help you get assistance.
> - If you are a victim of trafficking, you can receive help to rebuild your life safely in this country.
>
> From Department of Health and Human Services Fact Sheet – Resources: Messages for communicating with victims of human trafficking. Available at: www.acf.hhs.gov/sites/default/files/orr/communicating_with_victims_of_human_trafficking_0.pdf. Accessed April 30, 2017.

infections and HIV [3]. If the patient is accompanied, the provider should try to create an opportunity to interview the patient alone. A patient may be a potential victim if they have any of the "red flags" in Box 88.5, or have findings such as those in Boxes 88.2 and 88.3. Laboratory tests may indicate sexually transmitted infections and positive drug screens. Patients with these findings should be screened for CSE.

The Vera Screening Tool for Human Trafficking has been validated, but has 30 questions in its long form, and 16 in its short form. Interviewers found three questions from the tool particularly strong predictors of sex trafficking after controlling for demographics: (1) Did anyone you worked for or lived with trick or force you into doing anything you did not want you to do? (2) Did anyone ever pressure you to touch another person or have unwanted physical or sexual contact with another person? (3) Did you ever have sex in exchange for things of value, for example, money, housing, food, gifts, or favors? [7]. Screening questions like those suggested by the University of Kansas have not been validated, but are more practical to apply in a clinic setting.

This patient had multiple sexually transmitted infections. Her recurrent abortions are also concerning, as is the "daddy" tattoo, which may represent branding from her captor. When patients present with these types of problems, the possibility of the patient being a victim of CSE should be considered. In this instance, the patient was alone, but had the patient been accompanied, the clinician needs to create an opportunity to speak to the patient in private. While the

patient may not understand or be ready for help at this visit, building trust and incrementally providing information about victimization and opportunities for escape may help the patient be ready at a future visit. As victims are likely to be seen only in acute settings and by many different providers, documenting concerns in the chart may help another provider continue the counseling and discussion at future visits. At the same time, it is important to ask questions and provide opportunity for help, as many victims eventually reach the point that they are ready for help, and need opportunity and assistance to proceed.

This patient was evasive and uncomfortable revealing any aspect of her potential victimhood. The approach of asking questions about her life in a nonjudgmental way provides an opportunity for a patient to realize that her situation is not normal and help is available. The clinician should not expect the patient to reveal her victimhood. They should view the patient through the lens of her trauma history, self-blame that prevents her from seeing her exploitation, and her fear of retribution to herself, friends, or family. The visit should be viewed as an opportunity to move the patient closer toward seeking help. Although this patient would not discuss any problems, she appears to be becoming ready to seek assistance as evidenced by her taking the cards for the local shelter and NHTRC hotline. Resources like these should be made available in places the patients can access in private. The clinic bathroom is ideal, as it is likely the only place that the victim can go without the captor. Providing the information on small cards that can be easily hidden, for example in the patient's shoe, allows the patient to safely conceal the information until she is ready to use it. If the potential victim was

Box 88.5 "Red flags" during a medical encounter suggesting human trafficking

- Patient is not allowed to speak or make decisions.
- Patient claims to be just visiting or is unsure of where she is.
- Patient shows signs of physical or sexual abuse, medical neglect, multiple STIs, or torture.
- Patient is under 18 and engaging in commercial sex or trading sex for something of value.
- Multiple inconsistencies in story.
- Patient exhibits fear, anxiety, PTSD, submission, or tension.
- Patient is reluctant to explain her injury.

Sources: NHTRC Framework for a Human Trafficking Protocol in Healthcare Settings [8] and University of Kansas Human Trafficking Medical Assessment Tool. [9]

a minor, the provider has a legal obligation to report their concerns.

What to Do When a Victim Is Identified

Health-care providers should plan ahead for encountering a trafficking victim, and when possible, put protocols in place. Protocols should identify local service providers who can help victims get to safety and get the care they need as quickly as possible. The National Human Trafficking Resource Center is an important resource, and provides a hotline (1–888–373–7888) and framework for identifying and referring victims [8], which can be modified to create a local protocol. The University of Kansas Toolkit [9] was modified from this framework. In many ways, the initial response for human trafficking victims is similar to related crimes such as domestic violence or child abuse. Some providers incorporate human trafficking into existing protocol structures, while others have developed specific policies.

This patient left with the diagnosis uncertain, but took the hotline number. Had she identified herself during the visit in our center, we would have immediately involved our Sexual Assault Nurse Examiners, who have specialized training in trauma informed care, notified local law enforcement, and referred the patient to Safe Harbor, a local nonprofit that specializes in the care of human trafficking victims. In other settings, a call to the NHTRC hotline would give the provider guidance for next steps and local referral options. The hotline is also useful if the provider needs validation or help with their assessment. Had the patient called the hotline herself, the NHTRC would have provided her guidance and referral options.

Key Teaching Points

- Many gynecologists are unaware that they have treated victims of sex trafficking in their office, and clinicians need to have a high index of suspicion for potential victims of sex trafficking.
- Sex trafficking victims and survivors are reticent to disclose their victimization.
- Clinicians should have a plan for screening and referral of human trafficking victims.
- Clinician should respond to potential victims with trauma informed and victim-centered care.
- The National Human Trafficking Resource Center hotline (1-888-373-7888) is an important resource for potential victims and providers.

References

1. Human Trafficking. Committee Opinion No. 507. American College of Obstetricians and Gynecologists. *Obstet Gynecol* 2011;118:767–770.

2. Polaris Project. 2016 Hotline statistics. https://polarisproject.org/resources/2016-hotline-statistics. Accessed 4/23/17.

3. Lederer L, Wetzel C. The health consequences of sex trafficking and their implications for identifying victims in healthcare facilities. *Annals Health L* 2014;23(1):61–91. Web. 13 October 2014. Available at: www.annalsofhealthlaw.com/annalsofhealth law/vol_23_issue_1?pg=69#pg69. Accessed 4/23/17.

4. Family Violence Prevention Fund. Turning Pain into Power: Trafficking Survivors' Perspectives on Early Intervention Strategies. 2005. Available at: www.futureswithoutviolence.org/turning-pain-into-power-trafficking-survivors-perspectives-on-early-intervention-strategies/. Accessed 4/23/17

5. Macias-Konstantopoulos W. Human trafficking: The role of medicine in interrupting the cycle of abuse and violence. *Ann Intern Med* 2016;165:582–588.

6. Substance Abuse and Mental Health Services Administration. Trauma-Informed Care in Behavioral Health Services. Treatment Improvement Protocol (TIP) Series 57. HHS Publication No. (SMA) 13–4801. Rockville, MD: Substance Abuse and Mental Health Services Administration, 2014.

7. Simich L, Goyen L, Powell A, Mallozzi K. Improving human trafficking victim identification – Validation and dissemination of a screening tool. Final Report. Award No.: 2011-MU-MU-0066. National Institute of Justice. NCJ264712.

June 2014. Available at: http://archive.vera
.org/sites/default/files/resources/down
loads/human-trafficking-identification-tool
-technical-report.pdf. Accessed 4/30/17.

8. National Human Trafficking Resource
Center. Framework for a Human

Trafficking Protocol in Healthcare
Settings. Available at: https://humantraf
fickinghotline.org/sites/default/files/Fra
mework%20for%20a%20Human%20Tra
fficking%20Protocol%20in%20Healthcar
e%20Settings.pdf. Accessed 4/30/17.

9. Schwarz C, Unruh E, Cronin K et al.
Human trafficking identification
and service provision in the medical and
social service sectors. *Health Hum
Rights* 2016;18:
181–191.

A 41-Year-Old Woman with Loss of Interest in Having Sex

Tracy E. Irwin

History of Present Illness

A 41-year-old female, gravida 3, para 3, presents to your office with little interest in having sex over the past two years with her partner. This worsened over the past year, and it affects her relationship. She and her partner always use lubrication; however, lately she feels like it isn't enough and she has irritation for a few hours to one day after sex. She currently has sexual intercourse two times per month because of obligation to please her partner. She reports difficulty getting her partner to understand the pressures she feels regarding sex. She orgasms with clitoral stimulation with her partner and during masturbation. She has not masturbated in the past three months because she doesn't have time or interest. Her baseline sexual function was previously normal without difficulties with desire, lubrication, or orgasm. She uses depo-medroxyprogesterone (DMPA) for contraception and has had amenorrhea for three years. Her menses prior to using DMPA were every 21–23 days and lasted 2–4 days. She is hesitant to talk about past sexual experiences and denies any history of sexual trauma or abuse at this visit. She has had anxiety and depression intermittently since college for which she took SSRIs. She recently started a new job, which increased her stress level and led her to restart her antidepressant, paroxetine, three months ago. She is otherwise healthy and takes no other medications. Her children are aged 4, 6, and 10. Her mother underwent menopause at 43.

Physical Examination

General appearance	Well-developed woman in no acute distress
Vital signs	Within normal limits, Height 65 inches, weight 130 lb, BMI 21.6 kg/m^2
Abdomen	Thin, soft, non-tender, non-distended, no rebound, no guarding
External genitalia	Normal BUS, labia minora and majora, mild atrophy in posterior forchette
Vagina	Rugae diminished, mild atrophy
Cervix	Parous, no lesions or cervical motion tenderness
Uterus	Anteverted, mobile, normal size, non-tender
Adnexa	No masses or tenderness bilaterally
Laboratory studies	Not indicated
Imaging	Not indicated

How Would You Manage This Patient?

The causes of this patient's loss of interest in sex are multifactorial. While this patient has low sexual desire, she does not meet criteria for sexual interest/arousal disorder (SIAD) because she does not report reduced initiation of sexual activity, being unreceptive to her partner's attempts, nor does she mention reduced genital sensation, arousal, pleasure, or excitement during sexual encounters. Finally, her depression and SSRI use precludes the SIAD diagnosis. At this visit, her concerns regarding lubrication and her mood that were affecting her sexual function were addressed, as well as clarifying her definition of sexual satisfaction and what she considers normal sexual function.

Her physical causes include vaginal atrophy due to DMPA contraception, which inhibits ovulation. It is also possible that she has overall declining estrogen due to ovarian aging. She was switched to oral contraceptive pills and prescribed vaginal estrogen. For her anxiety and depression, she is currently taking paroxetine, which can have a negative effect on sexual function in up to 20 percent of women. She was changed to bupropion, which in some cases can enhance sexual function. Anxiety and depression put her at higher risk for SIAD; therefore she was encouraged to add cognitive behavioral therapy (CBT) to her treatment plan.

On an emotional level this patient is distracted and may have negative thoughts during sex. She has increased stress due to a job change and three small children. She was provided counseling on communication tips with her partner, limiting distractions by setting aside time for adults, and optimizing her mental health. She saw value in CBT for herself, and declined couples therapy at this time.

At follow-up visits, she felt more comfortable discussing past trauma and we strove to understand her past experiences/relationships and determine if there are cultural factors that play a role in her low desire. We discussed how pressure from her current partner could trigger emotions from a sexual assault she revealed that she experienced during college. She received counseling at the time and while she stated she was past it, she was open to discussing it in future therapy sessions. She had good understanding of her body and the biology behind sex; however, she struggled with the body composition changes in her 40s now that she is less active. We discussed the topics of attraction and attractiveness as well as diet and exercise as ways to bolster her self-confidence. In follow-up, she noted stable mood, small improvement with sexual desire, and improved vaginal lubrication.

Loss of Interest in Sex

Low sexual desire is the most common sexual complaint in women across all age groups, and is reported in up to 40 percent of individuals in cross-sectional studies [1]. Each patient has a unique context of their expectations, norms, and personal history regarding sex and intimacy. Practitioners should aim to see the patient's view of their sexual health through understanding the patient's cultural pressures, gender, sexual identity, and any history of trauma.

Sexual function is often simplified from a diagnostic standpoint as a linear process that goes from desire to arousal to orgasm. However, it is important to understand how emotional intimacy and sexual satisfaction play a role, as highlighted by Basson's model of sexual response (Figure 89.1). In this model, the sexual response is a positive feedback loop in which emotional intimacy is the driver of desire and arousal. Many women may not initially experience desire on initiation of intimacy. Further, emotional and physical satisfaction are sought after, which may or may not involve orgasm. Clinicians should be cognizant that "normal" sexual function varies among women, and also can vary within the same woman throughout different phases of her life.

The diagnosis of SIAD, according to the DSM-5, is made when a woman experiences three of the following for at least six months: (1) reduced or absent desire for sex, (2) reduced or absent sexual thoughts/fantasies, (3) reduced or absent initiation and receptivity of sexual activity, (4) reduced or absent sexual pleasure, (5) reduced desire triggered by sexual stimuli, and/or (6) reduced or absent genital or nongenital sensations [2]. These symptoms must cause significant distress and cannot be caused by severe relationship distress, emotional stress, the effects of a substance or medication, or the effect of another medical condition or other nonsexual mental disorder. The diagnostic criteria should be used cautiously, as women who experience less than three criteria or for a shorter duration may still have significant distress and warrant treatment, as is the case with this patient.

The most common physical factors that may be associated with a loss of interest in sex include comorbid medical conditions (hypertension, diabetes), pain with intercourse due to dryness or vaginismus, and medications (particularly antihypertensives and SSRIs) [3]. Neuroendocrine changes with aging, such as decreased testosterone and estrogen, can change intensity of sexual desire and sensation. Declining estrogen levels in the peri-menopausal period can result in vulvovaginal atrophy; however, this is not necessarily associated with loss of sexual desire. Progesterone-only methods of contraception can also contribute to atrophy. Of note, DMPA preferentially suppresses LH and ovulation. Up to one-third of users have normal estradiol; however, others, especially long-term users, can

experience low estradiol levels that result in vulvovaginal atrophy. Consider treating with estrogen cream preparations, estradiol (0.01 percent) or conjugated estrogen (0.625 mg/gram) 0.5 grams nightly for two weeks, then twice weekly or estradiol vaginal tablet (10 mcg) nightly for two weeks, then twice weekly for maintenance. Both topical estrogens and ospemifene 60 mg daily (a selective estrogen receptor modulator) are FDA-approved for vaginal atrophy and dyspareunia [3]. DMPA should not be overlooked as a factor contributing to low desire in this case.

Depression and anxiety are found in approximately 25 percent of women with low sexual desire [4]. In addition, SSRIs used to treat depression are common medications linked to sexual dysfunction. Decreasing the dosage or switching to another medication may alleviate some of the symptoms [3]. Serotonin pathways play a role in sexual inhibition, specifically the 2A receptors. Drugs that are more selective will activate stimulatory pathways or reduce inhibitory pathways to improve sexual side effects. Buprorion (150 mg–400 mg daily), a norepinephrine-dopamine reuptake inhibitor, has been shown in studies to improve sexual function in women with and without depression [4]. Multiple new medications such as gepirone, vilazadone, meclobamide, and agomelatine have been brought to market to decrease side effects noted with initial SSRIs. Post hoc analyses of phase IV clinical trials of these medications show improved sexual function in women though serotonin 5HT1A partial agonist properties. This patient has anxiety and depression and is taking paroxetine, both of which are likely factors in her symptoms.

CBT attempts to modify negative thoughts and behaviors that can interfere with desire. Discussion and education can reduce performance anxiety and shift focus to pleasure instead of sexual form and expectations. The use of CBT is recommended by the International Society for Sexual Medicine (grade B level of evidence) and is a widely used treatment for women with low sexual desire. This patient could benefit from CBT for both anxiety and depression as well as for low sexual desire. In a meta-analysis of 20 studies, CBT had a significant positive effect on desire and sexual satisfaction, with stronger

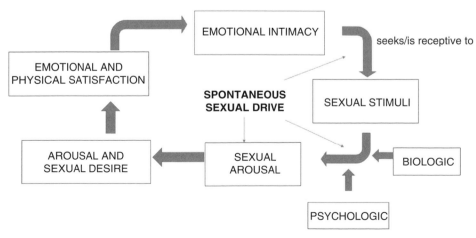

Figure 89.1 Basson's nonlinear model demonstrates how emotional intimacy, relationships, and sexual satisfaction affect female sexual response. Basson R. Human Sex-Response Cycles. *J Sex Mar Therapy* 2001; 27:1: 33–43

results in women diagnosed with hyposexual desire disorder (HSDD) [5]. Studies show CBT for sexual dysfunction also decreases frequency of comorbid mood disorders such as anxiety and depression.

Sex therapy for couples incorporates aspects of CBT, such as improved communication methods, sexual skills, and sensate focus exercises. It is most useful for vaginismus, aversions, and orgasm dysfunction. In the setting of low desire, sex therapy can educate couples, address misconceptions, identify distractions and provide couples tools to address relationship building and promote behavior change [1]. Couples therapy allows partners to boost trust, explore sensuality, and enhance and restore intimacy. Women are more likely to improve sexual desire using these modalities if both partners are highly motivated and there is underlying satisfaction with their relationship.

After addressing modifiable factors and psychosocial influences, patients may request pharmacotherapy. Flibanserin is the only FDA-approved medication for hypoactive sexual desire disorder in women. It is only approved for use in premenopausal women. It is thought to work by increasing the release of the neurotransmitter hormones dopamine and norepinephrine, while decreasing serotonin release in the area of the brain that regulates sexuality. It has only a modest effect on sexual desire, with an increase of 0.5–1 satisfactory sexual events (SSE) per month over placebo [6]. Side effects include hypotension, syncope, somnolence, and fatigue. Women should not drink alcohol or use birth control pills while taking it because they can worsen the side effects. Sildenafil citrate has not been shown to improve sexual function over placebo in women, but may have some utility in women with spinal cord injury (SCI) and multiple sclerosis (MS). In separate small studies of 19 women each, subjective arousal to visual and manual stimuli improved in women with SCI and lubrication improved in women with MS with no adverse events noted in either group.

Younger surgically menopausal women have a higher prevalence of hypoactive sexual desire disorder compared with women who undergo natural menopause. A recent systematic review and meta-analysis of short-term transdermal testosterone showed significant improvement in number of SSEs, number of orgasms, and sexual desire along with a reduction in personal distress in surgical and naturally menopausal women at the 300 mcg twice weekly dose [7]. While small studies on premenopausal women with low testosterone levels using topical testosterone over a short duration (3–4 months) show minimal improvement (0.8 SSE/month), the data are not adequate to recommend it [8]. Side effects included acne and hair growth, but none were rated as severe.

It is important to note there is no current FDA-approved testosterone treatment for low sexual desire and long-term data regarding breast cancer and coronary artery disease outcomes in premenopausal women, and duration of safe long-term use is lacking [1, 3]. If a decision is made to use topical testosterone, close follow-up is necessary and clear improvement in sexual function and satisfaction must occur. Data are limited on use longer than six months and does not support laboratory monitoring of free testosterone.

Key Teaching Points

- History is the primary diagnostic tool in determining contributing factors of low sexual desire, particularly past sexual experiences, cultural context, medical and psychological comorbidities, relationship factors, and personal expectations. These guide individualized management for each patient.
- Side effects of antidepressant medications as well as hypoactive sexual desire associated with depression can be a challenge. Buproprion has the lowest risk of diminishing sexual function as compared to other SSRIs and has been shown to improve sexual function in nondepressed patients.
- Individual therapy, cognitive behavioral therapy, and couples counseling can improve sexual desire.
- Medical therapies for low sexual desire may be useful in carefully selected and well-counseled patients. The utility of flibanserin is limited due to side effects, and can only be used in premenopausal women. Testosterone has been shown to be effective in surgically menopausal and postmenopausal women; however, it does not appear to benefit premenopausal women.

References

1. Kingsberg SA, Woodard T. Female sexual dysfunction: focus on low desire. *Obstet Gynecol* 2015;125:477–486.
2. American Psychiatric Association. *Diagnostic and Statistical Manual of Mental Disorders* (fifth edn.) American Psychiatric Association, 2013; Washington, DC.
3. American College of Obstetricians and Gynecologists. Female sexual dysfunction. *ACOG Practice Bulletin* 2017;119.
4. Taylor MJ, Rudkin L, Bullemor-Day P et al. Strategies for managing sexual dysfunction induced by antidepressant medication. *Cochrane Database Syst Rev* 2013,Issue 5.
5. Frühauf S, Gerger H, Schmidt HM, Munder T, Barth J. Efficacy of psychological interventions for sexual dysfunction: a systematic review and meta-analysis. *Arch Sex Behav* 2013;42 (6):915–933.
6. Jaspers, L, Feys F, Bramer WM et al. Efficacy and safety of flibanserin for the treatment of hypoactive sexual desire disorder in women: A systematic review and meta-analysis. *JAMA Internal Medicine* 2016;176:453–462.
7. Achilli C, Pundir J, Ramanathan P, Sabatini L, Hamoda H. Efficacy and safety of transdermal testosterone in postmenopausal women with hypoactive sexual desire disorder: a systematic review and meta-analysis. *Fertil Steril* 2017;107 (2):475–482.
8. Davis S, Papalia MA, Norman RJ et al. Safety and efficacy of a testosterone metered-dose transdermal spray for treating decreased sexual satisfaction in premenopausal women: a randomized trial. *Ann Intern Med* 2008;148 (8):569–577.

CASE 90 A 28-Year-Old Transgender Woman Requesting Well-Woman Visit

Ghazaleh Moayedi

History of Present Illness

A 28-year-old transgender woman presents requesting a well-woman examination. She takes unsupervised hormone therapy using multiple daily doses of oral contraceptives, and has done so off and on for the past several years. She describes significant nausea with this method and would like to discuss long-term management options. She engages in receptive vaginal sex and denies dyspareunia. In addition, she denies any symptoms of depression or gender dysphoria.

Her past medical history is significant only for adolescent gender dysphoria. She underwent psychosocial assessment and therapy by a qualified mental health professional with subsequent social, hormonal, and surgical gender transition. Her surgeries include vaginoplasty with concomitant orchiectomy one year ago and breast augmentation mammoplasty five years ago. Her family medical history is negative. The patient is currently employed, has a strong social support network, and is in a monogamous, heterosexual relationship with a cisgender man. She has no known drug allergies. Her only medication is drospirenone-ethinyl estradiol 3 mg–20 mcg TID.

Physical Examination

General appearance	Well-developed, well-nourished NAD

Vital Signs

Temperature	37.1°C
Pulse	76 bpm
Blood pressure	116/72 mmHg
BMI	23.1 kg/m^2
HEENT	Unremarkable
Cardiovascular	RRR
Pulmonary	CTAB
Breast	Symmetric without masses or tenderness, implants palpable, nipples without discharge, no axillary node enlargement
Abdomen	Non-distended, non-tender, no right upper quadrant tenderness
Genitalia	Asymmetric labia majora with minimal clitoral hooding; well-healed vaginal tissue; distal vaginal stenosis

Laboratory Studies

Serum estradiol	157 pg/mL
Serum testosterone	48 ng/dL
K+	4.1 mEq/L
Serum HBsAg, HCV, HIV, RPR	Negative
Urine GC/CT	Negative

How Would You Manage This Patient?

This is a healthy transgender woman requesting a well-woman exam. Given her history, she was offered immediate hormone supervision and advised to discontinue her drospirenone-ethinyl estradiol. Using the shared decision-making model, the patient was counseled on the various routes of estradiol and antiandrogen therapy. She chose oral therapy with estradiol 2 mg BID and spironolactone 50 mg BID. She was instructed to return for follow-up and repeat laboratory evaluation in one month.

With regard to her routine health maintenance, she was advised to continue a well-balanced diet and participate in at least 30 minutes of moderate-intensity exercise at least five days per week. She was advised to begin lipid and diabetes screening according to the United States Preventative Services Task Force (USPSTF) guidelines. She was counseled about the risks and benefits of cancer screening and was educated about breast self-awareness. She was advised that cervical cancer screening is not indicated and, although there are no clear guidelines for breast cancer screening in transgender women, mammography may be considered starting at the age of 50 years.

Well-Woman Visit for Transgender Women

Although assigned male at birth, the ongoing health care of transgender women and gender nonconforming people falls directly in the scope of the women's health-care provider [1]. Understanding the terminology of the transgender community and using the correct pronouns for individual patients conveys respect and lays the foundation for gender-affirming care. This terminology can vary by people, communities, regions, and cultures. Therefore, it is preferable to be familiar with general terms and ask patient preferences regarding pronouns rather than to make assumptions or memorize a list of definitions.

In general, every person has a sex assigned at birth, a gender identity, a gender expression, and a sexual orientation [2]. Sex assigned at birth is typically female, male, or intersex. Gender identity is a person's internal sense of gender whereas gender expression is how a person outwardly conveys their gender. This internal gender identity and external gender expression can be female, male, both, neither, or something else. Sexual orientation describes a person's sexual attraction and is independent of gender identity or expression. Gender identity and sexual orientation cannot be assumed or obtained from an exam; a patient must offer this information. Gender expression varies by cultural norms and a feminine gender expression in one culture could be considered masculine in another.

Gender nonconforming refers to people whose gender expression varies from a gender binary construct. Finally, gender dysphoria describes the psychological distress sometimes felt when sex assigned at birth conflicts with gender identity. Not all transgender and gender nonconforming people experience gender dysphoria. Social, hormonal, and surgical therapy are treatment options for gender dysphoria. Not all people require all therapies, and treatment is individualized [3].

The well-woman exam for transgender women should be carried out similarly to that of cisgender women with a few special considerations [1]. With regard to the pelvic examination, it is important to respectfully discuss prior surgeries with patients before making assumptions about genitalia. While there is no evidence to guide the need for routine pelvic examination in asymptomatic transgender women who have undergone feminizing surgery, it may be reasonable to perform a visual inspection on an annual basis to evaluate for lesions or granulation tissue and/or to assess vaginal caliber [4]. The most common surgery for vaginoplasty is penile inversion with orchiectomy. This technique creates a more posterior vagina than cisgender women, with the prostate anterior to the vagina. When inspecting the neovagina, traditional vaginal speculum may be uncomfortable; therefore, utilizing a pediatric speculum or an anoscope, similar to proctoscopy, may be preferable.

Unlike cisgender women, transgender women should be educated about periodic douching for hygiene, as sebaceous secretions, lubricant, and retained ejaculate can cause unpleasant discharge. Complications from penile inversion surgery that providers should evaluate include vaginal stenosis, webbing, asymmetric labia, widely spaced labia, inadequate clitoral hooding, and poorly defined labia minora. Use of progressive vaginal dilators are necessary for at least a year after penile inversion surgery. Early signs of vaginal stenosis can often be treated with increased frequency of dilation with a water-based, glycerine-free lubricant to prevent infection. Patients who are concerned about poor aesthetic results, stenosis, or webbing should be referred to a specialist in male-to-female genital surgery for consultation [4].

Women's health-care providers should feel comfortable initiating hormone therapy for transgender women because feminizing hormones are familiar medications. Typically, hormone therapy can be initiated using an informed consent model or with a referral from a qualified mental health professional. A referral from a mental health provider should not be a barrier to initiating hormone therapy, especially in people who are being bridged from unsupervised hormone use or who have previously been prescribed cross gender hormone therapy [3].

Hormone therapy for transgender women consists of an estrogen plus an antiandrogen. Medication and dosing recommendations are made by the Center of Excellence for Transgender Health, the World Professional Association for Transgender Health, the Endocrine Society, and Fenway Health. Ethinyl estradiol has historically been used for cross-gender therapy, but its use has been discouraged due to high rates of venous thromboembolism. The use of conjugated equine estrogen is also discouraged due to difficulty monitoring levels, possible increased risk of thromboembolism, and ethical concerns with procurement. Therefore, estradiol via oral, transdermal, or parenteral routes are the preferred methods of estrogen delivery. Studies have not compared which method is superior; therefore, the decision should be based on patient preferences using a shared decision-making model. Antiandrogens are used to reduce testosterone levels, even in the setting of orchiectomy. The most commonly used anti-androgen in the United States is spironolactone, but finasteride, dutasteride, and leuprolide may also be utilized [3, 5–7].

Transgender women on hormone therapy should undergo laboratory evaluation for routine age and risk-based screening as well as hormone monitoring. Testing for diabetes and hyperlipidemia should be in concordance with USPSTF guidelines for cisgender women, although some guidelines recommend annual lipid and glucose screening for those on hormone therapy. Several societies have published guidelines for laboratory monitoring of feminizing hormone therapy. In general, serum estradiol, total serum testosterone, and serum electrolytes should be checked one month after initiation, every 3–6 months for the first year, and 1–2 times per year thereafter [4–6]. Although prolactinomas have been described in transgender women on feminizing hormone therapy, they do not appear to be more common than in cisgender woman; therefore, routine serum prolactin screening is unnecessary. Prolactin levels should be checked, however, in transgender women with visual disturbances or significant galactorrhea and may be considered in those who report new onset headaches [4].

Recommendations on serum testing for sexually transmitted infections in transgender women do not differ from cisgender women. Gonorrhea and chlamydia are unlikely to be sampled from the neovagina; therefore, testing for these should be urine-based. Patients at risk should be educated on HIV pre-exposure prophylaxis per CDC guidelines [4].

Cancer and other health maintenance screening in transgender women should be age-based and address all present sexual organs. Since transgender women do not have a cervix, cervical cancer screening with cytology and/or HPV testing is not indicated. Breast cancer rates in transgender women are unknown and thought to be very low. The optimal age to initiate breast cancer screening in transgender women is unknown, and recommendations are conflicting. Using guidance from the American College of Obstetricians and Gynecologists for cisgender women, it may be reasonable to offer clinical breast examination every 1–3 years for transgender women ages 25–39 years and yearly thereafter [8], but the utility of this is unknown in this population, and a shared decision-making model should be utilized. The Center of Excellence for Transgender Health recommends biennial screening mammography, beginning at age 50 years and after at least 5–10 years of feminizing hormone therapy (or earlier in patients with risk factors) [4]. Colon cancer screening guidelines remain the same for transgender women as they do for the general population and are based on age and risk factors. Transgender women should undergo bone mineral density screening similar to cisgender women, beginning at age 65 years or sooner if they have established risk factors for osteoporosis [4, 9].

Consensus on prostate cancer screening in men or transgender women has not been reached. Few cases of prostate cancer have been described in transgender women, and risk is thought to be low. The most recent USPSTF guidelines recommend against the use of prostate-specific antigen for the screening of prostate cancer [10]. Guidelines for the screening of prostate cancer in transgender women should mirror those of cisgender men. Because women's health-care providers are generally not familiar with physical evaluation of the prostate, patients with prostatic complaints should be referred to a primary care physician or urologist. The referral should include information on the position of the prostate in relation to the neovagina (anterior) and recommendation of digital vaginal exam over digital rectal exam [4].

Key Teaching Points

- Women's health-care providers play a key role in the lifelong medical care of transgender and gender nonconforming people.
- Women's health-care providers are familiar with the administration and management of feminizing hormones and should manage hormone therapy for transgender women, which typically consists of estradiol with an antiandrogen, like spironolactone, as part of routine practice.
- Routine health care and screening tests for transgender women mirror those for cisgender women, with few exceptions.
- Chlamydia and gonorrhea testing in transgender women who have undergone vaginoplasty should be urine-based.
- Cervical cancer screening is not indicated in transgender female patients, and breast cancer screening with mammography should begin no earlier than age 50 years and after 5–10 years of feminizing hormone therapy in average-risk patients, utilizing a shared decision-making model.
- The neovagina is located between the prostate and rectum in the sagittal plane. When necessary, prostatic exams should be performed through the anterior vagina rather than the anterior rectum.

References

1. Committee on Health Care for Underserved Women. Committee Opinion no. 512: health care for transgender individuals. *Obstet Gynecol* 2011 December;118 (6):1454–1458.

2. Transgender Terminology [Internet]. National Center for Transgender Equality. 2015 [cited April 29, 2017]. Available from: www.transequality.org/issues/resources/transgender-terminology

3. Coleman E, Bockting W, Botzer M et al. Standards of care for the health of transsexual, transgender, and gender-nonconforming people, version 7. *International Journal of Transgenderism* 2012;13(4): 165–232.

4. Deutsch MB. Guidelines for the Primary and Gender-Affirming Care of Transgender and Gender Nonbinary People [Internet]. Center of Excellence for Transgender Health. 2016 [cited April 24, 2017]. Available from: www.transhealth.ucsf.edu/pdf/Transgender-PGACG-6-17-16.pdf

5. Hembree WC, Cohen-Kettenis P, de Waal HAD et al. Endocrine treatment of transsexual persons: an endocrine society clinical practice guideline. *J Clin Endocrinol Metab* 2009;94 (9):3132–3154.

6. Cavanaugh, T, Hopwood, R, Gonzalez, A, Thompson, J. The medical care of transgender persons [Internet]. Fenway Health; 2015 October. Available from: www.lgbthealtheducation.org/wp-content/uploads/COM-2245-The-Medical-Care-of-Transgender-Persons-v31816.pdf

7. Unger CA. Hormone therapy for transgender patients. *Transl Androl Urol* 2016 December;5(6):877–884.

8. American College of Obstetricians-Gynecologists. Breast cancer risk assessment and screening in average-risk women. Practice bulletin No. 179. *Obstet Gynecol.* 2017;130: e1–e16.

9. American College of Obstetricians and Gynecologists. Osteoporosis. Practice bulletin No. 129. *Obstet Gynecol* 2012 September;120(3):718–734.

10. Moyer VA, U.S. Preventive Services Task Force. Screening for prostate cancer: U.S. Preventive Services Task Force recommendation statement. *Ann Intern Med* 2012 July 17;157(2):120–134.

A 35-Year-Old Female-to-Male Transgender Patient with Vaginal Spotting on Testosterone

Beth Cronin

A 35-year-old transgender male patient presents to the office with a seven-month history of vaginal spotting. He reports a small amount of bleeding that stains his underwear every few weeks, and the bleeding is never heavy enough to soak through his clothes or require a pad. He denies any concurrent pain or discharge. He is sexually active with a cis-female partner (a woman) and reports some occasional spotting after penetrative intercourse with toys. He does not have pain or other problems with sex and has never had sex with a cis-male partner. His only medical problem is hypothyroidism. He had a mastectomy and chest reconstruction two years ago. He started testosterone five years ago, and has been amenorrheic on stable dosing for four years. He is not interested in further gender-affirming surgery at this time. His current medications include testosterone 50 mg subcutaneous injection weekly and levothyroxine 75 mcg daily. He has never been pregnant and does not desire pregnancy in the future. He has no history of sexually transmitted infections (STIs) or abnormal Pap smears, but he is unsure when his last Pap was done. He reports that he finds pelvic exams physically uncomfortable and emotionally challenging.

Physical Examination

General appearance	Well appearing, no acute distress; alert and oriented × 3
Vital Signs	
Temperature	37.3°C
Pulse	68 beats/min
Blood pressure	120/65 mmHg
Respiratory rate	16 breaths/min
Height	72 inches
Weight	175 lb
BMI	23.7
Cardiovascular	RRR, no murmurs
Lungs	Clear to auscultation bilaterally
Abdomen	Soft, non-tender, no palpable masses; no rebound or guarding. +bowel sounds
Genital exam	External genitalia with evidence of clitoromegaly, bilateral labia without lesions, nulliparous cervix without lesions, no discharge. Moderate vaginal atrophy. No active bleeding. Small mobile uterus without cervical motion tenderness. No adnexal fullness or tenderness
Extremities	Warm, non-tender

How Would You Manage This Patient?

This patient has vaginal spotting despite being on a stable dose of systemic testosterone therapy for the past four years. Given his history of hypothyroidism, a TSH and free T4 were ordered,

and during his examination, gonorrhea and chlamydia testing, as well as cervical cytology with HPV testing, were performed to evaluate for potential cervical causes of his spotting. In addition, transabdominal pelvic ultrasonography was scheduled to assess his endometrium. Given this patient's evidence of vaginal atrophy on examination, he was started on a short course of vaginal estrogen therapy and was advised to use lubricants during penetrative intercourse. He was scheduled to follow up in two weeks to discuss test results and reevaluate his symptoms.

His thyroid testing returned as normal, and his gonorrhea, chlamydia, cervical cytology, and HPV testing were all negative. The pelvic ultrasound revealed a normal uterus with no myometrial abnormalities, a 3 mm endometrial stripe, and small, normal ovaries bilaterally. At his follow-up visit, his spotting had resolved, and he was advised to continue twice weekly vaginal estrogen for an additional month and taper the dose as tolerated.

Transgender Male with Vaginal Bleeding on Testosterone Therapy

Presenting to the gynecology office, a place that is traditionally female-centric and focused on women's health, can be challenging for transgender men. Transgender individuals experience a significant amount of discrimination, with 63 percent of respondents to the 2015 Transgender Survey reporting having experienced a serious act of discrimination in their lifetime, and 33 percent reporting having had a negative experience with a health-care provider within the past year [1]. Signage that makes it clear that the office does not tolerate discrimination and intake forms that ask about sexual orientation and gender identity are important first steps in making the office welcoming and inclusive. It is also important to use gender-affirming terminology and query patients as to preferred name, pronouns, and terms to label body parts, as some will prefer a different term for the vagina, such as "front hole."

Persistent vaginal bleeding is a common yet troublesome symptom in the transgender male. After initiating testosterone therapy, menses will typically cease within six months secondary to ovarian suppression and endometrial atrophy; however, this is not always the case [2]. Ongoing bleeding despite being on testosterone therapy should be evaluated once a patient has been on a stable dose for 6–12 months. The differential diagnosis of bleeding on testosterone therapy is broad and includes persistent menses; pregnancy; cervical ectropion or infection; cervical polyps or malignancy; endometrial pathology including adenomyosis, polyps, leiomyomas, or prolapsing myomas; and vaginal atrophy. While testosterone greatly reduces the chances of becoming pregnant, it does not completely eliminate the possibility of ovulation; therefore, pregnancy must be ruled out in transgender males who are sexually active with sperm-producing partners. Although it is theoretically possible that unopposed estrogen secondary to aromatization of exogenous testosterone to estrogen may lead to an increased risk of endometrial cancer, this has been disproven. Transgender men do not need increased surveillance for endometrial cancer and should be evaluated solely based on symptoms and risk factors [3].

Taking a thorough history is the first step in evaluating vaginal bleeding in a transgender male. It is important to understand the frequency and volume of bleeding, along with thorough history of bleeding prior to initiating testosterone therapy. It is also important to ask about compliance with prescribed testosterone dosing, as breakthrough bleeding can occur if doses are being missed. In addition, patients should be queried about current sexual practices, history of STIs, and results of prior cervical cancer screening, if performed. Transgender men are much less likely than cis-women to obtain appropriate cervical cancer screening despite having the same recommended screening guidelines as cis-women.

After fully assessing potential risk factors and performing a urine pregnancy test when indicated, a pelvic examination is usually necessary. This may be postponed until a follow-up visit, after rapport is better established, in patients who are reluctant at the initial visit. Screening for gonorrhea and chlamydia can be performed using nucleic acid amplification tests (NAATs) with urine or self-collected vaginal swabs to avoid speculum exam in these patients. Offering benzodiazepines prior to the exam can help ease anxiety for some patients, and using a pediatric speculum with lubrication may aid in patient comfort during the examination.

On examination, it is important to include investigation for all potential causes of bleeding. Given the possibility of vaginal atrophy due to prolonged testosterone use, careful attention should be paid to evidence of atrophy as a source of bleeding. Typical findings of atrophy are pale epithelium with loss of rugae; there may also be erythema or petechiae present in severe cases. The cervix should be visualized, and specimens for gonorrhea and chlamydia testing as well as cervical cytology and HPV, if indicated, should be obtained. Pap smears in transgender men are ten times more likely to be unsatisfactory, which is generally secondary to testosterone usage. It is important to note testosterone use on the lab slip to alert the pathologist to possible changes in cell morphology [4].

In patients who have not achieved amenorrhea within 6–12 months of initiating testosterone therapy, testosterone levels should be checked to ensure the dosing is adequate to induce menstrual suppression. The target serum testosterone level is generally considered to be between 350 and 1,100 ng/dL. If testosterone levels are adequate and/or amenorrhea had previously been achieved, as in this patient, the PALM-COEIN classification should be used when considering causes of uterine bleeding and ordering further testing [5, 6]. Ruling out endometrial polyps, fibroids, hyperplasia, and malignancy is often simply completed with endometrial biopsy and/or a pelvic ultrasound. While endometrial biopsy and transvaginal ultrasound are often a routine part of the evaluation of abnormal uterine bleeding for cis-women, these procedures may be very challenging for some transgender men. Transabdominal ultrasound may be considered as a first-line step in the endometrial evaluation, especially in those at low risk for underlying pathology.

Once the cause of the vaginal bleeding has been established, appropriate treatment should be initiated. Infectious or structural causes should be managed as they would in cis-gender women. Patients with significant vaginal atrophy as the cause of the bleeding, like the patient described above, can be treated with a short course of vaginal estrogen therapy. This should be administered in whichever formulation the patient is most comfortable using. Although there are no universally accepted recommendations, starting with vaginal conjugated estrogens or estradiol cream, 0.5–1 g daily for 1–2 weeks, and tapering to 1–2 times per week for a total of 4–6 weeks is reasonable. In addition, lubricants should be recommended during penetrative intercourse and continued after completion of the estrogen therapy. Intermittent or maintenance vaginal estrogen therapy may be considered for recurrent symptoms despite the use of lubricants. One should reassure patients that vaginal estrogen is unlikely to reduce the masculinizing effects of testosterone therapy.

For patients with persistent menses as the source of vaginal bleeding, increasing the dose of testosterone may help induce amenorrhea [7]. The most common formulation used is testosterone cypionate, with subcutaneous or intramuscular dosing starting at 50 mg/week. This can be titrated to maximum dose of 100 mg/week. If the bleeding does not resolve on the maximum dose, it may be necessary to add a progestin to the regimen. This can be done using depot medroxyprogesterone acetate 150 mg/mL IM, daily norethindrone acetate 2.5–5 mg po, the etonogestrel 68 mg implant, or a 52 mg levonorgestrel-releasing intrauterine device, depending on patient preferences [3]. For individuals who do not desire pregnancy and are sexually active with cis-men or transgender women, options that are also effective contraceptives should be strongly considered. Aromatase inhibitors may also be used short term to help induce amenorrhea. There are no recommendations on specific dosing in these patients, but lower than typical doses may be effective given the decreased circulating estrogen levels in transgender men [3].

For transgender men with persistent uterine bleeding despite medical interventions, it is reasonable to discuss endometrial ablation or hysterectomy earlier than may be typical for a non-transgender patient, particularly in those who do not desire future childbearing. Many transgender men are interested in hysterectomy as part of their gender affirmation process, while others prefer to avoid surgery, if possible; therefore, management should be individualized utilizing a shared decision-making process.

Key Teaching Points

- Presenting to the gynecology office as a transgender male can be challenging. Making the office as welcoming as possible can help ease anxiety.
- Vaginal bleeding while on testosterone is not uncommon for transgender men but needs to be evaluated.
- The standard evaluation and workup of vaginal bleeding in transgender men is similar to that for cis-gender women,

and should include evaluation for vaginal atrophy, STI testing, cervical cancer screening, and evaluation for endometrial causes.

- Treatment of vaginal atrophy with topical estrogen can resolve symptoms and should not negate the masculinizing effects of testosterone therapy.

- Persistent menses while on testosterone therapy may be treated by increasing the testosterone dose, adding a progestin or aromatase inhibitor, or with surgical management via ablation or hysterectomy, depending on patient preference.

References

1. James SE, Herman JL, Rankin S et al. (2016). *The Report of the 2015 U.S. Transgender Survey*. Washington, DC: National Center for Transgender Equality.

2. Perrone AM, Cerpolini S, Maria Salfi NC et al. Effect of long-term testosterone administration on the endometrium of female-to-male (FtM) transsexuals. *J Sex Med* 2009 November;6(11):3193–3200.

3. Center of Excellence for Transgender Health, Department of Family and Community Medicine, University of California San Francisco. Guidelines for the Primary and Gender-Affirming Care of Transgender and Gender Nonbinary People; 2nd edition. Deutsch MB, ed. June 2016. Available at www.transhealth.ucsf.edu/ guidelines

4. Peitzmeier SM, Reisner SL, Harigopal P, Potter J. Female-to-male patients have high prevalence of unsatisfactory Paps compared to non-transgender females: implications for cervical cancer screening. *J Gen Intern Med* 2014 May;29(5):778–784.

5. Munro MG, Critchley HOD, Broder MS, Fraser IS, FIGO Working Group on Menstrual Disorders. FIGO classification system (PALM-COEIN) for causes of abnormal uterine bleeding in nongravid women of reproductive age. *Int J Gynaecol Obstet* 2011 April;113(1):3–13.

6. American College of Obstetricians and Gynecologists. Diagnosis of abnormal uterine bleeding in reproductive-aged women. Practice bulletin No. 128. *Obstet Gynecol* 2012;120:197–206.

7. Nakamura A, Watanabe M, Sugimoto M et al. Dose-response analysis of testosterone replacement therapy in patients with female to male gender identity disorder. *Endocr J* 2013;60(3): 275–281.

A 23-Year-Old Woman Who Reports Inability to Consummate Her Marriage Due to Vaginal Pain (Vaginismus Due to Sexual Abuse)

Cristina Wallace Huff

History of Present Illness

A 23-year-old, gravida 0, para 0, woman presents complaining of inability to consummate her marriage due to vaginal pain. She and her male partner have never been able to engage in coitus, and her partner has been unable to achieve penetration due to the vaginal pain she experiences. She feels anxious and tense about even the thought of having coitus. She denies vaginal discharge or pain outside of intercourse, and she reports regular, non-painful menses. She is also unable to insert tampons due to this vaginal pain and instead wears pads with her menses. She denies dysuria and reports having regular bowel movements without pain or straining.

She has no medical problems or previous surgeries. She denies a history of sexually transmitted diseases. She is not on any medications and has no food or drug allergies. She reports a history of being sexually abused by her uncle at the age of ten. She has not engaged in coitus with any other partners.

Physical Examination

General appearance	Awake, alert, and oriented and in no apparent distress
Vital Signs	
Temperature	37.0 °C
Pulse	80 beats/min
Respiratory rate	20 breaths/min
Oxygen saturation	99% on room air
Height	62 inches
Weight	110 lb
BMI	20.1 kg/m^2
Abdomen	Soft, non-tender, non-distended, no guarding, no rebound
External genitalia	Unremarkable
Vagina	Pain noted with pressure along the posterior fourchette. Unable to insert the speculum fully due to pain. On single-digit bimanual examination, pain appreciated by patient along the leviator ani muscles with hypertonus, no pain along the urethra noted.
Uterus and Adnexa	Limited ability to assess uterine size and adnexa due to patient discomfort at introitus

Laboratory Studies

Urine culture	No growth
KOH	Negative
Wet mount	Negative
Gc/chl	Negative

Imaging	Transabdominal pelvic ultrasound shows 7 cm uterus with no fibroids and normal-appearing bilateral ovaries

How Would You Manage This Patient?

This patient has an inability to participate in penetrative vaginal intercourse due to vaginismus. Vaginismus is frequently linked to hypoactive sexual desire disorder and sexual aversion. After a thorough history, physical examination, and imaging, other comorbidities were excluded. Given her history of sexual abuse, she was referred to a psychologist for cognitive therapy. A physical therapist was consulted to teach the patient pelvic floor exercises and deep muscle relaxation techniques and she was prescribed a lubricant with lidocaine. The patient started using vaginal dilators remote from sexual activity, with a lubricant, and was instructed to gradually increase the size of the dilators over time. After six months of therapy, the patient and her male partner were able to have comfortable intercourse.

Vaginal Pain due to Vaginismus

Women can experience sexual pain before, during, and after sexual intercourse. Estimates of general female sexual dysfunction have been reported in up to 40 to 50 percent of women [1]. The exact incidence of sexual pain is difficult to calculate, and the reported prevalence varies. Pain specifically during sex is a relatively common sexual problem that is reported to affect 8–22 percent of the population [2]. Inability to have sexual intercourse due to pain is uncommon, with a prevalence of between 1 and 6 percent. Sexual pain disorders, which include vulvodynia and vaginismus, are diagnosed when sexual pain causes "marked distress or interpersonal difficulty."

The term "vaginismus" specifically refers to an involuntary recurrent or persistent contracture of the vaginal musculature that may interfere with sexual intercourse. Dyspareunia is recurrent or persistent pain associated with sexual intercourse. Vulvodynia is another type of vulvar pain frequently discussed and is defined as an idiopathic vulvar pain. The *Diagnostic and Statistical Manual of Mental Disorders 5* now groups vaginismus, dyspareunia, and vulvodynia into a general disorder referred to as genito-pelvic pain/penetration disorder [3]. The diagnosis requires persistent symptoms for at least six months. Some women experience marked fear or anxiety in anticipation of pain resulting from vaginal penetration.

The exact etiology of vaginismus varies and may encompass both emotional symptoms and pain disorders. The DSM 5 emphasizes that any form of vaginal penetration can cause pain in these women, including insertion of tampons, fingers, vaginal dilators, speculum exams, and intercourse. Vaginismus can be subdivided into categories: primary, secondary, situational, spasmodic, partial, and complete vaginismus. Please see Table 92.1 for definitions.

Approaching patients with vaginismus can be challenging. These women often experience feelings of frustration, guilt, anger, and helplessness. They often have seen multiple providers and tried various interventions. For these patients to be properly treated, the physician must be comfortable talking with them about sexual dysfunction in a caring and compassionate way. Recording a thorough history of the patient is key. The physician must gain the patient's trust by asking for permission to obtain a sexual history and provide an environment where the patient feels comfortable discussing sexual problems. Patients who have been sexually assaulted can present with diffuse chronic abdominal or pelvic pain [5]. Often children who are sexually assaulted have disturbances of desire, arousal, and orgasm that impact them well into adulthood. All women, regardless of presenting complaint, need to be screened for sexual abuse annually. It is essential to acquire a history of medical conditions, surgeries, allergies, and previous treatments. It is also important to obtain information on the exact site, timing, and duration of the vaginal pain and elicit whether there were any inciting events such as physical/emotional abuse or trauma, or traumatic delivery. In the majority of cases, no inciting event is elicited.

A thorough physical exam should be performed with attention targeted to areas uncovered in history. Often patients with vaginal pain are quite anxious about examination. Discussion about the plan for the exam and verbal consent from the patient should be obtained. The exam can be broken down into components and does not need to be completed in one visit. The patient should be allowed to voice ways that will make the exam less traumatic or painful for her and be made aware she has the right to stop the exam at any time. The most important aspect of the exam is to delineate the exact location(s) of pain. During the gynecologic exam, light touch with a cotton swab can be used to identify areas of vulvar pain, beginning on the thighs and moving inward to the labia majora, labia minora, and interlabial sulci [6]. When pain is present, the patient can quantify the pain as mild, moderate, or severe. Quantification helps assess pain over time after treatment is initiated. The bimanual exam assesses the exact location of vaginal pain. Assessment includes whether the pain is located near the levator ani muscle, along the cervix, or around the urethra. Vaginal infection should be ruled out and uterine size and contour assessed. Pelvic imaging should be considered if there is concern for possible anatomic etiology.

The differential diagnosis for vaginismus includes endometriosis, pelvic congestion syndrome, interstitial cystitis, uterine leiomyomas, adenomyosis, pelvic inflammatory disease, pelvic adhesive disease, ovarian remnant syndrome, irritable bowel syndrome, vulvovaginitis, vulodynia, chronic vulvar dermatoses, condylomas, dermatologic diseases, and provoked vestibulodynia. Distinguishing vaginismus from a potential underlying disorder is important, as the treatment of vaginismus is different from treating a patient with an underlying associated disorder such as uterine leiomyomas or endometriosis. The exam and history can also help delineate potential underlying causes. Once other etiologies are ruled out, the diagnosis of vaginismus can be made. If another etiology is discovered, it should be treated first, prior to initiating treatment for vaginismus.

Treating vaginismus is complex. Removing a situational stimuli or psychosocial etiology often results in resolution of symptoms. According to a Cochrane review, there have been no studies comparing treatment versus nontreatment of vaginismus [7]. The effectiveness of various treatment options remains unclear. A combination of cognitive and behavioral psychotherapy is the best initial treatment. Patients should be referred to a psychiatrist or a behavioral health counselor who can focus on the underlying etiology of the vaginismus, and patients often require marriage counseling and sex therapy. Educating the patient and her partner about the physiology of the problem can also help the symptoms [8]. This approach may help dissociate the patient's emotional anxiety from the physical symptom. A key focus of treatment is learning to associate intercourse with pleasure rather than pain.

Desensitization techniques may help women manage their vaginal muscle tone. Physicians should refer patients to a physical therapist who specializes in the pelvic floor. In physical therapy, techniques like deep muscle relaxation, Kegel exercises, and reverse Kegel exercises, also known as pelvic floor drop exercises, are taught. Kegel exercises are performed by repeatedly contracting the levator ani muscles for one second and then relaxing the muscles for ten seconds. If initial treatment with pelvic floor exercises does not work, women should be given graded vaginal dilators [8] and instructed to voluntarily insert the dilators into their vagina. Topical anesthetics such as lidocaine gel are prescribed with the dilators and often make the dilator insertion more

Table 92.1 Types of vaginismus

Types of vaginismus	Definition
Primary (lifelong)	The inability to ever experience vaginal penetration
Secondary (acquired)	A woman, who previously was able to experience vaginal penetration, now is no longer able to due to muscular spasms
Situational	The inability to tolerate certain forms of vaginal penetration yet is able to tolerate some forms, like tampons or fingers
Spasmodic	A spasm of the vagina
Complete	The inability to tolerate any vaginal penetration
Partial	The ability to tolerate some degree of vaginal penetration

Data from Pacik [4]

tolerable. When a patient is ready, the lidocaine gel also helps decrease pain with vaginal penetration. The goal of dilator therapy is to help patients painlessly accommodate the dilators placed into the vagina, not to "dilate" the vagina. This process is slow and is performed nightly over weeks, slowly increasing the caliber of the dilator.

Pharmacotherapy has also been used in addition to psychotherapy. Anxiolytic medications are the most commonly used pharmacologic intervention and are typically reserved for patients with high levels of anxiety who do not respond to psychological therapies alone. Diazepam is the most common anxiolytic used and is the most effective pharmacologic agent. It is most effective when used in tandem with psychological therapy. Antidepressants and anticonvulsants have been used to treat vaginismus, but symptom resolution is less common and should be reserved for patients where other therapies have not worked. Specifically, venlafaxine or tricyclic antidepressants have been used, including amitriptyline. Typically, treatment with amitriptyline is started at a low dose of 10 mg and gradually increased up to a dose of 40–60 mg daily as tolerated.

Other therapies that have been tried but may not be helpful include hypnotherapy, relaxation therapy, and botulism toxin.

At this time, these therapies are not recommended as they have not been fully studied and have not been shown to demonstrate efficacy.

In conclusion, treating vaginismus is important due to the significant social and sexual implications for the patient. For many women, their self-worth is undermined by their inability to have intercourse, and they may report decreased self-esteem, lack of sustained relationships, and high rates of unconsummated marriage and divorce. Providing support and treatment for these patients can positively impact their lives.

Key Teaching Points

- Providers should provide an opportunity for patients to disclose problems of sexual dysfunction at routine gynecologic visits.
- Vaginismus is due to involuntary recurrent/persistent contracture of the vaginal musculature, which can interfere with sexual intercourse.
- A thorough history and physical exam is necessary to rule out other potential causes of vaginal pain.
- Combination cognitive and behavioral therapy is the best initial treatment for vaginismus.

References

1. Finding Solutions for Female Sexual Dysfunction. American College of Obstetricians and Gynecologists District II Resource Guide. 2010.

2. American College of Obstetricians and Gynecologists. Female sexual dysfunction. Practice bulletin No. 119. *Obstet Gynecol* 2011;117:996–1007.

3. American Psychiatric Association. *Diagnostic and Statistical Manual of Mental Disorders*, 5th edition, American Psychiatric Association, Arlington, VA 2013.

4. Pacik, P. Understanding and treating vaginismus: a multimodal approach. *Int Urogynecol J* 2014;25:1613–1620.

5. American College of Obstetricians and Gynecologists. Adult manifestations of childhood sexual abuse. Committee opinion No. 498. *Obstet Gynecol* 2011;118:392–395.

6. American College of Obstetricians and Gynecologists. Persistent vulvar pain. Committee opinion No. 673. *Obstet Gynecol* 2016;128: e78–e84.

7. Melnik T, Hawton K, McGuire H. Interventions for vaginismus. Cochrane *Database Syst Rev* 2012,**Issue** 12. Art. No.:CD001760. DOI: 10.1002/14651858.CD001760.pub2.

8. The Society of Obstetricians and Gynaecologists of Canada. Female sexual health consensus clinical guidelines No. 279: coital pain. *J Obstet Gynaecol Can* 2012;34(8): S41–S47.

A Tearful 32-Year-Old Woman Requesting a Sleeping Aid Two Weeks after Delivery (Postpartum Depression)

Enid Yvette Rivera-Chiauzzi

History of Present Illness

A 32-year-old female, gravida 1, para 1, presents two weeks after normal spontaneous vaginal delivery complaining of difficulty sleeping and requesting a sleep aid. Her pregnancy was uncomplicated. Her appetite is poor. She has had difficulty sleeping each night since delivery, as well as difficulty breastfeeding and guilt about formula supplementation. Although fatigued, she is unable to sleep while her infant is resting. She had no interest in seeing family or friends. The idea of leaving the baby with others causes anxiety. She is having difficulty caring for the baby. She feels "worthless" and says she thinks she is a "bad mother."

She has no medical problems or prior surgeries. She has a history of depression without treatment in her early 20s. She had no history of alcohol, tobacco, or drug use. She had no medication allergies and takes only prenatal vitamins.

Physical Examination

General appearance   Tearful, no acute distress

Vital Signs

Temperature:	36.9°C
Pulse	81 beats/min
Blood pressure	118/82 mmHg
Respiratory rate	18 respirations/min
Oxygen saturation	96% on room air
Neck	normal palpating thyroid
Abdomen	soft, non-tender
Heart	Regular rate and rhythm; no murmurs
Lungs	Clear to auscultation
Pelvic exam	Unremarkable
Edinburgh Postnatal Depression Scale	21 out of 30

How Would You Manage This Patient?

The patient screens positive for depression on the Edinburgh Postnatal Depression Scale [1] with a score of 21 (greater than 13 is consistent with depressive illness). She meets the clinical diagnosis of postpartum depression given her symptoms of insomnia, fatigue, changes in appetite, feelings of worthlessness, guilt, depression, and loss of interest. These symptoms have been present for 14 days, and she is having difficulty with maternal role functioning, making her symptoms less consistent with baby blues. She denies any suicidal, homicidal, or infanticide ideations.

The patient received counseling on normal postpartum mood changes and baby blues. She was informed that she has postpartum depression. Psychotherapy and medications were recommended. She was referred for cognitive-behavior therapy and prescribed sertraline 50 mg daily. After two weeks, she

had a 50 percent reduction in symptoms. Her medication dose was maintained for six months, and then her medication and therapy were stopped. She remains symptom free. She was counseled on the increased risk of recurrent postpartum depression in future pregnancies.

Postpartum Depression

Postpartum depression is defined as depression that occurs during the first year after delivery [2, 3]. Approximately 10–16 percent of pregnant women meet clinical criteria for postpartum depression. Depressive symptoms are very common postpartum; however, 70 percent of women with depressive symptoms do not meet clinical criteria for postpartum depression. Postpartum depression symptoms can be similar to normal postpartum mood changes, making it difficult for patients and providers to recognize [4]. Women with postpartum depression have anxiety symptoms more frequently than women with major depressive disorder. Risk factors for postpartum depression include depression (Cohen's $d = 0.75$) and anxiety ($d = 0.68$) during pregnancy, stressful life event during or early postpartum ($d = 0.61$), obstetric factors (traumatic birth experience, preterm birth, infant admission to neonatal intensive care, and breastfeeding problems) ($d = 0.26$), social support ($d = -0.64$), and past history of depression, including a prior pregnancy ($d = 0.58$) [2, 5]. Patients with history of depression have a higher risk of relapse postpartum, particularly if antidepressants were discontinued during pregnancy or if they have a history of four or more depressive relapses or depression lasting greater than five years [4, 6].

The entire family can be negatively impacted if peripartum or postpartum depression is not effectively managed. Newborn complications include low birth weight, increased crying, and inconsolability. Children of mothers with untreated depression at any point have increased risk for suicidal behaviors, conduct problems, emotional instability, and need for psychiatric care. Perinatal and postpartum maternal complications include increased life stress, decreased social support, poor maternal weight gain, smoking, alcohol, drug use, and suicide [4, 6]. Maternal suicide due to current or past mood disorders poses a greater risk of mortality than hemorrhage and hypertensive disorders [2].

The American College of Obstetricians and Gynecologists recommends the use of validated tools to screen for depression at least once during the perinatal period [2]. Close monitoring, evaluation, and assessment should be undertaken for women with risk factors for developing postpartum depression [2]. Several survey tools have been validated to screen for postpartum depression including the Edinburgh Postnatal Depression Scale, Beck Depression Inventory, Postpartum Depression Screening Scale, Patient Health

Table 93.1 Postpartum mood disorders [3, 8]

Diagnoses	Symptoms	Clinical characteristics
Postpartum baby blues	Emotional lability, frequent crying, anxiety, fatigue, insomnia, anger, sadness, irritability	Most common (50–80%) Begins to improve at 5 days Lasts 10–14 days No interference with maternal functioning Self-limited
Postpartum panic disorder	Palpitations, lightheadedness, numbness, fear of death, losing control	First panic attack Period of intense fear Attack peaks at 10 minutes
Postpartum obsessive compulsive disorder	Obsessive unwanted thoughts with accompanying behaviors	Is aware obsessions and action are wrong Avoids situation: e.g., removes all knives Compulsive ritual: e.g., changing dry baby
Postpartum post traumatic stress disorder	Nightmares, flashbacks, exaggerated startled response, anger, difficulty sleeping or concentrating	Occurs after birth trauma Threatened or actual injury or death to infant Threatened or actual injury to mother
Postpartum psychosis	Delusions, loss of touch with reality, hallucinations, extreme agitation, confusion, exhilaration, racing thoughts, rapid speech, rapid mood swings, paranoia, suicidal, infanticidal ideations	Most serious Least common 1–2/1,000 deliveries Occurs within first three months Associated with bipolar disorder Not aware obsessions/action are wrong 5% infanticide or suicide Diagnosis and treatment associated with good prognosis Frequently achieve remission

Questionnaire 9, Center for Epidemiologic Studies Depression Scale, and Zung Self-rating Depression Scale [2, 4]. The Edinburgh Postnatal Depression Scale is most frequently used because it can be completed in less than 5 minutes, has been validated in 12 languages, and can be scored easily. The Edinburgh Postnatal Depression Scale requires a low reading level and can assess anxiety symptoms [2]. Protocols should be designed to support screening, diagnosing, and treating women throughout the postpartum period. The American Academy of Pediatrics and US Preventive Services Task Force recommend screening for depression at well-child visits, given the high frequency at which they occur during the first year postpartum [7]. Obstetric and pediatric providers should work together to integrate appropriate screening and referral protocols. Long-term patient outcomes improve with collaborative care models [2].

Patients screening positive should be assessed to determine if they meet criteria for the diagnosis of postpartum depression. Particular attention should be paid to questions about harm to self and others (Question 10 on the Edinburgh Postnatal Depression Scale). Immediate hospitalization is required if signs of self-harm or suicidal or homicidal ideation are present or if there are infant safety concerns. Postpartum mood disorders have a broad differential diagnosis (Table 93.1). Postpartum depression is defined as a change from previous function, and lasting more than two weeks.

The patient must experience five or more symptoms. One of the symptoms must include depressed mood or loss of interest. The other symptoms can include changes in appetite, insomnia or hypersomnia, psychomotor agitation or retardation, fatigue or loss of energy, or feeling of worthlessness or guilt [8]. Once postpartum depression is diagnosed, the risks, benefits, and alternatives of behavioral and medical therapy in an outpatient setting should be discussed [2].

First-line treatment for women suffering from postpartum depression, regardless of severity, should begin with depression-focused psychotherapy such as interpersonal therapy or cognitive-behavioral therapy, which has been shown to be effective for short-term depressive symptoms. Therapy should be part of the treatment even if medication is prescribed. These psychotherapeutic modalities are ideal for women who have previously responded well to psychotherapy, or prefer not to take medication [6]. Therapy improves social isolation, depressive symptoms, and interpersonal relationships, and provides coping skills [2]. Collaboration and referral systems need to be in place to arrange timely access for these services since therapy needs to be provided by trained therapist.

In women with moderate or severe depression, medications are beneficial and should be recommended in conjunction with psychotherapy [4, 6]. For women who are breastfeeding, the best resource for medications is the Drugs and Lactation Database (LactMed) at National

Institutes of Health, which summaries the data for each medication and provides information about maternal and infant drug levels and effect on infant and lactation [9]. Although no long-term studies have determined the safe dosage or duration of treatment, available studies have shown that selective serotonin reuptake inhibitors (SSRIs) have minimal side effects and benefits outweigh the risk of no treatment for severe and moderate depression [2]. Infants of breastfeeding women on pharmacotherapy for depression should be observed for problems with feeding, weight gain, sleep, or other changes [2, 7].

When choosing an initial medication, the patient history and breastfeeding plan should be evaluated. If the patient has previously been successfully treated with a SSRI, the same medication should be prescribed [6]. Sertraline and paroxetine are first-line medications for treatment of postpartum depression due to effectiveness and safety for mother and infant, whether or not breastfeeding. Maternal risks from SSRI includes GI (nausea, vomiting, and diarrhea), activation (restlessness, agitation, akathisia, and sleep disturbances), sexual (decrease libido and anorgasmia), neurological (migraine and tension headaches), increased falls, changes in weight, and rarely, serotonin syndrome [6]. The recommended initial doses are Sertraline 50 mg and Paroxetine 20 mg daily [10]. Improvement in symptoms can be observed as early as week 1 to 2; however, average improvements occur between weeks 4 and 6. Timing of follow-up visits should be guided by the severity of the woman's symptoms. The dose should be increased incrementally until symptoms have improved by 50 percent, based on repeat screening tools such as Edinburgh Postnatal Depression Scale, with minimal side effects. The selected dose should be continued for at least six months to prevent recurrence [2, 6]. If a woman is taking the maximum dose for 4–8 weeks with less than 50 percent improvement of symptoms, then alternative medications should be considered and referral to psychiatry is warranted [6]. All medications have some potential for risk; however, in moderate to severe cases of postpartum depression, the benefits of medical therapy generally outweigh the possible risks [2].

Key Teaching Points

- Patients should be screened at least once during the perinatal period for depression and anxiety symptoms with a standardized, validated tool.
- Psychotherapy is an integral part of treatment, even when the patient is prescribed medication.
- For women with moderate and severe depression, the benefits of medical therapy outweigh the risk of going untreated.
- When possible, a medication to which the patient has previously responded well should be chosen.
- Women should be supported in their choice to breast- or formula feed while on antidepressant medication.
- Sertraline and paroxetine are excellent initial therapies, especially if considering breastfeeding.

References

1. Cox J, Holden J, Sagovsky R. Detection of postnatal depression. development of the 10-item Edinburgh Postnatal Depression Scale. *Br J Psychiatry* 1987;150(6):782–786.

2. American College of Obstetricians and Gynecologists. Screening for perinatal depression. Committee opinion No. 630. *Obstet Gynecol* 2015;125(5):1268–1271.

3. Diagnostic and statistical manual of mental disorders. 5th ed. Washington, DC: American Psychiatric Association; 2013.

4. American College of Obstetricians and Gynecologists. Use of psychiatric medications during pregnancy and lactation. ACOG Practice Bulletin No. 92. *Obstet Gynecol* 2008;111 (4):1001–1020.

5. Robertson E, Grace S, Wallington T, Stewart D. Antenatal risk factors for postpartum depression: a synthesis of recent literature. *Gen Hosp Psychiatry* 2004;26(4):289–295.

6. Gelenberg A, Freeman M, Markowitz J et al. *Practice guideline for the treatment of patients with major depressive disorder*. 3rd edn. Washington, DC: American Psychiatric Association; 2010.

7. Earls MF et al. Clinical report: incorporating recognition and management of perinatal and postpartum depression into pediatric practice. *Pediatrics* 2010;126 (5):1032–1039.

8. Thurgood S, Avery D, Williamson L. Postpartum depression (PPD). *Am J Clin Med* 2009;6(2):17–22.

9. Toxnet.nlm.nih.gov. (2017). Drugs and Lactation Database (LactMed). [online] Available at: https://toxnet.nlm.nih.gov /newtoxnet/lactmed.htm [Accessed June 26, 2017].

10. Sie S, Wennink J, van Driel J et al. Maternal use of SSRIs, SNRIs and NaSSAs: practical recommendations during pregnancy and lactation. Archives of Disease in Childhood – Fetal and Neonatal Edition. 2012;97(6): F472–F476.

A 50-Year-Old Breast Cancer Survivor with Severe Hot Flashes

Myrlene Jeudy

History of Present Illness

A 50-year-old, G3P2, with history of breast cancer presents to the office with severe hot flashes. Three years ago, she had right invasive ductal carcinoma that was estrogen and progestin receptor positive and Her2Neu negative. She was treated with breast conserving therapy and radiation. She is currently taking tamoxifen for endocrine therapy. She reports that she has hot flashes that occur frequently during the day and wake her up in the middle of the night and affect her sleep. Because of lack of sleep, she has less concentration at work. She has tried nonpharmacological methods of treating her symptoms, including dressing in layers, wearing loose-fitting clothes, using a portable fan, and keeping her window open at night, but her hot flashes continue to be severe and distressing to her. She also reports using black cohosh, which has not helped.

Her medical history is significant only for her breast cancer, with a surgical history that includes lumpectomy with sentinel lymph node biopsy. She has no known drug allergies. Her only medication is tamoxifen, which she has been taking daily for the past three years. She continues to have regular periods and denies any irregularities in menstruation. She denies genitourinary symptoms.

Physical Examination

General appearance	Well-developed, well-nourished woman

Vital Signs

Temperature	37.0°C
Pulse	80 beats/min
Blood pressure	110/72 mmHg
Respiratory rate	16 breaths/min
Oxygen saturation	100% on room air
Height	65 inches
Weight	130 lb
BMI	21.6 kg/m²
GYN	Normal external female genitalia. Normal vaginal mucosal. Parous cervix with no cervical lesions or cervical tenderness. Small anteverted uterus with no tenderness. No adnexal tenderness or masses palpated.

How Would You Manage This Patient?

This patient has severe vasomotor symptoms that are distressing and affecting her daily activities. She has a history of breast cancer and is currently on tamoxifen for treatment. Premenopausal women who undergo treatment for breast cancer are at increased risk of experiencing vasomotor symptoms due to the lower levels of estrogen from antiestrogen treatment. She has tried conservative measures such as wearing loose clothing, dressing in layers, and cooling with a portable fan, but her hot flashes are still bothersome. The patient does not have any genitourinary symptoms of menopause, which can also be associated with the treatment of breast cancer.

Due to her history of hormone receptor positive cancer, the patient was counseled on different nonhormonal medical treatments, including cognitive-behavioral therapy, exercise, and avoidance of triggers and alcohol, for her severe hot flashes. In addition, she was started on Effexor 37.5 mg daily. She was counseled that if she did not feel improvement of her symptoms to increase her dose after one week to 75 mg daily. The patient returned in three months and reported improvement of her symptoms on 37.5 mg daily. She was counseled to continue Effexor at this dose, and after 1–2 years to stop the medication to see if her hot flashes continue to be as bothersome.

Treatment of Hot Flashes in Breast Cancer Survivors

Breast cancer is the most common cancer in women in the United States, with a lifetime risk of one in eight (12.5 percent). In 2017, there were an estimated 252, 710 new breast cancer patients and approximately 3.1 million women currently living with breast cancer [1]. Hot flashes, a common symptom of all menopausal women (up to 80 percent), are even more common among breast cancer survivors, who are 5.3 times more likely than women in the general population to experience them [2]. Breast cancer survivors, especially those using tamoxifen, have more severe hot flashes that the general population. Thus, it is important to discuss this topic with women surviving breast cancer.

Hot flashes often begin in the perimenopausal period, and are described as a sudden sensation of intense heat felt in the face and upper body that are often recurrent and last from thirty seconds to five minutes. Hot flashes can vary in duration, frequency, and severity. They can be associated with perspiration, increases in heart rate, palpitations, and anxiety. Hot flashes which occur at night, also known as night sweats, can affect sleep. Hot flashes causing sleep deprivation can contribute to mood changes and/or irritability and can adversely affect quality of life. There have been many different proposed grading scales for the severity of hot flashes, and they are generally classified as mild, moderate, or severe. Mild hot flashes are noticeable but do not interfere with daily activities, while moderate hot flashes interfere somewhat with daily activities, and severe hot flashes are distressing and affect daily activities. Risk factors for hot flashes include sex, age, obesity, decreased physical activity, and smoking. Studies show hot flashes are more frequently reported by African American women and least reported by Asian women [3]. This could be due to cross-cultural perception, which may affect how hot flashes are reported by these women, or biologic differences.

Women with breast cancer have been reported to have more frequent and more severe hot flashes. One theory explaining this is the rapid estrogen withdrawal from therapies such as chemotherapy and endocrine therapy, surgical removal of the ovaries, or the need to abruptly stop hormone replacement therapy with the diagnosis of breast cancer. Endocrine therapies such as tamoxifen have been shown in women with hormone positive breast cancer to decrease their risk of recurrence by 50 percent. However, tamoxifen has also been shown to be a significant cause of hot flashes among breast cancer patients. There have been many studies in which women have discontinued tamoxifen due to its side effect of vasomotor symptoms despite its efficacy in decreasing breast cancer recurrence [4]. Therefore, it is important to discuss the management of hot flashes in women with breast cancer.

The options for treatment of hot flashes in breast cancer survivors include lifestyle modifications, nonhormonal pharmacologic agents, and alternative and complementary therapy. Hormonal therapy such as estrogen and progestin are not recommended in women with a history of breast cancer due to concerns about an increased risk of recurrence and cancer-related mortality. As a result, it is important to discuss nonhormonal treatment for hot flashes in breast cancer survivors.

Nonhormonal pharmacologic treatment options that have been effective in the treatment of vasomotor symptoms include selective serotonin reuptake inhibitors (SSRIs), selective norepinephrine reuptake inhibitors (SNRIs), and gabapentin. These medications are not as effective as hormonal replacement therapy but can be a first-line treatment option for breast cancer survivors. The choice of which agent to use should be individualized. SSRIs/SNRIs are the preferred initial medication for the treatment of hot flashes in breast cancer patients due to the variety of evidence for efficacy and provider comfort with prescribing. Depression is common in women with breast cancer and thus an SSRI/SNRI may have added benefit in addition to treating hot flashes in this population. Common side effects of SSRI/SNRI include dry mouth, nausea, constipation, loss of appetite, and loss of libido. These side effects are often dose-dependent. Gabapentin has been shown to improve sleep quality and therefore can be a desirable choice for women with insomnia due to hot flashes. Adverse side effects of this medication include dizziness, drowsiness, headaches, and disorientation.

Paroxetine can affect the metabolism of tamoxifen and thus can affect its efficacy. Although it is the only SSRI/SNRI approved by the US Food and Drug Administration (FDA) for the treatment of hot flashes, it should be avoided in breast cancer patients on tamoxifen because paroxetine is a potent inhibitor of CYP2D6, the enzyme that converts tamoxifen to its active metabolites [5]. First-line SSRIs/SNRIs for the treatment of hot flashes in breast cancer patients on tamoxifen include venlafaxine, citalopram, or escitalopram.

Clonidine is an antihypertensive agent that is an option for the treatment of hot flashes, but its effectiveness is less than that of SSRIs/SNRIs and gabapentin. It can be considered as a second-line approach if SSRIs/SNRIs and gabapentin are contraindicated or not effective. Table 94.1 outlines some

nonhormonal pharmacologic agents for the treatment of hot flashes in breast cancer survivors.

Since hot flashes are thought to be triggered by elevation of core body temperature, lifestyle modifications that either lower the core body temperature or prevent the rise in core body temperature have been proposed in the treatment of hot flashes. Some of the lifestyle modifications that are considered are clothing adjustments by dressing in layers that can easily be taken off and natural fibers that allow aeration. Other lifestyle modifications include use of a personal/portable fan, avoidance of triggers such as spicy/hot food or liquids, and avoidance of alcoholic beverages. However, there have not been any clinical trials that show significant decreases in hot flashes with these interventions. The North American Menopause Society (NAMS), while acknowledging that cooling techniques and avoidances of triggers appear risk free, does not recommend this as a form of treatment as it may delay more effective treatment options and there is no current evidence of improvement in hot flash symptoms [5].

Other nonmedical options are exercise, mindfulness-based stress reduction, paced respiration, relaxation, and acupuncture. There have been many randomized control trials that have looked at the effects of exercise and hot flashes. NAMS states that although there are many health benefits of exercise, randomized trials do not provide sufficient evidence to support exercise for treatment of hot flashes. Acupuncture also cannot be currently recommended for the use of hot flashes because of lack of evidence of its efficacy in reducing hot flashes. NAMS does state that cognitive-behavioral therapy has level 1 evidence showing efficacy in alleviating hot flashes and is a relatively risk-free therapy. It encourages women to be educated about this option but recognizes the barriers of time commitment as well as finding a credentialed provider in obtaining this therapy. NAMS also recommends weight loss, although with caution, as it might be beneficial.

Studies of herbal products have been contradictory in their efficacy in improving hot flashes. NAMS states that over-the-counter supplements and herbal therapies (including black cohosh, crinum, dioscorea, dong quai, evening primrose, flaxseed, ginseng, and others) are unlikely to be beneficial in alleviating hot flashes and should not be recommended for the treatment of hot flashes. The American College of Obstetricians and Gynecologists reports that the use of soy products is not advised in breast cancer survivors due to the lack of safety and efficacy in this population [6]. Behavior/lifestyle modifications should not delay other options that have been shown to be more effective for the treatment of hot flashes for breast cancer survivors.

Key Teaching Points

- Breast cancer survivors are at an increased risk of developing severe hot flashes and this may affect their ability to continue breast cancer treatments such as tamoxifen.
- Behavior/lifestyle modifications are reasonable treatment options in women with a history of breast cancer because they are minimal risk and cost-effective and may be

Table 94.1 Nonhormonal pharmacological treatment of hot flashes

Drug	Pharmacologic category	Dose	Suggested titration	Potential side effects
Venlafaxine (Effexor)	Antidepressant, SNRI	37.5–150 mg/d	37.5 mg daily or titrated by 37.5 mg per week to a dose of 75 mg or 150 mg daily	Dry mouth, nausea, decreased appetite, insomnia
Desvenlafaxine (Pristiq)	Antidepressant, SNRI	100–150 mg/d	25 mg daily and increase each day	Nausea, dry mouth, dizziness, fatigue, headache, insomnia
Citalopram (Celexa)	Antidepressant, SSRI	10–20 mg/d	10 mg daily and increase to 20 mg after 1–4 weeks if needed	Nausea, fatigue, sedation, palpitation, dry mouth, dizziness, headache, decreased libido
Escitalopram (Lexapro)	Antidepressant, SSRI	10–20 mg/d	10 mg daily, increase to 20 mg once daily after 4 weeks if needed	Nausea, fatigue, sedation, palpitation, dry mouth, dizziness, headache, decreased libido
Gabapentin (Neurotin)	Anticonvulsant	900–2,400 mg/d	300 mg once daily at bedtime on day 1, then 300 mg twice daily on day 2, then 300 mg 3 times daily	Dizziness, headache, unsteadiness, drowsiness
Pregabalin (Lyrica)	Anticonvulsant	150–300 mg/d	50 mg daily at bedtime; increase to 50 mg twice daily after 1 week and then increase to 75 mg twice daily after 1 week. Dose can be increased to 150 mg twice daily after 1 week	Dizziness, sedation, altered mental status, constipation
Clonidine (Catapres)	Antihypertensive, Alpha$_2$-Adrenergic Agonist	0.1–0.3 mg/d (patch) 0.1 mg/d (oral)	0.1 mg transdermal patch weekly	Nausea, dizziness, sedation, hypotension, insomnia, constipation, itchiness (with patch)

beneficial, but they should not delay other options that have been shown to be more effective for the treatment of hot flashes for breast cancer.

- SNRIs/SNRIs and gabapentin are effective nonhormonal treatment options for hot flashes in breast cancer survivors and should be considered first-line treatment options. Gabapentin has been shown to improve sleep quality and therefore can be a desirable choice for women with insomnia due to hot flashes.

- Clonidine is an antihypertensive agent that is an option for the treatment of hot flashes, but its effectiveness is less than that of SSRIs/SNRIs and gabapentin. It can be considered as a second-line approach if SSRIs/SNRIs and gabapentin are contraindicated or not effective.

- Due to limited data of efficacy and safety in this population, the use of over-the-counter supplements and herbal therapies is not recommended for the treatment of hot flashes.

References

1. American Cancer Society (ACS) How common is breast cancer. 2017; Available at: www.cancer.org/cancer/breastcancer/detailedguide/breast-cancer-key-statistics. Accessed April 29, 2017.

2. Harris PF, Remington PL, Trentham-Dietz A, Allen CI, Newcomb PA. Prevalence and treatment of menopausal symptoms among breast cancer survivors. *J Pain Symptom Manage* 2002 June;23(6):501–509.

3. Thurston RC, Joffe H. Vasomotor symptoms and menopause: findings from the Study of Women's Health across the nation. *Obstet Gynecol Clin North Am* 2011 September;38 (3):489–501.

4. Stan D, Loprinzi CL, Ruddy KJ. Breast cancer survivorship issues. *Hematol Oncol Clin North Am* 2013 August;27(4): 805–827, ix.

5. Nonhormonal management of menopause-associated vasomotor symptoms: 2015 position statement of the North American Menopause Society. *Menopause* 2015 November;22 (11):1155–1172.

6. ACOG Practice Bulletin No. 141: management of menopausal symptoms. *Obstet Gynecol* 2014 January;123(1):202–216.

A 56-Year-Old Woman with Dyspareunia

Nan G. O'Connell

History of Present Illness

A 56-year-old female presents to her gynecologist complaining of vaginal dryness and painful intercourse. Her last menstrual period was at age 52. She experienced bothersome vasomotor symptoms for about three years around the time of her final menstrual period, but this has resolved. She is in a monogamous relationship and she and her partner had been having intercourse 1–2 times weekly until about six months ago, when she began to experience a burning, sharp pain, especially with penetration. She reports that her vagina feels very dry and irritated during intercourse, and on a few occasions, she also noted a slight pinkish discharge afterward. These symptoms have persisted to the point of her having to refrain from intercourse. Urinary urgency has also become more of a problem for her. She is very worried about what is causing her symptoms and this problem is straining her relationship with her partner.

Her medical history is significant only for well-controlled hypothyroidism. She has had one cesarean and one vaginal delivery and no other major surgeries. She works for an accounting firm. Her family history is significant for breast cancer (mother) and Alzheimer's (maternal grandmother). Her medications include levothyroxine and a calcium supplement.

Physical Examination

General appearance	Anxious-appearing woman in no acute distress

Vital Signs

Temperature	36.8 C
Blood pressure	118/72
Pulse	78
Respiratory rate	16 per minute
BMI	25 kg/m^2
Abdomen:	Soft, non-distended, non-tender
Pelvic examination	Labia minora regressed, pale introitus, urethral eversion. Vaginal rugae significantly decreased, small amount thin yellow discharge. Cervix pale with some petechiae. Vagina admits two digits with some discomfort. The uterus and adnexa normal.

Laboratory Studies

Saline microscopy	Numerous leukocytes and parabasal (immature) cells, few superficial epithelial cells, no lactobacilli, pH=6.0. No clue cells, yeast, or trichomonads seen.
Urinalysis	Negative

How Would You Manage This Patient?

This patient has vulvovaginal atrophy related to the hypoestrogenic state of menopause. This is part of the constellation of symptoms now referred to as the genitourinary syndrome of menopause (GSM) [1]. The patient was unaware that her symptoms were related to menopause, and therefore, patient education was given about the changes that occur in a low-estrogen state. These changes can affect the vulva, vagina, and lower urinary tract, leading to urinary symptoms and dyspareunia from loss of lubrication and elasticity of the vagina, resulting in sexual dysfunction. This counseling helped alleviate some of the anxiety associated with her symptoms.

Management options were discussed, including use of a personal lubricant with sexual activity as well as local vaginal estrogen therapy. She was counseled about the options for local vaginal estrogen, which included cream, tablet, and ring formulations. She chose to begin the vaginal tablet and was instructed to use this nightly for 14 days and then to decrease dosing to twice weekly. This patient returned three months later and reported significant improvement in the dyspareunia and that she had been able to resume sexual intercourse. She denied any vaginal bleeding or discharge. She also related that her urinary urgency was better. She was encouraged to continue the treatment twice weekly, cautioning her that failure to do this would cause her symptoms to return. A recommendation for yearly follow-up was given.

Genitourinary Syndrome of Menopause

Symptoms of GSM, which include vaginal dryness, dyspareunia, itching, irritation, urinary frequency and urgency, and leucorrhea, affect 20–45 percent of perimenopausal and postmenopausal women. [1] They are related to the hypoestrogenic state associated with menopause. In contrast to vasomotor symptoms, which tend to improve with time, GSM often worsens without intervention and can lead to significant negative effects on a woman's sexual health and quality of life, as demonstrated in a number of surveys of postmenopausal women [2]. The timing of onset of these symptoms in the menopausal transition is quite variable, and many symptomatic women do not bring this problem to the attention of their providers unless providers routinely ask their patients about these symptoms.

During the reproductive years, in the presence of endogenous estrogen, the vagina has a well-vascularized, rugated surface that is usually well lubricated in response to sexual stimulation. Estrogen is a dominant regulator of vaginal physiology (alpha and beta receptors) and to a slightly lesser extent vulvar and lower genital tract physiology; therefore, chronically low estrogen levels associated with menopause cause significant physiologic and anatomic changes. These changes are attributable to diminished collagen, elastin, and hyaluronic acid content as well as impaired smooth muscle proliferation and loss of vascularity [2]. These physiologic and anatomic changes are apparent on physical examination.

The diagnosis of GSM can usually be made by history by assessing the patient's estrogen status (age, last menstrual period, cancer history, surgical history). It is important to ask all perimenopausal and postmenopausal women about symptoms of GSM, as a large percentage of patients are uncomfortable initiating a conversation about these issues with their provider. The history should assess whether the patient has symptoms of GSM and whether these symptoms are a problem and/or affecting her sexuality and quality of life.

Physical examination findings for GSM include small to absent labia minora, constricted introitus, and pale, dry vagina that lacks rugae. The vagina may also be shortened and narrowed. Particular care should be taken in performance of the pelvic examination as atrophic changes can make both the speculum and bimanual examinations painful for the patient, and petechiae and microtrauma may be present. Additional lubricant and a thinner caliber speculum can be helpful. The differential diagnosis includes autoimmune disorders, allergic and inflammatory conditions (e.g., desquamative inflammatory vaginitis, contact dermatitis, lichen planus, and lichen sclerosus), vaginal infections (candidiasis, trichomoniasis), trauma, and vaginismus. Findings on physical examination correlate with symptoms of vaginal dryness, dyspareunia, irritation, itching, and dysuria. Lack of lubrication, vaginal thinning, and loss of elasticity particularly lead to dyspareunia (Table 95.1). However, symptoms do not always correlate with findings on physical examination, with the discrepancy usually related to the sexual activity of the patient, as those who are sexually active tend to be more symptomatic. Other findings consistent with GSM are an elevated vaginal pH >4.5 and a saline microscopy demonstrating few superficial epithelial cells and lactobacilli and numerous parabasal cells and leukocytes. Parabasal or immature cells are smaller and rounder than superficial epithelial cells and have more prominent nuclei.

For some women, a personal lubricant with sexual activity may be all that is needed for treatment. Most over-the-counter lubricants are water- or silicone-based, with the silicone-based versions potentially being safer and more effective. Long-acting vaginal moisturizers can also be used, especially if the patient is bothered by dryness not associated with sexual activity.

If the patient's symptoms are not improved with the addition of lubrication or her presenting symptoms and physical findings are severe, vaginal estrogen therapy should be prescribed. This local therapy is preferred, especially in the absence of other menopausal complaints such as vasomotor symptoms. Three different delivery systems are currently available: estrogen cream (both estradiol and conjugated estrogens), a 10 mcg vaginal tablet, and an estrogen ring which delivers 7.5 mcg of estradiol per day. Choice of one of these therapies is dictated by patient preference, provider experience, and cost. The vaginal creams are administered with an applicator, which allows for adjustments in dosing. A typical dose is 0.5–1.0 g inserted nightly for 14 days and then decreased to twice weekly. Some patients find the creams to be messy, but the creams do have the advantage of more effective treatment of vulvar and introital symptoms. The vaginal tablet is administered with a disposable applicator. This is also used nightly for 14 days and then decreased to twice weekly for maintenance. The estrogen ring is inserted by the patient and replaced every three months [3, 4, 5].

Low-dose vaginal estrogen therapy is considered to have a lower risk profile than systemic hormone therapy, due to the very small changes in serum levels of estrogen. Of concern is the effect of unopposed estrogen on the endometrium and risk of endometrial cancer in patients with an intact uterus. Current evidence suggests that the administration of low-dose vaginal estrogen is safe for the endometrium; however, long-term data are lacking. Concomitant use of a progestogen is not currently recommended [3, 4]. If, however, a patient using one of these therapies reports any vaginal bleeding, this should be promptly evaluated with a transvaginal ultrasound and/or endometrial biopsy. In women with a history of estrogen-dependent breast cancer, the American College of Obstetricians and Gynecologists recommends that nonhormonal therapies be recommended first, but in those patients with more severe symptoms, data do not show an increased risk of cancer recurrence in patients prescribed low-dose vaginal estrogen. The tablet and the ring are preferred over the creams because there is less variability in dosing and potentially less systemic absorption. The patient's oncologist should be consulted before initiating treatment [6].

Vaginal estrogen therapy for GSM remains the gold standard but other therapies are now available. The selective estrogen receptor modulator (SERM) ospemifene is approved for the treatment of moderate-to-severe dyspareunia. It is a 60 mg oral tablet taken daily. It is not recommended that this be used in breast cancer patients due to lack of data in this population. As a SERM, ospemifene has the potential to increase the risk of venous thromboembolism and can increase vasomotor symptoms. Long-term data on endometrial safety are lacking. Another alternative therapy, recently approved by the FDA for the treatment of dyspareunia associated with menopause, is prasterone, otherwise known as dehydroepiandrosterone.

Table 95.1 Genitourinary syndrome of menopause

SYMPTOMS	FINDINGS
Vaginal dryness	Loss of vaginal rugae
Dyspareunia	Pallor of mucosa
Itching/irritation	Introital stenosis and shortening of Vagina
Leukorrhea	Decreased elasticity
Frequency and urgency	Petechiae
Incontinence	Regression of labia minora
Recurrent UTIs	Loss and graying of pubic hair
	Increased vaginal pH
	Increased parabasal cells on saline prep

This comes as a daily vaginal insert. Its efficacy was demonstrated in two placebo-controlled clinical trials. Prasterone is felt to exert its effects through stimulation of both testosterone and estrogen receptors [1]. Finally, a CO_2 laser procedure has been marketed for the treatment of vulvovaginal atrophy and dyspareunia. Used in the office setting, it involves three short procedures spaced six weeks apart. Research has demonstrated that the laser stimulates collagen synthesis but studies are small and of short duration and lack a control arm. More data on efficacy and safety need to be collected before embracing this new and expensive technology [5].

Vulvovaginal atrophy may occur in hypoestrogenic states other than natural menopause. Surgical removal of both ovaries, for example, in the case of a patient with a *BRCA* mutation who has risk-reducing bilateral salpingo-oophorectomy can cause abrupt onset of these symptoms. Cancer treatments (chemotherapy and radiation) and the use of GnRH agonists can result in early menopause (though sometimes temporary) and GSM. Patients with hypothalamic amenorrhea such as in cases of anorexia nervosa or hyperprolactinemia in the postpartum state can also be symptomatic. In these often younger patients with dyspareunia, there may be a higher level of distress in reaction to their impaired sexual function [1]. Aromatase inhibitors used as adjuvant therapy for breast cancer are especially associated with vulvovaginal atrophy.

Key Teaching Points

1. It is important to ask all perimenopausal and postmenopausal women about GSM as a large percentage of patients are uncomfortable initiating a conversation about these issues with their provider.

2. GSM often worsens without intervention, as opposed to vasomotor symptoms, which tend to improve with time, and can lead to significant negative effects on a woman's sexual health and quality of life.

3. Physical examination findings for GSM include small to absent labia minora, constricted introitus, pale and dry vagina that lacks rugae, and shortening and narrowing of the vagina.

4. Care should be taken in performing a pelvic examination, and there may be petechiae and microtrauma.

5. Vaginal estrogen therapy for GSM remains the gold standard, and low-dose vaginal estrogens can be safely used without a progestogen.

6. Nonestrogen alternatives are emerging, including the SERM ospemifene and prasterone, otherwise known as dehydroepiandrosterone.

7. Therapies for GSM must be continued indefinitely in order to maintain the therapeutic effects.

References

1. Portman DJ, Gass MLS, Vulvovaginal Atrophy Terminology Consensus Conference Panel. Genitourinary syndrome of menopause: new terminology for vulvovaginal atrophy from the International Society for the Study of Women's Sexual Health and the North American Menopause Society. *Menopause* 2014;**21**:1063–1068.

2. Gandhi J, Chen A, Dagur G et al. Genitourinary syndrome of menopause: an overview of clinical manifestations, pathophysiology, etiology, evaluation, and management. *Am J Obstet Gynecol* 2016;**215**:704–711.

3. Management of symptomatic vulvovaginal atrophy: 2013 position statement of the North American Menopause Society. *Menopause* 2013;**20**:888–902.

4. ACOG Practice bulletin No. 141: management of menopausal symptoms. *Obstet Gynecol* 2014;**123**:202–216.

5. Krychman ML, Shifren JL, Liu JH, Kingsberg SA, Utian WH. Menopause e-Consult, 2015;**11**(3), www.menopause.org/docs/default-source/professional/me061715.pdf?sfvrsn=10.pdf, accessed on May 4, 2017.

6. American College of Obstetricians and Gynecologists' Committee on Gynecologic Practice, Farrell R. ACOG Committee opinion No. 659 summary: The use of vaginal estrogen in women with a history of estrogen-dependent breast cancer. *Obstet Gynecol* 2016;**127**:618–619.

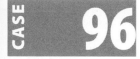

A 60-Year-Old Woman with FRAX® Score Indicating a 10 Percent Probability of Osteoporotic Fracture

Kathryn I. Marko

History of Present Illness

A 60-year-old female presents to her gynecologist for an annual examination. Her last menstrual period was 12 years ago. She denies hot flashes or night sweats. She experiences mild vaginal dryness with sex that is relieved with over-the-counter lubricants. She denies chest pain or shortness of breath.

Her past medical history is significant for mild hypertension controlled with weight control and exercise. She denies any surgical history. Her parents are both alive and well in their late 80s. Neither parent has a history of fracture. She is sedentary except for a one-mile walk on the weekends. She drinks one to two alcoholic beverages per week and has smoked a half pack per day of cigarettes for the last 30 years.

Her last pap test was normal five years ago. She had a mammogram last year that was normal. Her medications include calcium 500 mg daily and vitamin D 400 IU daily. She has no known drug allergies.

Physical Examination

General appearance	Well-developed, well-nourished woman who is in no distress

Vital Signs

Temperature	37.0°C
Pulse	80 beats/min
Blood pressure	125/82 mmHg
Respiratory rate	14 breaths/min
Height	63 inches
Weight	150 lb
BMI	26.6 kg/m^2
Heart	Regular rate and rhythm
Lungs	Clear to auscultation bilaterally
Abdomen	Soft, non-tender and non-distended
Musculoskeletal	No kyphosis
Pelvic exam	Mild vulvovaginal atrophy, otherwise unremarkable

Laboratory Tests

Pap test	Negative for intraepithelial lesion with a negative high-risk HPV test

Imaging

Mammogram	Bi-RADS 1 (Negative)
Bone mineral density with dual-energy X-ray absorptiometry (DXA)	T-score at femoral neck –2.0

FRAX Calculation

Ten-year probability of major osteoporotic fracture	10 percent
Ten-year probability of hip fracture	2.1 percent

How Would You Manage This Patient?

This patient is 60 years old, and in the absence of risk factors for osteoporosis would be too young for routine bone density screening. However, because she is postmenopausal and currently smoking, a DXA study is appropriate. A T-score of –2.0 indicates low bone mass. Therefore, a FRAX® score was calculated, which gives her a ten-year probability of 10 percent for major osteoporotic fracture and 2.1 percent probability of hip fracture. Given this level of risk, she does not require additional therapy at this time beyond counseling on lifestyle changes.

The patient was counseled regarding the importance of bone health and actions she can take to prevent osteoporosis and osteoporotic fracture in the future. She was informed that osteoporotic fracture is associated with significant morbidity and mortality with increasing risk as she ages. In order to maintain bone health, she was encouraged to stop smoking and to begin consistent exercise of at least 30 minutes of brisk walking five days a week. Additionally, she was advised to increase her total calcium intake to 1,200 mg/day and vitamin D to 600 IU daily. She will have a repeat DXA in five years.

Low Bone Mass in a Postmenopausal Woman

Bone health should be addressed in all women throughout their lives. Peak bone mass is achieved by age 30 [1]. In the year leading up to menopause and the immediate postmenopausal period, women have accelerated bone loss. Osteoporosis is a bone condition in which significant decreases in bone density predisposes women to fracture. Osteoporotic fractures have significant associated morbidity and increased mortality [2]. Both hip and vertebral fractures can lead to pain, loss of mobility, and decreased independence. Women with hip fracture have 25 percent increased mortality in the first year after the event [3]. In the United States, Caucasian women have the highest risk of hip fracture while African American women have the lowest [4]. Mexican American women fall in between. Although the risk of hip fracture is lower, Chinese American women tend to have lower bone density than Caucasian women. While there are significant differences in bone density and risk of fracture among different ethnic groups, the recommendations for counseling, screening, and treatment do not change.

When counseling women about bone health, several lifestyle changes should be recommended to all women, regardless of risk. These include managing modifiable clinical risk factors, such as smoking cessation and decreasing alcohol intake. Weight-bearing exercise improves bone density and reduces fracture risk [3]. For many patients this may be as simple as a brisk walk 3–5 times per week. Resistance exercises utilizing weight machines, resistance bands or free weights are also beneficial. Improving muscle strength and balance also decreases falls and therefore risk of fracture. Other fall prevention strategies include adequate lighting, clearing the floors of clutter, ensuring nonslip surfaces throughout the home, storing items within reach, and installing handrails in the bathroom and stairs.

Calcium and vitamin D are essential for bone health. The Institute of Medicine (IOM) recommends at least 1,200 mg of dietary calcium and 600 IU of vitamin D daily in a postmenopausal woman [5]. Calcium intake greater than the recommended amount can lead to gastrointestinal upset, including bloating and increased flatus. Additionally, excess calcium is associated with risk of developing renal calculi. There is some controversy as to the risk of cardiovascular events with increased calcium. Some investigators have noted an increase in cardiovascular events with calcium supplementation while others have not [4].

Starting at age 65, postmenopausal women should be routinely screened for osteoporosis using bone density measurement, most commonly with DXA. DXA should be repeated every 15 years in women with a normal bone density or with mild bone loss (T-score greater than or equal to −1.5). This screening interval is reduced to five years with more significant bone loss (T-score from −1.5 to −1.99) and yearly with a T-score between −2.0 and −2.49 [4]. Certain risk factors prompt earlier screening (age 50–65), including fragility fracture; medical causes of bone loss (steroid use, hyperparathyroidism); body weight <127 lb or BMI <21 kg/m^2; history of parental hip fracture; rheumatoid arthritis; current smoking; and alcohol intake of more than 3 units per day [3].

Bone density (T-score) is reported at the femoral neck, total hip, and spine. The T-score compares the patient's bone density to the mean average bone density for a young Caucasian woman. This is the value used for diagnosis and management decisions in postmenopausal women. A score of less than or equal to −2.5 indicates osteoporosis. A score between −2.5 and −1.0 indicates low bone mass (formerly called osteopenia). A score greater than or equal to −1.0 indicates a normal bone density [6]. The lowest T-score reported should dictate therapeutic decisions.

When a patient is diagnosed with osteoporosis, she should start medical therapy. If the DXA indicates low bone mass, therapy is based on the Fracture Risk Assessment Tool or FRAX* calculation [7]. FRAX* reports the patient's ten-year risk of major osteoporotic or hip fracture. It utilizes several clinical risk factors, including age, gender, height, weight, history of fracture, parental hip fracture, smoking, glucocorticoid use, rheumatoid arthritis, current smoking, >3 alcoholic units daily, secondary osteoporosis, and femoral neck T-score if available. There are different FRAX* calculators depending on the patient's geographic location and her ethnicity. If the ten-year risk of major osteoporotic fracture is >20 percent or hip fracture >3 percent, in patients with low bone mass, then therapy should be initiated. The patient in this case had a ten-year probability risk of 10 percent for major osteoporotic fracture and 2.1 percent probability of hip fracture, so medical therapy was not indicated.

Those with normal bone density do not require additional therapy beyond routine lifestyle recommendations. If a woman has a lower-than-expected bone density as indicated by a low Z-score, which compares her bone density to that of her peer group, it is critical to proceed with a workup for secondary causes of osteoporosis (including hyperthyroidism, type 1 diabetes, rheumatoid arthritis, and certain medications). Comprehensive lists of these conditions and basic workup have been published by NAMS and ACOG [3, 4]. Bone turnover markers have not been found to be helpful in routine practice [8]. Additionally, the IOM does not recommend universal vitamin D screening [5].

Medical therapy for osteoporosis focuses on reducing the risk of fracture (Table 96.1).[6] The first-line treatment is a bisphosphonate medication. These are antiresorptive medications that inhibit osteoclast resorption of bone. They reduce the risk of fracture by 35–65 percent. Bisphosphonates must be taken on an empty stomach with a full glass of water. The patient should be able to sit or stand for a full 30–60 minutes after the dose to avoid esophageal irritation. Those with anatomic esophageal abnormalities or syndromes of delayed esophageal emptying should avoid bisphosphonates. Side effects include esophageal and gastric irritation and musculoskeletal aches and pains. There have been some reports of osteonecrosis of the jaw (ONJ) and atypical femur fracture. These are rare and unlikely to occur at doses prescribed for osteoporosis therapy. However, some consider a drug holiday after 5–10 years of continuous use. Given the long half-life, bone density does not decrease significantly in the following 2–5 years. Repeat DXA should be performed after 2–5 years.

Other antiresorptive agents include raloxifene, calcitonin, and denosumab. Raloxifene is a partial estrogen agonist/antagonist that has been shown to decrease the risk of vertebral fractures as well as breast cancer. Adverse effects can include venous thromboembolism (VTE) and death from stroke. Calcitonin-salmon has been found to reduce vertebral fracture as well as pain due to vertebral fracture. It is recommended that patients be at least five years beyond menopause, as it has not been shown to be as effective in younger postmenopausal women. The subcutaneous injection can lead to flushing and nausea while the nasal spray can cause local irritation. Denosumab is a RANK ligand inhibitor that reduces both vertebral and hip fracture risk in high-risk patients. There is a concern for immune suppression and higher rates of infection in patients using this therapy. Hormone therapy (HT), including estrogen alone

Table 96.1 Therapeutic options for prevention and treatment of osteoporosis

Medication	Class	Route	Indication	Notes[*]
Antiresorptive Therapy				
Alendronate	Bisphosphonate	PO; daily or weekly	Prevention + Treatment	• Can lead to esophageal erosion • Take on an empty stomach with a full glass of water • Stay upright for at least 30 minutes after dose • Consider drug holiday after 5–10 years of therapy • Low adherence
Risedronate	Bisphosphonate	PO; daily, weekly or monthly	Prevention + Treatment	
Ibandronate	Bisphosphonate	PO; daily or monthly IV; q3mo	Prevention + Treatment Treatment	
Zoledronic acid	Bisphosphonate	IV; every 2 years IV; yearly	Prevention Treatment	• Contraindicated in patients with acute renal failure
Raloxifene	SERM	PO daily	Prevention + Treatment	• VTE • Reduced risk of invasive breast cancer
Calcitonin-salmon	Calcitonin	Nasal spray daily SQ QOD	Treatment	• Must be >5y from menopause • Reduces vertebral fracture pain
Denosumab	RANK ligand inhibitor	SQ every 6mo	Treatment	• Use in high-risk patients • Concern for increased infection risk
Estrogen or Estrogen and Progesterone	Hormone therapy	Various routes and dosing	Prevention	• Use in women with other menopausal symptoms • Can continue use for osteoporosis prevention if unable to tolerate or contraindications to other therapies • Potential risks of venous thromboembolism, breast cancer
Anabolic Therapy				
Teriparatide	Parathyroid hormone	SQ daily	Treatment	• Reserved for those with high fracture risk • Limit therapy to 24 months

Data from [4]
[*]This is not a comprehensive list of contraindications; please refer to package labeling.

or estrogen plus progestogen therapy, has been approved for prevention of osteoporosis. In multiple observational and randomized trials, HT reduces fracture risk. Unfortunately, when HT is stopped, bone density and fracture risk rapidly return to baseline. Sequential therapy with bisphosphonates following cessation of HT can mitigate this response.

The only anabolic therapy available is teriparatide or recombinant human parathyroid hormone. It stimulates osteoblastic activity and reduces fracture in both vertebral and nonvertebral sites. It is only recommended for patients at high risk of fracture and use should be limited to a total of 24 months of therapy due to an increased risk of osteosarcoma seen in lab rats on high-dose therapy. Side effects include nausea, dizziness, and hypercalcemia.

After therapy has been initiated, repeat DXA should be performed in 1–2 years, as this is the length of time required to see a change. If bone density is stable at that time, there is no need to repeat the DXA unless the patient develops new risk factors, there is concern for low adherence to therapy, or the patient stops therapy.

Key Teaching Points

- Women of all ages should be counseled regarding the importance of bone health.
- Postmenopausal women 65 years or older should be screened for low bone mass with a DXA.
- Postmenopausal women less than 65 years old should be screened if additional risk factors are present.
- Women are candidates for therapy if they have osteoporosis or low bone mass with a FRAX of >20 percent for major osteoporotic fracture or >3 percent for hip fracture.
- Treatment includes improving modifiable risk factors, lifestyle changes, adequate calcium, and vitamin D intake.
- Bisphosphonates are the first-line medical therapeutic agent.

References

1. Bonjour JP, Theintz G, Law F, Slosman D, Rizzoli R. Peak bone mass. *Osteoporos Int* 1994;4 (suppl 1):S7–13.

2. Cauley JA, Thompson DE, Ensrud KC, Scott JC, Black D. Risk of mortality following clinical fractures. *Osteoporos Int* 2000;11:556–561.

3. North American Menopause Society. Management of osteoporosis in postmenopausal women: 2010 position statement of The North American Menopause Society. *Menopause* 2010;17 (1):23–54.

4. American College of Obstetricians and Gynecologists. Osteoporosis. practice bulletin No. 129. *Obstet Gynecol* 2012;120:718–734.

5. Institute of Medicine. *Dietary reference intakes: calcium, vitamin D*. Washington, DC: National Academies Press;2011.

6. Kanis JA. Assessment of fracture risk and its application to screening for postmenopausal osteoporosis: synopsis of a WHO report. WHO study group. *Osteoporosis Int* 1994;4:368–381.

7. World Health Organization Collaborating Centre for Metabolic Bone Diseases, University of Sheffield, UK FRAX®: Fracture Risk Assessment Tool. Available at: www.shef.ac.uk/FRAX. Accessed April 29, 2017.

8. Miller PD, Hochberg MC, Wehren LE, Ross PD, Wasnich RD. How useful are measures of BMD and bone turnover? *Curr Med Res Opin* 2005;21:545–554.

A 45-Year-Old Woman with Menses Every 60–90 Days and Hot Flashes

Makeba Williams

History of Present Illness

A 45-year-old, G3P3, presents with a six-month history of irregular menses that occur every 60–90 days, last 7–10 days, and are increasingly heavy. She reports hot flashes and night sweats that are disrupting her performance at work and her sleep at night. She is sexually active and intermittently uses condoms. She does not desire pregnancy. Her past medical history and surgical history are negative. She denies tobacco use. She denies allergies to medications.

Physical Examination

General appearance	Well-developed, well-nourished, alert and oriented

Vital Signs

Temperature	37.0°C
Pulse	90 beats/min
Blood pressure	122/80 mmHg
Respiratory rate	16 breaths/min
Oxygen saturation	100 percent on room air
Height	67 inches
Weight	175 lb
BMI	27.4 kg/m^2
Abdomen	Soft, non-tender, non-distended, no guarding, no rebound
External genitalia	Unremarkable
Vagina	Normal in appearance, scant dark blood in posterior fornix
Cervix	Parous, closed, no active bleeding or passage of tissue
Uterus	Anteverted, mobile, normal size, mild tenderness on bimanual examination
Adnexa	Non-tender, unremarkable

Laboratory Studies

Urine pregnancy test	Negative
Hemoglobin	11.0 g/dL
Hematocrit	33.2 percent
Endometrial biopsy	Secretory phase endometrium

Imaging

Transvaginal ultrasound	Uterus measures 7.9 × 4.6 × 5.1 cm. No uterine fibroids. Endometrial stripe thickness measures 6 mm.

How Would You Manage This Patient?

The changes in the patient's volume and frequency of menstrual flow along with new onset of vasomotor symptoms (hot flashes and night sweats) suggest she is perimenopausal. Because the patient is sexually active and not consistently using contraception, an initial urine pregnancy test was performed, which was negative. Next, other commonly recognized causes of abnormal uterine bleeding were considered, including polyp, adenomyosis, leiomyoma, malignancy and hyperplasia, coagulopathy, ovulatory dysfunction, endometrial, iatrogenic, and not yet classified (PALM-COEIN). The normal-appearing endometrium and uterus on ultrasonography suggest that there was no underlying structural cause for the irregular bleeding such as fibroids or polyps. While an endometrial thickness of less than 5 mm is considered normal for the postmenopausal patient, a specific cutoff has not been established for the perimenopausal woman since it will vary in thickness under the influence of fluctuating hormone levels. In this 45-year-old patient with abnormal uterine bleeding, endometrial sampling was performed to assess for malignancy or endometrial hyperplasia. The result of secretory phase endometrium on the endometrial biopsy suggests recent ovulation and reduces the possibility that a malignant or premalignant lesion is responsible for the change in bleeding pattern.

Regulation of menstrual bleeding, control of vasomotor symptoms and contraception were all priorities for this patient. Systemic estrogen is the most effective treatment of perimenopausal and menopausal vasomotor symptoms, and therefore an oral contraceptive pill containing 30 micrograms of estrogen combined with progestogen was recommended. She was instructed to skip the placebo pills to reduce the frequency of heavy withdrawal bleeding and to minimize vasomotor symptoms during the hormone-free interval. The patient was counseled that she should continue the oral contraceptive pill until age 50, at which time it could be stopped to assess for the persistence of vasomotor symptoms and amenorrhea, which could indicate menopause.

Oral Contraceptive and Perimenopause

The menopausal transition, also known as perimenopause, is the period of time that begins with menstrual cycle irregularities and ends one year after the final menstrual period. The average age of onset of perimenopause in the United States is 45 years, and this transition period may last as long as six years. Menstrual cycles are characterized by a persistent difference of seven days or more in length of consecutive menstrual cycles [1] and variable follicle-stimulating hormone levels (FSH). During this time, vasomotor symptoms such as hot flashes and night sweats as well as bleeding irregularities may develop because of declining ovarian follicular function and decreased estrogen production [2]. Vasomotor symptoms are the most common symptom, with a prevalence of 50–82 percent in the United States. They tend to peak approximately one year after the final menstrual period [3]. Perimenopause culminates after 12 months of amenorrhea, at which time menopause is diagnosed, on average at age 51.

Although ovulation is unpredictable during the menopausal transition, women remain potentially fertile until menopause and are at risk for unplanned pregnancy. Seventy-five percent of women between the ages of 40 and 44 report sexual activity, while only four percent are actively trying to conceive. Forty-eight percent of pregnancies conceived among women age 40 or older are unintended [4]. Pregnancies conceived during this period are at increased risk for fetal aneuploidy and spontaneous abortion, and women in this age group are at increased risk for gestational diabetes and hypertensive disorders [4]. Counseling sexually active perimenopausal women about contraceptive options and the associated risks of pregnancy is important.

The late reproductive-aged woman who presents with symptoms suggestive of perimenopause should be evaluated with a thorough history to assess the frequency and severity of symptoms and impact on quality of life. A pelvic examination should be performed in all perimenopausal patients who experience abnormal uterine bleeding, and evaluation may include pelvic ultrasound and endometrial biopsy. All women older than 45 years with abnormal uterine bleeding should have an endometrial sampling performed (after pregnancy is excluded). Thyroid-stimulating hormone level should be considered to rule out underlying thyroid disease as a cause of both vasomotor symptoms and abnormal uterine bleeding. Perimenopause is a clinical diagnosis of exclusion made after other causes have been ruled out.

Treatment options for the symptomatic perimenopausal woman are guided by the patient's preferences and goals, which may include bleeding management, contraception, and vasomotor symptom relief. Expectant management is appropriate for the patients in whom hormonal cycle control is either not desired or contraindicated by medical conditions. For patients who have vasomotor symptoms, irregular bleeding, and need contraception, combined hormonal contraception in the form of transdermal patches, vaginal rings, or estrogen-progestin oral contraceptive pills may be used. Non-contraceptive benefits of combined oral contraceptives for perimenopausal women include regulation of menstrual cycles, reduced heavy menstrual bleeding, suppression of vasomotor symptoms, enhanced bone mineral density, risk reduction of epithelial ovarian and endometrial cancer, and decreased dysmenorrhea and pelvic pain associated with endometriosis [2]. For patients with irregular bleeding without major vasomotor symptoms who may also desire contraception, the levonogestrel intrauterine system and depot medroxyprogesterone acetate may be used. Cyclical progestin therapy may also be used to manage irregular bleeding; however, it does not offer reliable contraception.

Combined oral contraceptives may be particularly useful during this highly symptomatic period to address the bleeding irregularities and vasomotor symptoms. Low-dose combined oral contraceptive pills can decrease the heavy menstrual volume associated with anovulatory cycles. Estrogen in these combined hormonal formulations is the most efficacious therapy for the treatment of vasomotor symptoms. The recommendation is to use the lowest dose of estrogen that provides symptom relief and cycle control [2]. Low-dose monophasic pills containing 30 mcg or less of ethinyl estradiol are a good first-line option for women without contraindications to combined oral contraceptives.

Formulations containing 20 mcg may be associated with higher rates of breakthrough bleeding and poorer cycle control, and there is no evidence that these formulations are safer [5]. The progestogens combined with estradiol vary among the available combined oral contraceptive formulations, and there is currently no definitive evidence supporting a preferred progestogen for perimenopausal women.

When selecting a regimen, individualized patient preferences and symptoms should be considered. Traditional regimens include 21 days of active hormones and a seven-day hormone-free interval (21/7) that provides a consistent menstrual-like withdrawal bleed. Reducing the hormone-free interval to four days or using extended interval dosing (84/7) may decrease vasomotor symptoms during the hormone-free interval and minimize heavy menstrual bleeding [4, 2, 6].

In addition to the contraceptive benefits and relief of vasomotor symptoms, combined oral contraceptives have been associated with decreased risk of ovarian cancer, endometrial cancer, and colorectal cancer [7]. The relative risk of ovarian cancer after 5–9 years of use is 0.64; after more than 15 years of use the risk is reduced to 0.42 [5]. Use of combined oral contraception in the perimenopausal period is associated with increased bone density and preserved bone mass with the use of a combined oral contraceptive pill containing at least 20 mcg of ethinyl estradiol [5, 7, 8].

Combined oral contraception may be associated with increased risk of venous thromboembolism (VTE) and stroke (CVA). These risks also inherently increase with age [9]. The baseline risk of venous thromboembolism increases significantly with age, and use of combined hormonal contraceptives results in a two- to fourfold increased risk of venous thromboembolism. This risk increases threefold in the setting of obesity compared to combined oral contraceptive users who are of normal weight [9]. Pregnancy in the older pregnant patient, however, confers a more than four- to tenfold increased risk of VTE [4].

The incidence of breast cancer increases as women age and the fear of developing breast cancer may lead many women to avoid combined oral contraception. There is no consistent evidence to suggest that combined oral contraceptive use has an adverse impact on breast cancer development. The Collaborative Group on Hormonal Factors and Breast Cancer found a slightly increased risk of breast cancer with five years or more combined hormonal contraceptive use among women over age 45. The risk normalized five to nine years after discontinuing combined hormonal contraceptive use. Other studies failed to show an increased risk of breast cancer among past, recent, current, or even long-term users of combined hormonal contraceptives [9]. Patients should be counseled that combined oral contraceptive pills are only contraindicated in the patient with a personal history of breast cancer; family history alone is not a contraindication.

No method of contraception is contraindicated solely based upon age alone. Smoking and comorbidities that increase in prevalence as a woman ages may alter the benefit-risk profile of contraceptive options [9, 10]. Unless there is a clear contraindication to the use of combined oral contraception, such as tobacco use, personal history of stroke, migraine with aura, or breast cancer, combined oral contraceptives are a good option for the perimenopausal patient [10].

Combined oral contraceptive pills can be continued in the early menopause years and then discontinued when inhibition of ovulation is no longer needed. Because combined oral contraception can induce amenorrhea and mask the final menstrual period, it is important to be certain that menopause has been achieved prior to discontinuing combined oral contraception (Figure 97.1) [6]. Starting at age 50, it is reasonable to assess whether hormonal contraception can be discontinued. One method is to discontinue combined hormonal contraception for 1–2 months to determine if amenorrhea ensues and if hot flashes resume. Nonhormonal back-up contraception is advised during this diagnostic period. Alternatively, for the patient who is unwilling or unable to discontinue combined oral contraception and use back-up contraception, serum FSH levels can be assessed. An FSH level greater than or equal to 30 IU/l on two occasions 6–8 weeks apart, tested 7–14 days after use of combined oral contraception may be used to diagnose menopause [6].

Once menopause has been diagnosed, combined oral contraception should be discontinued. Patients who continue to experience bothersome vasomotor symptoms can be transitioned to a lower-dose hormone therapy for treatment. The dose of ethinyl estradiol in the lowest formulations of combined oral contraception is four times higher than hormone therapy doses of estradiol [9]. It is recommended that the lowest dose of hormone therapy be used to relieve vasomotor symptoms of menopause [2]. Estrogen used for the treatment of menopausal symptoms is available in a variety of oral, transdermal, or vaginal preparations. Transdermal preparations may be associated with reduced risk of VTE and stroke [3]. Standard doses of estrogen include conjugated estrogen .625 mg/d, micronized estradiol-17β 1 mg/d, and transdermal estradiol-17β 0.0375–0.05 mg/d. Low doses of estrogen include conjugated estrogen 0.3–0.45 mg/d, micronized estradiol-17β .5 mg/d, and transdermal estradiol-17β 0.025 mg/d. For women with a uterus in place, estrogen should be combined with progestin to protect the uterus from potentially harmful effects of unopposed estrogen [3].

Key Teaching Points

- The menopausal transition, also known as perimenopause, is the period of time that begins with menstrual cycle irregularities and ends one year after the final menstrual period.
- The potential for ovulation and pregnancy continues during the perimenopausal period and the unintended pregnancy rate among this population is high.
- While an EMS measurement of less than 5 mm is considered normal for the postmenopausal patient, a specific cutoff has not been established for the perimenopausal woman since it will vary in thickness under the influence of fluctuating hormone levels.

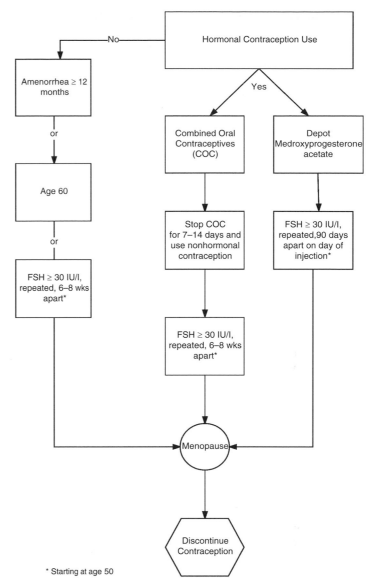

Figure 97.1 Confirming menopause and determining when to discontinue contraception.

- All women older than 45 years with abnormal uterine bleeding should have an endometrial sampling performed (after pregnancy is excluded).
- No method of contraception is contraindicated solely based upon age alone. Unless there is a contraindication to the use of combined oral contraception, such as tobacco use, personal history of stroke, migraine with aura, or breast cancer, combined oral contraceptives are a good option for the perimenopausal patient.
- Combined oral contraception can also provide cycle control, relieve vasomotor symptoms, decrease cancer risk, and increase bone mineral density.
- Starting at age 50, it is reasonable to assess whether hormonal contraception can be discontinued. One method is to discontinue combined hormonal contraception for 1–2 months to determine if amenorrhea ensues and if hot flashes resume.

References

1. Harlow SD, Gass M, Hall JE et al. Executive summary of the stages of reproductive aging workshop + 10: addressing the unfinished agenda of staging reproductive aging. *Menopause* 2012 April;19(4):387–395.

2. North American Menopause Society. Menopause practice: a clinician's guide. 2014.

3. ACOG Practice bulletin No. 141: management of menopausal symptoms. *Obstet Gynecol* 2014 January;123 (1):202–216.

4. Linton A, Golobof A, Shulman LP. Contraception for the perimenopausal woman. *Climacteric* 2016 November;19 (6):526–534.

5. Hardman SMR, Gebbie AE. Hormonal contraceptive regimens in the perimenopause. *Maturitas* 2009 July;63 (3):204–212.

6. Baldwin MK, Jensen JT. Contraception during the perimenopause. *Maturitas* 2013 November;76(3):235–242.

7. ACOG Practice bulletin No. 110: noncontraceptive uses of hormonal contraceptives. *Obstet Gynecol.* 2010 January;115(1):206–218.

8. de Bastos M, Stegeman BH, Rosendaal FR et al. Combined oral contraceptives: venous thrombosis. In: *The Cochrane Collaboration*, editor. Cochrane Database of Systematic Reviews [Internet]. Chichester, UK: John Wiley & Sons, Ltd; 2014 [cited April 18, 2017]. Available from: http://doi.wiley.com/10.1002/14651858 .CD010813.pub2

9. Mendoza N, Soto E, Sánchez-Borrego R. Do women aged over 40 need different counseling on combined hormonal contraception? *Maturitas* 2016 May;87:79–83.

10. Curtis KM, Tepper NK, Jatlaoui TC et al. U.S. medical eligibility criteria for contraceptive use, 2016. *MMWR Recomm Rep* 2016 July 29;65(3):1–103.

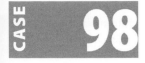
A 70-Year-Old Victim of Elder Abuse

Nguyet A. Nguyen

History of Present Illness

A 70-year-old, gravida 1, para 1, woman presents for her well-woman exam. She reports that she is overall doing "fine" and has no complaints today. Her husband died several years ago. She is accompanied by her 56-year-old daughter, who was recently divorced, and has lived with the patient for several years to provide care. She is a long-time patient of your multispecialty practice and you note that she has not been seen in over five years. During your evaluation, the patient is not her usual cheerful self and makes limited eye contact with you. Her daughter answers most of your questions with limited involvement of the patient.

The patient has a history of hypertension, hypercholesterolemia, and osteoporosis. When asked about her medications, her daughter states she is unsure of what medications her mother is on but she will "pick them up later." She has no significant surgical history and denies smoking or drinking alcohol. When asked about her diet, her daughter states that her mother is "too finicky and she won't eat what I give her." The daughter is reluctant to leave the room when you ask the patient if she would like privacy during her physical exam.

Physical Examination

General appearance	Thin, frail woman with disheveled hair. Slightly malodorous

Vital Signs

Temperature	37.2°C
Pulse	84 beats/min
Blood pressure	160/98 mmHg
Respiratory rate	12 breaths/min
Oxygen saturation	97 percent on room air
Body mass index (BMI)	18 kg/m^2 (BMI 23 kg/m^2 at last visit 5 years ago)
HEENT	Neck soft, no thyromegaly or cervical lymphadenopathy
Cardiovascular	Regular rate and rhythm
Pulmonary	Clear to auscultation bilaterally, no wheezes or rhonchi
Abdomen	Thin abdomen, prominent costal margins, no hepatospenomegaly
External genitalia	Moist appearing with mild erythema along perineum, urine odor noted
Vagina	Atrophic vaginal mucosa, no blood in vault, stenotic cervix
Uterus	Small uterus, nonpalpable adnexa, no tenderness on bimanual examination
Rectum	Weak tone, no masses palpated
Extremities	1+ pitting edema midway to calf in bilateral lower extremities, different states of ecchymosis noted along bilateral upper arms along wrists
Skin	Warm, dry abrasions noted along forearms, small 3 cm laceration noted along right upper arm with ecchymosis surrounding the area, nails with debris

Laboratory Studies

WBCs	9,500/µL
Platelet count	298,000/µL
Hgb	8 g/dL
Sodium	132 mmol/L
Potassium	3.4 mmol/L
Chloride	100 mmol/L
CO$_2$	22 mmol/L
Anion Gap	10 mmol/L
Creatinine	1.1 mg/dL
Calcium	7.9 mg/dL
Total Protein	4 g/DL
Albumin	2.3 g/dL
Liver function tests	Within normal limits

How Would You Manage This Patient?

The patient may be a victim of elder abuse. Her disheveled appearance, change in demeanor, and evidence of malnutrition along with her daughter's behavior raise significant concerns. The patient and daughter were interviewed separately. The patient's medical history and medications were reviewed and no medical or pharmacologic problems explained the observed changes. The interview started with open-ended questions such as "How has it been living with your daughter?", then slowly progressed to more direct questioning, such as "Do you feel safe in your home?" and "Has anyone hurt or abused you in any way?" The patient reported her daughter moved into her home, and is helping her. She is reluctant to share additional details with you. Her answers supported suspicion of elder abuse. The Elder Abuse Suspicion Index (EASI) was used and results were positive, further supporting elder abuse [1]. The patient's history and findings on physical examination were documented in detail. Referral to a neuropsychologist was made to assess the patient's cognitive status for any signs of dementia or psychologic etiology that may explain her weight or behavior changes.

The National Center on Elder Abuse (NCEA) state resource page was referenced for the state in which the care was provided (Colorado) and noted the Colorado Adult Protective Services (APS) requires mandatory reporting of any suspicion or knowledge of elder abuse to local law enforcement within 24 hours. The law states "any person providing healthcare or healthcare related services" to an at-risk elder (a person 70 years or older) is considered a "mandatory reporter" [2–3]. A detailed list of mandatory reporters is prepared, which includes physicians. Colorado law clarifies it is sufficient to

315

have reasonable suspicion to report elder abuse and the reporter is immune from any criminal charges or civil law disputes.

The provider contacted her local law enforcement to assist in making the report and for guidance on determining if it was safe for the patient to go home with her caregiver. After consultation, the provider shared her concerns with the patient and that a report has been filed. The provider did not share this information with the patient's daughter due to concern that this would put the patient in danger of retaliation by her daughter. The patient was allowed to go home and was aware that the authorities will make a visit to her home.

Two weeks later, APS visited the patient's home and discovered that the house was cluttered and filthy. There was little food in the home and multiple empty medicine bottles were noted. After further investigation, the patient reports that her daughter has been verbally abusive, pushed the patient during a verbal altercation, and at times forces her to stay in her room while her daughter has friends over to her home. She states that she does not want to lose her home and independence and "really wants to be left alone."

Your office was contacted by APS to provide further information regarding the case. You share that her cognitive function assessment is still pending. APS found evidence of neglect, as well as financial, psychological, and physical abuse. APS began working with the patient to provide support from local resources and continued medical care to help regain her health and independence. The investigation is still in progress and no formal charges have been filed against the daughter. The patient's daughter is still living in the home; however, APS has reached out to her to offer resources and social support to aid in coping with stressors as an elder caregiver until the case has come to a conclusion.

Elder Abuse and Mistreatment

The geriatric population is one of the fastest growing age groups in the United States. It is projected to double from 900 million in 2015 to about 2 billion people in 2050 [4]. Women will compose over half of this population. Elder abuse affects about 1 in 10 older adults [4–5]. About 20 percent of elders who present to the emergency room experience neglect [5]. Elder abuse is defined by the US National Academy of Sciences with definition supported by other world organizations as:

> (a) intentional actions that cause harm or create a serious risk of harm (whether or not harm is intended), to a vulnerable elder by a caregiver or other person who stands in a trust relationship to the elder, or
> (b) failure by a caregiver to satisfy the elder's basic needs or to protect the elder from harm [6].

The two key factors in this definition are that the elder is harmed in some way and that the caregiver responsible either caused this harm or failed to prevent it. The major risk factors for elder abuse are cognitive impairment, depression or anxiety, social isolation, and a shared living situation [7]. Financial abuse is more prevalent in older patients who live alone [7]. Perpetrators are usually people who are heavily dependent on

the elderly victim. Research on elder abuse is limited due to different definitions of elder abuse and mistreatment resulting in differing recommendation from major societies on screening and treatment outcomes.

Given the growth in this population, medical providers should be educated and trained on clinical signs and symptoms of elder abuse. Many medical providers report little to no education on elder abuse in their training. Cognitive impairment also complicates this area of research and training. The US Preventative Service Task Force (USPSTF) states there is no clear evidence that routine screening for elder abuse improves outcomes. The American College of Obstetricians and Gynecologists (ACOG), the American Medical Association, and the American Academy for Neurology recommend annual screening in the elder population (usually greater than age 65). ACOG recommends screening women ages 65 years and older at each well-woman visit and provides tools for screening along with resources for providers who are unclear about the organizations available locally for assistance [8].

It is important to interview the patient and caretaker separately, if possible. Providers should start with open-ended questions such as, "Can you tell me how this occurred?" or "Are you able to recall what happened?" then progress to more direct questioning. Providers should also thoroughly review the patient's medical and surgical history, determine who is responsible for managing and providing the elder patient their medications, and perform a brief assessment of the patient's baseline functional status [9]. If providers are unable to establish the patient's baseline cognition, then a referral to a neuropsychologist is indicated. If no organic etiology is found, these signs may suggest elder abuse. Physical findings of elder abuse are uncommon. If present, they should be documented in detail to aid in an investigation should it be necessary. Photographs or body charts are helpful when an elder patient's case is being reviewed [7, 9].

If the patient appears to be cognitively intact, the EASI can be used to help determine if a report is needed. The EASI is a tool validated for screening cognitively intact patients who are 65 years and older for elder abuse. It is a six-question tool which can take 2–5 minutes to administer. The first five questions ask for "YES/NO" answers from the patient and the last question is answered by the provider. Any "yes" answers to questions 2–6 establish potential concern and should prompt possible referral [1].

Resources, reporting requirements, legal protections for providers, and agencies with jurisdiction vary from state to state. A suspicion of elder abuse is sufficient, even in the absence of strong evidence, to warrant an APS report or notifying your local organization for further assistance. The Administration on Aging's NCEA website is a central site with state-specific guidelines on legal requirements and local resources to aid in reporting suspicion of elder abuse (https://ncea.acl.gov/resources/state .html) [2]. The Eldercare Locator (telephone: 800–677-1116) is another resource that provides state-specific organizations and laws, available for weekday use. Most states mandate reporting in cases where elder abuse is suspected. Reporting typically requires at a minimum the name and address of the at-risk elder, description of the incident or findings that led to the report, documentation of any injury in detail, and, if possible, the alleged perpetrator's name and address. The provider should also provide any additional information they feel is relevant such as what prompted the call, any medical or physical condition that may impair the elder's activities of daily living, and whether the elder is working with services or organizations that help the elder with their care [3]. Once APS is involved, providers are still responsible for ensuring that follow-up medical care is provided as the elder patient recovers from their traumatic experiences. The goal for APS is to allow patient autonomy to make decisions regarding the resources they are willing to accept and to try to keep families together by providing aid to reduce stressors that can lead to elder abuse.

Key Teaching Points

- Elder abuse is common and likely underreported. Providers should have a low threshold to screen.
- The patient and caregiver should be interviewed separately, starting with open-ended questions to help guide the conversation.
- History and physical findings should be documented in detail to assist in elder abuse cases.
- Any level of suspicion for elder abuse should prompt a report to APS or other local agency with legal jurisdiction.

References

1. Yaffe MJ, Tazkarji B. Understanding elder abuse in family practice. *Can Fam Physician* 2012;58(12):1336–1340, e695–e698.

2. Resources [Internet]. NCEA National Center on Elder Abuse. [cited June 30, 2017]. Available from: https://ncea.acl.gov/resources/state.html

3. Who are mandatory reporters? [Internet]. Colorado Department of Human Services. [cited June 30, 2017]. Available from: www.coloradoaps.com/about-mandatory-reporting-update.html

4. Krug E, Dahlber LL, Mercy JA, Zwi AB, Lozano R. eds. Abuse of the Elderly [Internet] WHO. World Report on Violence and Health. Geneva. 2002. Available from: www.who.int/mediacentre/factsheets/fs357/en. Retrieved April 10, 2017.

5. Cooper C, Selwood A, Livingston G, The prevalence of elder abuse and neglect: a systematic review. *Age Ageing* 2008;37(2):151–160.

6. Acierno R et al., Prevalence and correlates of emotional, physical, sexual, and financial abuse and potential neglect in the United States: the National Elder Mistreatment Study. *Am J Public Health* 2010;**100**(2):292–297.

7. Lachs MS, Pillemer K. Elder abuse. *Lancet* 2004;364(9441):1263–1272.

8. American College of Obstetricians and Gynecologists. Elder Abuse and Women's Health. Committee Opinion 568. *Obstet Gynecol* 2013;122:187–191.

9. Hoover RM, Polson M. Detecting elder abuse and neglect: assessment and intervention. *Am Fam Physician* 2014;89 (6):453–460.

Index

abdominal pain, imperforate hymen and, 221
abnormal nipple discharge, 108
abnormal uterine bleeding (AUB), 20
  classification of, 61
  FIGO and, 61
accidental bowel leakage, 254
ACE. *See* angiotensin-converting enzyme
ACIP. *See* Advisory Committee for Immunization Practices
acne, irregular menses and, 200–2
  oral contraceptive use and, 200
  PCOS and, 200–2
    COCs and, 201–2
    hyperandrogenism and, 201
    laboratory testing, 201
    lifestyle management for, 202
ACOG. *See* American College of Obstetricians and Gynecologists
actinomyces, 71–72
  history of illness, 71
  with IUD, 71
    bacterial colonization, 72
    detection rates for, 72
    diagnosis of, 72
    patient management, 71–72
    prevalence rates for, 72
    therapy strategies for, 72
acupuncture
  for chronic pelvic pain, 13
  for over active bladder (OAB), 264–65
acute genital ulcers. *See* genital ulcers
add-back therapy, 17
adnexal masses, in postmenopausal women, 230–32
  malignancy risks, 230
  surgical management of, 231–32
  tumor marker testing for, 231
  ultrasound for, 231

adolescent endometriosis, 7–9
  diagnostic considerations, 8–9
  laparoscopic imaging in, 9
  OHVIRA syndrome, 7
  prevalence rate of, 7
  therapeutic considerations, 8
    with NSAIDs, 7–8, 9
adolescents. *See also* chlamydia; labial hypertrophy
  PCOS in, 200–2
    COCs and, 201–2
    hyperandrogenism and, 201
    lifestyle management for, 202
  with secondary amenorrhea, 224–26
advanced maternal age (AMA)
  chronic hypertension and, 190
  miscarriage rates, 192
  pregnancy planning and, 190
    aneuploidy risks, 192
    comorbidity risks, 192
    Down Syndrome, 192
Advisory Committee for Immunization Practices (ACIP), 137
albicans species, 156
AMA. *See* advanced maternal age
amenorrhea. *See also* hypothalamic amenorrhea; secondary amenorrhea
  transgender males and, 292
American College of Obstetricians and Gynecologists (ACOG), 130, 187, 316
American Society for Colposcopy and Cervical Pathology (ASCCP)
  HSIL guidelines, 130
  LSIL and, 116
    positive margins for, 123–24
American Society for Reproductive Medicine (ASRM), 9
AMH. *See* anti-Mullerian hormone
Amino-cerv, 46
amiodarone, 1
amitriptyline, 14, 267

Amsterdam criteria, for Lynch syndrome, 119
anabolic therapy, 309–9
anastrozole, 134
aneuploidy, 192
angiotensin II receptor blockers, 192
angiotensin-converting enzyme (ACE), 192
anogenital warts, 143
anorexia nervosa
  bone density and, 225–26
  diagnosis of, 225
    SCOFF screening questionnaire, 224, 225
  menstrual dysfunction with, 225
  prevalence of, 225
  prognosis rates for, 226
  secondary amenorrhea from, 224–26
    hormonal treatment for, 225
  treatment of, 225
antiandrogens, 289
antibacterial therapy, for non-specific vulvovaginitis, 207
antibiotic therapy
  for Bartholin's cyst, 160
  for lactational mastitis, 105
  oral, 105
  periprocedural, 160
antidepressants. *See* tricyclic antidepressants
anti-Mullerian hormone (AMH), endometriomas and, 171
antiphospholipid antibody syndrome, 174
antiresorptive agents, 308
antiretroviral drugs (ARVs), 68–69
antithrombin III deficiency, 174
anxiety, loss of sexual desire and, 286
aphthae/aphthosis of the vulva, 209–12
  clinical presentation, 210
    acute ulcers, 210, 211
  diagnostic evaluation, 210
  STIs and, 210
    testing for, 212

treatment therapies, 211–12
  corticosteroid therapy, 211–12
  topical analgesics, 211–12
ART. *See* assisted reproductive technology
ARVs. *See* antiretroviral drugs
ASCCP. *See* American Society for Colposcopy and Cervical Pathology
ASC-US. *See* atypical squamous cells of undetermined significance
Ashkenazi Jewish women, pregnancy planning for, 187–89
  genetic counseling, 187–88
    ACOG guidelines, 187, 188
    costs of, 188
    for genetic disorders, 187–88
Aspercreme, 112
ASRM. *See* American Society for Reproductive Medicine
assisted reproductive technology (ART), in HIV-positive women, 87
asymptomatic ovarian cysts, 233–34
  benign, 234
  cystadenomas, 234
  in premenopausal women, 233–34
atenolol, 192
atrophic vaginitis, 42–44
  causes of, 43
  clinical presentation, 43
  diagnosis of, 43
  hypoestrogenism and, 43
  treatment therapies for, 43–44
    alternative non-estrogen approaches, 44
    contraindications to, 44
    local vaginal estrogen therapy, 42, 44
atypical ductal hyperplasia, 100
atypical squamous cells of undetermined significance (ASC-US), 115

ASCCP management
    guidelines, 116
    in young adult females, 115–16
AUB. See abnormal uterine
    bleeding
axillary dissection, 103
azithromycin, 1, 27, 30

bacterial vaginosis, 27–28
bariatric surgery. See gastric
    bypass
barrier methods, as contraceptive
    option, 74
Bartholin's cyst, 158–60
    diagnosis of, 158–59
    diagram of, 159
    MRSA and, 160
    recurrence of, 160
    treatment therapies, 158, 159
        with periprocedural
            antibiotics, 160
    Word catheter placement, 159
Bartholin's Gland Cancers, 160
Basson's model of sexual
    response, 285–86
benign ovarian cysts, 234
benign precocious puberty, 219
benzodiazepines, 1
β-hCG testing, 250–52
bichloroacetic acid, 150
bilateral clear nipple discharge,
    95–96
    categorization of, 95
    laboratory studies for, 95, 96
    LNG-IUD and, 95
    malignancy rates in, 96
    mammogram in evaluation, 95
    milky, 95, 99
    pathologic, 95, 99
    pregnancy testing and, 96
    prevalence rates, 95
bilateral hydrosalpinx, 164
    HSG for, 164
    pelvic ultrasound for, 165
bilateral salpingo-oophorectomy,
    246
biofeedback therapy, 254
    for posterior wall defects, 277
body mass index (BMI)
    etonogestrel implant and, 80
    precocious puberty and, 217
    weight categories by, 91
bone density issues, 53, 307–10
    with anorexia nervosa, 225–26
    dual-energy X-ray
        absorptiometry, 307, 308,
        309
    FRAX calculation for, 307, 308
    lifestyle modifications, 308–8
    physical examination, 307
    in post-menopausal women,
        307–9
bosentan, 83
Botulinum Toxin A, 264–65, 296
BRCA genetic mutations
    breast cancers and, 125–27
    Cowden syndrome, 125
    Li Fraumeni syndrome, 125

Lynch syndrome and, 125
ovarian cancer and, 125–27
PTEN Hamartoma Tumor
    Syndrome, 125
breast cancers, 132–34
    BRCA genetic mutations and,
        125–27
    risk-reducing bilateral
        salpingo-oopherectomy
        (RRSO) and, 126–27
    risk-reducing options,
        126–27
    screening and prevention
        options, 127
    chemoprevention for, 134
    high-risk screening, 132–34
        Gail model, 133
        with MRI, 134
        NCCN guidelines, 133–34
        Tyrer-Cuzick model, 133
    perimenopause and, 312
    prevalence rates, 132
    risk reduction surgery for, 134
        mastectomy, 134
        risk-reducing bilateral
            salpingo-oopherectomy
            (RRSO), 134
    unilateral bloody nipple
        discharge and, 99
breast erythema, 104–5
breast exams, with unilateral
    bloody nipple discharge,
    98, 99
breast masses, 101–3
    DCIS, 101
    lactational mastitis and, 105
    during pregnancy, 101–3
        clinical presentation
            of, 102
        diagnosis and prognosis of,
            102
        lesions, 102
        mammography for, 102–3
        pharmacokinetics for, 103
        surgery for, 103
        treatment options for, 103
        ultrasound imaging for, 101,
            102, 103
breast pain. See also cyclic breast
    pain
    classification of, 111–12
    extra mammary, 111–12
    noncyclical, 111–12
breastfeeding, after lactational
    mastitis, 106
bromocriptine, 112–13
BSO. See bilateral salpingo-
    oophorectomy

calcitonin, 308
calcium intake, for osteoporosis,
    308
cancer risks, Lynch syndrome,
    118, 119
    chemoprevention, 119–20
    hysterectomy and, 120
Candida albicans, 32–33
    fluconazole treatment, 34

Candida glabrata, 34
Candida krusei, 34
Candida Saccharomyces, 34
candida vaginitis, 155–57. See
    also recurrent vulvovagi-
    nal candidiasis
    treatment therapies, with OTC
        medication, 155
carbamazepine, 83
carcinomas. See also breast can-
    cers; breast masses; ovar-
    ian cancer
    DCIS, 101
    intraductal, 99
cascade testing, for Lynch
    syndrome, 118, 120
CBT. See cognitive behavioral
    therapy
CDC. See Centers for Disease
    Control
cefixime, 30
ceftriaxone, 27, 30
Centers for Disease Control
    (CDC)
    chlamydia guidelines, 39–40
    on condyloma acuminata
        treatments, 150
    HIV treatment therapy
        guidelines, 69–70
    Zika virus testing guidelines,
        178
central precocious puberty, 217,
    219
cephalosporins, 270
cervical biopsy, 122
cervical dysplasia, 115
cervical intraepithelial neoplasia
    (CIN)
    HPV and, 136, 137
    prevalence rates, 136
cervicitis, 26–28
    chlamydia and, 26
        prevalence rates for, 27
    gonorrhea and, 26
        nucleic acid amplification
            tests, 27
        prevalence rates for, 27
    mucopurulent, 26–28
        treatment for, 27
    noninfectious, 26
    PID and, 26
    testing for, 26–27
cesarean delivery, 255
CHC. See combined hormonal
    contraception
chemoprevention, 119–20, 134
chlamydia, 26
    among adolescents, 39–40
        CDC guidelines for, 39–40
        clinical considerations for,
            39–40
        confidentiality and privacy
            considerations, 40
        history of illness, 39
        nucleic acid amplification
            tests for, 39
    expedited partner therapy
        (EPT) for, 29–30

PID and, 244
after sexual assault, testing for,
    89
chronic hypertension. See
    hypertension
cimetidine, 1, 267
CIN. See cervical intraepithelial
    neoplasia
cisplatin, 103
citalopram, 181
clindamycin, 243–44
clobetasol, 141
clomiphene citrate, 167, 168
clonidine, 302
clotrimazole, 24
COCs. See combined oral
    contraceptive pills
cognitive behavioral therapy
    (CBT)
    for chronic pelvic pain, 14
    for levator ani spasm
        syndrome, 6
    for loss of sexual desire, 285,
        286–87
    for postpartum depression,
        297
    for vulvodynia, 147
colorectal cancer, 118, 119
colposcopy, for HSIL
    ASCCP guidelines, 130
    for young adult women,
        129–30
combined hormonal
    contraception (CHC), 92
combined oral contraceptive pills
    (COCs), 68
    obesity and, 91–92
    for PCOS, in adolescents,
        201–2
    perimenopause and,
        312, 313
commercial sexual exploitation
    (CSE), 279–83. See also
    human sex trafficking
complicated stress urinary
    incontinence (SUI), 257
condyloma acuminata, 142–43,
    149–51
    classification of, 143
    clinical presentation of, 143
    diagnosis of, 149–50
    HPV and, 149, 150
    risk factors for, 149
    STI screenings and, 149
    treatment therapies for, 143,
        150–51
        CDC recommendations,
            150
        efficacy of, 151
        recurrence rates for, 151
confidentiality issues, for
    chlamydia among
    adolescents, 40
contraceptive counseling
    with DVT, 73–74
    etonogestrel implant, removal
        of, 80
    for HIV-positive women, 86

contraceptive counseling (cont.)
  for LARC, in postpartum
      period, 77
  obesity and
      for combined hormonal
          contraception, 92
      contraceptive patch, 92
      shared decision-making in,
          91
      US MEC guidelines, 91–92
  pulmonary embolus (PE) and,
      73–74
      barrier methods, 74
      patient management, 73
      range of contraceptive
          options, 73
      risk factors in, 73, 74
      STI screening as part of, 73
      US MEC guidelines, 73, 74
contraceptive implants. See also
      etonogestrel implant
  guidelines for, 83
  medications with, 83
  pregnancy tests before, 82–83
  pregnancy with, 82–84
      ectopic, 83
      intrauterine, 83–84
      protease inhibitors
          and, 83
      timing of, 83
contraceptive use. See also
      levonorgestrel
      intrauterine device; oral
      contraceptive use
  with pulmonary embolus (PE),
      73–74
      barrier methods, 74
      range of contraceptive
          options, 73
      risk factors in, 73, 74
      STI screening as part of, 73
      US MEC guidelines, 73, 74
corticosteroids, for vulvar lichen
      sclerosus, 141
Cowden syndrome, BRCA
      genetic mutations and,
      125
cramping. See menstrual
      cramping
cryotherapy
  for condyloma acuminata,
      143, 150
  for friable cervix, 46
cyclic breast pain, 111–13
  classification of, 111–12
  etiology of, 111–12
  with mastodynia, 111–13
      classification of, 112
      evaluation and diagnosis,
          112
      imaging, 112
      treatment strategies,
          112–13
cyclic medroxyprogesterone. See
      medroxyprogesterone
cyclophosphamide, 103
cystadenomas, 234
cystectomy, 241

cystic teratoma, mature,
      227–28
  complications from, 228
      malignancies, 228
  development of, 227
  evaluation of, 227
  in postmenopausal women,
      227–28
  Rokitansky nodule, 227
  treatment for, 228
  ultrasound imaging, 227–28
cystitis. See uncomplicated
      cystitis
cysts. See breast masses; cystic
      teratoma; ovarian cysts
cytolytic vaginitis, 156

DCIS. See ductal carcinoma
      in situ
deep dyspareunia, 4–6
  examination for, 4
  oral contraceptive use and, 4
deep vein thrombosis (DVT),
      73–74
  barrier methods and, 74
  contraceptive counseling with,
      73–74
  diagnosis and testing for,
      185–86
  estrogen therapy risks, 73–74
  pregnancy planning with,
      184–86
  thromboprophylaxis and,
      185
  prevalence rates for, 184–85
  risk factors for, 73, 74
  treatment therapies, 186
      enoxaparin, 184, 186
      low-molecular weight
          heparin, 186
      unfractionated heparin, 184
  VTE and, 91–92, 184–86
denosumab, 308
Depot Leuprolide, 16
depot medroxyprogesterone
      acetate (DMPA), 17, 18,
      92–93
depression. See also postpartum
      depression
  citalopram, 181
  loss of sexual desire and, 286
  patient management, 181
      relapse issues, 182
      with SSRIs, 181, 182
  pregnancy planning and,
      181–83
      decision aids, 182–83
      relapse, 182
      treatment therapies as part
          of, 182
  prevalence rates, 181
dermoid cysts. See cystic
      teratoma
desensitization techniques, for
      vaginismus, 295–96
diabetes
  GDM, 194
  history of illness, 194

patient management,
      194
pre-gestational diabetes
      mellitus
  comorbidities with, 195
  exercise and, 195
  medications for, 195
  pregnancy planning, 194–95
  pregnancy planning and,
      194–96
      complication risks, 195
      evaluation of, 194–95
      pre-gestational diabetes
          mellitus counseling,
          194–95
  recurrent pregnancy loss and,
      174
dicloxacillin, 104
diet therapies
  for painful bladder syndrome,
      267
  for postpartum flatal
      incontinence, 254
dihydrotesterone, 141
displaced IUDs, 65–67
  consultation for
      replacement, 66
  evaluation of, 65
  prior patient medical
      history, 65
  ultrasound imaging for, 65
distal rectoceles, 276. See also
      posterior wall defects
  diagnosis of, 277
  management of, 277
  risk factors for, 277
DMPA. See depot
      medroxyprogesterone
      acetate
Doderlein's cytolysis, 156
Down Syndrome, 192
doxycycline, 27, 243
dual-energy X-ray
      absorptiometry (DXA),
      307, 308, 309
ductal carcinoma in situ (DCIS),
      101
ductal ectasia, 99
  unilateral green nipple
      discharge with, 107–8
      clinical presentation, 107
      diagnosis of, 107
duloxetine, 14
DVT. See deep vein thrombosis
DXA. See dual-energy X-ray
      absorptiometry
dysmenorrhea, 7–9
  adolescent endometriosis, 7–9
      diagnostic considerations,
          8–9
      NSAIDs for, 7–8, 9
      OHVIRA syndrome, 7
      prevalence rate of, 7
      therapeutic considerations,
          7–8, 9
  diagnostic criteria for, 8
  patient management, 7
      LNG-IUD, 7

secondary, 8,
      17
  symptoms of, 8
  treatment strategies
      with NSAIDs, 7–8
      therapeutic considerations
          in, 8
dyspareunia. See also deep dys-
      pareunia; genitourinary
      syndrome of menopause
  vaginismus and, 294

early breast development. See
      precocious puberty
EASI. See Elder Abuse Suspicion
      Index
ectopic pregnancy
  with contraceptive implants,
      83
  pregnancy of unknown
      location (PUL) and, 252
Edinburgh Postnatal Depression
      Scale (EPDS), 297, 298,
      299
efavirenz, 68, 70
elder abuse, 315–17
  assessment interviews for, 316
  definition of, 316
  Elder Abuse Suspicion Index
      (EASI), 315
  mistreatment and, 316–17
  national and state
      organizations and,
      315–17
  reporting requirements,
      316–17
  screening for, 316
Elmiron. See pentosan
      polysulfate
emollient therapy, 141
endometrial cancer, 118, 119
endometrial polyps, 61–62
  detection rates for, 62
  diagnosis and evaluation of,
      61, 62
  prevalence rates, 61
  sonohysterogram, 62
  ultrasound imaging for, 61, 62
endometriomas, 170–72. See also
      ovarian endometriomas
  AMH levels and, 171
  clinical presentation, 171
  infertility and, 171
  laparoscopy for, 170–71
  medical treatment therapies,
      171
  prevalence rates, 171
  surgical excision of, 171
  ultrasound imaging of, 170
endometriosis, 16–18. See also
      dysmenorrhea
  adolescent, 7–9
      diagnostic considerations,
          281, 8–9
      OHVIRA syndrome, 7
      prevalence rate of, 7
      therapeutic considerations,
          7–8, 9

diagnosis of, 17, 171
evaluation of, 16–17
infertility and, 162
ovarian endometriomas with, 236
ovarian remnant syndrome and, 246–47
patient management with, 16
with oral contraceptive use, 16
prevalence rates, 16–17, 171
secondary dysmenorrhea, 8, 17
teaching points, 18
treatment therapies, 17–18
with add-back therapy, 17
with GnRH agonists, 17, 18
with NSAIDs, 17, 18
with surgery, 17–18
endometrium, LNG-IUD in, 57
energy imbalance, correction of, 53
enoxaparin, 184, 186
Environmental Protection Agency (EPA), 179
EPDS. See Edinburgh Postnatal Depression Scale
EPT. See expedited partner therapy
erythema
breast, 104–5
vestibulodynia and, 147
estrogen therapy
with DVT, 73–74
for hypothalamic amenorrhea, 51
local vaginal, 42, 44, 305–6
for POI, 49
through oral contraceptive use, 49
with pulmonary embolus (PE), 73–74
for transgender women, 289
ethinyl estradiol, 68, 92, 289
etonogestrel implant, removal of, 79–81
contraceptive counseling for, 80
after deep placement, 80–81
BMI factors, 80
location of implant, 80–81
imaging, 79
management of, 79–80
medical history prior to, 79
pop-out technique for, 80
exemestane, 134
expedited partner therapy (EPT), 29–30
for chlamydia, 29–30
for gonorrhea, 29–30
legal status of, 30
with patient-delivered partner therapy, 29
pregnancy and, 30
for syphilis, 30

Factor V Leiden, 174
fecal incontinence, 253–55
accidental bowel leakage, 254

diagnosis of, 254
etiology of, 253–54
OASIS and, 253–54
pelvic anatomy and, 254
prevalence of, 253
risk factors for, 254
felbamate, 83
Female Athlete Triad Coalition, 52–53
first-line therapies, for PCOS, 168–69
Flector patch, 112
flibanserin, 287
fluconazole, 32, 34, 156
fluorouracil, 103
fluoxetine, 1
fragile X mental retardation protein (FMRP), 48
Fragile X mutation gene (FMR1), 47
Fragile X permutation, primary ovarian insufficiency (POI) from, 48–49
fragile X mental retardation protein and, 48
Fragile X mutation gene, 48, 49
reproductive counseling for, 49
FRAX calculations, for bone density, 307, 308
Freidrich's criteria, for vestibulodynia, 145
friable cervix, 45–46
clinical presentation of, 45
postcoital bleeding, 45–46
diagnosis of, 46
history of illness, 45
imaging for, 45
LNG IUD use and, 45
with negative evaluation, 45–46
patient management with, 45
LEEP in, 45
treatment therapies for, 46
with cryotherapy, 46
with topical agents, 46
fusion of labia, 152

gabapentin, 14, 267
Gail model, for breast cancer screening, 133
galactorrhea, 108
gastric bypass
malabsorptive procedures, 55
obesity criteria and, 54
pregnancy and, 54–56
complications with, 56
nutritional deficiencies with, 55
prenatal care, 55
recommended weight gain guidelines, 55
restrictive procedures, 55
secondary amenorrhea after
after gastric bypass, 54–56
imaging guidelines, 54
patient counseling for, 54

GDM. See gestational diabetes
gender dysphoria, 288–89
gender identity and expression, 288–89
generalized vulvodynia, 146
genetic counseling, for Ashkenazi Jewish women, in pregnancy planning, 187–88
ACOG guidelines, 187, 188
costs of, 188
for genetic disorders, 187–88
Genetic Information Nondiscrimination Act, 125
genital ulcers, acute, 210, 211
genitourinary syndrome of menopause (GSM), 42–44, 304–6
causes of, 43
cervical ectropion, 46
clinical presentation, 43
diagnosis of, 43, 305
hypoestrogenism and, 43
symptoms of, 304, 305
treatment therapies for, 43–44, 305–6
alternative non-estrogen approaches, 44
contraindications to, 44
local vaginal estrogen therapy, 42, 44, 305–6
with lubricants, 305
vulvovaginal atrophy and, 306
gestational diabetes (GDM), 194
gestational sac, 251
gland cancers, Bartholin's cyst and, 160
glyburide, 195
gonadotropin-releasing hormone (GnRH), for endometriosis, 17, 18
gonadotropins, for PCOS, 169
gonorrhea, 26
expedited partner therapy for, 29–30
PID and, 244
after sexual assault, testing for, 89
griseofulvin, 83
GSM. See genitourinary syndrome of menopause
Guillain-Barré Syndrome (GBS), 178

heavy menstrual bleeding (HMB), 19
symptomatic adenomyosis and, 20
hepatitis B, 90
high-grade squamous intraepithelial lesion (HSIL), 129–31. See also vulvar HSIL
colposcopy
ASCCP guidelines, 130
for young adult women, 129–30

with colposcopy, 129
LEEP, 129
in young adult women, 129–31
biopsy recommendations, 130
colposcopy for, 129–30
HPV and, 129
treatment guidelines, 130–31
hirsutism, irregular menses and, 200–2
oral contraceptive use and, 200
PCOS and, 200–2
COCs and, 201–2
hyperandrogenism and, 201
laboratory testing, 201
lifestyle management for, 202
HIV. See human immunodeficiency virus
HMB. See heavy menstrual bleeding
hormonal therapy. See also gonadotropin-releasing hormone
for anorexia nervosa, 225
for chronic pelvic pain, 14
for hot flashes, in breast cancer survivors, 302
for loss of sexual desire, 287
for mastodynia, 112
for osteoporosis, 308
for transgender women, 289
antiandrogens, 289
estrogen, 289
ethinyl estradiol, 289
medication and dosing regimens, 289
for vulvar lichen sclerosus, 141
hot flashes, in breast cancer survivors, 301–3
clinical presentation, 301
risk factors, 301
treatment options, 302
hormonal therapy, 302
lifestyle modifications, 302
nonhormonal pharmacological, 302, 303
SSRIs/SNRIs, 302
HPV disorders. See human papilloma virus disorders
HSG. See hysterosalpingogram
HSIL. See high-grade squamous intraepithelial lesion
Human Fibroblast Lysate cream, 141
human immunodeficiency virus (HIV), 68–70
contraception and, 85–87
through ART, 87
protease inhibitors and, 87
through sterilization, 85
TB assessments, 85
types of, 86–87

(HIV) (cont.)
US MEC guidelines, 86
history of illness, 68
IUD management with, 85–87
LNG-IUDs, 86
pelvic inflammatory
diseases and, 86
oral contraceptive use and,
68–70
drug interactions with, 69
patient management and,
68–70
recommended guidelines
for, 68–70
US MEC guidelines for, 69
after sexual assault, testing for,
89–90
treatment therapies
antiretroviral drugs,
68–69
CDC recommendations,
69–70
efavirenz, 68, 70
ethinyl estradiol, 68
non-nucleoside reverse
transcriptase inhibitors,
68
nucleoside reverse
transcriptase inhibitors,
68
protease inhibitors, 68
Stavudine, 68
Zidovudine, 68
human papilloma virus (HPV)
disorders, 90, 136–38
CIN and, 136, 137
condyloma acuminata and,
149, 150
etiology of, 136
HSIL and, 129
LSIL and, 115–16
LEEP with, 122
patient management with,
136
screening for, 138
prevalence rates, 136, 137
vaccines, 136–38
Advisory Committee for
Immunization Practice
(ACIP)
recommendations, 137
efficacy rates, 137, 138
for women, 137
vulvar HSIL and, 142
human sex trafficking, 279–83
age demographics, 279–80
definition of, 279
health consequences of, 281
identification of victims,
281–83
local service providers, 283
by medical professionals,
283, 280–81
STIs, 282
physical manifestations of, 281
reproductive health problems
as result of, 281

screening questions for,
280
under Trafficking Victims
Protection Act, 279
trauma informed care
approach, 281
communication with
victims, 282
Hunner's ulcer, 268
hydrosalpinges, 165
treatment for, 165
hymen abnormalities, 213–15.
See also imperforate
hymen
diagnosis of, 214
non-obstructing, 214
prevalence of, 214
septate hymen, 213–15
classification of, 214
diagnosis of, 214
nonsurgical treatment of,
215
patient management,
213–15
surgical treatment of, 215
hymenectomy, 221
hyperandrogenism, 201
hyperlipidemia, 195
hyperprolactinemia, 108
recurrent pregnancy loss and,
174
hypertension, chronic, 190–93
diagnosis of, 190
through laboratory
assessment, 190
pre-gestational diabetes
mellitus and, 195
pregnancy planning with, 190
AMA issues and, 190, 192
medication therapies for,
192
preeclampsia, 190
risk group classification,
191–92
secondary, 191
common causes of, 191
target organ damage, 190
hypnotherapy, 296
hypoestrogenism, 43
hypothalamic amenorrhea,
51–53
clinical presentation of, 52
diagnosis and screening for,
52, 52
estrogen therapy for, 51
prevalence rates for, 52
risks with, 52
treatment therapies for, 53
bone density issues, 53
energy imbalance
correction, 53
with oral contraceptives, 53
hypothalamic-pituitary-ovarian
(HPO) axis, 68
hypothyroidism, 174, 195
hysterectomy
for chronic pelvic pain, 15

for endometriosis,
18
for Lynch syndrome, 120
for symptomatic adenomyosis,
21
hysterosalpingogram (HSG), 162
for bilateral hydrosalpinx, 164

IBCLC. See International Board
Certified Lactation
Consultant
ICSI. See intracytoplasmic sperm
injection
iliohypogastric nerve, 10, 11
iliolingual nerve, 10, 11
iliolingual-iliohypogastric nerve
entrapment, 10–12
diagnostic evaluation of, 11
neurectomy for, 11
prevalence rates for, 10
therapeutic approaches to, 11
treatment strategies, 11–12
Imiquimod cream, 150
imperforate hymen, 221–23
clinical presentation, 221
cyclic abdominal pain, 221
diagnosis of, 222
physical examination for, 221,
222
prevalence rates, 221
surgical treatment of, 222
hymenectomy, 221
postoperative care after,
222
ultrasound imaging for, 221
incontinence. See fecal
incontinence;
postpartum flatal
incontinence; stress
urinary incontinence
infertility. See also bilateral
hydrosalpinx; polycystic
ovary syndrome
alternative approaches to,
165–66
diagnostic evaluation of,
161–62
endometriomas and, 171
endometriosis and, 162
hydrosalpinges and, 165
treatment for, 165
male factor, 162
ovarian reserve testing
for, 162
after salpingectomy, 165
ovulatory dysfunction and,
161–62, 168
prevalence rates for, 168
TSH therapy for, 161
tubal factor, 164–65
tubal patency and, 162
through HSG, 162
inherited thrombophilias. See
thrombophilias
in vitro fertilization (IVF)
Fragile X permutation
and, 49

with ovarian endometrioma,
237
PCOS and, 169
Institute of Medicine, 55
weight gain recommendations
for pregnancy, 55
insulin, 195
intercourse. See painful
intercourse
interferon, 143
International Board Certified
Lactation Consultant
(IBCLC), 105
International Society for the
Study of Vulvovaginal
Disease (ISSVD), 143, 145
interstitial cystitis. See painful
bladder syndrome
intracytoplasmic sperm injection
(ICSI), 237
intraductal carcinomas, 99
intrauterine devices (IUDs). See
also copper intrauterine
device; displaced IUDs;
levonorgestrel intrauter-
ine device
actinomyces with, 71
bacterial colonization, 72
detection rates for, 72
diagnosis of, 72
prevalence rates for, 72
therapy strategies for, 72
for HIV-positive women, 85–87
copper IUDs, 86
LNG-IUDs, 86
pelvic inflammatory
diseases and, 86
PID and, 244
tubo-ovarian abscess (TOA)
and, 244
intrauterine pregnancy, with
contraceptive implants,
83–84
intravaginal
dehydroepiandrosterone,
44
irregular menstruation, 59
ISSVD. See International Society
for the Study of
Vulvovaginal Disease
IUDs. See intrauterine devices
IVF. See in vitro fertilization

Kegel exercises
for posterior wall defects, 276
for stress urinary incontinence
(SUI), 257
for urinary incontinence, 256
for vaginismus, 295–96

labetalol, 192
labia. See fusion of labia
labial hypertrophy, 197–98
definition, 197
mild, 197
severe, 198
surgical treatment for, 198

complications as result of, 198
postoperative appearance, 198
risks of, 198
vulvar irritation and, 197
lactation, nipple discharge and, 108
lactational mastitis, 104–6
abscess and
open incision and drainage, disadvantages of, 106
oral antibiotics for treatment of, 105
ultrasound imaging for diagnosis of, 104
ultrasound-guided aspiration for treatment of, 105
breast erythema and, 104–5
breast masses and, 105
breastfeeding after, 106
International Board Certified Lactation Consultant and, 105
pain management with, 106
persistent fever and, 104–5
symptoms of, 105
treatment therapies, 105–6
failure of, 105
optimal duration of, 105–6
laparoscopic evaluation
for adolescent endometriosis, 9
for chronic pelvic pain, 14
laparoscopic ovarian drilling, 169
laparoscopic surgery
for endometriomas, 170–71
for endometriosis, 17–18
for ovarian torsion, 240–41
LARC. See long-acting reversible contraception
laser therapy, 44
Le Fort's Colpocleisis, 274
LEEP. See loop electrosurgical excision procedure
lesions, breast, 102
letrozole, 168–69
levator ani spasm syndrome, 4–6
definition of, 4–5
diagnostic criteria, 5
evaluation for, 5
examination for, 5
pathogenesis, 4–5
presentation criteria, 5
prevalence rates, 4–5
treatment strategies, 5–6
with alternative therapies, 6
with cognitive behavioral therapy, 6
with physical therapy, 5–6
Levetiracetam, 19
levofloxacin, 27
levonorgestrel intrauterine device (LNG-IUD), 7, 45
acoustic shadowing, 66
actinomyces with, 71
bacterial colonization of, 72
detection rates for, 72

diagnosis of, 72
prevalence rates for, 72
therapy strategies for, 72
approval length for, 66
bilateral clear nipple discharge and, 95
displaced, 65–67
consultation for replacement, 66
evaluation of, 65
ultrasound imaging for, 65, 66
within endometrium, 57
expulsion rates for, 66
for HIV-positive women, 86
as LARC, 77
painful intercourse and, 19
perforation risks, 66
pregnancy with, 57–58
history of, 57
laboratory studies, 57
removal of, 57
severe menstrual cramping and, 19
side effects of, 66
symptomatic adenomyosis and, 21
usage rates, 66
vaginal spotting with, 57–58
history of, 57
physical examination for, 57
levothyroxine therapy, 60
Li Fraumeni syndrome, BRCA genetic mutations, 125
lichen sclerosus (LS), 203–5.
in childhood, 204–5
clinical presentation of, 204
corticosteroid therapy for, 204
diagnosis of, 203, 204
recurrence rates, 205
surgical management, 204–5
topical calcineurin inhibitor therapy, 204
treatment goals for, 204–5
etiology of, 204
patient management, 203–4
linoleic acid, 112
Lipschutz ulcer. See aphthae/ aphthosis of the vulva
LMWH. See low-molecular weight heparin
LNG-IUD. See levonorgestrel intrauterine device
local vaginal estrogen therapy, 42, 44, 305–6
long-acting reversible contraception (LARC), in postpartum period
contraceptive counseling for, 77
with LNG-IUD, 77
physical placement of, 77–78
manual insertion technique, 78

ring forcep technique, 78
selection criteria for, 77
US MEC guidelines, 76, 77
usage rates for, 76–77
loop electrosurgical excision procedure (LEEP)
with HSIL, 129
with LSIL, 45, 122–24
HPV and, 122
positive margins, 122, 123–24
loperamide, 254
loss of sexual desire, 285–87
anxiety and, 286
Basson's model of sexual response, 285–86
causes of, 285
emotional, 285, 286
physical, 285, 286
depression and, 286
history of illness, 285
sexual interest/arousal disorder, 285, 286
treatment therapies, 287
cognitive behavioral therapy for, 285, 286–87
hormonal, 287
pharmacological, 287
Lovenox, 73
low grade squamous intraepithelial lesion (LSIL), 115–17
ASC-US, 115
ASCCP management guidelines, 116
in young adult females, 115–16
history of illness, 115, 136
HPV and, 136–38
LEEP and, 122
screening for, 138
with HPV vaccine, 136
laboratory studies, 136
LEEP with, 122–24
HPV and, 122
positive margins, 122, 123–24
negative for intraepithelial lesion or malignancy, 115
screening for, 115
in young adult females, 115–16
ASCCP guidelines, 116
ASC-US, 115–16
cervical dysplasia, 115
HPV infection, 115–16
management of, 115–16, 117
metaplasia, 115
regression over time, 116
low-molecular weight heparin (LMWH), 186
LSIL. See low grade squamous intraepithelial lesion
lubricants, for GSM, 305
lumpectomy, 103
luteal phase deficiency, 174
Lynch syndrome, 118–21
BRCA genetic mutations, 125

cancer risks, 118, 119
chemoprevention, 119–20
hysterectomy and, 120
risk reduction strategies, 119–20
prevalence rates, 118
risk assessment, 119
testing, 119
Amsterdam criteria, 119
cascade, 118, 120
Revised Bethesda guidelines, 119

magnetic resonance imaging (MRI)
for breast cancer screening, 134
in ovarian remnant syndrome, 248
for precocious puberty, 219
for uterine septum, 63
malabsorptive procedures, in gastric bypass, 55
male factor infertility, 162
mammograms
for bilateral clear nipple discharge, 95
for breast masses, 102–3
for unilateral bloody nipple discharge, 98
manual insertion technique, with LARC, 78
massage therapy, for levator ani spasm syndrome, 6
mastectomy
for breast cancer treatments, 134
modified radical, 103
mastodynia, 111–13
classification of, 112
evaluation and diagnosis, 112
imaging, 112
treatment strategies, 112–13
mature cystic teratoma. See cystic teratoma
median perineotomy, 153
medroxyprogesterone, cyclic, 51
menopause. See genitourinary syndrome of menopause; hot flashes; perimenopause
menstrual cramping, severe, 19–21. See also symptomatic adenomyosis
AUB and, 20
heavy menstrual bleeding, 19
symptomatic adenomyosis and, 20
LNG-IUD and, 19
oral contraceptive use and, 19
physical examination for, 19
pictorial blood loss assessment chart for, 19
ultrasound imaging, 19
uterine artery embolization (UAE) for, 21
menstruation
irregular, 59

menstruation (cont.)
evaluation of, 59
obesity and, irregular patterns and, 55
primary hypothyroidism and, 59–60
diagnosis of, 59
reproductive physiology influenced by, 59
treatment therapies, 60
TSH and, 59, 60
metaplasia, LSIL and, 115
metformin, 195
methicillin resistant staff aureus (MRSA), Bartholin's cyst and, 160
methyldopa, 192
metronidazole, 24, 89
for PID, 243
for *Trichomonas vaginalis*, during pregnancy, 37
for tubo-ovarian abscess (TOA), 243–44
metronidazole allergy, 24–25
desensitization strategies, 24–25
with trichomonas infection, 23–24
diagnosis of, 24
nucleic acid amplification tests and, 24
microcephaly, 178
microscopic hematuria with negative urine culture, 260–62
common causes of, 261
definition, 261
evaluation of, 261
imaging for, 261
prevalence of, 260
risk factors for, 261
screening for, 262
USPSTF recommendations, 262
midcycle vaginal spotting, 61
evaluation of, 61
laboratory analysis of, 61
ultrasound imaging, 61
mild labial hypertrophy, 197
milky bilateral nipple discharge, 95, 99
mirabegron, 264–65
miscarriage rates, with AMA, 192
MMEs. *See* morphine milligram equivalents
modified radical mastectomy. *See* radical mastectomy
Monsel's solution, 46
morphine milligram equivalents (MMEs), 1
MRI. *See* magnetic resonance imaging
mucopurulent cervicitis, 26–28
treatment for, 27

NAATs. *See* nucleic acid amplification tests

National Comprehensive Cancer Network (NCCN), 126, 133–34
NCCN. *See* National Comprehensive Cancer Network
negative for intraepithelial lesion or malignancy (NILM), 115
nerve modulators, 264–65
neurectomy, 11
neuropathic pain monitors, 147
nifedipine, 192
NILM. *See* negative for intrae-pithelial lesion or malignancy
nipple discharge. *See also* bilateral clear nipple discharge; unilateral bloody nipple discharge; unilateral green nipple discharge
abnormal, 108
clinical presentation, 108
evaluation of, 108
galactorrhea and, 108
lactation and, 108
management of, 108, 109
nitrofurantoin, 270
nitroimidazoles, 24
non-nucleoside reverse transcriptase inhibitors (NNRTIs), 68
non-obstructing hymen abnormalities, 214
non-specific vulvovaginitis. *See* vulvovaginitis
non-steroidal anti-inflammatory drugs (NSAIDs)
for dysmenorrhea, 7–8
for mastodynia, 112
for pelvic pain
chronic, 14
severe, 1–2
for severe pelvic pain, 1–2
norelgestromin, 92
norethindrone, 17
normal (physiologic) nipple discharge, 108
nortriptyline, 14
NRTIs. *See* nucleoside reverse transcriptase inhibitors
NSAIDs. *See* non-steroidal anti-inflammatory drugs
nucleic acid amplification tests (NAATs), 24, 27
for chlamydia, 39
after sexual assault, 89
for transgender males, 292
nucleic acid tests, for Zika virus, 178
nucleoside reverse transcriptase inhibitors (NRTIs), 68
Nuprin, 112

OAB. *See* overactive bladder
OASIS. *See* obstetric anal sphincter injuries

obesity. *See also* body mass index
contraceptive counseling
for CHC, 92
for contraceptive patch, 92
shared decision-making in, 91
US MEC guidelines, 91–92
gastric bypass and, 54
global prevalence of, 91
menstrual patterns and, irregularity of, 55
oral contraceptive use and, 91–93
COCs, 91–92
PCOS and, 168
stress urinary incontinence (SUI) and, 257
VTE and, 91–92
WHO definition of, 91
obstetric anal sphincter injuries (OASIS), 253–54
obstructed hemivagina and ipsilateral renal anomaly (OHVIRA) syndrome, 7
ofloxacin, 27
OHVIRA syndrome. *See* obstructed hemivagina and ipsilateral renal anomaly syndrome
oophoropexy, 241
opioids
for pelvic pain
chronic, 14–15
severe, 1–2
oral antibiotic therapy, 105
oral contraceptive use
acne and, in adolescents, 200
COCs, 68
obesity and, 91–92
perimenopause and, 312, 313
deep dyspareunia and, 4
endometriosis and, 16
hirsutism and, in adolescents, 200
HIV treatment therapies and, 68–70
drug interactions with, 69
patient management and, 68–70
US MEC guidelines, 69
hormones in, 68
for hypothalamic amenorrhea, 53
obesity and, 91–93
COCs, 91–92
ovarian cancer and, 125
painful intercourse and, 19
perimenopause and, 311–13
cancer risks with, 312
COCs, 312, 313
stroke risks, 312
VTE risks, 312
POPs, 68
in premature ovarian insufficiency (POI)
treatment therapies, 49

severe menstrual cramping and, 19
with symptomatic adenomyosis, 20–21
ormeloxifene, 113
Ospemifene, 44
osteoporosis, 307–9
calcium intake and, 308
lifestyle modifications, 308–8
treatment options, 308–9
with anabolic therapy, 309–9
with antiresorptive agents, 308
with hormone therapy, 308
vitamin D intake and, 308
OTC medication. *See* over-the-counter medication
ovarian cancer, 118, 119
BRCA genetic mutations and, 125–27
risk-reducing options, 126–27
screening and prevention options, 127
genetic counseling for, 126
under Genetic Information Nondiscrimination Act, 125
NCCN guidelines, 126
oral contraceptive use, 125
patient management with, 125
perimenopause and, 312
ovarian cysts, 230–32. *See also* asymptomatic ovarian cysts
adnexal masses, in postmenopausal women, 230–32
malignancy risks, 230
surgical management of, 231–32
tumor marker testing for, 231
ultrasound imaging for, 231
ovarian endometriomas, 236–38
diagnosis of, 237
with endometriosis, 236
history of illness, 236
laboratory studies, 236
with ultrasound imaging, 236, 237
prevalence rates, 236–37
recurrence rates, 238
treatment strategies, 237
complications of, 238
individualization of, 237
IVF/ICSI issues, 237
postoperative long-term suppression, 237–38
surgery in, 237
ovarian remnant syndrome, 246–48
clinical presentation, 247
diagnosis of, 246–47
through imaging, 247
with MRI, 248

with endometriosis, 246–47
evaluation of, 246
laboratory studies, 246
treatment strategies for,
247–48
medical therapies, 247
radiotherapy, 247
surgical approach, 247–48
ovarian reserve testing, for
infertility, 162
after salpingectomy, 165
ovarian torsion, 239–41
history of illness, 239
lymphatic/venous outflow
with, 240
with pelvic pain, 239
physical examination
for, 239
prevalence rates for, 239–40
treatment strategies for,
240–41
cystectomy, 241
laparoscopy in, 240–41
oophoropexy, 241
ultrasound imaging,
239, 240
overactive bladder (OAB),
263–65
evaluation of, 263
laboratory studies, 264
process of, 263
quality of life with, 263
treatment options, 264–65
first-line medications in, 264
pelvic floor therapy, 264
pharmacotherapy, 264–65
over-the-counter (OTC)
medication, for candida
vaginitis, 155
ovulation, during
perimenopause, 311–12
ovulatory dysfunction, 161–62,
168
oxcarbazepine, 83
oxycodone, for severe pelvic
pain, 1
oxytocin gel, 44

pain management, with
lactational mastitis, 106
pain-centered approach, to
chronic pelvic pain, 13
painful bladder syndrome,
266–68
definition, 266
diagnosis of, 266–67
through urinalysis, 267
Hunner's ulcer, 268
treatment options, 267–68
cystoscopy, 268
through diet, 267
pharmacologic, 267
painful intercourse, 19–21. See
also symptomatic
adenomyosis
AUB and, 20
in elderly women, 42. See also
atrophic vaginitis

heavy menstrual bleeding, 19
symptomatic adenomyosis
and, 20
LNG-IUD and, 19
oral contraceptive use and, 19
patient management with, 19
physical examination for, 19
pictorial blood loss assessment
chart for, 19
ultrasound imaging for, 19
uterine artery embolization
(UAE) for, 21
PALM-COEIN. See polyp, adenomyosis, leiomyoma,
malignancy and hyper-
plasia, coagulopathy,
ovulatory dysfunction,
endometrial, iatrogenic
and not yet classified
paroxetine, 302
pathologic bilateral nipple
discharge, 95, 99
patient-delivered partner therapy
(PDT), 29
PCOS. See polycystic ovary
syndrome
PDT. See patient-delivered partner therapy
PE. See pulmonary embolism
pediatric diseases. See
vulvovaginitis
pelvic exams, for deep
dyspareunia, 4
pelvic floor dysfunction, 15
pelvic floor therapy, for OAB,
264
pelvic inflammatory disease
(PID), 26, 242–44
chlamydia and, 244
diagnostic criteria, 243
gonorrhea and, 244
IUD use and, 244
treatment therapies for,
243–44
pharmacologic, 243
with tubo-ovarian abscess,
242–44
pelvic inflammatory diseases,
IUDs and, 86
pelvic organ prolapse, 273. See
also uterine procidentia
pelvic pain, chronic, 13–15
diagnostic evaluation of, 14
with laparoscopy, 14
negative, 14
etiology of, 13
ovarian torsion and, 239
patient management, 13
pain-centered approach, 13
pelvic floor dysfunction and,
15
physical exam for, 13, 14
treatment therapies, 14
acupuncture, 13
with cognitive behavioral
therapy, 14
with hormones, 14
with hysterectomy, 15

with NSAIDs, 14
opioids, 14–15
pharmacological, 14
with TENS, 15
tricyclic antidepressants, 14
pelvic pain, severe, 1–3
medication treatments
for, 2–3
contracts and agreements
for, 2–3
with MMEs, 1
with NSAIDs, 1–2
with opioids, 1–2
with oxycodone, 1
patient management, 1–2
with physical therapy, 2
screening and monitoring of, 2
risk stratification, 2
urine drug screen (UDS), 2
teaching points for, 3
pentosan polysulfate (Elmiron),
267
perimenopause, 311–13
age of onset for, 311
confirmation of, 313
laboratory studies, 311
oral contraceptive use and,
311–13
cancer risks with, 312
COCs, 312, 313
stroke risks, 312
VTE risks, 312
ovulation during, 311–12
PALM-COEIN and, 311
symptoms of, 312
treatment options, 312
ultrasound imaging, 311
perineal pain. See vestibulodynia
peripheral precocious puberty,
218, 219
periprocedural antibiotics, 160
persistent fever, 104–5
persistent vulvovaginal
candidiasis, 33
pessary trials, 258
for posterior wall defects,
277–78
for uterine procidentia, 274
Pfannenstiel incision, pain at,
10–12
history of illness, 10
iliolingual-iliohypogastric
nerve entrapment, 10–12
diagnostic evaluation of, 11
neurectomy for, 11
physical examination for, 11
prevalence rates for, 10
therapeutic approaches to,
11
treatment strategies, 11–12
PGD. See pre-implantation
genetic diagnosis
PGDM. See pre-gestational
diabetes mellitus
phenytoin, 83
photodynamic therapy, 141
PHTS. See PTEN Hamartoma
Tumor Syndrome

physiologic nipple discharge. See
normal nipple discharge
pictorial blood loss assessment
chart, 19
PID. See pelvic inflammatory
disease
PIs. See protease inhibitors
plaque reduction neutralization
test, 178
podofilox, 150
podophyllin, 143
POI. See primary ovarian
insufficiency
polycystic ovary syndrome
(PCOS), 167–69
in adolescents, 200–2
COCs and, 201–2
hyperandrogenism and,
201
laboratory testing, 201
lifestyle management for,
202
gonadotropins for, 169
infertility and, 167–69
laparoscopic ovarian drilling
for, 169
obesity and, 168
treatment therapies
clomiphene citrate, 167,
168
first-line, 168–69
IVF and, 169
second-line, 169
stratification of, 168
polyp, adenomyosis, leiomyoma,
malignancy and
hyperplasia,
coagulopathy, ovulatory
dysfunction,
endometrial, iatrogenic
and not yet classified
(PALM-COEIN), 311
pop-out technique, for
etonogestrel implant
removal, 80
POP-Q assessment, 272, 273
POPs. See progestin-only pills
postcoital bleeding, with friable
cervix, 45–46
posterior wall defects, 276–78
Kegel exercises, 276
physical examination, 276
of pelvis with maximum
valsalva, 276
symptoms of, 277
treatment therapies for, 277
pessaries, 277–78
through surgery, 278
postpartum contraceptive use,
76–78
LARC, patient management
with, 76
during pregnancy, 76
laboratory studies, 76
medical history, 76
physical examinations, 76
postpartum depression, 297–99
clinical presentation, 297

postpartum depression (cont.)
definition, 297
mood disorders, 298
screening tools for, 297–98
Edinburgh Postnatal
Depression Scale (EPDS),
297, 298, 299
treatment options, 298–99
cognitive behavioral
therapy, 297
first-line, 298
through medications,
298–99
SSRIs, 299
postpartum flatal incontinence,
253–55
accidental bowel leakage, 254
cesarean delivery with, 255
diagnosis of, 254
etiology of, 253–54
OASIS and, 253–54
pelvic anatomy and, 254
prevalence of, 253
risk factors for, 254
treatment therapies, 254–55
biofeedback, 254
through diet, 254
pharmacologic, 254
precocious puberty, 216–19
benign, 219
causes of, 216–17
BMI, 217
hormonal, 216–17
race and ethnic factors, 217
central, 217, 219
classification of, 217
etiology of, 217–18
evaluation, 216–17
clinical characteristics, 219
flow sheet, 218
through MRI, 219
peripheral, 218, 219
physical examination for, 216,
217–19
laboratory studies, 216,
218–19
sexual maturity rating in,
217–18
preconception counseling. See
also pregnancy planning
Zika virus and, 179
prednisone, 267
preeclampsia, 190
pre-gestational diabetes mellitus
(PGDM)
comorbidities with, 195
exercise and, 195
medications for, 195
pregnancy planning, 194–95
pregnancy. See also breast
masses; pregnancy
planning
axillary dissection during, 103
with contraceptive implants,
82–84
ectopic, 83
intrauterine, 83–84
laboratory studies for, 82

expedited partner therapy
(EPT) and, 30
gastric bypass and, 54–56
complications with, 56
nutritional deficiencies
with, 55
prenatal care, 55
recommended weight gain
guidelines, 55
with LNG-IUD, 57–58
history of, 57
laboratory studies, 57
lumpectomy during, 103
modified radical mastectomy
during, 103
trichomonas infection during,
36–38
laboratory studies, 36
Trichomonas vaginalis during,
36–37
diagnosis of, 37
metronidazole for, 37
pre-term birth risks, 37
prevalence rates for, 36
sexual partner counseling, 37
treatment strategies, 37
Zika virus during, 178
pregnancy loss, recurrent,
173–75
definition, 173
diagnosis of, 173–74
hormone production and, 174
lifestyle risk factors, 174
luteal phase deficiency, 174
physical examination, 173
evaluation criteria, 174
testing for, 175
treatable causes of, 174, 175
antiphospholipid antibody
syndrome, 174
diabetes, 174
hyperprolactinemia, 174
testing for, 175
thyroid dysfunction, 174
uterine abnormalities and, 174
pregnancy of undetermined
location (PUL)
ectopic pregnancy and, 252
evaluation of, 250
through β-hCG testing,
250–52
of gestational sac, 251
through US, 250
nomenclature for, 250
pregnancy planning
AMA and, 190
aneuploidy risks, 192
comorbidity risks, 192
Down Syndrome, 192
for Ashkenazi Jewish women,
187–89
genetic counseling, 187–88
with chronic hypertension,
190
AMA issues and, 190, 192
medication therapies for,
192
preeclampsia, 190

risk group classification,
191–92
with depression, 181–83
decision aids, 182–83
relapse issues, 182
treatment therapies as part
of, 182
with diabetes, 194–96
complication risks, 195
evaluation of, 194–95
pre-gestational diabetes
mellitus counseling,
194–95
with DVT, 184–86
thromboprophylaxis and,
185
with Zika virus, 177–79
preconception counseling,
179
pregnancy tests, 82–83
bilateral clear nipple discharge
and, 96
after sexual assault, 88–89
pre-implantation genetic
diagnosis (PGD), 47
for Fragile X permutation, 49
premature menopause, 48. See
also primary ovarian
insufficiency
premature ovarian dysfunction,
48. See also primary
ovarian insufficiency
premature ovarian failure, 48
prenatal care, after gastric
bypass, 55
primary hypothyroidism,
menstruation and, 59–60
diagnosis of, 59
reproductive physiology
influenced by, 59
treatment therapies, 60
TSH and, 59, 60
primary ovarian insufficiency
(POI)
causes of, 48
estrogen replacement therapy
for, 49
through oral contraceptive
use, 49
from Fragile X permutation,
48–49
cytosine-guanine-guanine
repeats, 48–49
fragile X mental retardation
protein and, 48
Fragile X mutation genes,
48, 49
reproductive counseling for,
49
screening for, 48–49
prevalence rates for, 48
secondary amenorrhea
and, 47
privacy issues, for chlamydia
among adolescents, 40
progesterone, 141
pregnancy loss and, 174
progestin-only pills (POPs), 68

prostate cancer screening, 290
protease inhibitors (PIs), 68
contraception influenced by,
87
contraceptive implants and, 83
Protein C activity, 174
Protein S activity, 174
prothrombin gene mutations,
174
provoked vulvodynia, 146
pseudocyst of the clitoris, 153
PTEN Hamartoma Tumor
Syndrome (PHTS), 125
puberty. See precocious puberty;
sexual maturity rating
PUL. See pregnancy of undetermined location
pulmonary embolism (PE),
73–74
contraceptive counseling with,
73–74
barrier methods, 74
range of contraceptive
options, 73
risk factors in, 73, 74
STI screening as part of, 73
US MEC criteria guidelines,
73, 74
DVT and, 73–74
barrier methods and, 74
contraceptive counseling
with, 73–74
estrogen therapy risks,
73–74
risk factors for, 73, 74
estrogen therapy risks, 73–74
risk factors for, 73

quality of life
with OAB, 263
with stress urinary
incontinence (SUI),
256–57

race and ethnicity, precocious
puberty and, 217
radical mastectomy, modified, 103
radiotherapy, for ovarian
remnant syndrome, 247
raloxifene, 134, 308
randomized controlled trials
(RCTs)
for Bartholin's cyst, 159
for endometriosis, 17
recalcitrant disease, 153–54
treatment therapies for,
153–54
rectal flora, UTIs and, 269–70
rectoceles. See distal rectoceles
recurrent pregnancy loss. See
pregnancy loss
recurrent UTIs, 269–71
diagnosis of, 269–70
evaluation of, 271
prevention strategies, 270
rectal flora and, 269–70
risk factors for, 269
treatment options for, 270

recurrent VVC (RVVC), 33, 34–35, 155–57
  albicans species and, 156
  cytolytic vaginitis and, 156
  diagnostic criteria for, 156
  Doderlein's cytolysis, 156
  evaluation of, 155, 156
  non-*albicans* species and, 156
  optimal therapy for, 33–34
  patient management, 155
  prevalence rates for, 155–56
  treatment therapies
    drug-resistance issues, 156
    fluconazole, 156
  vulvar pruritis and, 156
relaxation therapy, 296
reproduction
  human sex trafficking as influence on, 281
  primary hypothyroidism as influence on, 59
reproductive counseling, for Fragile X permutation, 49
restrictive procedures, in gastric bypass, 55
Revised Bethesda guidelines, for Lynch syndrome, 119
rifampin, 83
ring forcep technique, for postpartum IUD placement, 78
risk assessment
  for severe pelvic pain, 2
  for unilateral bloody nipple discharge, 99
  for breast cancer, 99
risk-reducing bilateral salpingo-oopherectomy (RRSO), 126–27, 134
Ritonavir, 68
Rokitansky nodule, 227
RRSO. *See* risk-reducing bilateral salpingo-oopherectomy
RVVC. *See* recurrent VVC

saline infusion sonogram (SIS), 61
salpingectomy, 165
SANE. *See* sexual assault nurse examiner
SCOFF screening questionnaire, for eating disorders, 224, 225
secondary amenorrhea, 47–48, 51–53. *See also* hypothalamic amenorrhea
  from anorexia nervosa, 224–26
  hormonal treatment for, 225
  causes of, 47–48
  Fragile X mutation gene and, 47
  after gastric bypass, 54–56
  imaging guidelines, 54
  history of illness, 47, 51
  PGD and, 47
  physical examination for, 47, 51

primary ovarian insufficiency (POI) and, 47
secondary dysmenorrhea, 8
secondary hypertension, 191
  common causes of, 191
second-line therapies, for PCOS, 169
selective norepinephrine reuptake inhibitors (SNRIs), 302
selective serotonin reuptake inhibitors (SSRIs), 181, 182
  for hot flashes in breast cancer survivors, 302
  for postpartum depression, 299
septate hymen, 213–15
  classification of, 214
  diagnosis of, 214
  non-surgical treatment of, 215
  patient management, 213–15
  surgical treatment of, 215
sertraline, 297
severe labial hypertrophy, 198
sexual assault, 88–90
  emergency department evaluation of, 88
  follow-up counseling after, 90
  hospital evaluation of, 88
  patient management after, 88
  patient medical history and, 88
  physical examination after, 88
  pregnancy tests after, 88–89
  prevalence rates for, 88
  STI assessments after, 89–90
    for chlamydia, 89
    for gonorrhea, 89
    for hepatitis B, 90
    for HIV, 89–90
    for HPV, 90
    with nucleic acid amplification tests, 89
    for syphilis, 90
    for trichomonas infection, 89
sexual assault nurse examiner (SANE), 88
sexual desire. *See* loss of sexual desire
sexual interest/arousal disorder (SIAD), 285, 286
sexual maturity rating, 217–18
sexual partners, counseling for, 37
sexually transmitted infections (STIs), 29. *See also* sexual assault; trichomonas infection; trichomonas vaginitis
  acute genital ulcers and, 210
  testing for STIs and, 212
  chlamydia, 26
    expedited partner therapy (EPT) for, 29–30
    condyloma acuminata and, 149
    in contraceptive counseling and, 73

gonorrhea, 26
  expedited partner therapy (EPT) for, 29–30
  in human sex trafficking victims, 282
  in transgender men, screening for, 292
  in WWE for transgender women, 289
sexually-transmitted diseases (STDs), 279
  history of illness, 279
  laboratory studies, 279
SIAD. *See* sexual interest/arousal disorder
sildenafil citrate, 287
sinecatechins, 143, 150
SIS. *See* saline infusion sonogram
SNRIs. *See* selective norepinephrine reuptake inhibitors
sonohysterogram, for endometrial polyps, 62
squamous intraepithelial lesion. *See* high-grade squamous intraepithelial lesion; low-grade squamous intraepithelial lesion
SSRIs. *See* selective serotonin reuptake inhibitors
St. John's wort, 83
Stavudine, 68
STDs. *See* sexually-transmitted diseases
sterilization, 85
STIs. *See* sexually transmitted infections
stress urinary incontinence (SUI), 256–58
  behavioral therapy for, 257–58
  clinical presentation, 257
  complicated, 257
  diagnosis of, 256
  evaluation of, 257
  Kegel exercises for, 257
  obesity and, 257
  patient management, 256, 257–58
  pessary trials, 258
  physical examination, 256, 257
  prevalence of, 256
  quality of life issues with, 256–57
  screening tools for, 256–57
  surgical treatment, 258
    urethral slings, 258
  uncomplicated, 257
stroke risks, 312
SUI. *See* stress urinary incontinence
sulfamethoxazole, 270
symptomatic adenomyosis, 19–21
  diagnosis of, 20
  heavy menstrual bleeding and, 20
  risk factors for, 20
  tamoxifen therapy, 20

treatment therapies for, 20–21
  through hysterectomy, 21
  LNG-IUD, 21
  through oral contraceptive use, 20–21
syphilis, 30
  after sexual assault, testing for, 90

tamoxifen therapy, 20
  for breast cancers, 134
  for mastodynia, 112
TB. *See* tuberculosis
TCA. *See* trichloroacetic acid
TENS. *See* transcutaneous electrical nerve stimulation
testosterone, 141
  for loss of sexual desire, 287
  for transgender males, 291–92
    amenorrhea as result of, 292
3D ultrasound imaging, 61
thromboembolic disease. *See* deep vein thrombosis; venous thromboembolism
thrombophilias, inherited, 174
thyroid dysfunction, recurrent pregnancy loss and, 174
thyroid-stimulating hormone (TSH), 59, 60
  for infertility, 161
Tibolone, 44
tinidazole, 24, 89
TOA. *See* tubo-ovarian abscess
topical calcineurin inhibitor, 204
topiramate, 83
Trafficking Victims Protection Act (TVPA), 279
transcutaneous electrical nerve stimulation (TENS), 15
  for vulvodynia, 147
transgender males, vaginal spotting for, 291–93
  evaluation of, 292
  nucleic acid amplification tests, 292
  patient management, 291
  physical examination, 291
  prevalence of, 291–92
  STI screening, 292
  on testosterone therapy, 291–92
    amenorrhea as result of, 292
  treatment options for, 292
transgender women. *See also* well-woman examination
  gender dysphoria and, 288–89
  gender identity for, 288–89
  hormone therapy for, 289
    antiandrogens, 289
    estrogen, 289
    ethinyl estradiol, 289
    medication and dosing regimens, 289

transvaginal ultrasound (TVUS), 61
    for adnexal masses, in postmenopausal women, 231
    for displaced IUD, 65
    for ovarian endometriomas, 237
trauma informed care approach, to human sex trafficking, 281
    communication with victims, 282
trichloroacetic acid (TCA), 143, 150
trichomonas infection, 23–24, 29–31. *See also* chlamydia; gonorrhea
    diagnosis of, 24
    history of illness, 23, 29
    laboratory studies, 23
    with metronidazole allergy, 23–24
        diagnosis of, 24
        nucleic acid amplification tests and, 24
    during pregnancy, 36–38
        history of illness, 36
        laboratory studies, 36
        prevalence rates for, 27
    after sexual assault, testing for, 89
    symptoms of, 23
    treatment for, 23
Trichomonas vaginalis, 23
    during pregnancy, 36–37
        diagnosis of, 37
        metronidazole for, 37
        pre-term birth risks, 37
        prevalence rates for, 36
        sexual partner counseling, 37
        treatment strategies, 37
    trichomonas vaginitis, 29–31
        expedited partner therapy (EPT), 29–30
        legal status of, 30
        with patient-delivered partnet therapy (PDPT), 29
        pregnancy and, 30
        metronidazole treatment, 29
trichomoniasis, 30
tricyclic antidepressants, 14. *See also specific drugs*
trimethoprim, 270
TSH. *See* thyroid-stimulating hormone
tubal factor infertility, 164–65
tubal patency, 162
    through HSG, 162
tuberculosis (TB), HIV and, 85
tubo-ovarian abscess (TOA)
    bacterial comorbidities, 244
    clinical presentation, 243
    IUDs and, 244
    PID and, 242–44

treatment strategies for, 243–44
    parenteral, 243–44
TVPA. *See* Trafficking Victims Protection Act
TVUS. *See* transvaginal ultrasound
2D ultrasound imaging
    for painful intercourse, 19
    for severe menstrual cramping, 19
Tyrer-Cuzick model, for breast cancer screening, 133

UAE. *See* uterine artery embolization
UDS. *See* urine drug screen
UFH. *See* unfractionated heparin
ulcers. *See also* aphthae/ aphthosis of the vulva
    acute genital, 210, 211
    vulvar, 209–12

ultrasound (US) imaging
    for asymptomatic ovarian cysts, 234
    for bilateral hydrosalpinx, 165
    for breast masses, during pregnancy, 101, 102, 103
    for displaced IUD, 66
        TVUS, 65
    of endometriomas, 170
    for friable cervix, 45
    for imperforate hymen, 221
    for lactational mastitis, 104
        for oral antibiotics, 105
    for mature cystic teratoma, 227–28
    of ovarian cysts, 230
    for ovarian endometriomas, 236, 237
    for ovarian torsion, 239, 240
    for perimenopause, 311
    of pregnancy of unknown location (PUL), 250
    ultrasound imaging, 61
        for adnexal masses, in postmenopausal women, 231
        for displaced/misplaced IUD, 65
        for ovarian endometriomas, 236, 237
        for painful intercourse, 19
        for severe menstrual cramping, 19
    of unilateral bloody nipple discharge, 98
uncomplicated Bartholin's cyst, 158–60
uncomplicated cystitis, 270
uncomplicated stress urinary incontinence (SUI), 257
uncomplicated urethritis, 270
unfractionated heparin (UFH), 184
unilateral bloody nipple discharge, 98–100

atypical ductal hyperplasia and, 100
causes of, 99
    ductal ectasia, 99
    intraductal carcinomas, 99
diagnostic evaluation of, 99–100
laboratory studies for, 98
mammograms for, 98
patient management, 98–99
physical examination of, 98
    with breast exam, 98, 99
risk assessment for, 99
    for breast cancer, 99
ultrasound imaging of, 98
unilateral green nipple discharge, 107–9
    with ductal ectasia, 107–8
        clinical presentation, 107
        diagnosis of, 107
        imaging for, 107
        laboratory studies, 107
        patient management, 107
United States Medical Eligibility Criteria (US MEC), 73, 74
    for contraceptive counseling for HIV-positive women, 86
    with obesity, 91–92
    for LARC, 76, 77
United States Preventive Services Task Force (USPSTF), 262
urethral slings, for stress urinary incontinence, 258
urethritis. *See* uncomplicated urethritis
urge incontinence. *See* overactive bladder
urinary tract infections (UTIs), 269–71
    recurrent, 269–71
        diagnosis of, 269–70
        evaluation of, 271
        prevention strategies, 270
        rectal flora and, 269–70
        risk factors for, 269
        treatment options for, 270
    uncomplicated cystitis, 270
    uncomplicated urethritis, 270
urine drug screen (UDS), for severe pelvic pain, 2
US imaging. *See* ultrasound imaging
US MEC. *See* United States Medical Eligibility Criteria
USPSTF. *See* United States Preventive Services Task Force
uterine abnormalities, recurrent pregnancy loss and, 174
uterine artery embolization (UAE), 21
uterine procidentia, 272–74
    evaluation of, 273
        through POP-Q assessment, 272, 273
    imaging of, 272

patient management, 272–74
    complications of, 274
        through pessaries, 274
    surgical options, 274
    symptoms of, 273
uterine septum, 62
    clinical presentation of, 62
    hysteroscopic imaging, 62, 63
    MRI imaging of, 63
UTIs. *See* urinary tract infections

vaginal discharge and itching, 42–44. *See also* atrophic vaginitis; vulvovaginal candidiasis
    in non-specific vulvovaginitis, 206–7
vaginal pain. *See* vaginismus
vaginal spotting
    AUB, 20
        classification of, 61
        FIGO and, 61
    endometrial polyps and, 61–62
        detection rates for, 62
        diagnosis and evaluation of, 61, 62
        prevalence rates, 61
        sonohysterogram, 62
        ultrasound imaging for, 61, 62
    with LNG-IUD, 57–58
    midcycle, 61
        evaluation of, 61
        laboratory analysis of, 61
        patient management for, 61
        3D ultrasound imaging, 61
    with uterine septum, 62
        clinical presentation of, 62
        hysteroscopic imaging, 62, 63
        MRI imaging of, 63
vaginismus, 294–96
    diagnosis of, 295
    dyspareunia and, 294
    etiology of, 294–95
    incidence rates, 294
    patient management, 294
    physical examination, 294, 295
    treatment options, 295–96
        alternative, 296
        desensitization techniques, 295–96
        Kegel exercises, 295–96
        pharmacotherapy, 296
        types of, 295
    vulvodynia and, 294
vaginitis. *See also* atrophic vaginitis; candida vaginitis
    cytolytic vaginitis, 156
vaginoscopy, 207–8
venlafaxine, 14
venous thromboembolism (VTE), 91–92, 184–86
    perimenopause and, 312
vestibulodynia, 145–48. *See also* vulvodynia
    erythema and, 147

Freidrich's criteria in, 145
treatment therapies for, 145
vulvar lichen sclerosus and, 153
vitamin D intake, for osteoporosis, 308
VTE. *See* venous thromboembolism
vulvar HSIL, 142–44
  condyloma acuminata and, 142–43
    anogenital warts, 143
    classification of, 143
    clinical presentation of, 143
    treatment therapies for, 143
  evaluation of, 142
  history of illness, 142
  HPV and, 142
  ISSVD terminology for, 143
  recurrence rates, 143
  treatment for, 142–43
vulvar irritation and itching, 203–5. *See also* lichen sclerosus
  labia hypertrophy and, 197
  physical examination for, 203
vulvar lichen sclerosus, 139–41, 152–54
  clinical presentation of, 140
  complications of, 152–54
    adhesions and scarring, 152
    malignancies, 152
    pseudocyst of the clitoris, 153
  diagnosis of, 139, 140
  with fusion of labia, 152
  history of illness, 139, 152
  median perineotomy and, 153
  patient management, 139, 152
  physical examination, 139, 152
    biopsies in, 140
  recalcitrant disease and, 153–54

treatment therapies for, 153–54
treatment therapies for, 140–41
  with corticosteroids, 141
  emollient therapy, 141
  with hormones, 141
  Human Fibroblast Lysate cream, 141
  photodynamic therapy, 141
  surgery as, 141, 153
  vestibulodynia and, 153
  vulvar hygiene, 140
  vulvodynia and, 153
  vulvoperineoplasty, 154
vulvar pruritis, 156
vulvar ulcers, 209–12. *See also* aphthae/aphthosis of the vulva
  physical examination, 209
    through laboratory studies, 209
vulvodynia, 145–47
  causes of, 145–46
  generalized, 146
  ISSVD classification of, 145
  management and treatment of, 146–47
    cognitive behavioral therapy, 147
    neuropathic pain monitors, 147
    surgical excision, 147
    TENS, 147
  prevalence rates for, 145
  provoked, 146
  vaginismus and, 294
  vulvar lichen sclerosus and, 153
vulvovaginal atrophy, 306
vulvovaginal candidiasis (VVC), 32–35. *See also* recurrent VVC

Candida albicans, 32–33
  fluconazole treatment, 34
Candida glabrata, 34
Candida krusei, 34
Candida Saccharomyces, 34
  clinical presentation of, 33
  diagnosis of, 33
  evaluation of, 33
  lab studies for, 32
  patient management with, 32, 33–34
    with fluconazole, 32, 34
  persistent, 33
  recurrent, 33, 34–35
    optimal therapy for, 33–34
  risk factors, 33
  symptoms of, 32–33
vulvovaginal diseases. *See* vulvar HSIL; vulvar lichen sclerosus
vulvovaginitis, non-specific, in children, 206–8
  antibacterial therapy, 207
  clinical presentation, 206–7
  diagnosis of, 206, 207
  physical examination, 206, 207
    bacterial isolation, 207
    with vaginoscopy, 207–8
  vaginal discharge and itching, 206–7
VVC. *See* vulvovaginal candidiasis

weight categories, by BMI, 91
weight gain guidelines, 55
well-woman examination (WWE) for transgender women
  cancer screening, 289–90
    for prostate cancer, 290
  gender identity and expression, 288–89
  patient management, 288

patient medical history, 288
physical examination, 288
sexual orientation, 288–89
STI testing, 289
vaginal education and care, 289
WHO. *See* World Health Organization
Word catheter placement, 159
World Health Organization (WHO)
  obesity definitions, 91
  on Zika virus, 178

Zidovudine, 68
Zika virus, 177–79
  clinical features of, 178
  discovery of, 177
  Environmental Protection Agency and, 179
  Guillain-Barré Syndrome and, 178
  microcephaly and, 178
  during pregnancy, 178
  pregnancy planning with, 177–79
    patient management and, 177
    physical examination for, 177
    preconception counseling, 179
  symptoms of, 177–78
  testing for, 178
    CDC guidelines for, 178
    nucleic acid tests, 178
    plaque reduction neutralization test, 178
  transmission of, 177
  treatment for, 178
  WHO on, 178